Pioneers of Cardiac Surgery

Pioneers of Cardiac Surgery

William S. Stoney, MD

Vanderbilt University Press • Nashville

First printing 2008
Third printing 2014

This book is printed on acid-free paper.

Design by Dariel Mayer

Library of Congress Cataloging-in-Publication Data

Stoney, William S., 1928–
Pioneers of cardiac surgery / William S. Stoney. — 1st ed.
p. ; cm.
ISBN 978-0-8265-1594-0 (cloth : alk. paper)
1. Heart—Surgery—History. 2. Heart surgeons—Interviews. 3. Heart surgeons—Biography. I. Title.
[DNLM: 1. Cardiac Surgical Procedures—Biography. 2. Cardiac Surgical Procedures—Interview. 3. Cardiac Surgical Procedures—history. 4. History, 19th Century. 5. History, 20th Century. WZ 112.5.C2 S881p 2007]
RD598.S789 2007
617.4'12059—dc22 2007032190

For Marian Tilley Stoney

Contents

Acknowledgments

This began as a project to interview some of the first-generation cardiac surgeons and to record the interviews on videotape for the Special Collections of the Eskind Medical School Library at Vanderbilt. It was supported by a grant from the Department of Cardiac and Thoracic Surgery of Vanderbilt University School of Medicine. Dr. Harvey Bender was the department chairman and made a number of suggestions as to participants and management of the grant. After his retirement, the grant was administrated by his successor, Dr. John Byrne. This grant made it possible to use professional video photographers for recording and editing the various interviews. Additional support was provided by Cardiovascular Surgery Associates at St. Thomas Hospital in Nashville, Tennessee, who supplied office space and a variety of other services during the preparation of the manuscript, and for their generous support I am grateful.

Eventually it became apparent that these interviews would be more accessible if published as a book. In the beginning I was somewhat intimidated by the time and commitment necessary to convert interviews with thirty-eight cardiac surgeons into a manuscript. Without the enthusiasm, encouragement, and support of my wife, Marian, it would not have happened. She talked me into starting and inspired me to finish.

Early in the process of editing the audiotapes into a more readable narrative format, I enlisted the assistance of my daughter, Elizabeth Shannon Stoney, BA, MFA. She worked an entire summer editing and retyping the interviews and at the same time preserving the conversational style of the original recordings. She is the major editor of this book.

Robert D. Collins, MD, the John L. Shapiro Professor of Pathology at Vanderbilt, is one of the most senior and most revered faculty members at Vanderbilt Medical School. He has published several scientific books and also a biography of Dr. Ernest Goodpasture, plus a history of the origins of Vanderbilt University. He has helped me with valuable advice about the process of writing and publishing through what became an almost weekly telephone conference. He was the first person to review and evaluate the manuscript, and his help and cheerful encouragement has led to the completion of the project.

I asked several of my colleagues and fishing companions to read the manuscript and to make suggestions. They each took this seriously and added a number of suggestions as to format, facts, style, and some stories from the past that were better kept in oral form rather than in print. Those readers were: William C. Alford, MD; Harvey W. Bender,

MD; John N. Hammon, MD; Robert K. Brawley, MD; R. Darryl Fisher, MD; and Jackson Harris, MD. They each knew the surgeons interviewed in one way or another and their suggestions helped the manuscript reach its present form.

William T. Cocke III, BA, PhD, is a former classmate from our undergraduate days. He is now an emeritus professor at the University of the South at Sewanee, Tennessee. He edited the final version of the manuscript and made numerous corrections of faulty punctuation plus many useful suggestions about word usage and style. It was his advice to try to preserve, as much as possible, the individual voice of each of the speakers.

During the last month of preparation, William E. Walker, MD, went through the entire manuscript checking facts, dates, spelling, and redundancies. He added additional insights from his years as a cardiac surgeon at Vanderbilt and later in Houston. For this, I will always be in his debt.

I extend heartfelt gratitude to my loyal secretary, Ann K. Smith, who came to work on a promise that this would only take three or four months and has remained for the two years that it actually required. She cheerfully typed the manuscript several times over, gathered photographs, kept files and notes, wrote letters, and made countless helpful suggestions, a job well done.

A final acknowledgment must go to the surgeons themselves for agreeing to be interviewed, and to them and their families for generously allowing those interviews to be published.

Preface

Cardiac surgery is a relatively young specialty having evolved for the most part in the second half of the twentieth century. However, the history of that evolution has been well documented in a number of excellent sources, reflecting the fact that surgeons in general are interested in the history of medicine and especially in the history of their respective operations. Three books recently published provide an accurate account of the way cardiac surgery developed. They are; Harris Shumacker's book *The Evolution of Cardiac Surgery*, Stephen Westaby's *Landmarks in Cardiac Surgery*, and Larry Stephenson's *Heart Surgery Classics*. In addition there are biographies of Alfred Blalock, Denton Cooley, C. Walton Lillehei, and John Gibbon plus autobiographies by René Favaloro, Christiaan Barnard, James Hardy, Geoffrey Wooler, and Vivien Thomas. Also here and there in various surgical journals are a variety of historical and biographical articles concerning the people and events that have contributed to the progress of cardiac surgery.

This book is an addition to the history of cardiac surgery and is a collection of interviews with some of the first-generation cardiac surgeons. Each of them tells us some details of his education, his entry into medicine, and the mentors and institutions that helped shape his career and also describes many of the contributions that made cardiac surgery possible. It starts with the Blalock-Taussig shunt in November 1944 and ends with the total artificial heart operations of 1982 to 1984.

These operations and procedures depended on the development of new surgical techniques and also on the development of a variety of new drugs and materials. For example, the development of the Gibbon heart-lung machine in 1953 required a safe and reliable method of preventing coagulation of the blood when it was exposed to the various manipulations and surfaces of an artificial oxygenator. The anticoagulant heparin had become available in the mid-1930s, but in spite of heparin, rubber and glass surfaces rapidly removed all of the platelets of an experimental laboratory animal, creating severe coagulopathy and bleeding. The plastic tubing that was developed for the beer and food industry after World War II proved to be much less traumatic to the clotting mechanism and therefore was adapted to be used in heart-lung machines. This and a hundred other similar advances in technology have made cardiac surgery possible.

In the beginning of cardiac surgery there was also an element of learning by trial and error. Early cardiac catheterization techniques were comparatively simple and diagnostic errors were not uncommon. Vascular surgical instruments and techniques were still evolving. The idea of a critical care area with nurses trained to recognize and treat postoperative problems had not yet emerged. Many of the first cardiac operations were done with a transverse thoracic incision, crossing the sternum at the third or fourth interspace. This turned out to have limitations of exposure and produced a very painful and sometimes unstable wound. It was replaced by a midline sternal splitting incision which gave much better exposure of the heart and was less painful. Air embolization from intracardiac air was another problem of many early cardiac operations and was the cause of unexpected neurological injury until surgeons learned how to eliminate air from the system before the heart resumed its pumping activity. The use of pacemakers, postoperative antibiotics, postoperative ventilators, and various cardiac and antiarrhythmic drugs gradually became common. Most of these various new techniques evolved in the early years of cardiac surgery between 1955 and 1965 and brought about a profound drop in the risk of cardiac operations from a 30 to 40 percent risk of death in 1955 to less than a 5 to 10 percent risk by 1965.

As cardiac surgical procedures became safer in the mid-1960s, numerous medical centers acquired a catherization laboratory and a heart-lung machine and developed a cardiac surgical service. Because of the large initial investment, most of these early programs were in academic centers. A few centers such as the University of Minnesota, Methodist Hospital in Houston, and Johns Hopkins Hospital had a relatively large number of patients with a daily cardiac surgery schedule, but the average cardiac program at that time did only two or three heart operations each week. No one anticipated the explosive growth of cardiac surgery that followed the first successful coronary bypass operations of 1967. Cardiac surgical programs rapidly opened in hundreds of community hospitals, and many of these programs would eventually do over a thousand operations a year. The hospital with the largest volume of all, the Texas Heart Institute, at one time was doing five thousand cardiac operations a year. Cardiac surgery rapidly changed from a very small specialty to become one of the most common and most profitable operations performed in many hospitals.

In the early days of cardiac surgery, we all expected outcomes to improve and the risks to decline, but at that time no one would have believed how safe cardiac surgery has become today. Recently a cardiac surgical group reported five hundred off-pump coronary artery bypass operations with only three postoperative deaths, a mortality rate of 0.6 percent. This was accomplished in spite of the fact that many of the patients were considered to be high risk with various other complicating problems.

My serious interest in the history of cardiac surgery began about fifteen years ago. One of my friends asked me to prepare a talk for one of the fall meetings of our local surgical society. He suggested that I talk about surgical history so I prepared a talk about the development of the five most pivotal operations in the evolution of cardiac surgery: (1) the Blue Baby operation, (2) the first successful use of a heart-lung machine, (3) the first artificial heart valve, (4) the first coronary artery bypass, and (5) the first heart transplant. Each of these operations marked a giant step forward in the development of cardiac surgery.

After getting this information together,

it occurred to me that since many of the surgeons involved in these important operations were still active, it would be interesting to record their recollections of how these procedures were developed. It would be a valuable addition to the history of medicine collections of our medical library.

At that time Harvey Bender was the chairman of the Department of Cardiac and Thoracic Surgery at Vanderbilt University Medical School. He was enthusiastic about the idea of an oral history collection for the medical library, so with the generosity of a donor, a grant was arranged through his department that would cover the cost of filming and editing the interviews. The first interview was done in 1996 in Philadelphia with Dr. John Templeton, who was John Gibbon's associate during the development of the first heart-lung machine. During the next six or seven years, I interviewed thirty-eight cardiac surgeons, some at national meetings and some at their home or hospital.

Unfortunately, several of the first-generation cardiac surgeons had died before this project got underway: Alfred Blalock, Dwight Harken, Lord Brock, John Gibbon, Glenn Morrow, Robert Gross, and others. Two important early pioneers that I did not interview were John Kirklin and David Sabiston. When asked to participate both expressed interest in the project but meetings were delayed or postponed for one reason or another until declining health made an interview with each impractical.

One obvious feature of the collection of interviews is the absence of women. In the first two decades of cardiac surgery (1940–1950) there were no female cardiac surgeons. Helen Taussig at Johns Hopkins was a pediatric cardiologist, not a surgeon, but her knowledge of congenital heart disease was an enormous factor in the development and success of the first operations done for children with cyanotic heart disease, the Blue Baby operations. Her influence was also a major factor in the subsequent development of one of the first cardiac surgical training programs. However, it was not until 1961 that a woman was certified by the Board of Thoracic Surgery. That person was Nina Braunwald. She received her cardiac surgical training at the National Institute of Health under Glenn Morrow and later joined the faculty of Harvard Medical School. She is credited with the first total replacement of a mitral valve with a prosthetic valve. It was a valve that she designed, but it had only limited success. She later designed a cloth-covered caged-ball valve that was more practical and was used in over five thousand patients. Dr. Braunwald died in 1992 of breast cancer. Dr. Taussig died in an automobile accident in 1986 at age eighty. Today cardiac surgery is still a male dominated specialty. However, there are now 173 women certified by the Board of Thoracic and Cardiac Surgery, and it is estimated that two-thirds of those women confine their work to cardiac surgery, the other one third is involved with thoracic surgical procedures. At the present time the Chairman of the Board of Thoracic (and Cardiac) Surgery is Carolyn E. Reed, MD.

Looking back, there are two others that would have been interesting to include, Willem Kolff and Robert Jarvik. Both can best be described as physician biomedical engineers. Since the original plan of the project was to interview surgeons, these two names never came up as potential participants, but either one or both would have been an interesting and valuable addition.

The video interviews are each about one hour or more and are now kept in the special collections of the Annette and Irwin Eskind Biomedical Library at Vanderbilt University Medical School. They are available for review by students, residents, faculty, and others interested in the history of cardiac surgery. The videos tell the life story of the various surgeons, and also they bring out the personality and spirit of the person interviewed which is not always apparent from reading a transcript.

Recently I collected transcripts of these interviews and began reviewing them as a possible foundation for a book about the origins of the various operations used in cardiac surgery today. The question and answer format of an interview works nicely as a visual presentation but for a reader it tends to interrupt the story and the message. For this reason the transcripts were edited into a narrative format and the interviewer's questions were either eliminated or were woven into the story being told.

To help keep these events in sequence, the first part of this volume has two guides. The first is a year-by-year list of various events in the progress of cardiac surgery during the twentieth century. The second narrative is a history of cardiac surgery which introduces the major participants and techniques of cardiac surgery in the order that they occurred.

These interviews give insight into the problems that these pioneer cardiac surgeons and their patients had to face and how those problems were solved. Missing from most of the interviews is personal history about marriage, children, and activities outside of medicine. If I could start over, I would include more information about personal life and the obvious problems that the commitment to cardiac surgery must bring to a family.

The culture of the surgeon's work and the rigors of residency training is another area that was only briefly explored in these interviews. From internship through residency training young medical school graduates in the past were immersed in the culture of surgery. This system was inherited from European training programs of the late nineteenth century and were imitated in this country by William Halsted of Johns Hopkins and Harvey Cushing of the Peter Bent Brigham and were perpetuated by the generation of Alfred Blalock and Michael DeBakey. The men represented in these interviews came of age and received their training in a time when this culture of endurance was common. Surgeons in training were expected to be the first doctors on the hospital wards each morning and the last to leave in the evening. They were expected to stay in the hospital every other night. This meant thirty-six hours in the hospital with twelve hours off in each forty-eight hour period. The chief of surgery had absolute power and all of his decisions were final. Above all, there was total commitment to the welfare and care of the patient. Some programs were more strenuous than others. For example, at Vanderbilt for many years surgical residents were not allowed to be married. At Johns Hopkins, residents were expected to be always on call and could leave the hospital only by arranging to sign out to another resident. The most brutal program of all was that of Dr. DeBakey at Baylor in Houston. When a resident first came on Dr. DeBakey's service, he was required to stay in the hospital, responsible for the care of patients in the postoperative recovery room, for three straight months without ever leaving the hospital. Grady Hallman, who later became one of Dr. Cooley's associates, described his time on Dr. DeBakey's service this way:

> My car was stolen while I was on the unbroken 90-day shift, and I couldn't even get out to see about it. I lived on sandwiches, fried pies, and Fritos. I got a vitamin deficiency and my tongue turned fire red. I figure what I went through was the supreme test of human endurance.[1]

Another example of the work ethic of the surgeon of that era is that of a nationally known liver transplant surgeon who would come to work with a backpack and bedroll and would frequently sleep on the floor in the intensive care area next to the bed of his critically ill patient. He also had a habit of completing his own work and then taking on the work of the other surgeons in his group that he thought should not be postponed until the next day, much to their aggravation.

The surgeons represented in these interviews all grew up in the old training system of strict discipline, hard work, long hours, and receiving almost no income. And yet, these hardships are rarely mentioned in the stories that they tell and never with any bitterness. It was accepted as the price that was required to become a surgeon.

This culture has now been modified by numerous changes in postgraduate surgical education and today's young surgeon has reasonable working hours, receives adequate compensation during residency, and can discuss his progress and his future with the chief of surgery.

The biggest change of all in surgical training has been the recent requirement that residents are not allowed to work longer than eighty hours a week and must have one full day off each week. This came about after it was demonstrated that residents' performance and decisions began to seriously deteriorate after working long hours with little or no sleep.

The days of the surgical equivalent of "iron men in wooden ships" are now gone. These interviews recall those days and are preserved here as a reminder of how the specialty of cardiac surgery began.

References

1. Thomas Thompson, *Hearts: Of Surgeons and Transplants, Miracles and Disasters along the Cardiac Frontier.* New York: McCall; 1971. 242.

Significant Events in Cardiac Surgery

1896 Ludwig Rehn—First successful suture repair of a stab wound of the heart.

1904–1906 Alexis Carrel and Charles Guthrie—Described vascular suture techniques and experimental organ transplants.

1907 Friedrich Trendelenburg—First attempt to remove a pulmonary embolus.

1916 Jay McLean—Discovered heparin while still a medical student.

1923 Elliott Cutler—First attempt to improve mitral stenosis by valvotomy.

1924 Martin Kirschner—First successful pulmonary embolectomy.

1925 Henry Souttar—First mitral commissurotomy by way of left atrial appendage.

1929 Werner Forssmann—First right heart catheterization (on himself).

1938 Robert Gross—First successful ligation of a patent ductus arteriosus.

1944 Clarence Crafoord—First successful repair of coarctation of the aorta.

1944 Alfred Blalock—First subclavian-pulmonary anastomosis for tetralogy of Fallot, the Blue Baby operation.

1943–1945 Dwight Harken—Successful removal of foreign bodies from the heart.

1945 Charles Bailey—First modern successful mitral commissurotomy.

1947 Claude Beck—Successful conversion of ventricular fibrillation using electric shock.

1947 Thomas Sellors—First successful pulmonary valvotomy for pulmonary stenosis.

1950 Arthur Vineberg—First mammary artery implant for ischemic heart disease.

1951 Clarence Dennis—First attempt to close an atrial septal defect using a pump-oxygenator. (Patient did not survive.)

1952 Robert Gross—Successful closure of an atrial septal defect using the "Gross well."

1952 John Lewis—First successful open-heart closure of an atrial septal defect using hypothermia.

1952 Charles Hufnagel—Placed an artificial valve in the descending thoracic aorta for aortic regurgitation.

1953 John Gibbon—First successful closure of an atrial septal defect using a heart-lung machine.

1954 C. Walton Lillehei—First closure of a ventricular septal defect using cross-circulation.

1955 John Kirklin—Closure of a ventricular septal defect using the Mayo-Gibbon heart lung machine.

1955 C. Walton Lillehei—Closure of a ventricular septal defect using a heart-lung machine (bubble oxygenator).

1957 William Longmire—First successful coronary artery endarterectomy.

1958 Ake Senning—Correction of transposition of great vessels (atrial).

1958 Ake Senning—First totally implanted cardiac pacemaker.

1958 Mason Sones—First selective coronary arteriogram.

1960 Denton Cooley and Michael DeBakey—First total replacement of an ascending aortic aneurysm with a homograft using a heart-lung machine.

1960 Albert Starr—First successful replacement of the mitral valve with an artificial valve.

1960 James Jude and William Kouwenhoven—First closed-chest resuscitation for cardiac arrest—CPR.

1961 Edward Sharp—First pulmonary embolectomy using a heart-lung machine.

1962 Donald Ross—First aortic valve replacement using a homograft valve.

1962 David Sabiston—First aortocoronary vein bypass graft. (Patient did not survive.)

1964 James Hardy—First heart transplant. Donor heart was from a chimpanzee. (Patient did not survive.)

1965 Carlos Duran—First porcine valve used to replace the aortic valve.

1966 Edward Garrett and Michael DeBakey—First successful saphenous vein aortocoronary bypass graft. (Not reported until 1973.)

1967 Alain Carpentier—First use of gluteraldehyde-preserved heterografts for aortic and mitral valve replacement.

1967 Gain Rastelli and Dwight McGoon—Report of successful repair and classification of common atrioventricular canal.

1967 Adrian Kantrowitz—First use of the intra-aortic balloon.

1967 Donald Ross—First aortic valve replacement using the patient's own pulmonary valve (Ross procedure).

1967 Christiaan Barnard—First heart transplant. Patient, Louis Washkansky, died eighteen days later.

1967 Adrian Kantrowitz—First heart transplant in the United States. Second in the world. Patient died after six hours.

1968 Christiaan Barnard—First successful heart transplant. Patient, Philip Blaiberg, lived 593 days.

1968 Norman Shumway—First heart transplant by the leading cardiac transplant investigator. Patient, Mike Kasperak, died fifteen days later of sepsis.

1968 George Green—First series of patients with internal thoracic artery grafts to the left anterior descending coronary artery.

1968 Francis Fontan—Surgical repair of tricuspid atresia.

1968 Will Sealy—First surgical ablation of recurrent atrial tachycardia.

1968 René Favaloro—First reported series of successful aortocoronary bypass grafts using saphenous vein.

1969 Denton Cooley—First use of an artificial heart as a bridge to transplant. (Patient did not survive.)

1973 William Gay and Paul Ebert—Use of potassium-induced cardioplegia for myocardial protection.

1975 Adib Jatene—Repair of transposition of the great vessels. Arterial switch.

1980 Leiczyslaw Mirowski—First implantable automatic cardiac defibrillator.

1981 Bruce Reitz and Norman Shumway–First heart-lung transplant.

1982 William DeVries—First total artificial heart operation using the Jarvik 7. Patient, Barney Clark, lived 112 days.

1983 Alain Carpentier—Report of mitral valve repair for mitral insufficiency.

1983 William Norwood—Repair of hypoplastic left heart syndrome.

1987 James Cox—Surgical treatment of atrial fibrillation.

2001 Laman Gray—First totally implantable artificial heart. Patient, Bob Tools, lived four months.

Pioneers of Cardiac Surgery

A Short History of Cardiac Surgery

Since the time of Hippocrates, there has been a difference between those who practice medicine and those who practice surgery. Internists practice the "art" of medicine, while surgeons lean more to the "craft." These two divisions have taken different paths over time. Medicine has slowly, but steadily, progressed as new information has been published, scientific discoveries have been made, and pharmacology has advanced. Surgical progress, on the other hand, has been held in slow motion by the long absence of anesthesia and the problem of postoperative infections. Although there have been many inventive and gifted surgeons in the past, operations remained relatively rare because of the horror of pain and the risk of infection. When an operation was necessary before the discovery of anesthetic agents, all efforts were concentrated on speed and speed alone. Major amputations could be done in one or two minutes, and the celebrated London lithotomists of the early nineteenth century could remove a bladder stone in one minute flat.[1] Even so, most operations that are common today were totally out of the question until 1846 when a dentist, William Morton, successfully demonstrated the use of ether as an anesthetic at the Massachusetts General Hospital. Suddenly, an operation could be carried out in an orderly manner without pain. Abdominal operations, obstetrical procedures, eye surgery, and numerous other operations became practical. However, there was still a problem: the risk of postoperative infection. A practical anesthetic came into use twenty years before the recognition and understanding of microorganisms.

In the late 1860s, Joseph Lister, Regius Professor of Surgery at the University of Glasgow, began using a dilute solution of carbolic acid to clean and irrigate the wounds of compound fractures after reading the reports of Louis Pasteur. In 1867 Lister reported in the *Lancet* his success in treating eleven compound fractures. Nine of the eleven patients healed with no infection. The use of carbolic acid to sterilize wounds was called "antisepsis." He next began using a continuous carbolic spray over incisions and the hands of the surgeon during elective operations, with astonishing results. Instead of the usual postoperative infections, his patients recovered without fever or purulent drainage. It took time for this new technique of antiseptic surgery to be adopted by others, especially the older generation of surgeons, but within the next ten years the craft of surgery began to blossom. In the 1880s, surgeons in Germany took this concept a step further and began boiling all gowns, drapes, instruments, sutures, and anything that would come in contact with the surgical field. Aseptic surgery replaced carbolic acid.

Once anesthesia and asepsis were in place, surgery finally became a full partner with internal medicine.

Huge advances in abdominal surgical techniques occurred in the 1880s and 1890s. Advances in ophthalmology and ear, nose, and throat surgery developed in the first part of the twentieth century, and they became the first surgical specialties in 1916 and 1924.[2]

For the most part, advances in medicine and surgery followed new technology, new pharmacology, and new surgical procedures first worked out in experimental laboratories. Since the beginning, surgery, more than any other branch of medicine, advanced only as new technology evolved. Of the surgical subspecialties, cardiac surgery has been the most dependent on evolving technology; hence its development did not really begin until one hundred years after the introduction of anesthesia.

Stab Wounds of the Heart

In 1896 Ludwig Rehn of Frankfurt, Germany, successfully closed a stab wound of the left ventricle with three silk sutures. After Rehn's case report, other surgeons adopted his technique. The first successful repair of a stab wound of the heart in the United States was done by Luther L. Hill of Montgomery, Alabama, in 1902.[3] He had presented a review of the reported cases of wounds of the heart to his local medical society, advocating surgical closure, and, as a result, was called to the home of a young man who had been stabbed in the chest and was in shock. Anticipating that some type of surgery would be needed, Dr. Hill took with him an anesthetist and an assistant. The operation was done on a kitchen table with a kerosene lantern for light. The pericardium was opened, clots were evacuated, and the patient's condition improved. A wound of the right ventricle was closed with a single catgut suture and the patient survived. An interesting footnote to this story is that Hill had named his son, Lister, for Lord Lister, the founder of antiseptic surgery. Lister Hill later became a U.S. senator from Alabama and was responsible for the Hill-Burton Act in 1946, which provided federal funds to community hospitals for modernization. Over six thousand hospitals received such funds and, in return, were required to provide a certain amount of charity care.

Alexis Carrel and Charles Guthrie

The publication in 1904 of a series of articles on vascular surgical techniques and experimental organ transplantation by Alexis Carrel and Charles Guthrie laid some of the foundation that would be used in the future by vascular and cardiac surgeons.

Alexis Carrel was born in Lyons, France, in 1873. He graduated from the University of Lyons medical school in 1900 and remained on the faculty as a junior member of the Department of Surgery. His interest in vascular surgery began with the death of the French president from a stab wound of the abdomen that lacerated the portal vein. The president's surgeons had no experience with vascular repair, and no attempt was made to suture the portal vein. Carrel began a study of experimental vascular surgical techniques, but, disappointed by his failure to attain a permanent academic appointment in Lyons, he moved first to Montreal and, later in 1904, to the Department of Physiology at the University of Chicago, where he first met Charles Guthrie. Carrel and Guthrie worked out a variety of techniques for vascular surgery, including meticulous asepsis, noncrushing instruments, small tapered needles, very fine silk lubricated with Vaseline, and a triangulation technique that kept tension on a continuous vascular suture line, thus avoiding a purse-string effect. They described interposition arterial grafts, vein grafts as an arterial substitute, end-to-end and end-to-side anastomoses, autografts (using the animal's own tissue), homografts (using tissue from another animal of the same species), and xenografts (using tissue from an animal of a different species). They performed successful kidney autografts and limb transplants in cats and dogs, and an orthotopic (added on rather than replacing the heart) heart transplant. Recognizing that autografted kidneys could function indefinitely but that homograft kidneys always failed, they postulated that it might be possible to "discover a means of recognizing the individuals, if such exist, between whom organs can be interchanged with impunity." What is most remarkable about these experiments is that they were accomplished without the use of an anticoagulant. Heparin was only discovered in 1916, by a preclinical Johns Hopkins medical student named Jay McLean, but it was not available clinically until the mid-1930s.

Carrel and Guthrie published a series of articles between 1904 and 1906 describing these vascular techniques and experiments.[4] They then separated, with Guthrie becoming chairman of the Department of Physiology at Washington University, and Carrel moving to the Rockefeller Institute for Medical Research in New York, where he continued his

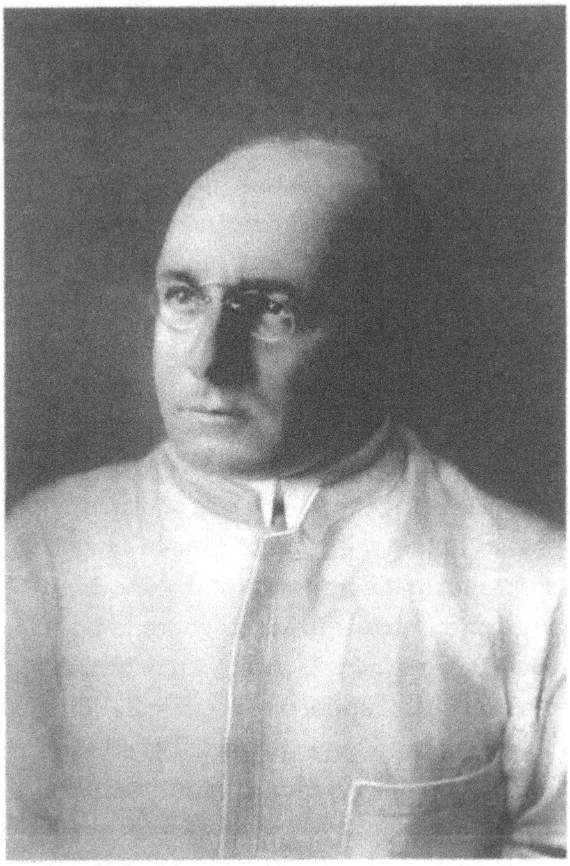

Alexis Carrel

organ and tissue transplant experiments for the next twenty-seven years.

Carrel was awarded the Nobel Prize for Physiology or Medicine in 1912 for this marvelous work. It was the first Nobel Prize given for research done in the United States; Carrel, however, remained a French citizen for the rest of his life. His Nobel lecture summarizes the techniques for vascular anastomosis and the various limb and organ transplant procedures that he developed.[5] The Nobel committee did not include Guthrie in the award.

Carrel joined the French army at the beginning of the First World War in 1914. He became the head of a small military hospital that was dedicated to the treatment of wounds and, in particular, wound infections. Along with his colleague, Henry Dakin, a chemist, he developed the use of dilute sodium hypochlorite, an antiseptic that proved to be extremely useful in dealing with the grossly contaminated wounds during that conflict.[6] Dakin's solution is still used today.

He returned to the Rockefeller Institute after World War I and worked there during the 1920s and 1930s, spending the summer months on an island off the coast of France. During the 1930s he associated with Charles Lindbergh, whose sister-in-law had severe rheumatic mitral valve disease. Lindbergh postulated that her valve could be repaired or replaced if there were a method of temporarily supporting the circulation, such as a heart-lung machine. Together, he and Carrel began working on a tissue perfusion device, which was successful for small organs such as the thyroid, but the project never advanced beyond that stage.[7] Their work is frequently mentioned, probably because of the fame of Lindbergh, but it was not important to the actual development of the heart-lung machine.

In 1939 Carrel returned to France, and, after the German occupation, he joined the pro-German Vichy government as director of the Carrel Foundation for the Study of Human Problems. He died of an acute myocardial infarct in Paris in 1944, his reputation somewhat tarnished by his association with the German army of occupation and by a book he authored, *Man, the Unknown*, which advocated eugenics.

Trendelenburg and Pulmonary Embolectomy

Today, the sudden collapse and death of a postoperative patient from a pulmonary embolus (blood clot) is relatively rare, but this was not always so. In the first half of the twentieth century it was fairly common. The reduction in postoperative venous thromboembolism has been brought about by a variety of changes, the most important being early ambulation and attention to proper hydration and fluid therapy during and after operations. Also, the ubiquitous use of aspirin and aspirin-like substances today must have played some part in altering the risk. Today, patients are commonly started on anticoagulation drugs after hip replacement and other selected procedures to avoid postoperative venous thrombosis.

Starting in 1905, Freidrich Trendelenburg of Leipzig began a study of this problem. At that time, peripheral arterial embolism was well-known, and femoral embolectomy had been successfully carried out. He proposed that the same procedure could be done for a pulmonary embolus. His research showed that death from a massive pulmonary embolus was usually not instant. There was often an interval of fifteen minutes or more, sometimes an hour or more, from the onset of symptoms to death. He proposed that the clinical picture was frequently clear enough to recognize the problem, and the interval between onset and death was long enough to attempt an embolectomy. The biggest problem was that there was no infallible way to diagnose pulmonary embolism. Acute myocardial infarction could produce a similar clinical picture. Indeed, in later years, more than once a patient was rushed to the operating room with a suspected pulmonary embolus, only to find that there was no clot and that the problem was a myocardial infarct. In spite of this uncertainty, Trendelenburg worked out a surgical technique in the experimental laboratory. Through a parasternal incision he would occlude the main pulmonary artery, with a tourniquet, as close to the heart as possible. He would next open the pulmonary artery distal to the tourniquet, remove the pulmonary embolus, close the pulmonary artery temporarily with a clamp, and release the tourniquet. To avoid operating on a patient that might otherwise survive, he planned to take the patient to the operating room, have him prepared and draped, and not begin the operation until the patient was at the point of death. Trendelenburg attempted this operation on three patients in 1906 and 1907, but all three patients died, the first two in the operating room, and the third patient several hours later of bleeding from the internal thoracic artery.[8] Attempts by others also failed until Trendelenburg's trainee, Martin Kirschner, did a successful pulmonary embolectomy in 1924. Still, it was never a procedure with much hope of success.

Years later, however, this operation was the stimulus for John Gibbon to begin his research to develop a heart-lung machine. In 1934, as an intern, Gibbon was involved with an unsuccessful pulmonary embolectomy in Boston. He recognized that temporary extracorporeal circulatory support would make this procedure practical. After nineteen years of research, he developed a heart-lung machine in 1953. While the Trendelenburg operation has fallen into disrepute because of the reported 90 percent mortality, the present-day use of radioisotope studies, pulmonary arteriograms, and open-heart surgery have made pulmonary embolectomy a reasonable strategy for massive pulmonary embolism.

Trendelenburg's idea that embolectomy would be beneficial for massive pulmonary embolism was exactly right. It failed at that time because vascular surgery was in its infancy. The only safe and realistic way to remove a pulmonary embolus involves cardiopulmonary bypass. The Trendelenburg operation is an example of a procedure that was proposed and carried out long before the technology necessary for success was available.

Mitral Stenosis in the 1920s

Another cardiac disorder, mitral stenosis (narrowing of the mitral valve), also appeared to have a surgical solution. Although it was known to be caused by rheumatic fever, many physicians at that time believed that the symptoms of shortness of breath, cardiac enlargement, and heart failure were due to rheumatic injury to the myocardium and not due to stenosis or leakage of the valves. Elliott Cutler at the Peter Bent Brigham Hospital in Boston was one of the first to challenge this view; he reviewed autopsy specimens of patients who had died of mitral valve disease and concluded that valvular stenosis was frequently the principal cause of the symptoms. His theory was that mitral regurgitation was less important than mitral stenosis. He proposed an operation to incise both leaflets of the mitral valve to convert mitral stenosis to "mild" regurgitation. His first operation was done in 1923. He inserted a valvulotome through a stab wound in the apex of the left ventricle of a twelve-year-old

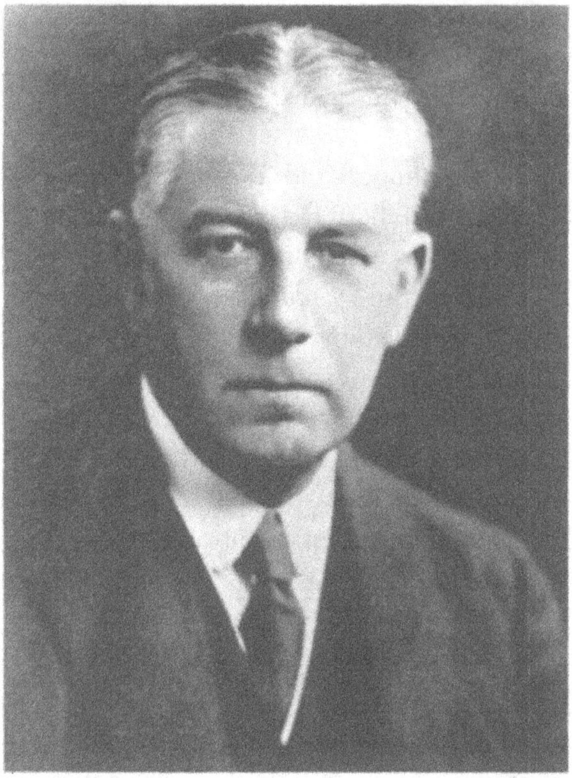

Sir Henry Souttar

female patient with severe mitral stenosis and successfully incised both leaflets. The patient survived and was improved but eventually died of additional cardiac problems four years later.[9] Cutler operated on six patients for mitral stenosis, but the only survivor was the first.[10]

In 1925 in London, Sir Henry Souttar also operated on a patient with mitral stenosis. He used the left atrial appendage to approach the valve and inserted his finger through a purse-string suture. Although there was some regurgitation, he was able to open the valve along the commissures and the operation was considered a success.[11] This method of opening the valve along the commissures rather than cutting the leaflets at right angles to the commissures would prove to be the most satisfactory operation twenty years later. However, Souttar's medical colleagues remained convinced that the myocardium was the problem and that valve disease was only of secondary importance. Although Souttar's patient did well and lived for several years, no other patient was referred. Years later, when asked by Dwight Harken why he did only one operation, he said, "It is of no use to be ahead of one's time."

Patent Ductus Arteriosus

In the 1930s the possibility of surgical closure of a patent ductus began to attract attention, not only because of heart failure and pulmonary hypertension, but also because of the possibility of bacterial "endocarditis" at the site of the ductus. The ductus arteriosus is a communication between the pulmonary artery and the aorta that remains open during fetal development but closes spontaneously at birth. If it remains open, it is called a patent ductus. The first such operation was done by John Strieder at Massachusetts General Hospital in 1937, in a patient with acute progressive bacterial endocarditis. The ductus was partially closed by sutures, and the murmur was gone postoperatively. Unfortunately, the patient died on the fourth postoperative day, of acute gastric dilatation.[12]

A year later, in August 1938, Robert Gross successfully ligated a patent ductus at the Boston Children's Hospital. Gross had prepared for this operation by careful study of autopsy specimens. His chief, Dr. William Ladd, was unwilling to give Gross permission to proceed, but Ladd always took a month-long vacation in August, so Gross scheduled the operation when Ladd was out of town. It was a success, and was soon repeated at Boston Children's and elsewhere. Despite the success, Gross had proceeded against Ladd's advice, and the resulting strained relationship between the two was never completely resolved.[13]

Coarctation of the Aorta

During the early 1940s, surgeons began to consider the possibility of correcting coarctation of the aorta. This congenital abnormality is a localized, very tight narrowing of the aorta just beyond the left subclavian artery at the site of the ligamentum arteriosum (the remnant of the ductus arteriosus). Coarctation produces high blood pressure and in adulthood can also be associated with aneurysmal dilatation of the aorta. It was correctly thought that if coarctation could be repaired, the high blood pressure would abate. Today, coarctation is usually repaired in childhood, but in 1940 there were a large number of adults with coarctation of the aorta and severe hypertension.

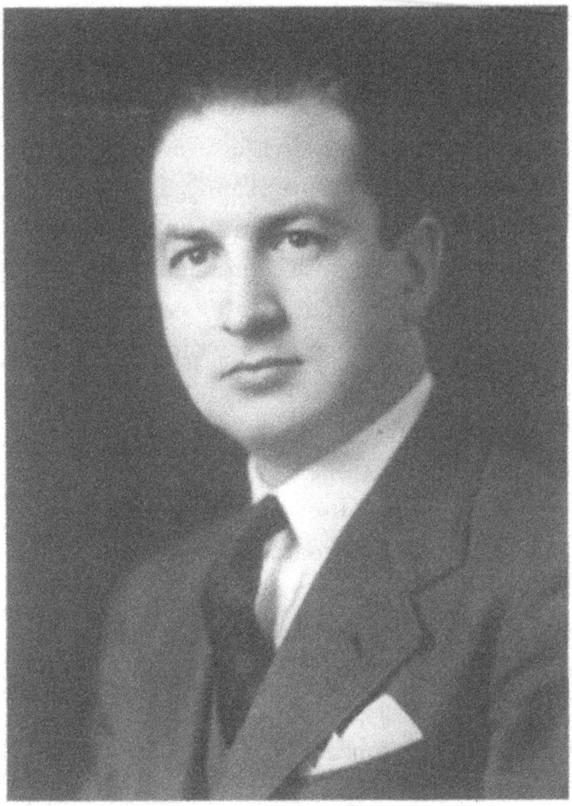

Robert E. Gross

Three different investigators were in the forefront of attempting to develop a surgical solution for this abnormality: Alfred Blalock at Johns Hopkins, Robert Gross at the Boston Children's Hospital, and Clarence Crafoord at Sabbatsberg Hospital in Stockholm.

Vascular surgical techniques had advanced in the experimental laboratory to the point that it was clear that the aorta could be clamped, divided, and then sutured together, with the assurance that the aorta would heal without disruption, leaking, or forming an aneurysm. Two theoretical problems existed. First, it was thought that if the aorta were clamped long enough to remove the segment containing the coarctation and re-anastomose the aorta (thirty minutes or more), ischemic damage to the spinal cord would result, leaving the patient paraplegic. Clamping the thoracic aorta of an experimental animal for more than thirty minutes frequently produced paralysis. The second problem was the perceived difficulty of bringing the two aortic ends back together after the excision of the stenotic segment. Could enough aorta be mobilized to avoid excessive tension in the anastomosis? Blalock, Gross, and Crafoord were each investigating this problem, and each had a different idea as to how the operation should be done.

Blalock's plan was to mobilize the left subclavian artery, divide it distally, and then turn this artery down to the aorta beyond the coarctation, creating a bypass. He planned to use a partial clamp on the aorta, thereby avoiding the hazard of complete occlusion.[14]

After working out the details of this operation in the experimental laboratory, he used this technique on a patient in 1944, but found it necessary to divide several pairs of intercostal arteries in placing the clamp. Unfortunately, the loss of these intercostals produced spinal cord ischemia, and the patient developed partial paralysis of the legs, just what Blalock hoped to avoid. This tragic outcome discouraged him,[15] but it has been used successfully by others in later years with various modifications.[16]

Robert Gross observed the extensive collateral vessels in coarctation patients at autopsy and thought correctly that this collateral network would provide enough circulation to the spinal cord that it would be possible to clamp the aorta long enough to excise the localized narrow segment and suture the ends together.[17] He was concerned that after removing two to three centimeters of aorta he might not be able to bring the two ends of the aorta together, but he discovered in dogs that he could mobilize the upper thoracic aorta, excise a short segment, and reconnect the ends without tension.[18] He also began investigating methods of preserving segments of aorta that could be kept in a tissue bank for use in those patients in whom the coarctation involved a longer segment of the aorta, too long for excision and direct re-anastomosis. The method he finally selected was graft dehydration, sterilization with ethylene oxide, and frozen storage.[19] During the1950s, such freeze-dried homografts were used extensively to replace both abdominal and thoracic aortic aneurysms, but they were not very durable and eventually many had to be replaced with Dacron grafts.

Clarence Crafoord in Stockholm was also interested in the surgical treatment of coarctation of the aorta. While operating on a patient with a patent ductus arteriosus, he had encountered bleeding from the thin wall of the ductus that he could not easily control. He therefore clamped the aorta above and below the site of the ductus, and was able to divide the ductus and suture the laceration. He used this technique on several occasions, clamping the aorta for as long as twenty minutes, and postulated that a coarctation patent could tolerate a longer period of aortic clamping because of the extensive collaterals bridging the aorta above and below the coarctation.

In October 1944 Crafoord did a successful excision and repair of a coarctation on a twelve-year-old boy,[20] and Gross followed suit in the United States eight months later. For some time, Gross thought that Crafoord had been made aware of his experimental work in Boston and that Crafoord had used the information in his decision to proceed. It appears now that Crafoord was not aware of the work Gross had done and that Crafoord arrived at the technique through his experience of clamping the aorta during repair of a patent ductus. Like many other medical "firsts," the operations occurred in two widely separate locations almost at the same time. Advancing technology and medical progress made coarctation repair possible. Gross and Crafoord arrived at the same solution at about the same time by a different route.

Tetralogy of Fallot and the Blue Baby Operation

The successful operations for patent ductus and coarctation were significant, but were not thought of as the beginning of a new era in surgery. However, an operation done by Alfred Blalock in November 1944 at Johns Hopkins changed the surgical world, and it is reasonable to say that the specialty of cardiac surgery was born that day. The patient was Eileen Saxon, an eighteen-month-old, very ill girl with severe cyanotic heart disease. The operation was a subclavian-pulmonary artery anastomosis, known now as the Blalock-Taussig shunt, and labeled by the press thereafter as the "Blue Baby operation."

The term "blue baby" describes a patient with a congenital cardiac abnormality that circulates desaturated arterial blood. This produces a bluish discoloration of the child, most noticeable in the lips, eyes, and nail beds. While there are many different cardiac defects that cause this "cyanotic heart disease," the most common after infancy is the "tetralogy of Fallot," named for the French physician Etienne Fallot, who first accurately described it in 1888.[21] While tetralogy of Fallot has four distinct anatomical abnormalities, the two important features are obstruction of blood flow to the lungs (pulmonary stenosis) and a large ventricular septal defect (an opening between the two pumping chambers of the heart) that allows blue venous blood to be shunted into the systemic circulation. Patients with tetralogy have low exercise tolerance, fail to grow normally, and may have frequent fainting spells. Before the Blalock-Taussig shunt, most of them had a very limited life expectancy, and many died in infancy or childhood; few lived beyond age fourteen.

Five people were pivotal in the successful development of the Blue Baby operation at Johns Hopkins. The two major figures were Blalock, the chief of surgery, and Helen Taussig, the director of the Children's Car-

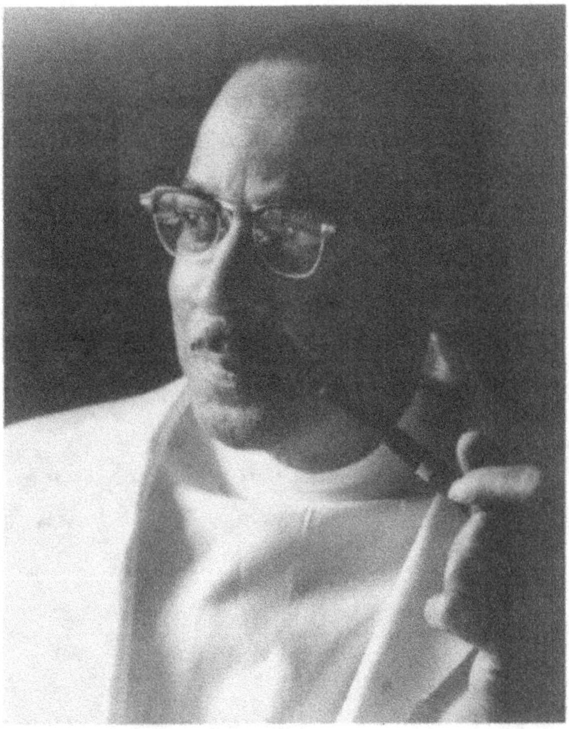

Vivien T. Thomas when he was director of the Surgical Research Laboratories, Johns Hopkins University School of Medicine

diac Clinic. Next in importance was Vivien Thomas, a very talented and skilled African American who had worked for Blalock as his laboratory assistant for fourteen years, initially at Vanderbilt. The final two were Edwards Park and Sanford Leeds. Park was chairman of pediatrics, and worked with Blalock to develop an operation for coarctation of the aorta. Park knew of Taussig's interest in surgery for tetralogy of Fallot, and arranged for her to meet Blalock to explore the possibility.[22] Leeds was a young surgical resident from the University of California who had worked in Dr. Blalock's experimental laboratory at Vanderbilt for two years in 1938 and 1939, not long after Leeds's graduation from medical school. During that time, they published together fifteen articles on a

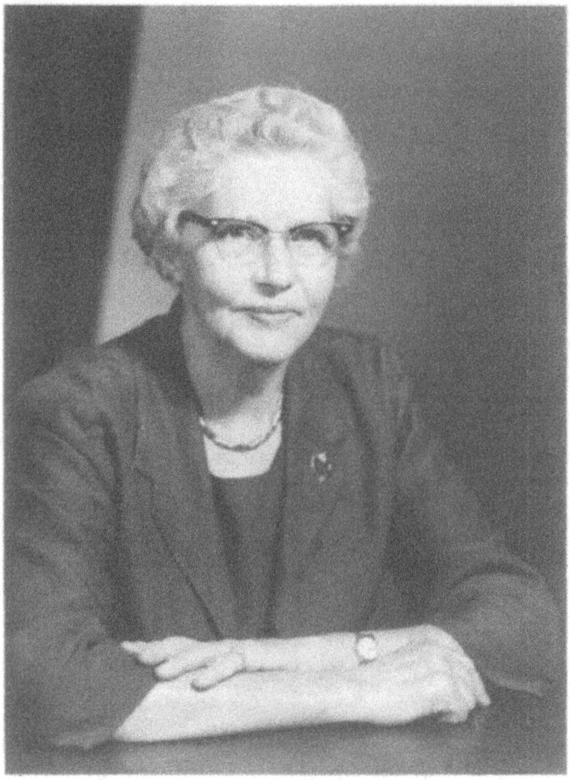

Helen B. Taussig

variety of experimental procedures, one of which was a left subclavian artery to left pulmonary artery anastomosis in dogs, intended to produce pulmonary hypertension.[23] This was reported in the *Journal of Thoracic Surgery* in 1939.[24] While pulmonary hypertension did not result, several of the dogs were followed for up to six years, yielding the fundamental information that made the Blue Baby operation possible: that subclavian-pulmonary anastomosis had no long-term adverse effects.

There is one other item of note in that brief article. The first author was Sanford Levy and the second author was Alfred Blalock. Sanford Levy was the resident from the University of California working with Dr. Blalock. At about the time of his return to California in 1939, Levy had his name changed to Sanford Leeds. Leeds and Levy are the same person. This name change has led to some confusion in later publications about the experimental origins of the Blue Baby operation. Many years later, Sanford Leeds was interviewed by Dr. Peter Olch for the oral history archives of the National Library of Medicine, and Dr. Leeds spoke at length, and heatedly, of the anti-Semitic attitudes that were still present in surgical departments and societies in the 1930s.[25] He did not say so, but it seems likely that he changed his name to avoid some of these prejudices. After serving in the medical corps for five years during World War II, he returned to San Francisco and had a long and distinguished career there as a thoracic surgeon.

Helen Taussig was the daughter of a professor of economics at Harvard, but her application to Harvard Medical School was rejected, since only men were taken until 1945. She then applied to and was accepted by the Johns Hopkins School of Medicine, graduating in 1927. The Johns Hopkins medical school had accepted a few women in each class since its opening in 1893.

After two years of pediatric residency, Taussig was assigned by her chief, Dr. Edwards Park, to take charge of the cardiac clinic at the Harriet Lane Home, the children's "hospital within a hospital" at Hopkins. Over the next ten years she became a leading authority on congenital heart disease, despite impaired hearing that eventually required an amplified stethoscope and hearing aids. Cardiac catheterization was rarely utilized at that time, and she much preferred diagnostic fluoroscopy. Long periods of follow-up allowed her to understand the natural history of the conditions and various anatomical abnormalities. She gradually became aware that some children with cyanotic heart disease did well as long as the ductus arteriosus remained open, but if it closed, rapid decline and death tended to occur. If infants with tetralogy of Fallot did well until the ductus closed, she reasoned that the primary problem with this disorder must be decreased pulmonary blood flow, rather than the coexisting ventricular septal defect. "Why not develop an operation to create an artificial ductus?" she reasoned.

Medical discoveries and new medical techniques usually arise after an investigator makes an original observation or original insight into a problem that had remained unnoticed by others. A classic example occurred in 1798 when Edward Jenner was told by a milkmaid that those in her occupation who had contracted cowpox, a mild skin infection, were thereafter protected against smallpox. His investigations supported this observation, and he eventually put this theory to an experiment. He inoculated a boy with cowpox, and after the skin infection cleared, he inoculated him again, this time with smallpox. Fortunately, the boy remained healthy and the practice of vaccination was born. The final result, of course, was the total elimination of smallpox two hundred years later. Helen Taussig's observation eventually led to the Blue Baby operation and the beginning of modern cardiac surgery. A characteristic of some medical discoveries is that they are worked out not by one person working alone, but by two investigators working together. There are many examples of this: Banting and Best discovered insulin, Florey and Chain brought penicillin into clinical use, Watson and Crick first described the structure of DNA, Carrel and Guthrie investigated vascular surgery, Shumway and Lower worked out the techniques of cardiac transplantation, and there are many more. Blalock and Taussig should be included in this category; they fit nicely into this concept. It has been pointed out by others that Blalock and Taussig really did not work together smoothly, but it was clearly the combination of Taussig's knowledge of congenital heart disease and Blalock's understanding of experimental vascular surgery that made the Blue Baby operation successful. Blalock's work with Taussig was just one of two examples of Blalock's working closely with another investigator. In addition to Blalock and Taussig's development of the Blue Baby operation in the 1940s, Blalock and Vivien Thomas worked out the understanding of shock in the 1930s.

Sometime in 1940 or 1941 Dr. Taussig was in Boston and made an appointment to meet Robert Gross at the Boston Children's Hospital. Gross had first successfully closed a patent ductus in a child in 1939. Taussig thought that Gross was the most likely surgeon to try her theory. Dr. Gross listened to her proposal but is said to have told her that he was interested in operations to close a patent ductus, not to create one, and nothing came of the meeting.[26]

Park encouraged her to present her idea to Blalock, who recalled the experiments at Vanderbilt with Sanford Leeds and recognized immediately that a subclavian-pulmonary artery anastomosis would accomplish exactly what she was proposing. Taussig presented a unique original observation to the one person in the country who had the experimental background and surgical experience to see immediately that it could be done. Taussig and Blalock had separate skills and information that, when brought together, forever changed the future for patients with tetralogy of Fallot. This was a combination of ideas and information that led to the solution of a difficult health problem, similar to but not as great as Jenner and the milkmaid.

Alfred Blalock grew up in Jonesboro, Georgia, and graduated first from the University of Georgia in 1918, and then from the Johns Hopkins School of Medicine in 1922. After two years on the Hopkins surgical service and a year on the ENT service, he was appointed chief resident in surgery at the Vanderbilt School of Medicine in 1925. His close friend Tinsley Harrison was chief resident in medicine at Vanderbilt at the same time. They both were appointed to the full-time faculty the following year and began working together in the experimental laboratory on a daily basis. At that time there was not a clear understanding of shock, and through a number of experiments and publications over the next fifteen years, Blalock was able to show that it was not caused by some unrecognized toxic agent but was secondary to loss of blood volume. This proved to be a very important contribution, and it was put to good use initially in the management of military injuries during World War II.

When Dean Lewis, the chief of surgery at Johns Hopkins, had a stroke in 1939, Evarts Graham of Washington University was first offered the position, but he declined the offer and advised them to consider Alfred Blalock. Blalock accepted and moved to Baltimore in 1941, taking with him his secretary, Frances Grebel; his laboratory assistant, Vivien Thomas; and one surgical resident, George W. Duncan. Dr. Blalock's salary was to be $16,000 per year,[27] and the total annual budget for the Department of Surgery was $85,000.[28]

Blalock's first years at Johns Hopkins were difficult, both because of local antipathy to a young surgeon "from the outside," and because he undertook the unpopular steps of reducing the number of residents and the length of their training. He spent his mornings in the operating room, and his afternoons in the experimental laboratory. When Helen Taussig made her proposal, he and Vivien Thomas set out to create an animal with cyanosis to test Taussig's theory. This proved difficult, but they did eventually develop a cyanotic model and found that a subclavian-pulmonary shunt would improve the blood oxygen saturation.[29]

Their first patient was a critically ill, deeply cyanotic child who was fourteen months old but weighed only 8.8 pounds. She required an oxygen tent, and "after eating she would become deeply cyanotic, roll up her eyes, lose consciousness, and appear extremely ill." When she was scheduled for a subclavian-pulmonary artery shunt in November 1944, the chief of anesthesia took one look at her and cancelled the case. His resident, Merel Harmel, agreed to give the anesthesia, and the operation was rescheduled a day or two later. The first assistant was the chief resident, William Longmire, and the second assistant was Denton Cooley. Vivien Thomas stood behind Dr. Blalock, and Helen Taussig was also present in the operating room.

This was an operation that was done before most of the technology to make it easier and safer was available. For example, they did not have an endotracheal tube small enough, so the ether anesthetic was

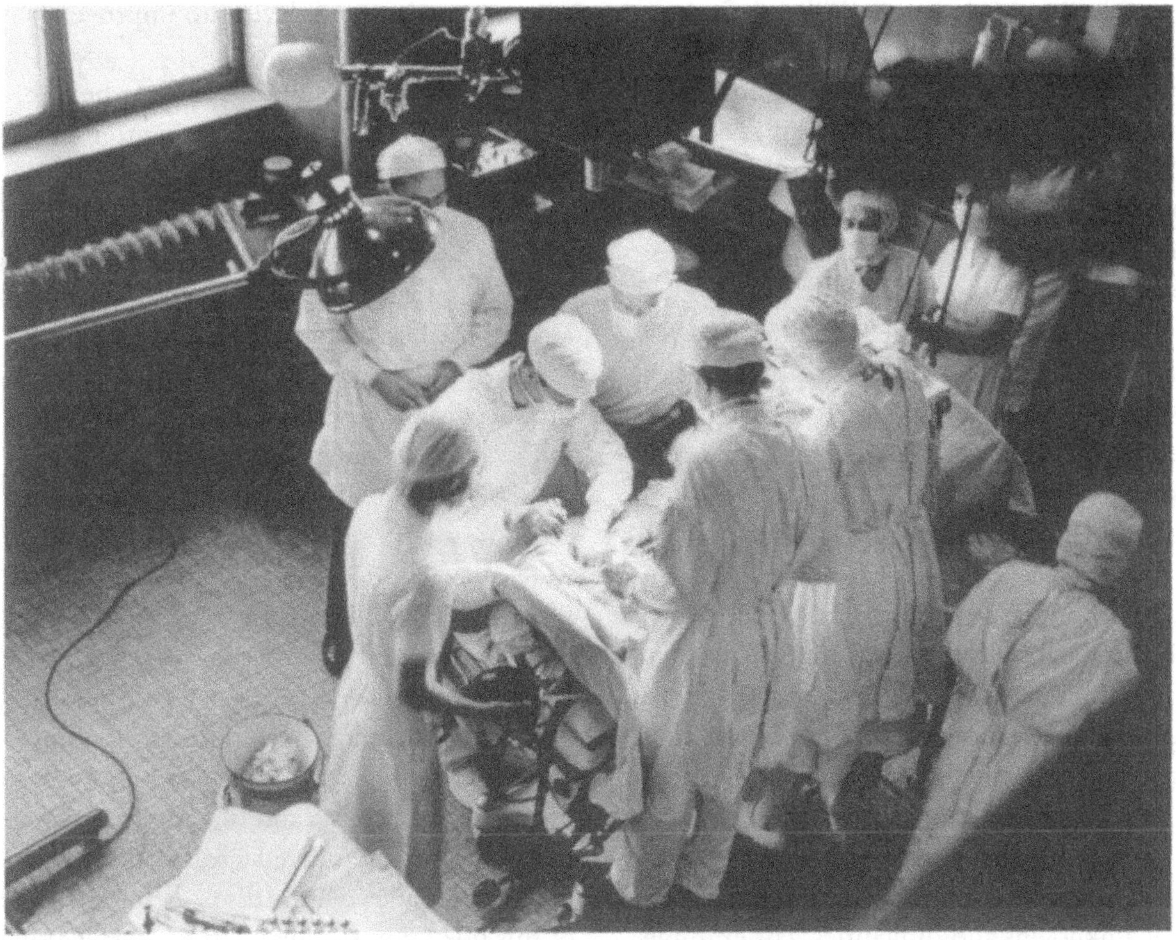

Blue Baby operation at Johns Hopkins in 1947: Dr. Blalock is on the left, Denton Cooley on the right, Olive L. Berger is the nurse anesthetist, and Vivien Thomas stands behind Blalock.

given with a mask. The vascular clamps were rubber-shod bulldog clamps, which were tied in place to prevent slipping. The sutures were 5/0 beaded china silk, threaded on fine straight needles and lubricated with mineral oil. In spite of these handicaps, the operation was completed in an hour and a half and was a success. The patient developed a postoperative pneumothorax but eventually left the hospital improved. Two additional patients followed, and in May 1945 Blalock and Taussig published their experience in the *Journal of the American Medical Association.* In many ways, it is a unique article. The title proclaimed for the first time that surgery was to be the treatment for congenital heart disease—"The Surgical Treatment of Malformations of the Heart in which There Is Pulmonary Stenosis or Pulmonary Atresia."[30] It noted the insufficient pulmonary blood flow in patients with tetralogy and recalled Taussig's observation that those with an open ductus continued to do well. It cited Leeds and Blalock's article describing subclavian-pulmonary artery anastomosis in dogs and described in great detail the case reports and operative technique in the three patients, each of whom had a slightly different operation due in part to anatomical variations. The article ended with a discussion of the various congenital malformations in which a shunt should or should not be of benefit.

All three patients recovered and were improved. The first, who was very small, stayed in the hospital for two months, but was less cyanotic and grew from 8.8 to 12 pounds. The improvement in the two others was much more dramatic, with greatly increased exercise tolerance, decreased cyanosis, and recession of the clubbing of the fingers and toes.

When he completed his training, Longmire was asked by Blalock to join the faculty as chief of plastic surgery, and he became Blalock's closest friend and confidant. Many years later he wrote that Blalock considered the work on shock his most important contribution, not the Blue Baby operation.

Today, however, one might differ and say that the Blue Baby operation was his most important contribution, considering all of the unknowns and difficulties. For example, Dr. Taussig's observation of the increase of cyanosis in infants with tetralogy of Fallot when the ductus closed was based only on clinical findings and fluoroscopy. Without cardiac catheterization, the diagnosis could have been incorrect. The first patient was critically ill, malnourished and grossly underweight, and requiring continuous oxygen. Could such a patient tolerate a general anesthetic and, if so, could she tolerate clamping the left main pulmonary artery for thirty minutes or more, long enough to construct the anastomosis? Would dividing the subclavian artery produce ischemia of the arm and hand? The answers were unknown. Also, one cannot overstate the difficulties of doing vascular surgery without today's instruments, suture materials, and devices to improve vision.

Why did this operation mark the beginning of cardiac surgery? Before it, attempts to improve a patient's cardiac condition by an operation had either failed or, if successful, had not been thought of as heralding a new surgical specialty. The prior operations in and around the heart had been isolated single events at different locations. This operation produced sudden, intense interest, not only in the surgical community but also in the media. This actually caused Blalock some embarrassment, since physicians of the day were expected to keep a low public profile and any hint at advertisement was considered unethical.

There was, thereafter, both a continuous succession of cardiac operations at Hopkins and a program of surgical education in heart disease. Cardiologists and the public recognized that surgery offered a solution for children with cyanotic heart disease. The success of this operation stimulated the investigation of other cardiac anomalies and their natural histories, and the result was a significant improvement in diagnostic and prognostic accuracy, and a steady decrease in surgical risk.

Children with heart disease came to Baltimore from all over the country. Other medical centers started cardiac surgical programs that offered at least three operations: closure of a patent ductus, repair of coarctation, and the Blalock-Taussig shunt. Gradually other procedures evolved, but it was the success of the initial Blue Baby operation that was the foundation of this early period of cardiac surgery.

Dr. Blalock received invitations from several European surgical centers to visit and demonstrate the operation, which had not been attempted as yet outside the United States. On August 22, 1947, he and his wife Mary departed New York on the *Mauretania* for four weeks in London working at Guy's Hospital with Mr. Russell Brock (later Sir Russell and, later still, Lord Brock), one week in Stockholm with Clarence Crafoord, and two weeks in Paris with Professor Francois d'Allaines at the Hospital Broussais. Blalock asked his third-year resident, Hank Bahnson, and Bahnson's wife, Louise, to go with them. Bahnson would be Blalock's first assistant. During the next few weeks, they did ten Blalock-Taussig operations at Guy's, all of which went well. Their trip had been planned to coincide with the first postwar meeting of the International Society of Surgeons and Dr. Blalock was asked to speak on the surgical treatment of congenital heart disease. He was also asked to give a lecture at the British Medical Association.

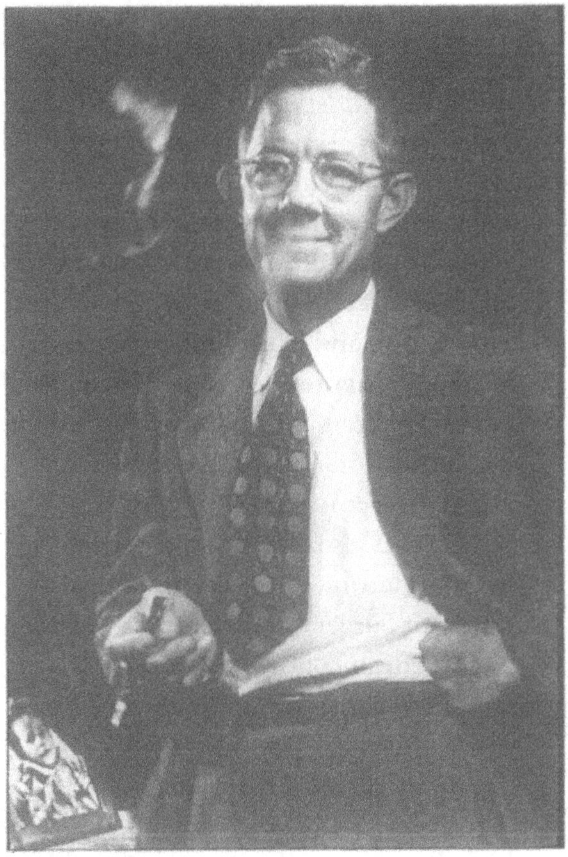

Alfred Blalock

When Dr. Mark Ravitch was preparing a short biography of Blalock for the preface of his two volume-work, *The Papers of Alfred Blalock*, in 1966, he wrote to Lord Brock and asked him for information about Blalock's London visit. This is Lord Brock's letter as published in Ravitch's book:

> Intense interest had already been aroused throughout Great Britain by the reports of his successful work on previously hopeless cases of cyanotic heart disease, and everyone was eager to see and hear him. There were two notable occasions that must be unforgettable to anyone who was present.
>
> The first was when he and Dr. Helen Taussig gave a combined lecture in the Great Hall of the British Medical Association; the huge hall was packed. Dr. Taussig delivered her address impeccably and was followed by Dr. Blalock who presented his surgical contribution with his characteristic, apparently casual, drawl but really a forceful and incisive presentation of his brilliant and impressive results. The silence of the audience betokened their rapt attention and appreciation. The hall was quite dark for projection of his slides which had been illustrating patients before and after operation, when suddenly a long searchlight beam traversed the whole length of the hall and unerringly picked out on the platform a Guy's nursing sister, dressed in her attractive blue uniform, sitting on a chair and holding a small cherub-like

girl of 2½ years with a halo of blonde curly hair and looking pink and well; she had been operated on at Guy's by Blalock a week earlier. The effect was dramatic and theatrical and the applause from the audience was tumultuous. It was a Madonna-like tableau, a perfect climax to an impressive lecture on an epoch-making contribution and left nothing more to be said by the lecturer. No audience could fail to have been convinced or satisfied by this summation and no one there could possibly forget it.

This was also the occasion of the London meeting of the International Society of Surgery; the first since the war. The American contingent included many of the top names of the American College of Surgeons. On each afternoon a lecture was given at the College, the lecturers being Dr. Evarts Graham, Dr. Arthur Allen, Dr. Dallas Phemister, and Dr. Naffziger, all before packed audiences. On Friday afternoon Blalock lectured on the surgical treatment of congenital heart disease. The scene was astonishing; it was literally impossible to enter the building of the College by the time his lecture was due to start; not only was the lecture hall packed but so were all adjacent corridors and spaces, in which fortunately loud speakers had been installed. Many who came to listen could not get beyond the portico. The occasion, quite unparalleled, was made even more remarkable in that after delivering his lecture, Blalock repeated it in a second sitting for the benefit of those who had been unable to get in! Could there ever be a second demonstration of the admiration and profound interest in his pioneer work? These feelings were also fortified by the general feeling of appreciation for the friendliness, modesty, and attractiveness of his character.

His clinical and operative sessions at Guy's were equally popular and impressive. He had brought Dr. Hank Bahnson with him as his first assistant and together they operated on 10 patients with Fallot's tetralogy. Obviously, it was a difficult assignment to do these pioneer procedures in unfamiliar surroundings, before large audiences, and on anxious cases. Success was complete; all 10 patients did well and indirectly many more patients must have benefited by the invaluable technical information many surgeons obtained from these incomparable demonstrations. Blalock's sangfroid and imperturbability were remarkable; he patiently answered innumerable questions and I remember the special impression he made when someone asked him if he had ever encountered a particular technical difficulty. He looked at his questioner with his characteristic glance and drawled "Well, doctor, everything has happened to me." This frank remark was fully appreciated in all its contexts by all.

. . . [T]he outstanding important result of his visit was the firm introduction and launching of his operation in Great Britain and the Continent, acceptance of the immense possibilities of surgery in the alleviation of congenital heart disease in centres previously unconvinced and reluctant. The large numbers of visitors from the Continent and London for the International Meeting meant that they were also able to benefit and so the gospel was spread even more widely.[31]

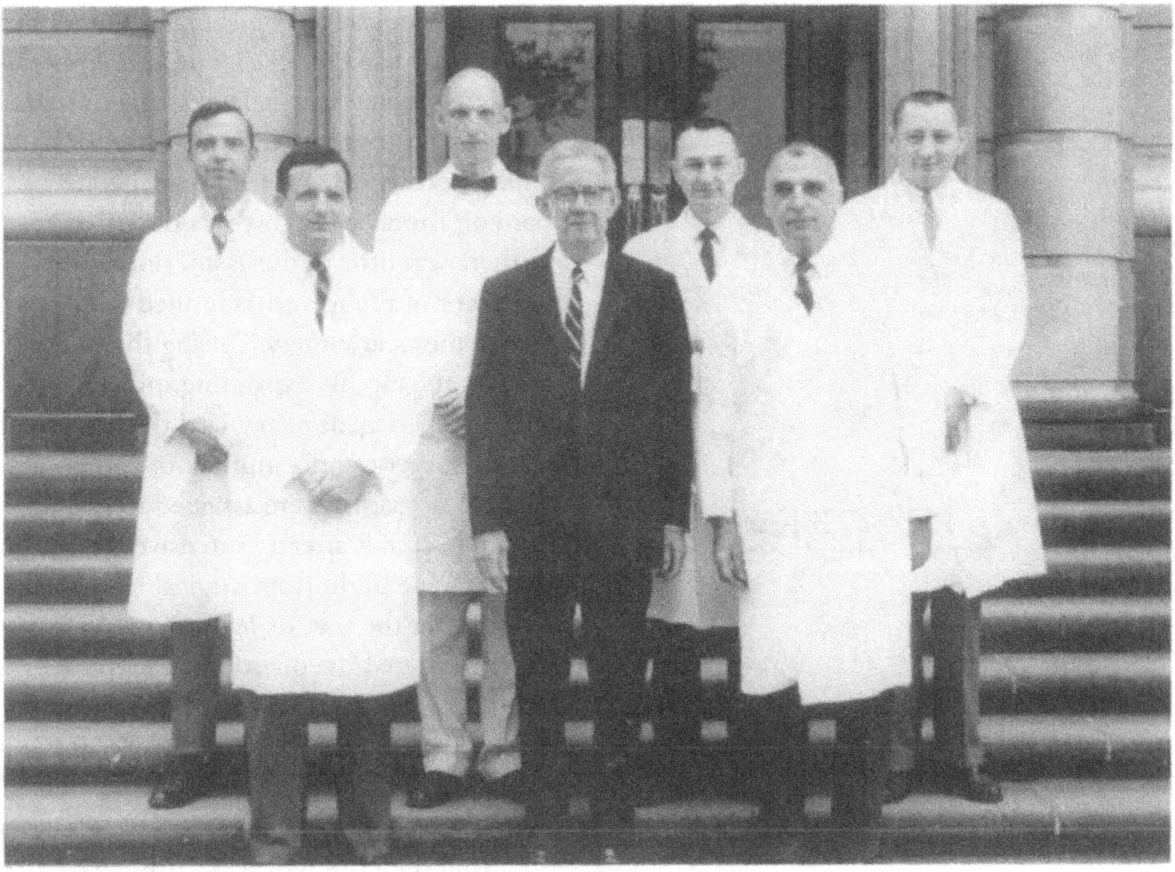

Johns Hopkins University Medical School Surgical Faculty, 1964.
First Row: David C. Sabiston Jr., Alfred Blalock, Mark M. Ravitch.
Second Row: Clarence S. Weldon, J. Alex Haller Jr., James R. Jude, Robert A. Gaertner.

The Blalocks and Bahnsons went on to Stockholm on September 27 to visit Clarence Crafoord at the Sabbetsburg Hospital. There they did no operations since Dr. Crafoord had previously visited Dr. Blalock in Baltimore and had observed several Blalock-Taussig procedures. They flew from Stockholm to Paris on October 5 to meet Professor Francois d'Allaines and performed several operations at the Hospital Broussais. The final patient was an adult with a large patent ductus who had recently had an episode of bacterial endocarditis, a difficult problem under any circumstances. Blalock asked Bahnson to do the operation while he and Mrs. Blalock went sightseeing. This was the first closure of a patent ductus done in France, and the operation was difficult with unexpected bleeding but finally a complete success, a great testament to the surgical skill of Hank Bahnson. Professor D'Allaines had assigned his junior colleague Charles Dubost to be the official translator for Dr. Blalock and also to be the scrub nurse for the seven Blalock-Taussig operations in Paris. Later, Dubost said of Dr. Blalock's visit: "Blalock impressed me so much that then and there I decided to forget about surgery of stomachs, colons, and rectums, and to devote my career to what was to become an entirely new specialty."[32]

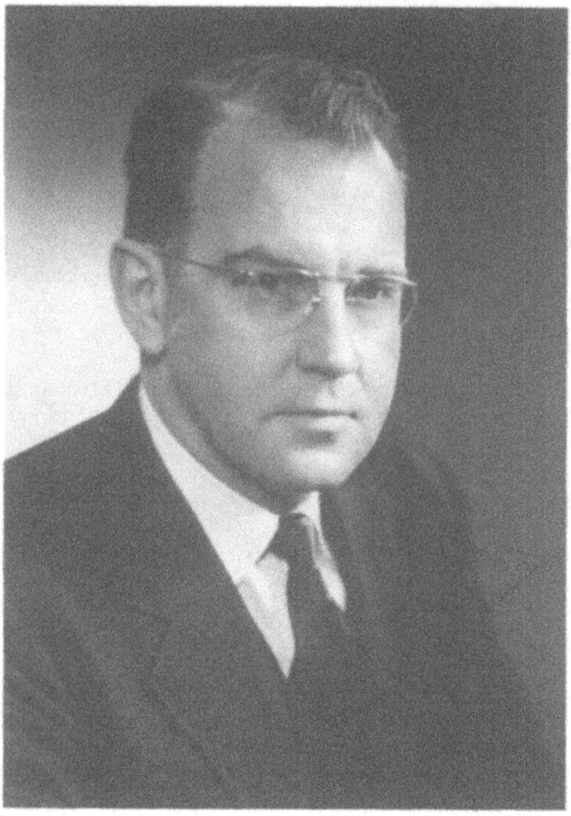

Dwight E. Harken

The impact of the Blue Baby operation on Hopkins was more than a flood of patients with congenital heart disease. It also brought a succession of talented and creative young surgical residents, most of whom went on to distinguished careers in other medical schools. The Blue Baby operation and all that came with it reestablished the Hopkins program as the premier surgical training program of that era.

World War II

The Second World War played a significant role in the advancement of thoracic surgery as a separate discipline, rather than a part of general surgery. (The American Board of Surgery had been established in 1936.) The American Association for Thoracic Surgery had been founded in 1917, but its members considered themselves general surgeons with an interest in thoracic surgery. At the 1937 annual meeting, the subject of a separate Board of Thoracic Surgery was discussed, but there was little enthusiasm, since only 18 percent of the members limited their work to thoracic surgery. During the war, however, the rapidly expanding military medical department recognized the need for thoracic surgery, and a number of young "thoracic surgeons" were assigned to various military hospitals after an intensive three-month course in thoracic surgical techniques. After the war, in 1946, the AATS again considered the question of a separate board. As a result, the Board of Thoracic Surgery was established, and thoracic and cardiac surgery became a bona fide separate specialty.

During the First World War, thoracotomy was unusual for penetrating chest wounds, and the mortality was very high. Thoracic surgery was then in its infancy and was usually confined to procedures dealing with empyema. However, during the Second World War things were quite different, and thoracic injuries were treated by appropriate surgical procedures. This led to some of the very first cardiac operations for foreign body removal. Dwight Harken was a young surgeon on the staff of the Peter Bent Brigham Hospital when he entered military service in 1942. He had completed three years of surgical residency in New York and a one-year fellowship in thoracic surgery with the leading British thoracic surgeon, Tudor Edwards, in London. Harken was placed in charge of thoracic surgery for the American Army in England and eventually was chief of thoracic surgery at a military hospital in Cirencester. Over a three-year period, he operated on 134 patients who had shrapnel or bullets in and around the heart. In 13 of these, he removed a foreign body from inside one of the cardiac chambers.[33] To accomplish this, Harken made a stab wound between stay sutures in the myocardial wall, through which he grasped the foreign body with an instrument and removed it. Then the incision was quickly closed using the previously placed sutures. Blood loss was rapidly replaced by pumping cross-matched blood into the venous system through large-bore needles. In addition, 43 other fragments were removed from the pericardium, 19 from the mediastinum, and 59 from in and around the great vessels. Miraculously, all 134 patients survived.

An interesting side benefit came from this experience. The Army cardiologist at the Cirencester Hospital was Paul Zoll, also from Boston. He frequently came to the operating room to help with the management of his patients. Watching Harken operate, he made an interesting observation. He noticed that frequently if an instrument touched the heart it would stimulate a heartbeat, an extrasystole. Also, a flick of the surgeon's finger on the heart could precipitate an extra beat. After returning home to Boston, Zoll began to investigate various methods of electrical stimulation of the heart, first as an attempt to resuscitate patients following cardiac arrest and then to treat patients with Stokes-Adams attacks due to heart block. This led to the earliest use of external pacing and to Zoll's many contributions to the development of pacemakers and defibrillators.

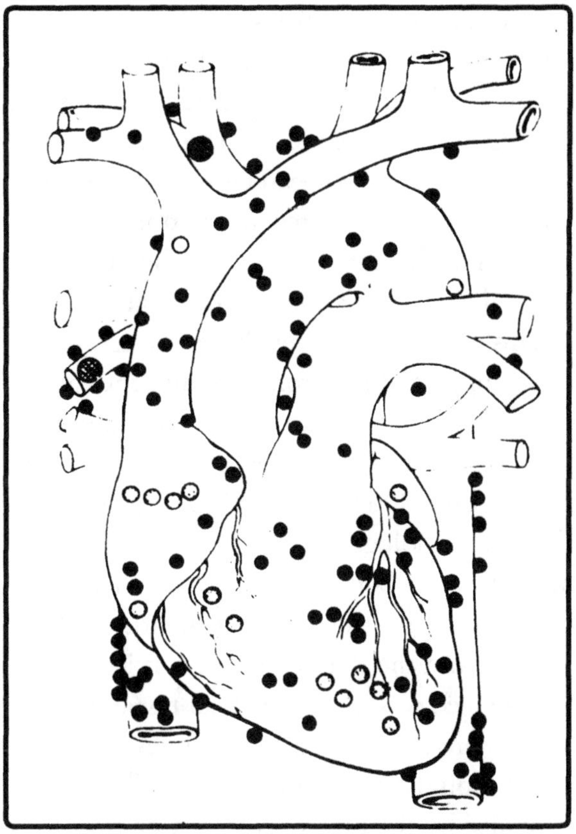

Position of foreign bodies removed from within and around the heart by Dwight Harken, 1944–1945. Black, inpinging; cross-hatching, embolic; stippled, within the structure.

Before the Second World War, Europe, particularly Germany, was considered to have the best science and medicine in the world. While medical education in the United States had gone through a revolutionary reform for the better after the 1910 Flexner Report, it was still thought that the best medical training and research were in Europe. It had been common since colonial times for young American physicians and surgeons to visit Vienna, Paris, London, or Berlin as a final part of their education. This was particularly true in the 1920s and 1930s. Sir William Osler was a great advocate of an extended summer visit to several different

European medical centers every three or four years as a refresher course for himself and his fellow faculty members at Johns Hopkins.

When the war ended in 1945, the devastation of many European cities and the problems of recovery and reconstruction greatly affected health care services. At the same time, the war had stimulated a great deal of scientific research in the United States: the development of the atomic bomb, the early computers used to break German codes, the success in mass production of penicillin, and the wartime development of various other drugs and biological products. Immediately after the war, Congress approved generous funding for the National Institutes of Health, and the Public Health Service was encouraged to support medical research. The states were encouraged to build new community hospitals with matching federal funds provided by the Hill-Burton Act of 1946. Veterans' hospitals were asked to affiliate with nearby medical schools, and their medical staffs were funded by the government but appointed by the parent medical school. From 1955 to 1960 the NIH annual budget increased from $81 million to $400 million. Finally, on July 30, 1965, Congress passed the Medicare and Medicaid Acts, which provided health insurance for the elderly and for the poor. This vast increase in funding produced a rapid expansion of medical schools and community hospitals, with a dramatic increase in medical research. The Nobel Prize in Physiology or Medicine was first awarded in 1901. During the next forty years, up to the beginning of World War II, there were five Nobel Prize winners from the United States. After the war, the United States dominated the Nobel Prize for medicine. In forty-three of the next sixty years, an American won or shared the prize. The center of medical education and research had shifted from Europe to the United States, and, as a result, young physicians from Europe came to the United States for additional training or, in many cases, to stay. The transatlantic medical information traffic had reversed its direction.

Post–World War II Developments

After the war, Dwight Harken returned to Boston and selected mitral stenosis as the next potential area to advance cardiac surgery. At the same time, Charles Bailey in Philadelphia and Russell Brock in London also took up the same project. Harken talked to Elliott Cutler about his operations for mitral stenosis in the 1920s and reasoned that the left atrial approach would be preferable to the apical ventriculotomy approach used by Cutler. Charles Bailey came to the same conclusion and devised a sheathed knife that could be attached to the index finger of the surgeon. After introducing the knife and finger into the left atrium, the valve could first be palpated, and then the knife would be unsheathed to incise the commissures.

Bailey met with considerable criticism after three successive patients died in the operating room during attempts to open the mitral valve. He was threatened with loss of hospital privileges if he continued. For this reason, he scheduled two patients on June 10, 1945, at separate hospitals in Philadelphia. The first patient had a cardiac arrest soon after being anesthetized, could not be resuscitated, and died. Because of this death and his previous failures, Bailey was concerned that the hospital administrator would cancel his afternoon operation, so he and his surgical team quickly went across town to start the second operation before the administration heard the bad news about the first. After four failures, this fifth attempt to open a stenotic valve was a total success—the patient lived another thirty-eight years.[34] Six days later in Boston, Dwight Harken did a successful mitral valvuloplasty, after four previous operations that resulted in death. Harken's patient was reported in the *New England Journal of Medicine* in 1948.[35] Bailey did the first modern successful mitral commissurotomy, and Harken was the first to report a success. Later in 1948, in London, Russell Brock did a successful mitral commissurotomy using finger pressure to open the commissures.[36] This turned out to be preferable to the technique of blindly incising the commissures. Further refinement involved the use of a dilator introduced through a purse string at the apex of the left ventricle and guided into the mitral valve by a finger in the left atrium, accomplished first by Charles Dubost. Oswald Tubbs of London devised an improved dilator, and during the next ten years this relatively simple and low-risk operation benefited large numbers of patients. It was not abandoned until the heart-lung machine became well established, and even then remained a safe and cost-effective procedure, particularly in developing countries.

Mitral commissurotomy was the first new cardiac operation to be developed after the Second World War. Three other unusual cardiac operative procedures were added in the early 1950s before the heart-lung machine became a part of cardiac surgery: closure of atrial septal defects using the Gross atrial well,[38] closure of atrial septal defects using hypothermia and inflow occlusion (an atrial septal defect is an abnormal hole between

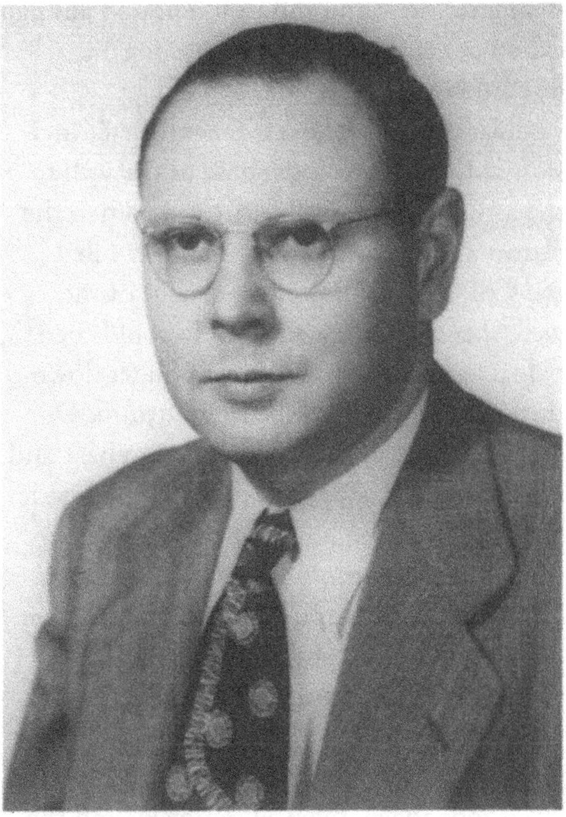

Charles P. Bailey

the two collecting chambers of the heart),[39] and the Hufnagel prosthetic aortic valve.[40] Each of these operations was first done in 1952, and each was discontinued around 1957 when the use of heart-lung machines provided a much safer surgical method. Each was a nerve-racking operation that required precise timing with little or no margin for error and that presented a thin line between success and disaster.

Dissatisfied with previous methods attempting "closed" repair of atrial septal defects, Robert Gross at the Boston Children's Hospital devised an ingenious method using a funnel-shaped rubber well, fifteen centimeters tall, with a wide upper mouth of thirteen centimeters' diameter, and a smaller mouth at the bottom of five centimeters' diameter. He found through repeated animal experiments (over one hundred dogs) that he could isolate the atrial appendage with a vascular clamp, make a five-centimeter incision in it, and attach the base of the well to the atrium with multiple sutures. When the clamp was removed, blood partially filled the well, but because of the height of the well, there was no overflow. He could then palpate the defect by putting a finger down through the well into the right atrium. During this time the heart continued to beat and normal cardiac activity was not interrupted. Sutures were then blindly placed by palpation around the rim of the defect and then brought outside through a patch held above the well. When all sutures were placed, the patch was lowered through the well down to the defect, and the sutures were tied. The clamp was then again placed across the atrial appendage, the well removed, and the atriotomy closed.[41] The main hazard of this technique was air embolism. If the right atrial pressure was low and the patient suddenly took an unexpected deep breath, air could be sucked into the right atrium.

Actually, the early results of the Gross well technique were pretty bad. To shorten the operating time, Gross used a Hufnagel double-disc button for the first three patients. This was a plastic device that came with two discs. One disc was placed on the left atrial side of the septum and the other on the right atrial side, and then the two were snapped together, which closed the septal defect. Unfortunately, in the first three patients the buttons became dislodged during the early postoperative course and all three patients died. Direct suture closure or a patch was used for four additional patients. Of the first seven operations using the atrial well there were only three survivors, each of whom had direct suture closure of the defect. In a later series of twenty-one patients, there were four deaths, two of which occurred in patients who were found to have atrioventricular defects. In addition to a relatively high operative mortality, a significant number of patients had incomplete closure of the atrial defect. John Kirklin at the Mayo Clinic adopted this technique, as did others, and in time it became a reasonably safe operation with satisfactory results.

The second technique for repairing atrial septal defects prior to the development of the heart-lung machine was total body hypothermia and inflow occlusion. It had been shown by Wilfred Bigelow at the University of Toronto that lowering body temperature reduced the metabolic rate and oxygen consumption of all tissue. In experimental animals cooled to 20 degrees Celsius, the circulation could be interrupted for as long as twenty minutes with no evidence of brain damage. Similar investigations were done by Charles Bailey and Henry Swan. With this cerebral protection, clamping the venae cavae made it possible to open the heart and close an atrial septal defect with sutures. The main hazard of this technique was that the heart rhythm is unstable when cooled below 30 degrees Celsius, and ventricular fibrillation may occur. When it did occur, it was difficult to defibrillate the heart at low temperatures. Rapid rewarming was necessary, but a method of rapid rewarming was not yet available. Therefore, it was recognized that cooling should not go below 30 degrees Celsius. This limited the time of total circulatory arrest to a maximum of about ten minutes, enough for rapid repair of atrial septal defect or pulmonary stenosis, but not enough for other more complex defects such as ventricular septal defects or tetralogy of Fallot. Charles Bailey was the first to try this technique on a patient. In August 1952 he closed an atrial septal defect in a thirty-year-old female. Unfortunately, irreversible ventricular fibrillation occurred. At autopsy, it was thought that the ventricular fibrillation was caused by coronary artery air embolism.

In September 1952 John Lewis at the University of Minnesota successfully used hypothermia and inflow occlusion to close an atrial septal defect in a five-year-old girl. To avoid air embolism into the aorta and coronary arteries, Lewis clamped not only the venae cavae but also the pulmonary artery and the aorta. The aortic clamp was placed just above the aortic valve, proximal to the origin of the coronary arteries. Cooling the patient was accomplished by wrapping the patient in a cooling blanket that circulated cold alcohol. Rectal and esophageal temperature probes were used. Rewarming was done by immersion of the patient in a tub of warm water, which rewarmed faster than an electric blanket. This was the first successful open-heart operation.

Hypothermia and inflow occlusion were used by a large number of surgical groups, and some enthusiasts thought that eventually deep hypothermia would become practical and would be used for longer and more complex procedures. However, hypothermia was not without hazards. The patient could be overcooled, air embolism could occur, or the circulatory arrest time could be unexpectedly prolonged, leading to brain damage.

Fortunately, the technique of hypothermia with inflow occlusion was used for only four or five years and was eventually completely replaced by the more reliable heart-lung machines. However, in later years hypothermia combined with the heart-lung machine added additional safety to cardiac operations and became an important part of myocardial preservation techniques. The time would come when some of the more complicated congenital heart abnormalities were best corrected using profound hypothermia in the 10 to 15 degree Celsius range with fairly long periods of total circulatory arrest, combined with the use of a heart-lung machine during the cooling and warming periods.

The third unique operation of the pre-heart-lung period was the use of the Hufnagel caged-ball valve. Charles Hufnagel graduated from Harvard Medical School in 1941 and trained at the Peter Bent Brigham Hospital. He spent a year with Robert Gross at the Boston Children's Hospital and was involved in the first successful coarctation operations. He then joined the surgical faculty at Georgetown; throughout his career he was interested in experimental surgery and involved in the development of new techniques and materials for cardiac and vascular surgery.

In 1950 Hufnagel began experiments to develop an artificial aortic valve to be placed in the descending aorta of patients with severe aortic valve insufficiency (leakage).[42] Ideally, the defective aortic valve should be replaced at its natural site, but this was impossible without heart-lung machine support. He developed a caged-ball valve that could be placed in the descending aorta, that could be clamped safely for up to twenty minutes before the likelihood of spinal cord ischemia ensued. Twenty minutes is not long enough to sew a valve in place, so he developed a valve suitable for rapid insertion. It

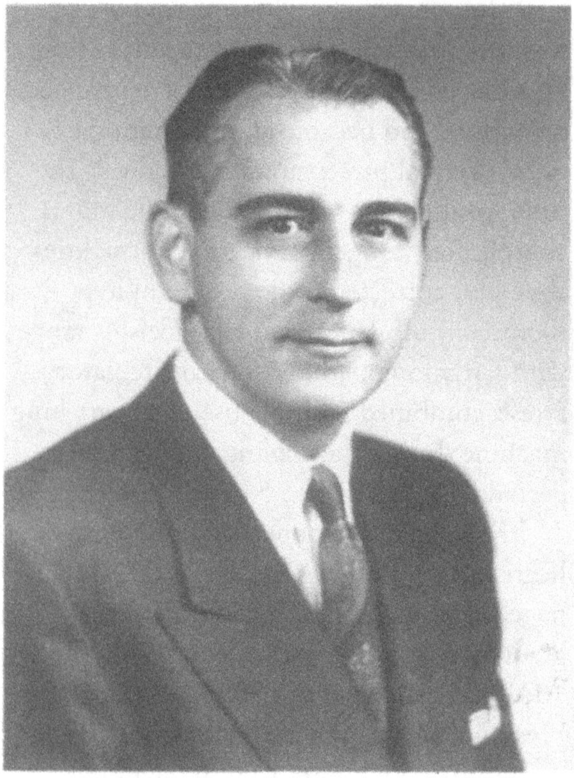

Charles A. Hufnagel

was encased in a clear methyl methacrylate cylinder about eight centimeters in length and of the same diameter as the aorta. At each end was a circular groove. With the aorta clamped just beyond the left subclavian artery, Hufnagel would excise a short segment of aorta and place a nylon ring with multiple teeth outside each end. He would then insert the lip of the cylinder first into the upper and then the lower aorta. The nylon rings were tied down so that the inner teeth gripped the aorta and fitted into the circular groove at each end of the cylinder, similar to an automobile hose clamp. All of this could be accomplished in five or six minutes of cross-clamp time. This would only partially solve the problem. The patient would still have a leaking aortic valve affecting the upper half of the body, but from the new valve down there was normal diastolic pressure and no sign of aortic insufficiency. For most, this was a great improvement. Initially, the valve noise was very loud, and each heartbeat could be heard several feet away. To improve this problem, the ball was changed to polyethylene, a softer material. Hufnagel placed this valve in ninety patients. For those not in severe congestive heart failure, the operative mortality was about 10 percent. The problem of aortic valve incompetence was not really solved until the Starr-Edwards valve came into use in the early 1960s. It, too, used the caged-ball principle and owed some gratitude to its earlier and less-refined cousin, the Hufnagel valve.

These three operations were done without the safety net of the heart-lung machine. If something went wrong, there was very little time for recovery, and as a result the operative mortality rate was relatively high.

Development of the Heart-Lung Machine

Dr. John H. Gibbon was the developer of the first successful heart-lung machine. In May 1953, at Jefferson Medical College, he was able to close an atrial septal defect using a heart-lung machine for temporary total support of the circulation.[43] It was one of the most important medical advances in the second half of the twentieth century.

The idea of a heart-lung machine first occurred to Gibbon in 1930. At that time he was two years out of Jefferson Medical College and a surgical house officer at the University of Pennsylvania Hospital. During those two clinical years he developed an interest in research and had obtained a fellowship under Dr. Edward Churchill for the following year at the Massachusetts General Hospital. Churchill was interested in pulmonary embolism and the operation used to remove an embolus, the Trendelenburg procedure. In Churchill's laboratory, Gibbon began to measure the effects of gradual occlusion of the pulmonary artery, which would simulate the changes brought about by a massive pulmonary embolus.

In the fall of 1930, the year of Gibbon's fellowship in Boston, Dr. Churchill was asked to see a patient who was thought to have had a pulmonary embolus two weeks after a cholecystectomy. The patient was in sudden distress with shortness of breath, chest pain, cyanosis, vasoconstriction, and a drop in blood pressure. Churchill agreed that the most likely diagnosis was a large pulmonary embolus and proposed to do a Trendelenburg operation. Since there was no way to confirm the diagnosis, the Trendelenburg protocol was to take the patient to the operating room and have everything ready for a thoracotomy but not to start the operation until the patient appeared to be at the point of death. Then a parasternal incision would be quickly made, the pulmonary artery would be occluded at its origin, the main pulmonary artery quickly opened, and the clot removed. It was hoped that the heart would recover enough to restore circulation. At that time only a handful of such operations had been successful. Most of the patients had died, and there had not been a successful pulmonary embolectomy done in the United States. Gibbon was assigned the job of sitting with the patient during the night, recording the blood pressure and heart rate every fifteen minutes. He was to notify the surgical team when death seemed imminent.

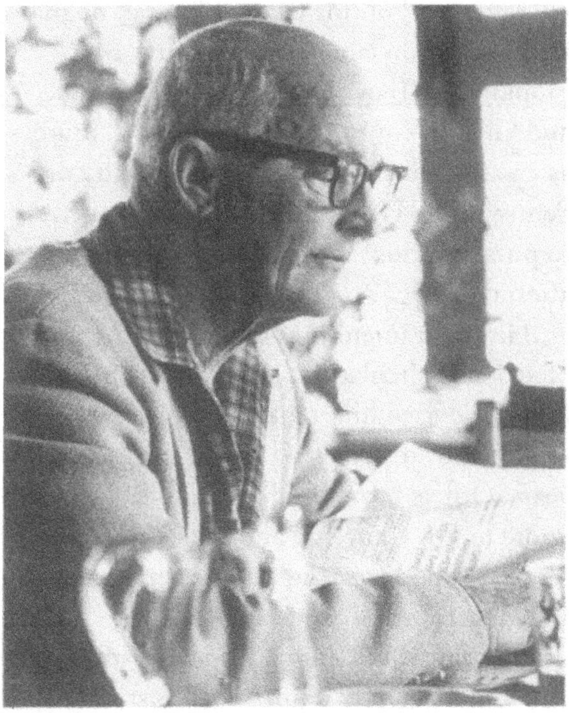

John H. Gibbon

It was during that night, as he watched this patient struggle with increased venous pressure, increasing cyanosis, and decreasing cardiac output, that Gibbon realized some form of temporary circulatory assistance was needed to solve this problem. A machine that could temporarily take the venous blood, oxygenate it, and return it to the arterial system would allow time to remove the pulmonary embolus and restore normal pulmonary artery flow.[44] Early the next morning the condition of the patient became critical, and Dr. Churchill attempted a Trendelenburg procedure. A large clot was removed, but the patient had been hypotensive for too long and did not survive. During the next few weeks, as he continued his research on the effects of occluding the pulmonary artery in experimental animals, Gibbon became convinced that the idea of a circulatory assist device would be a worthwhile research project.

At the end of this fellowship year, he married his Boston laboratory assistant, Mary Hopkinson. They returned to Philadelphia, and Gibbon continued his surgical training as an assistant surgeon at the University of Pennsylvania Hospital. He also continued to pursue various research projects in the afternoons.

His main interest, however, was the idea of artificial circulation. Most of his colleagues advised him that this project was too difficult to solve and might take several years. Others thought it impossible. Gibbon wrote to Dr. Churchill and asked if he could return to the Massachusetts General Hospital for another year as a research fellow to work on this problem. Churchill agreed, and Gibbon and his family returned to Boston in 1934. During that year Gibbon succeeded in developing a heart-lung machine that could sustain the circulation of small experimental animals (cats) for as long as thirty minutes, during which time the pulmonary artery was completely occluded.[45] His oxygenator was a rotating steel cylinder. Blood was introduced at the top of the cylinder and formed a film over the inner surface, where it was exposed to oxygen. The pumps used were secondhand Dale-Shuster pumps. There were numerous problems of hemolysis, anemia, and bleeding, but eventually he was able to sustain the circulation of a cat long enough for a pulmonary embolectomy to succeed.

Gibbon and his family returned to Philadelphia in 1935. He was appointed the surgical research fellow at the Harrison Research Laboratory at the University of Pennsylvania Medical School, and the following year he was appointed to the surgical staff of the University of Pennsylvania Hospital. He continued his experiments with artificial circulation and began to have some long-term survivors of cats that had been totally supported by his heart-lung machine for thirty minutes or more.[46] This work was put on hold in 1942 when he entered the Army Medical Corps as a major and served two years in the Pacific and another two years at Galesburg Military Hospital in Illinois. After discharge from the army he returned to the University of Pennsylvania and shortly afterward was offered the position of professor of surgery and director of surgical research at Jefferson Medical College. At Jefferson he resumed his work developing a heart-lung machine in addition to his increasing responsibilities as a thoracic surgeon.

Gibbon now needed a larger oxygenator for dogs rather than cats. Through a fortunate set of circumstances, Gibbon met Thomas Watson, the president of IBM, who was immediately taken with the idea of providing both financial and engineering support to the project. In 1947 Gibbon's former chief resident, Dr. J. Y. Templeton, was appointed to the surgical faculty at Jefferson and was working for Gibbon in the laboratory on the heart-lung project. Also working in the laboratory with Templeton was a medical student named E. J. Clark. Clark had been a pilot in World War II and had served with the Military Air Transport Service in India. He was engaged to be married to the daughter of the president of Lafayette College who was a close friend of Thomas Watson. Clark asked his future father-in-law to tell Watson about their progress on the heart-lung machine to see if he might be interested in meeting Dr. Gibbon. The meeting was arranged, and Watson became an enthusiastic supporter.[47] He assigned Gustov Malmros, his chief engineer, to assist Gibbon and Templeton.

Over the next six years, at their own expense, IBM built three pump-oxygenators. The first was for animal use only; Model II was used for the first successful human open-heart operation in 1953; and Model III was an improved design that was eventually manufactured by Med-Science Medtronics. Gibbon and Watson agreed that the heart-lung machine design would be shared with other surgeons and institutions, that the patents would be owned by Jefferson Medical School, and that the company selected to manufacture the pump in the future would pay only a small royalty to Jefferson Medical School. Eventually IBM provided more than $200,000 in expenses and invaluable mechanical and electrical engineering support. The machine they developed had an elegant stainless-steel cabinet. With switches, pumps, gauges, and an upright vertical screen oxygenator, it weighed over two thousand pounds. Although there were still problems with postoperative bleeding and air embolism, the success rate with dogs gradually improved to the point that Gibbon was prepared to begin trials with human patients in 1952.

Blood was pumped by DeBakey roller pumps. The Gibbon oxygenator contained a series of stainless-steel screens. Each screen had a small reservoir, or weir, at the top, which fed blood in a film down the screen. Model II (used in the first successful operation) had six screens, and Model III had eight. The screens were enclosed in a clear plastic case that was flooded with oxygen. Carbon dioxide could be added if the pH became too alkalotic. There were two pumping circuits. The primary circuit fed the oxygenator at a fixed rate so that the weirs at the top of each screen were always full. This ensured that blood flowed down the screens as a film and did not coalesce into a stream. If the film was lost and the blood came down as a stream, most of the blood would not be exposed to oxygen, and the O_2 saturation would drop precipitously. A second circuit took oxygenated blood from the reservoir at the bottom of the oxygenator and pumped it into the patient. The output of this circuit had to be kept at a lower flow rate than the oxygenator circuit so that the weirs were always kept full. Venous blood was pumped into the oxygenator by a third pump. Most present-day systems use gravity-siphon for the venous return from the patient. The Gibbon machine pumped the venous blood into the oxygenator since the oxygenator was mounted on top of the cabinet and was higher than the patient. The venous pump required a special monitor and automatic shutoff because the patient's vena cava occasionally was sucked up against the venous cannula, occluding the flow. An electronic sensor was mounted in the reservoir at the bottom of the oxygenator that controlled the venous pump. If the blood level in the reservoir went up, the venous pump slowed, and if the level went down, the venous pump increased its speed.

Gibbon and the engineers at IBM had made an almost robotic pump-oxygenator, which could monitor and adjust the flow and the pH. They had gone to great lengths to develop a machine that was as safe as they could make it, and for them it worked well, but it was far too complex and expensive for the majority of potential users. They did not realize that the variables occurring in each operation could be managed better by a technician than by an electronic device; they did not fully anticipate the role of the perfusionist. In the near future a small specialty would evolve for managing the heart-lung machine, with its own training programs, organization, credentialing, and journal. The cardiac perfusionist would become an integral part of every cardiac surgical team.

The first patient was a fifteen-month-old child in heart failure with what was thought to be an atrial septal defect. Because the child was so sick, cardiac catheterization was not done. At operation, the patient was connected to the heart-lung machine and the right atrium was opened, but no atrial septal defect could be found. The patient's heart failed and death occurred in the operating room. At autopsy the child was found to have a very large patent ductus arteriosus rather than an atrial septal defect. The diagnosis was wrong.

The second procedure was done on May 6, 1953, over a year later. This patient was an eighteen-year-old college student, Cecelia Bavolek. She had shortness of breath on exertion, and at cardiac catheterization an atrial septal defect was confirmed. At operation she was placed on the heart-lung machine for forty-five minutes, and for twenty-six minutes the total circulation was provided by the heart-lung machine. The atrial septal defect was closed with a continuous suture. A catheter had been placed in the left ventricle to remove any intracavitary air before coming off bypass. During the closure of the atrial septal defect, the oxygen saturation of the blood from the pump gradually decreased. This was caused by small blood clots forming in the oxygenator that interfered with the filming of blood on the screens. The pump had been primed with fresh heparinized blood obtained from donors early that morning. The clotting problem was due to the fact that each five hundred cubic centimeters of blood had received only ten units of heparin for anticoagulation, which was an inadequate dose. Fortunately, the decrease in oxygenation of the blood did not cause a problem, and the patient recovered with no complications. After that experience, twenty-five units of heparin were used for each five hundred cubic centimeters of blood. Cecelia Bavolek was the first person in the world to survive an open-heart operation using a heart-lung machine. She is alive and well today.

Dr. Gibbon operated on two additional patients in 1953. Both were thought to have atrial septal defects and both were five years old. The first patient had cardiac arrest during the early part of the operation, and, although placed on the heart-lung machine, he could not sustain an adequate cardiac output and died in the operating room. The second patient, thought to have an atrial septal defect, turned out to have an atrioventricular canal defect plus a patent ductus. An attempt to correct this complex defect was not successful, and this patient also died in the operating room. Once again the preoperative diagnosis was wrong.

It is easy to understand why John Gibbon became discouraged. He decided that they would do no more operations with the heart-lung machine for a year, and during that time they would develop a cardiology service with a cardiologist experienced in cardiac catheterization to avoid the diagnostic mistakes that they had already encountered. Also, they would return to the laboratory, work with an improved heart-lung machine (Model III), and work on the problems of postoperative bleeding. Finally, he turned over the responsibility for the cardiac surgery service to his younger associate, John Y. Templeton. Gibbon spent the rest of his surgical career dealing with diseases of the lungs and esophagus. He did no more cardiac operations.

Although the Gibbon machine produced

excellent results, it did not achieve wide acceptance. It was very expensive, had to be custom made, was very complex requiring hours to set up, and it required two to four technicians to run it.

Dr. Bernard Miller was Gibbon's laboratory assistant from 1951 to 1955 during the development of the heart-lung machine at Jefferson Medical College. In an interview in 1996 he described the Model II heart-lung machine in this way:

> It was a very large stainless-steel cabinet that measured four-and-a-half feet in height, perhaps five feet in length, and about two feet in width. The oxygenator was mounted above the level of the top deck on the left side of the machine. The top deck contained the four pumps. On the front panel were four recorders: one recorded rectal temperature, one recorded oxygen saturation, one recorded flow, and the fourth recorded pH. The machine weighed in excess of two thousand pounds. When we would move it over from the laboratory on the morning of surgery to take it down the elevator to the hospital, the elevator would always sink an inch or two as we loaded it, from stretching the cables, I guess. This was always a brief episode of concern for us. There was also a second steel cabinet, which contained the emergency electrical backup in the event the main electrical service to the hospital was lost during an operation. This was a generator run by batteries that could operate the pumps for at least twenty minutes, which was thought to be sufficient time for the surgeon to close the cardiac incision and come off bypass. The emergency generator with batteries must have weighed an additional five hundred to six hundred pounds. There were four tachometers for the four pumps and two additional meters that provided information concerning the venous flow. If a sudden occlusion of the venous flow occurred, the pumps were automatically stopped so that the problem could be corrected. The cabinet was sealed and was flooded with nitrogen a few centimeters above room pressure to prevent the chance of an explosion, since both ether and cyclopropane were commonly in use and both were highly flammable. In all, it was a relatively safe but a very complex machine.[48]

In the late 1940s, the Mayo Clinic became interested in developing a cardiology and cardiac surgical service. This plan was led by Dr. John Kirklin, who had graduated from Harvard Medical School in 1942. He had completed an accelerated wartime surgical residency at the Mayo Clinic and at the University of Pennsylvania, and during the latter part of World War II he was a military neurosurgeon at the O'Reilly General Hospital in Missouri. After the war he returned to the Mayo Clinic and completed his surgical residency. He then did a six-month fellowship with Robert Gross at the Boston Children's Hospital. After returning to the Mayo Clinic, he joined cardiologist James DuShane, pathologist Jesse Edwards, and physiologist Earl Wood in establishing a cardiac surgical service. Kirklin and his associates realized that the future of cardiac surgery required the use of a reliable heart-lung machine to allow sufficient time and exposure to correct the majority of congenital heart abnormalities. To see what was available in 1952, he visited the four physicians whose teams were developing heart-lung machines: William Mustard in Toronto, Forest Dodrill in Detroit, Clarence Dennis in Minneapolis, and John Gibbon in Philadelphia. He and his colleagues decided that the Gibbon machine was the most promising, and Gibbon graciously shared all of his information with them, including the blueprints for the heart-lung machine built by IBM. Using these plans, the engineering laboratory at the Mayo Clinic built a similar machine with some modifications. After extensive work in the experimental laboratory, they began a clinical trial in 1955. They planned to operate on eight successive patients with various congenital heart abnormalities and to do all eight operations even if the patients did not survive. Actually, four of the eight survived, and Kirklin went on to establish one of the most outstanding cardiac surgical centers in the world, known for its low mortality and its honest and scholarly reports.[49]

I had the good fortune to visit the Mayo Clinic in 1956 and watch Dr. Kirklin close a ventricular septal defect using the Mayo-Gibbon machine. The most delicate manipulation of the machine occurred prior to connecting the lines to the patient. First, saline was used to fill the oxygenator circuit. When it was evident that saline was flowing down each screen in a thin film, the technicians then rapidly added the fresh heparinized blood to the venous line and discarded the saline from the arterial side. Once the oxygenator circuit was primed with blood, it ran continuously. When Dr. Kirklin had finished placing the cannulas in the patient, the machine was carefully moved closer to the operating table. The arterial and venous lines were connected to the patient and the arterial and venous pumps were activated. All this time the oxygenator pump kept a constant flow of blood down the screens. Great care was taken not to bump or otherwise disturb the apparatus so that filming would be constant and not suddenly coalesce into rivulets or a single stream. There were four technicians whose job was to run the pump. It all worked with precision, and it was very impressive. However, most visiting surgeons were daunted by the complexity and the expense of the Mayo-Gibbon heart-lung machine and concluded that it was beyond their means.

Lillehei and Cross-Circulation

At exactly the same time, a second cardiac surgical center evolved at the University of Minnesota under the leadership of Dr. Owen Wangensteen but guided and inspired by the brilliant surgeon C. Walton Lillehei. Lillehei had finished medical school during the early years of World War II and after an accelerated internship entered the army as a medical officer in 1942. He was immediately sent overseas and participated in the invasions of North Africa, Sicily, Italy, and finally Anzio, ending the war as a lieutenant colonel. He returned to Minneapolis, completed his training, and joined the faculty.

Two other young surgeons on the faculty had begun to investigate various methods that might be used to correct congenital heart defects. Dr. Clarence Dennis had visited John Gibbon and had developed a heart-lung machine that used rotating screen discs as the oxygenator. Unfortunately, his first two operations on children in 1952 had been failures.[50] John Lewis, another Wangensteen protégé, developed the hypothermia-inflow stasis technique, referred to above, that had been first advocated by Dr. Wilfred Bigelow in Toronto. In 1952 Lewis did the first successful open-heart operation: closure of an atrial septal defect during six or seven minutes of hypothermic circulatory arrest, in a five-year-old girl named Jacqueline Johnson. Her postoperative course was uneventful, and she made a complete recovery. The technique of hypothermia and inflow occlusion was used by several different surgeons at that time, including John Kirklin at the Mayo Clinic and Henry Swan in Denver. However, it was limited to operations that could be completed in five to eight minutes. The two most common operations suitable for hypothermia at that time were closure of an atrial septal defect and pulmonary valvotomy. There was just not enough time to complete the more complex operations using hypothermia. When John Lewis tried, in two successive operations, to use this method for closure of a ventricular septal defect (an abnormal opening between the two pumping chambers of the heart), both patients died.[51] Lillehei, Kirklin, and others recognized that complex operations would require much more time. The solution had to be a heart-lung machine.

In 1952 an article by Andreasen and Watson, published in the *British Journal of Surgery*, described experiments in which the total circulation of experimental animals could be reduced by 90 percent for up to two hours, followed by recovery.[52] This was accomplished by total occlusion of both the superior and inferior vena cava, but leaving open the azygos vein. This allowed a small flow of blood through the body at a very low blood pressure. They found that dogs could tolerate this low flow for at least thirty minutes or more if the circulation at the end of that time was restored to normal. What was especially significant was that with low flow there was no injury to the brain or other organs. The surgical resident working in the experimental laboratory for Lillehei at that time was Morley Cohen. He began investigating the possibility of open-heart surgery using very low flows, in contrast to the established technique being used by Gibbon and Kirklin that utilized high-volume blood flow from the pump-oxygenator. Cohen developed a technique in which he used one lobe of the lung of a dog as its own oxygenator. This proved to be successful but was a difficult and complex technique, and, if everything was not just exactly right, it led to edema of the lung. However, one evening while he was discussing this with fellow resident Herbert Warden, they began talking about the circulation of the fetus during pregnancy.[53] Cohen's wife was expecting a baby within the following few weeks. It suddenly occurred to Cohen that the mother was acting as the oxygenator for the fetus. Why not use a large dog as the oxygenator for a smaller one, utilizing the low-flow azygos principle? Lillehei immediately approved an experimental trial, and after several months they found that they could do experimental open-heart operations, taking oxygenated blood from a large donor dog, pumping it into the arterial system of a much smaller recipient dog, and returning venous blood from the recipient back to the donor for oxygenation. A Sigmamotor pump was set up between the two animals and the blood was pumped through plastic tubing obtained from a local company. They called this "controlled cross-circulation." Their experiments showed that both the donor dogs and the recipient dogs recovered with

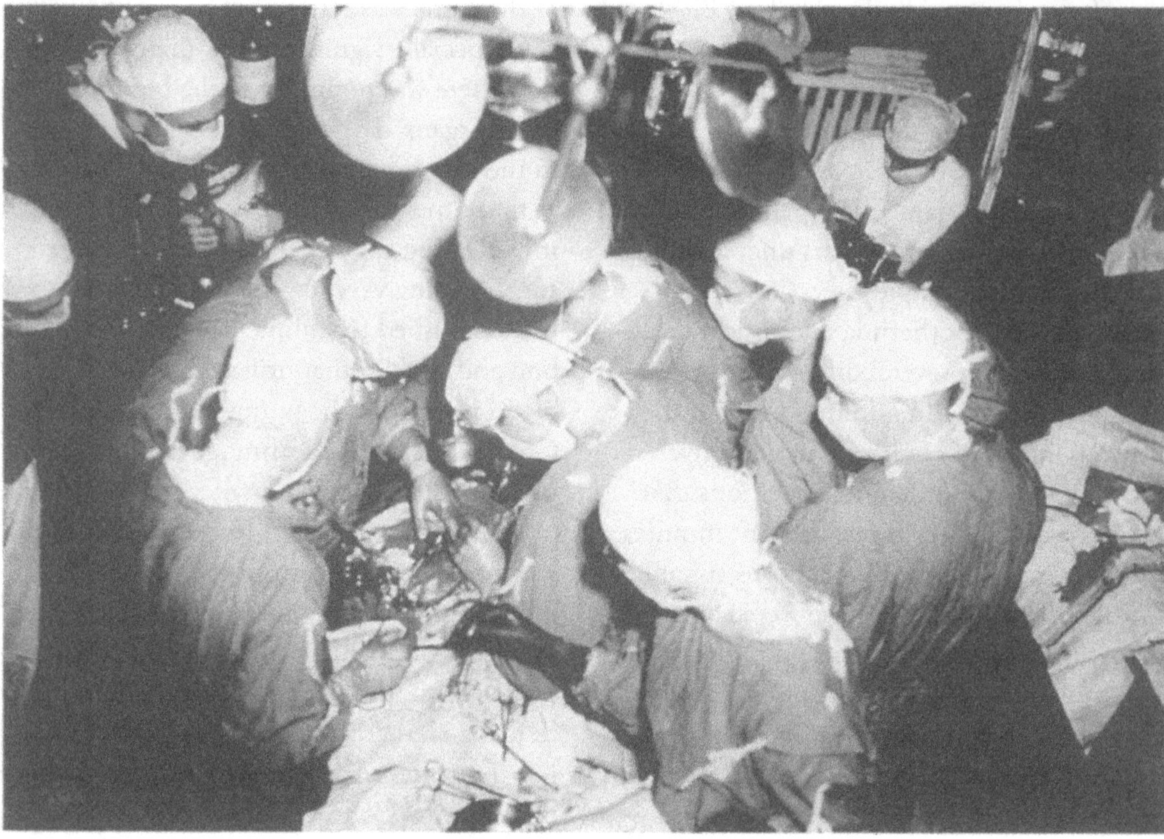

Cross-circulation procedure. Dr. Lillehei is in the center of the photograph with the large headlight.

no evidence of neurological injury. After extensive investigation, they developed confidence in this system and proposed to Dr. Wangensteen, the chief of surgery, that they begin a trial using this technique for patients. The mother or father would be the donor for the child who needed surgical correction of a heart defect. Wangensteen eventually gave his approval: "By all means, go ahead."

The first cross-circulation operation was done in March 1954. A ventricular septal defect was closed in a one-year-old boy; his father was the donor for the cross-circulation. The operation went well, but the patient developed pneumonia in the postoperative period and died several days later. Within a month Lillehei operated successfully on a four-year-old girl with a ventricular septal defect and a three-year-old boy with a similar problem. His report of these three patients using cross-circulation was given at the meeting of the American Association for Thoracic Surgery in Montreal in the spring of 1954 and received wide publicity, interest, curiosity, and some criticism.[54] There were those who thought that a mechanical pump-oxygenator would be the preferred technique and that the cross-circulation technique involved too much risk for the donor parent. More than one critic pointed out that this was the only operation that could have a 200-percent mortality rate.

Walt Lillehei went on to use this cross-circulation technique for the next eighteen months. He operated on a total of forty-five patients; twenty-eight survived the operation and the majority of the survivors were still alive thirty years later.[55] He was the first surgeon to successfully close a ventricular septal defect, the first to do a total repair of tetralogy of Fallot, and the first to repair an atrioventricular canal (a complex combination of defects between the chambers of the heart involving the mitral and tricuspid valves).

However, there had been two severe complications involving donor parents during the cross-circulation experience at the University of Minnesota. The first was a severe neurological injury to a mother caused by the anesthesiologist, who pumped air into an empty IV bottle, mistakenly thinking it was full. Air under pressure went into the patient. This occurred during the early stage of the operation, so the procedure was cancelled. The mother survived but was left with permanent cognitive loss that eventually required long-term care in a mental hospital.[56] A second accident occurred, also to a mother, just at the end of a short cross-circulation operation. The mother became hypotensive and had sudden cardiac arrest. Her chest was immediately opened and her circulation was restored by cardiac resuscitation and immediate transfusion. This accident was caused by a ligature on the child's venous cannula that had been tied so tightly that it had restricted venous flow back to the mother, creating loss of blood volume and hypotension of the mother. Fortunately, the mother recovered with no permanent injury.

Lillehei was aware of the risks and limitations of the cross-circulation technique. It could only be used for small children, and because of the low-flow azygos principle it would be risky for operations that might require perfusion times of an hour or more. For long procedures and for adults, a heart-lung machine would be necessary.

DeWall and a Practical Heart-Lung Machine

Richard DeWall was an assistant resident working in Lillehei's laboratory and operating room. Lillehei asked him if he could develop an oxygenator and heart-lung machine that could replace the cross-circulation system and also be used for larger children and adults. In a matter of a few months DeWall developed a simple bubble oxygenator that could be assembled with inexpensive plastic tubing.[57] He used the same Sigmamotor "finger" pump adopted from the dairy industry that had been used for the cross-circulation operations. The main problem of bubble oxygenators had been excessive foaming of the blood and the risk of air embolism if bubbles entered the arterial circuit. DeWall solved this problem by adding a silicone defoaming agent made by Dow-Corning to the defoaming chamber and then letting the blood descend through a length of plastic tubing arranged in a helix. He found that debubbling was more efficient if large bubbles were used. If the bubbles were very small, such as those produced by a micropore nozzle, then debubbling was almost impossible. His bubbles were created by fifteen size-22 hypodermic needles stuck through a rubber stopper at the bottom of the oxygenator column, each connected to an oxygen source. This very simple oxygenator used a pump that could be bought for $500 plus several feet of disposable polyvinyl tubing made for the beer

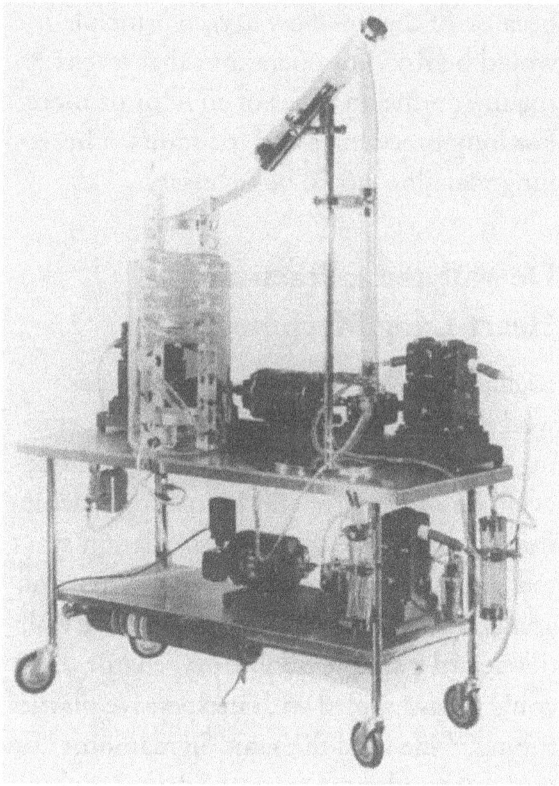

DeWall bubble oxygenator and Sigmamotor pump, 1956

industry by the Mayon Company in Minneapolis. In mid-1955 a bubble oxygenator was used for the first time on a patient and was so successful that cross-circulation was rapidly replaced by this homemade bubble oxygenator and pump.

The advantages of this relatively simple system were immediately recognized by the many medical visitors who came to Minneapolis during that time to observe and learn about open-heart surgery. Visitors could watch Lillehei and his surgical team in the morning, and in the afternoon they could visit the experimental lab where DeWall would show them how to assemble and use the bubble oxygenator. Before leaving they would stop at the Mayon Company and order tubing, and also order a pump from the Sigmamotor Company. They carried home with them a diagram of the exact specifications for a working heart-lung machine. Within a year the Travenol Company was able to market a preassembled bubble oxygenator made of plastic sheeting. The device was based on the DeWall design; was inexpensive, sterile, and disposable; and could be primed with saline. This 1957 DeWall disposable bubble oxygenator made it possible for surgeons all over the world to begin cardiac surgical programs. The initial doubts about the hazards of a bubble oxygenator were soon put to rest by the success of this device. Many years later at a national meeting, Walt Lillehei presented the long-term results of the patients who had survived the first operations at the University of Minnesota. Denton Cooley congratulated Lillehei at the end of his discussion and then added, "Walt Lillehei brought the can opener to the cardiac surgery picnic."[55] The can opener that opened cardiac surgery to surgical groups all over the world was the DeWall-Lillehei bubble oxygenator.

The word spread among surgical centers. The two places in the world where open-heart operations were being done on a daily basis were both in Minnesota. In Minneapolis in 1954 and 1955, Lillehei was using hypothermia and inflow occlusion for brief operations, such as those for atrial septal defects and pulmonary stenosis. For more complex operations, he was using the cross-circulation procedure. At the Mayo Clinic in Rochester, Dr. Kirklin used the Gross atrial well for atrial septal defects and the Mayo-Gibbon pump-oxygenator for more complex procedures.

The initial experience of other surgical groups with cardiac surgery supported by

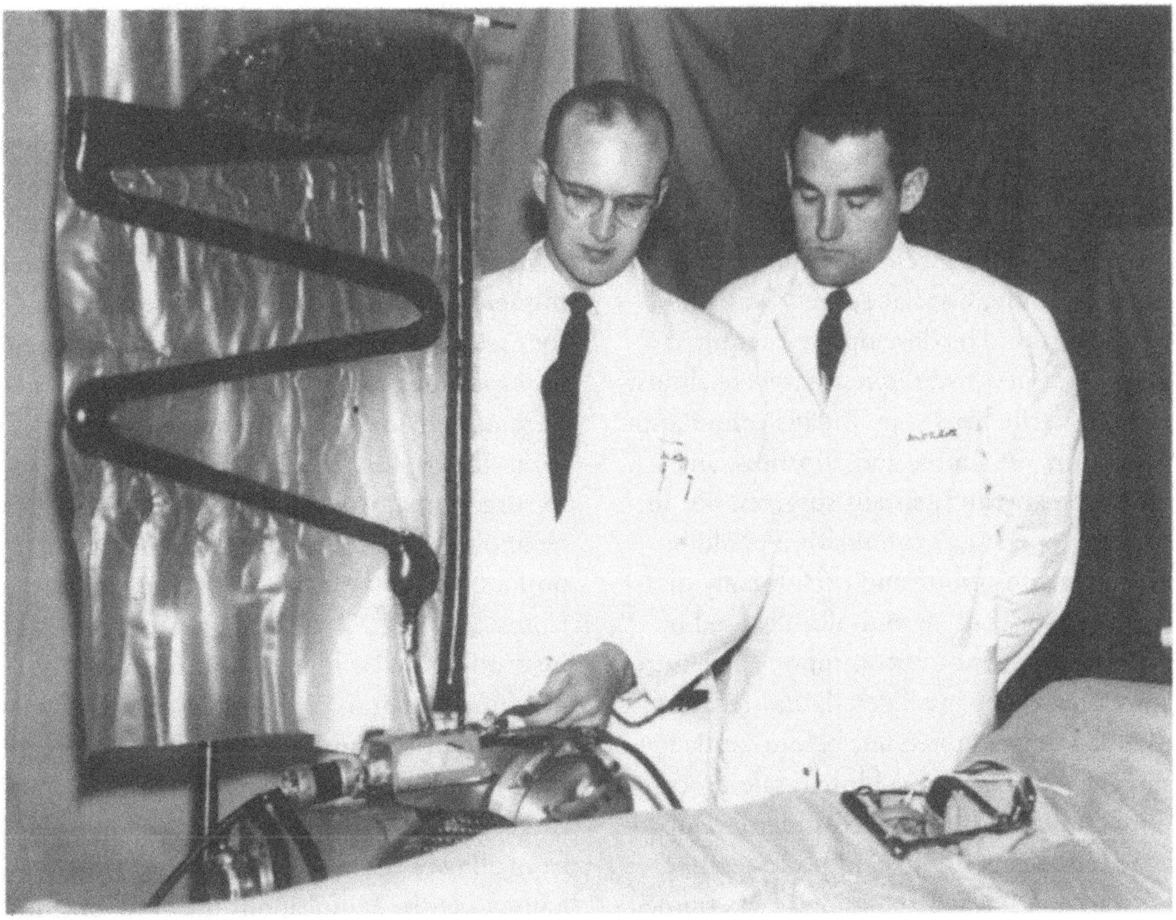

Dick DeWall and Vince Gott with the Travenol disposable bubble oxygenator

pump-oxygenators had been so disastrous that it produced great discouragement. The leading investigator, John Gibbon, used his machine to operate on four patients, three of whom died in the operating room; he had only one success. He was so discouraged that he gave up cardiac surgery altogether. Lillehei later reviewed the earliest reported operations using a heart-lung machine for the introduction of *Cardiopulmonary Bypass*, a book edited by Joe Utley. His review started with Dennis in 1951 and ended in 1955.[58] Of eighteen open-heart operations at six different institutions during that interval, all but three patients were infants or children. The oxygenators used were film and bubble oxygenators, one autogenous lung, and one monkey lung. Seventeen of the eighteen patients had died, the majority in the operating room. The one survivor was the eighteen-year-old patient of John Gibbon in whom he had closed an atrial septal defect. In all probability there were a few additional similar procedures that were never reported and that had equally discouraging results.

The outcomes were dismal for several reasons. The heart-lung machines were still imperfect, and the best method of oxygenation of the blood was not yet established. Bubble oxygenators produced too much froth, film oxygenators were temperamental, sterilization was difficult, and the use of the patient's own lung or an animal lung had severe technical disadvantages.

Another factor was also at work: Because the risk of cardiac surgery was so great, patients, particularly those with mitral and aortic valve disease, were not referred to the surgeon until they were in advanced stages of heart failure. Cardiac surgery was a new technology and its development required a long list of new techniques that were almost all learned the hard way. Today's cannulation techniques are simple and effortless, and often done by the assistant surgeon, but in the early operations cannulation could be very time consuming and occasionally disastrous. Episodes of air embolism caused by the pump were not uncommon. There were a hundred other small details and techniques that had to be worked out before cardiac surgery was transformed into a safe procedure. Other areas that were underdeveloped were cardiac anesthesia and postoperative critical care. No anesthesiologist was trained specifically for cardiac surgery. Postoperative patients went to a recovery room for a few hours and then usually back to their room. There were no critical care areas, few monitors, and very few postoperative ventilators.

Also, it was not unusual for the preoperative diagnosis to be incorrect. Cardiac catheterization was in its infancy and imaging techniques were primitive. Echocardiography, image intensifiers, and cineangiography did not exist. Cardiac catheterization usually involved measuring pressures and oxygen saturations in the right atrium, right ventricle, and pulmonary artery; left-heart catheterization was rare. Cardiac output could be calculated by a dye-dilution technique. For the first ten years of cardiac surgery, the first thing each surgeon did as soon as the heart was exposed was to examine the heart and the great vessels carefully to look for additional problems that might have been missed at the time of catheterization. Finding unexpected congenital abnormalities or unrecognized valve disease was not uncommon.

Looking back, we can easily identify the numerous obstacles that had to be overcome for cardiac surgery to become a safe and useful procedure, but at the time the obstacles were not obvious. Some people began to think that it was the heart's poor response to surgery that was the problem, not the technology and techniques. This negative outlook was totally changed in the years from 1955 to 1957 by two men and two institutions: Walt Lillehei at the University of Minnesota and John Kirklin at the Mayo Clinic. During those two years, these were the only two places on earth where cardiac surgery was done on a daily basis. Surgeons from all over the world came to see what was happening. In Minneapolis they saw Lillehei use controlled cross-circulation during 1954 and into 1955. After the first few months of 1955 they watched him use a relatively simple heart-lung machine with a bubble oxygenator. At the Mayo Clinic, they saw John Kirklin and his colleagues do similar operations using a copy of John Gibbon's device, the Mayo-Gibbon heart-lung machine.

The success of the heart-lung machines at the University of Minnesota and at the Mayo Clinic led to the rapid spread of open-heart surgery to hospitals all over the world. Many of these hospitals had already developed experience with operations for coarctation of the aorta and patent ductus arteriosus, and with Blalock-Taussig shunt procedures. However, the early open-heart experience with atrial septal defects, ventricular septal defects, and tetralogy of Fallot was not without problems. For example, ventricular defects were often closed by sutures without using a patch, and in some of these the sutures were under too much stress and the repair failed. Surgeons did not recognize initially that the conduction tissue was usually near the rim of the ventricular septal defect and could be permanently injured if a suture was placed across this area. This produced complete heart block with a very slow heart rate and eventual cardiac arrest. The solution was based on a better understanding of the anatomy of the conduction system so that injury could be avoided and the development and use of cardiac pacing. The first pacemakers were large and used standard alternating current, but battery-operated models were developed and eventually miniaturized. By the early 1960s, they were small enough for permanent implantation. Over the next ten years the risk of surgical repair of complex congenital abnormalities such as tetralogy of Fallot, transposition of the great vessels, and common atrioventricular canal became reasonable.

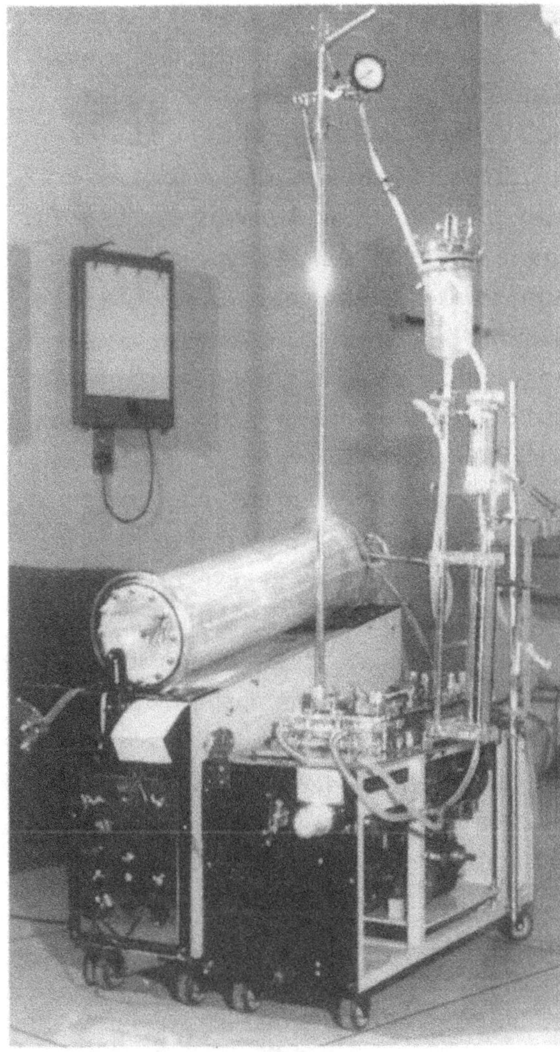

Melrose rotating-disc oxygenator

In the mid-1950s, as open-heart surgery began to spread beyond the University of Minnesota and the Mayo Clinic, a third type of oxygenator became available. First described by Clarence Crafoord in 1949 and Viking Björk in 1948, this oxygenator used a series of stainless-steel discs, eight or nine inches in diameter, mounted closely together on a spindle.[59] When the discs were rapidly rotated with the lower third of the disc immersed in blood, the blood would be brought up as a film over the discs and would then be exposed to a flow of oxygen. The rotating-disc oxygenator, as it was called in the United States, was further developed by Kay and Cross in Cleveland, and by 1958 the Kay-Cross heart-lung machines were being sold at a reasonable price.[60] During the late 1950s and early 1960s, rotating-disc oxygenators were used by Frank Gerbode at Stanford, Albert Starr in Portland, Robert Gross in Boston, and at many other centers. Dennis Melrose developed a modification of this oxygenator that was used in England and several European hospitals. The principal disadvantages of the rotating-disc oxygenator were its large priming volume and the long time required both to set it up and also to clean and sterilize it for its next use. It was gradually displaced by the improved hard-shell bubble oxygenators of the mid-1960s.

Three types of heart-lung machines evolved in the 1950s. All eventually used the simple and reliable DeBakey roller pumps, but each used a different method of oxygenating the blood—the Gibbon film oxygenator, the Kay-Cross rotating-disc oxygenator, or the DeWall bubble oxygenator. Gibbon's machine never became popular. A few custom-built copies were made and a company was licensed to produce them, but not very many were sold. It was too expensive, too complicated, and too temperamental. The DeWall bubble oxygenator demonstrated that a simple heart-lung machine operated by a trained perfusionist was the most practical technology for open-heart surgery. The rotating-disc oxygenators, which worked well enough, were in turn replaced by the more efficient and disposable hard-shell bubble oxygenators.

The ideal oxygenator had always been thought to consist of a membrane that would allow oxygen to cross it but would separate the blood from the gaseous mixture. The most practical of this type is the disposable micropore-membrane oxygenator, which became available in the mid-1970s and is used by most cardiac surgical centers today, replacing all of the old bubble, disc, and film oxygenators.

Today's heart-lung machine is a greatly improved and reliable system when compared to the devices used during the early open-heart operations, but the exposure of the blood to various foreign surfaces can still produce unwelcome results. Every patient has at least a temporary alteration of the coagulation system, a decline in platelet function, and various poorly understood alterations of the immune system. An hour or two of cardiopulmonary bypass is easily tolerated by almost all patients, but if that time is prolonged, the possibility of poor coagulation, infection, or postoperative cognitive loss goes up. It is a very good system, but it is not yet perfectly safe.

The Starr-Edwards Valve

The 1960s brought the most exciting and innovative time for cardiac surgery. The technology of the heart-lung machine was established with two very dependable systems. Surgical groups used either a rotating-disc oxygenator or a disposable bubble oxygenator, and there were several companies that sold heart-lung machines. During this ten-year period, the average mortality rate for cardiac surgery for most institutions went down from about 30 percent to about 5 percent. There were several reasons. First of all, cardiac surgeons learned the various techniques and basics of cardiac surgery, including incisions, cannulation, prevention of air embolism, prevention of postoperative bleeding, myocardial preservation, and control and treatment of arrhythmias. National meetings were particularly stimulating with all sorts of useful new information being presented. Secondly, as results improved, cardiologists began to recommend surgical treatment for patients at an earlier stage of their disease, and fewer patients reached the operating room in extremis from end-stage heart disease and profound heart failure.

Then a huge event occurred in 1961. At the annual meeting of the American Surgical Association in Boca Raton, Florida,

Albert Starr described the successful use of a caged-ball prosthetic mitral valve in six patients.[61] It was by far the meeting's most important paper: For the first time, a dependable prosthetic valve was available for mitral valve replacement. Previous attempts to repair the mitral valve had been made with inconsistent results. For calcific aortic stenosis, repair had been aimed at decalcifying the valve, but such repair sometimes left the leaflets too thin and fragile to function properly. Various Dacron fabric leaflets were used to replace those that were damaged, but the results were unsatisfactory. For example, at the National Institutes of Health in the early 1960s, Dr. Morrow repaired or decalcified the aortic valve on ten successive patients with aortic stenosis, and each one died in the early postoperative period. When the Starr-Edwards aortic valve became available, nine out of the next ten patients survived.[62] The results were as different as day is to night. During this same time at the Vanderbilt University Hospital, the operative mortality for aortic valve replacement was as follows: 1962 through 1964, 51 percent; 1965 through 1966, 32 percent; 1967 through 1968, 15 percent; and 1969 through 1970, 2 percent. During that same time, this rapid decline in operative mortality occurred in every institution where cardiac surgery was being done and was due to improved equipment, better postoperative care, better myocardial preservation during operations, and a hundred other factors.[63]

The development of the Starr-Edwards valve was the first big event of the 1960s. Albert Starr had finished his thoracic and cardiac training at Columbia and was recruited in 1957 by the pediatric service of

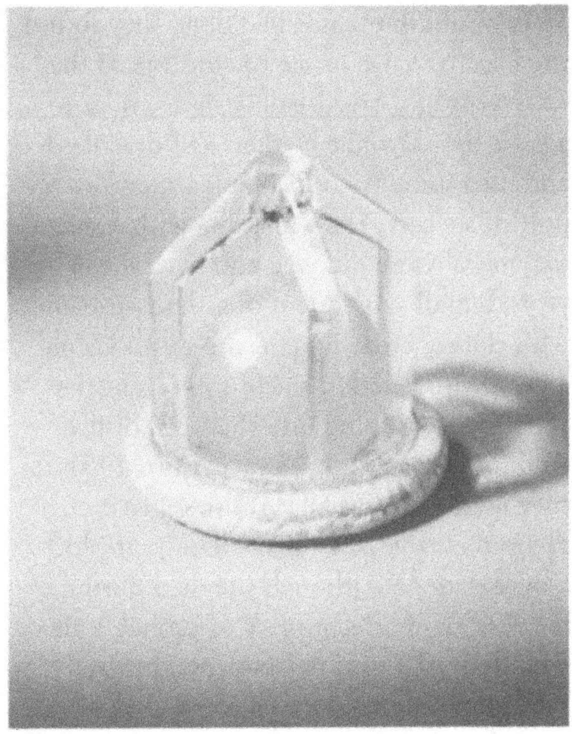

The first Starr-Edwards valve

the University of Oregon to start a cardiac surgery program there. He began a clinical cardiac surgical program after spending the first six months in the experimental laboratory getting everybody acquainted with a rotating-disc heart-lung machine.

A retired engineer named Lowell Edwards made an appointment to see Dr. Starr in 1958. He wanted to discuss the possibility of developing an artificial mechanical heart, and he needed a cardiac surgeon to help him. Starr told Edwards that there was not even a satisfactory artificial valve available, much less an artificial heart, so maybe they should first try to develop a valve. Edwards asked, "Which one?" Starr said he thought the mitral valve would be the most difficult, so they should start with that. Their first model was a bileaflet valve. Edwards would construct the new valve in his machine shop, and then

Starr would implant it in a dog. They found the bileaflet valve prone to clotting, so they next went to a caged-ball design similar to a valve that Dwight Harken had described and used for aortic valve replacement with limited success. Their first dog with a caged-ball mitral valve did well and lived for many years, but all subsequent dogs had problems with clots encroaching on the valve. Using a valve with a Teflon shield to prevent the clot from advancing into the valve orifice, they then began to have success. In 1961 they used a caged-ball valve to replace the mitral valve of a thirty-three-year-old female patient. Although she died during the first night after surgery of probable air embolism, the next five patients survived. Edwards and Starr formed a company—the Edwards Laboratories—to produce the valve, and in a very short time both mitral and aortic valves became available to others. It was by far the most successful and useful valve for aortic or mitral valve replacement for the next fifteen to twenty years and was the standard to which other valve designs were compared. It was used all over the world.[64]

As might be expected, suddenly a large number of artificial valves of various designs were developed and produced, usually identified by the principal surgeon's name. FDA medical-device regulation did not begin until 1976, so it was not difficult to produce and market a new valve design. Some of the artificial valves of the 1960s and early 1970s were the Kay-Cross valve, the DeBakey, the Beall, the McGovern, the Wada, the Smeloff, the Hufnagel, the Cooley, the Cape Town, and many others.[65] Some of these valves did have ingenious features and materials that in time proved to be of lasting benefit, but none was as reliable as the Starr-Edwards valve, and most of them had only brief popularity. A few had such serious flaws or poor durability that they were withdrawn from the market. The medical-device regulations of 1976 greatly reduced the variety of new valves being produced, but even with these regulations and with controlled clinical trials prior to general use, valve failures have occurred. Early in the history of the Starr-Edwards valve, patients experienced an unforeseen late problem in which the Silastic poppet gradually absorbed lipids from the blood stream, causing slight swelling of the poppet. This produced asymmetrical wear and in some cases actual fracture of the poppet. This problem was resolved by using a different curing method for the silicone poppet so that it would not absorb lipids.[66] Although the postoperative complication rates and operative mortality rates were high compared to today's results, at the time the majority of patients were greatly improved after valve replacement.

A second category of patients that had miserable outcomes in the earliest days of cardiac surgery were those with complex congenital cardiac abnormalities such as common atrioventricular canal, transposition of the great vessels, and tricuspid atresia. The mid-1960s brought new and innovative techniques such as the Rastelli[67] operation, the Mustard[68] and Senning[69] operations, and the Fontan[70] operation. These procedures were possible because of a better understanding of the anatomy of congenital heart disease and the advance in open-heart techniques that made a quiet, relatively dry, and unhurried operative field possible so that precise repair could be accomplished. During the 1960s, cardiac surgery evolved from a very high-risk operation to a relatively safe and reliable choice for patients with both complex congenital cardiac problems and for patients with aortic and mitral valve disease.

Coronary Artery Surgery

In 1912 James Herrick presented a talk at the annual meeting of the American Medical Association with the title: "Clinical Features of Sudden Occlusion of the Coronary Arteries."[71] He described the symptoms and signs of acute myocardial infarction and showed that this syndrome was caused by thrombosis of a coronary artery with subsequent myocardial injury. Before that time the relationship between angina and coronary artery calcification and narrowing had been recognized, but the symptom complex of acute myocardial infarction was not understood and was sometimes called apoplexy or thought to be a gastrointestinal problem. At the time of the AMA meeting, Herrick's presentation did not bring about much interest, but gradually, over the next few years, the relationship between coronary thrombosis and the symptoms of an acute myocardial infarct were recognized, especially after electrocardiograms became more common.

As it became generally recognized that the symptoms of angina were caused by coronary disease and inadequate coronary blood flow, various surgical procedures were proposed to decrease the symptoms. During the 1920s, it was thought that cervical and thoracic sympathectomy might be beneficial, but the results were unpredictable.[72] Another theory was that the symptoms could be alleviated by reducing the metabolic demand of the patient by thyroidectomy. This procedure was used in the 1930s.[73] It did reduce angina attacks, but the patients were reduced to a hypothyroid state, which was about as bad as the problem of angina. The third surgical solution was to increase the blood supply to the myocardium. The principal advocate of this approach was Claude Beck of Case Western Reserve in Cleveland. His first procedures involved bringing flaps of pectoral muscle onto the epicardial surface and abrading the pericardium to promote vascular adhesions.[74] He also used other substances, such as talc and asbestos, in the pericardium. These operations were done in the late 1930s. He then shifted to trying to create a higher myocardial venous pressure by creating a stenosis of the coronary sinus.[75] Finally, he combined this with an autologous arterial graft from the descending aorta to the coronary sinus to produce retrograde coronary flow.[76] Pericardial abrasion and poudrage with talc, combined with surgical narrowing of the coronary sinus to three millimeters, was called the Beck I operation. The Beck II was coronary sinus narrowing combined with an arterial graft to the coronary sinus to promote retrograde flow. The Beck I was cautiously adopted by various other surgeons and was used off and on until the advent of coronary bypass grafts in 1967.

In the immediate post–World War II period, Arthur Vineberg of McGill University in Montreal began extensive investigation of the possible benefit of implanting a mammary artery into the myocardium with the idea that it would develop collateral circulation with the coronary arteries. He found that if the multiple side branches of the mobilized mammary artery were left open and the distal end ligated, collaterals would develop.[77] After extensive laboratory investigation, he began a clinical program and reported that several months after this procedure his patients were improved. His operative mortality was 6 percent. His first procedure was done in 1950, and he continued utilizing this operation for the next twenty years.[78] It was never really accepted by other surgical groups until 1963 when Mason Sones studied two patients that had previously had Vineberg operations in Montreal. In one patient, Sones found little evidence of collaterals between the mammary artery and the coronary arteries, but in the second patient he found extensive filling of the left anterior descending from the previously implanted internal mammary.[79] With this finding, Donald Effler began utilizing the Vineberg operation at the Cleveland Clinic, and his optimistic reports led others to begin using this procedure in the mid-1960s.

All of these early attempts to improve the symptoms and life expectancy of patients with coronary artery disease were done well before selective coronary arteriography was available. In the 1950s when peripheral arteriography became fairly common, selective coronary arteriography was thought dangerous because of the risk of cardiac arrest or an acute myocardial infarct. The technique used at that time was to inject a large bolus of dye into the aortic root and take multiple films as the dye went through the coronary system, but cardiac motion and dilution of the dye produced very poor images of the coronary arteries.

An accident produced the first selective coronary arteriogram. Mason Sones was a pediatric cardiologist at the Cleveland Clinic. In 1958 he was planning to do an aortogram on a twenty-seven-year-old patient named Otis Dickey. The catheter was carefully positioned in the aortic root using fluoroscopy. The patient was then moved up the table a few feet to be positioned over a film changer that made one or two films per second. Unknown to Sones, the catheter moved during this change in position and the tip of the catheter went into the right coronary artery so that thirty cubic centimeters of dye was injected directly into the right coronary artery instead of into the aortic root. As soon as Sones realized what had happened, he began preparation for some sort of acute myocardial event or cardiac arrest, but nothing happened. The EKG and cardiac rhythm remained normal. After a brief period of asystole, the films showed a beautifully detailed arteriogram of the right coronary artery with resolution that had never been seen. When it became clear that no damage had been done, Sones repeated the procedure on a second patient. This success led to the birth of coronary arteriography and eventually to the birth of coronary artery surgery.

Sones perfected the details of selective coronary arteriography over the next two to three years. Through a small purse-string suture in the exposed brachial artery, he made a stab wound and inserted a small catheter with a flexible tip. The catheter was then advanced into the ascending aorta and maneuvered into the ostium of each coronary artery. The position of the catheter was verified by injecting small amounts of dye, being careful not to completely obstruct the artery with the catheter. Then ten cubic centimeters of dye was hand injected. He helped develop a cine camera to record the images at thirty frames a second, made possible by the use of an image intensifier. From that time on cinearteriograms replaced the old cumbersome direct X-ray film changer.

This system gave precise, clear, and detailed images of the coronary arteries and the collateral pathways in those patients with previously occluded vessels.[80]

Along with his colleagues and fellow cardiologists William Proudfit and E. K. Shirey, Mason Sones did coronary arteriograms on hundreds of patients. He and Proudfit, and later he and Favaloro, developed a totally new perspective of the pathology and natural history of coronary artery disease. Up until that time, coronary artery disease was evaluated by the history of the patient plus the electrocardiogram and whatever laboratory data that might be pertinent. Usually the symptoms of the patient were the most important element in the assessment. In most medical problems, as the symptoms and signs become more severe, so does the pathology of the problem. For example, in appendicitis the pain and tenderness in the abdomen at first is not too severe, but increases as the inflammation progresses toward rupture. In coronary artery disease, the symptoms of exertional angina may follow this same pattern and progress as the severity of the coronary disease gets worse, but quite often this is not the case. In some patients, angina may be prominent but the risk small, if the coronary disease is confined to the right coronary artery. In others, the symptoms may be unimpressive but the risk substantial, if the coronary disease involves a large anterior descending, or the left main coronary artery. Finally, at least 20 percent of patients have no warning symptoms at all and the first event is an acute heart attack or even sudden death. The coronary arteriogram made it possible to evaluate the severity of coronary disease and the relative risk of such sudden complications. The arteriogram replaced symptoms as the most important element in evaluating the disease. Sones, Proudfit, Shirey, and Favaloro recognized that the patient's history and EKG did not tell the whole story and that a coronary arteriogram was necessary to evaluate the prognosis accurately. Through presentations at meetings and publication of their data, they began to propose a change in the evaluation of patients with coronary artery disease, and that change involved a coronary arteriogram.

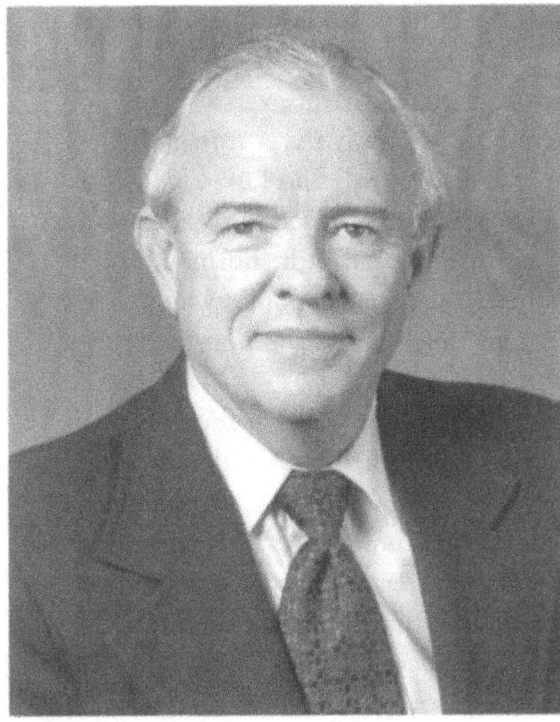

Frank Mason Sones

This news was received in two different ways. Many cardiologists and internists recognized the logic and value of a coronary arteriogram, but a minority of more conservative physicians failed to recognize this as progress, and several years of controversy ensued.[81] The first dispute was whether coronary arteriography should be done as part of the evaluation of patients with chest pain. Later came the more contentious argument over the value of surgical intervention for coronary artery disease. It took several years before enough evidence was available to demonstrate clearly that coronary bypass operations really did prolong life.[82] Those controversies have faded into the past, and today intervention is the norm, although catheter-mediated angioplasty and stenting are now much more common than surgical procedures.

It was René Favaloro at the Cleveland Clinic who worked out the details and techniques of the first successful coronary artery bypass procedures in 1966 and 1967. It should be remembered that Favaloro was not the first to operate on diseased coronary arteries. Claude Beck and Arthur Vineberg both devised indirect operations that were designed to bring a new source of blood to the myocardium. Neither of these procedures was particularly effective, and they were not widely used. Endarterectomy was a surgical procedure that had been found to be useful in the carotid artery and in various other locations of the arterial system. In 1958 William Longmire and Jack Cannon reported a small series of patients in whom they had done an endarterectomy of one or more of the coronary arteries.[83] These operations were done without cardiopulmonary bypass, so they were handicapped by the constant motion of the beating heart. The results were not impressive. In 1967 V. L. Kolessov from Leningrad reported five patients in whom he had used the internal thoracic artery as a graft to the coronary artery system. None of his patients had preoperative or postoperative arteriograms. The patients all had severe angina, and at the time of surgery the location of the site of coronary disease was determined by simple palpation of the artery. In four patients the internal thoracic coronary artery anastomosis was done in the middle third of the anterior descending coronary artery, and in one patient the graft was to the circumflex coronary artery. One patient died in the operating room, and the other four survived and were improved. Cardiopulmonary bypass was not used. Postoperative coronary arteriograms were not obtained because of "fear that it might result in fibrillation of the heart ventricles."[84]

In Houston in 1966 Edward Garrett and Michael DeBakey did an off-pump coronary endarterectomy on a patient with severe exertional angina. When the endarterectomy was completed, the remaining arterial wall was too flimsy to be reconstructed. They then used a segment of the patient's saphenous vein to restore circulation to the left coronary artery by constructing an aorta-coronary bypass graft. The patient recovered, and seven years later (in 1973) a follow-up arteriogram was obtained, which showed a very healthy vein bypass graft filling the left anterior descending coronary artery.[85] This was the first successful vein coronary bypass graft. It is curious that Garrett and DeBakey did not realize that the operation they had used to salvage an artery damaged by endarterectomy could be used as a primary operation for patients with severe coronary disease. The publication in 1973 was significant, not so much to give them precedence but because it showed that vein grafts to the coronary arteries could function for at least seven years and probably much longer.

Another early coronary artery bypass operation was done by David Sabiston at Duke in 1962.[86] He used a saphenous vein to bypass the right coronary artery. Unfortunately, the patient had a massive stroke three days after the operation and subsequently died. It was thought that the stroke occurred as a result of a thrombus at the site of the aortic anastomosis that had subsequently embolized.

René Favaloro established coronary artery surgery as primary treatment for ischemic heart disease. He was born in La Plata, Argentina, attended school there, and graduated first in his class from the La Plata University Medical School in 1949. He was interested in thoracic surgery, and after his internship he was offered a position as a surgical resident. This was during the presidency of Juan Peron, and Favaloro was asked to join the Peronist Party as a requirement to continuing his surgical training. He did not agree with the Perón government, so instead he dropped out of the training program and became a general practitioner and surgeon in Jacinto Arauz, a small town in the Pampas. He and his brother built a small hospital, and he worked there for the next twelve years, but he still wanted to be a thoracic surgeon. On the advice of his mentor, Professor Mainetti, who had recently visited several medical centers in the United States, he decided to go to the Cleveland Clinic to complete his training. He had to overcome some difficulties with his English and had to pass the Education Commission for Foreign Medical Graduates examination, but eventually he was accepted as a surgical resident at the Cleveland Clinic. He finished his training in 1964 and then joined the staff. During this time Mason Sones had done hundreds of coronary arteriograms, and Favaloro developed an interest in the possibility of surgical intervention for ischemic heart disease. In the beginning they did Vineberg procedures, but by 1967 to 1968 they rapidly progressed from patch grafts to interposition vein grafts, and finally to aorta to coronary end-to-side bypass grafts using saphenous vein.[87] Most of the early operations were done on right coronary arteries, and with success in those grafts they progressed to multiple grafts of the anterior descending and circumflex branches. The mortality rate was low, and their patients were carefully followed. Postoperative arteriograms showed that the grafts continued to function in both the short and long term. The Cleveland Clinic started an entirely new way of evaluating and treating patients with coronary artery disease that was accepted all over the world. Revascularization procedures either by catheter intervention or by surgical techniques are now carried out on more than one million patients each year.

Favaloro and Sones were the catalysts that changed the way everyone looked at patients with coronary artery disease. Watchful waiting was replaced by intervention, with the result of greatly improved lives and longevity.

Above all else, Favaloro was an Argentine patriot. He could have stayed at the Cleveland Clinic or accepted one of many lucrative offers at other institutions, but instead he returned to Argentina in 1971. He worked in a private clinic at first but eventually established the Favaloro Foundation, which is a large hospital and a multispecialty clinic in Buenos Aires. The policy of the Favaloro Foundation is that no patient will be turned away because of inability to pay. His hospital had a large and active cardiac surgical service but also was a leader in liver, kidney, and heart transplantation. Argentina and the surgical world was shocked and saddened when he died at age seventy-seven of a self-inflicted gunshot wound. The Favaloro Foundation was deep in debt, and he also had personal problems.

Cardiac Transplantation

Some of the first experiments in organ transplantation were done by Alexis Carrel and Charles Guthrie at the University of Chicago between 1904 and 1906. After developing techniques for vascular anastomosis, they went on to do a variety of autografts (taking an organ or tissue out and then putting it back in the same animal) and homografts (replacing an organ or tissue with an organ from another animal of the same species) in dogs and cats of arteries, veins, kidneys, ovaries, spleens, thyroids, and hearts. A heart transplant experiment was reported in *American Medicine* in December 1905 and describes transplanting a small dog's heart into the neck of a larger dog. The description of the configuration of the vascular connections is not precise, but the recipient aorta was connected to the donor carotid artery for perfusion of the coronary arteries, and the pulmonary artery was anastomosed to the jugular vein. Ischemic time of the recipient heart was one hour and fifteen minutes. After reperfusion was established in the recipient heart, Carrel writes:

> Strong fibrillar contractions were seen. Afterward contractions of the auricles appeared and about an hour after the operation, effective contractions of the ventricles began. The transplanted heart beat at the rate of 88 per minute while the rate of the normal heart was 100 per minute. A little later, tracings were taken. Owing to the fact that the operation was made without aseptic technique, coagulation occurred in the cavities of the heart after about two hours and the experiment was interrupted.[88]

It would be helpful if Carrel had included a more detailed description of the vascular connections used for this experiment and also had explained the meaning of "fibrillar contractions." One would expect that after an hour and fifteen minutes of ischemia, the transplanted heart would fibrillate when reperfused. Defibrillation had been described by 1905, but defibrillation was not mentioned in the article.

Carrel recognized that kidney autografts functioned long term, but that kidney homografts functioned for only a few days and then failed. He suggested correctly that there was an unrecognized biological problem with homografted organs that would have to be identified and eliminated before organ transplants could become useful.

In the late 1950s and early 1960s, interest in experimental heart transplantation occurred in a number of different institutions. Norman Shumway and Richard Lower began a long series of experiments at Stanford that established the basic surgical techniques and the detection and management of tissue rejection.[89] They used azathioprine and steroids to treat rejection and identified rejection episodes by loss of amplitude of the R wave of the EKG.

During the 1960s, heart transplantation in experimental animals was being investigated in Moscow; Chicago; New Orleans; Jackson, Mississippi; Philadelphia; Bombay, India; and several other places. In January 1964 James Hardy at the University of Mississippi decided that his group was ready to attempt a human heart transplant. The recipient was to be a patient who was within hours of death from heart failure that could not be improved by surgical or medical treatment. Their plan was to stabilize the recipient patient by placing him on the heart-lung machine and then proceed to transplantation.

At that time, in 1964, the concept of brain death was not accepted in most countries. Death was defined as the moment the heart stopped. This meant that the donor heart would have to be from a death in the same hospital at about the same time. As soon as the donor patient died, Hardy planned to put that person on cardiopulmonary bypass, take him to the operating room where the recipient patient was already on cardiopulmonary bypass, and transplant the heart from donor to recipient. They realized that it would be unusual for two such patients to reach the point of death at the same time, so they had a backup plan. Two patients at Tulane had received chimpanzee kidney transplants, which had functioned well for several months. They thought that a chimpanzee heart could be used if a human donor heart was not available, and that is exactly what happened. The patient selected to be the recipient gradually became worse, requiring a tracheotomy and ventilator support. For several hours he had a very low blood pressure and cardiac output and was near death. He was taken to the operating room in shock and was connected to a heart-lung machine and started on cardiopulmonary bypass. A donor was not readily available, so the chimpanzee heart was used. It functioned for about an hour and a half and then gradually failed. It may have failed in part because of the overall poor condition of the patient and the effects of preoperative hypotension. Since it was the first heart transplant that had been attempted in a human being, this operation received a lot of media attention and a great deal of criticism. At that time, kidney transplants were gaining acceptance, but almost all liver transplant patients had died, and some in the medical profession thought that organ transplants should be discontinued. The fact that Hardy and his group had used a "monkey" heart added to the criticism. Also at that time there was a great deal of racial conflict in Mississippi, which was brought into the debate. Altogether it was a particularly unpleasant aftermath for Dr. Hardy and the University of Mississippi Medical School. The criticism from the press and from the medical profession was so severe and painful that Hardy and his associates decided to give up any further attempts at heart transplantation. However, later that same year Hardy published their experience, "Heart Transplantation in Man: Developmental Studies and Report of a Case," in the *Journal of the American Medical Association*.[90]

Four years later, when the first human-to-human heart transplant was done in South Africa by Christiaan Barnard, responses from the media and the medical profession were overwhelmingly positive and supportive. Fortunately, as heart transplantation has taken its place as part of the treatment for end-stage heart disease, Dr. Hardy's contribution has been accepted as a significant and positive part of the evolution of this procedure; this acceptance may have erased some of the painful memories of that first operation.

By the fall of 1967 Norman Shumway and his group at Stanford had achieved a succession of long-term survivors of dog heart transplants using azathioprine and prednisone for episodes of rejection. He announced that they were prepared to proceed with a human heart transplant but pointed out the difficulty of selecting a recipient, since the procedure had never been done and the outcome was uncertain.[91]

At the same time Christiaan Barnard, the chief of cardiac surgery at Groote Schuur Hospital in Cape Town, South Africa, had come to Richmond, Virginia, for a few months. He came to work with David Hume who had developed a successful kidney transplant service at the Medical College of Virginia. Barnard was there to learn the techniques of kidney transplantation and the postoperative management of transplant patients, with a plan to develop a kidney transplant service in Cape Town. Richard Lower, who had worked for several years with Shumway during the evolution of experimental heart transplantation, had been asked to join the faculty at the Medical College of Virginia, and by that time he was doing heart transplant procedures in the experimental laboratory, with plans to develop a clinical program. It was inevitable that the visiting surgeon, Barnard, observed Lower doing heart transplant procedures on dogs during his visit. Barnard returned to Cape Town in the early fall determined to do a heart transplant, and he set about working in the experimental lab with his surgical team.

In the United States and most other countries, "death" occurred when the heart stopped beating, but in South Africa, death was determined by the declaration of two physicians that the patient was dead. This meant that brain death was acceptable. Barnard and his cardiologist colleague, Val Schrire, planned to select a recipient who was in the final stages of heart failure and who could not be improved by either additional medical or surgical treatment. If the patient was agreeable to transplant, they would keep him or her in the hospital and wait until a second patient with irreversible brain damage was brought to the hospital. When it was certain that this patient was brain dead without hope for recovery, they would then ask the family for permission to use the heart for a transplant operation. The patient Schrire selected for the first transplant was Louis Washkansky, fifty-three years old and in congestive heart failure from coronary artery disease. In early December 1967 a young girl, Denise Darvall, was struck by a car while crossing the street and was brought to Groote Schuur in a coma. When it became apparent that the coma was irreversible, her father gave permission for the surgeons to use her heart; her mother had been killed in the same accident. The way it was managed, they first took Washkansky to the operating room. He was anesthetized, the chest was opened, and everything was prepared to place him on a heart-lung machine. After preparing Darvall for surgery in an adjacent operating room, they turned off her ventilator; she quickly became anoxic and her heart fibrillated. When the heart stopped altogether, they put her on a second heart-lung machine to perfuse her heart with oxygenated blood. Her heart was then removed and taken into the first operating room where Washkansky was now also on a heart-lung machine. They perfused the donor heart from the same circuit until Washkansky's heart could be removed and replaced with the much smaller heart of Darvall. When all was secure, they defibrillated the heart and, after a short time, were able to come off the heart-lung machine with Washkansky's circulation being maintained by the transplanted heart.[92] Initially everything worked well and the early postoperative course was not difficult, but after two weeks Washkansky developed a fever. Thinking that rejection was the cause, they increased the azathioprine and cortisone, but the fever was caused by Klebsiella pneumonia, and after a total of eighteen days Washkansky died.

This operation set off an enormous amount of interest in the media of every country in the world. Barnard became an international celebrity overnight, was invited to come to the United States, and was interviewed on *Face the Nation* and various other television programs. He was also on the cover of *Time* magazine. Almost immediately another heart transplant operation was done on an infant in New York by Adrian Kantrowitz, but it was not successful.[93]

Twelve days after Louis Washkansky died, Barnard did a second heart transplant in Cape Town. The patient was Philip Blaiberg, a fifty-eight-year-old dentist. This transplant was a success and Blaiberg lived for nineteen months. Norman Shumway did the fourth heart transplant in the world one month after Barnard's first operation. Shumway's first patient died after two weeks.

It seems rather strange to us now, but these operations set off a wave of intense interest in cardiac transplantation at almost every cardiac surgical center in the world. Everybody wanted to do one. During the next fourteen months, heart transplant operations were done in hospitals all over the world—in India, Turkey, Russia, Poland, Brazil, Spain, Venezuela, Israel, Switzerland, Chile, France, and Argentina—altogether in twenty different countries and by twenty-nine different surgical teams in the United States. Someone at the time said, "Heart transplants were done in locations where you might be concerned about having an appendectomy." The results were terrible. During those first fourteen months, 167 patients had a heart transplant, and 143 of them died, most of them in the early postoperative course. The overall mortality was 84 percent. A small number of patients survived for one to two years. Most surgical groups did one or two transplants and then gave it up because the results were so poor.

The operation itself requires planning and organization, but the surgical technique is straightforward. The problem was rejection. No one knew exactly how to recognize and deal with rejection. Loss of amplitude of the R wave was not a very sensitive marker of early rejection, and it was difficult to discriminate between rejection and infection. The wrong choice here would usually lead to a disastrous result. Clearly, it was a problem of surgical technique evolving too far ahead of the science of transplantation and rejection. The operation was too easy; managing the problems of rejection was too difficult.

After those first few months of excitement and enthusiasm, reality and a return of common sense prevailed, and heart transplantation was discontinued by almost everyone except Norman Shumway at Stanford. Barnard continued to do a few more transplants in South Africa, as did Christian Cabrol in Paris, but it was Shumway and his associates who continued to do transplants in a small number of patients each year with the plan to learn as much as possible from each patient. They developed a flexible transvenous instrument to biopsy a tiny segment of myocardium from the right ventricle, using only local anesthesia, making it possible to recognize rejection in its earliest stages.[94] They worked out the process of remote retrieval of donor hearts, eliminating the need for the donor patient to be transported to the recipient's hospital, and in 1980 they began the use of cyclosporine, a new and much better immunological agent. These advances in the recognition and treatment of rejection encouraged various surgical groups to return to cardiac transplantation as a viable treatment for patients with end-stage heart disease. By 1988, 2,450 heart transplants were performed in that single year, with a mortality rate of only 8.9 percent, and over one hundred cardiac centers in the United States were performing cardiac transplantation. Science had finally caught up with the surgical technology.

The success of cardiac transplantation fills an important role for patients with certain forms of end-stage heart disease. Unfortunately, there are still problems for the transplant patient. Immunosuppression is not without its difficulties. In some respects the patient has exchanged the problem of heart failure for a life with the new problems of immunosuppression. However, when you meet someone who is a ten- or fifteen-year survivor of organ transplantation, there is no doubt that it is a magnificent procedure.

Total Artificial Heart

Cardiac transplantation began with enormous enthusiasm and excitement in 1968, but this began to fade rapidly after the many early tragic failures. Fortunately, by the mid-1980s, cardiac transplantation had gradually become a relatively safe, reliable, and less sensational procedure. It offered a good solution for patients with end-stage heart failure, but the waiting time for a donor heart gradually increased to six months or longer, and there were far more transplant candidates than there were donors. More deaths occurred in patients waiting for a donor than during or after the transplant procedure.

Although cardiac transplantation was now a useful operation, most transplant surgeons thought that eventually we would use an artificial heart for patients with heart failure. Most of us in the 1980s thought that in eight or ten years a suitable artificial heart would be available and transplants would no longer be necessary. After all, we already had a variety of mechanical and biological heart valves as well as cardiac pacemakers. It would just be a matter of time until an artificial heart could be taken right off the shelf, sutured in place, and started up. The restrictive factor of not enough heart donors would be over.

One of the earliest pioneers in the development of artificial hearts was Willem Kolff. During World War II in Holland, Kolff recognized the possibility of using cellophane as a membrane for dialysis for patients with renal failure, and although at first he had a succession of failures, by the end of the war he had developed a workable dialysis machine. After the war he immigrated to the United States, became a citizen, and was the head of the Department of Artificial Organs at the Cleveland Clinic. In the 1950s he built the first heart-lung machine used at the Cleveland Clinic and in 1960 set out to develop an artificial heart. At the same time an Argentine surgeon named Domingo Liotta had developed an experimental artificial heart in Cordoba, Argentina. Kolff brought Liotta to the Cleveland Clinic, and the following year (1961) they reported the implantation in dogs of three different types of orthotopic total artificial hearts.[95] It was the first time that an air-driven pneumatic artificial heart had been described.

Dr. Michael DeBakey was enthusiastic about this work and offered Liotta a position at Baylor Medical School in Houston to continue his investigations, with a promise of strong financial backing for his research. He started with an emphasis on a left ventricular assist device rather than a total artificial heart. Myocardial protection during cardiac operations was not well understood in the 1960s. Sometimes after a long procedure such as a double valve replacement, the heart would not be able to sustain an adequate output due to anoxic injury of the myocardium. DeBakey and others had found that if they used the heart-lung machine to assist circulation for an hour or two, this would sometimes be enough for the heart to recover, but it was also obvious that prolonged assistance for several days would be necessary for most patients. Dr. DeBakey wanted Liotta to develop a left ventricular assist device for that situation or for patients who might recover if assisted through temporary cardiogenic shock following an acute myocardial infarct. DeBakey thought that a total artificial heart was still possible but for the present wanted to concentrate on a left ventricular assist device. Liotta developed a suitable left ventricular assist device, and it was first used in 1962 for a patient who had experienced cardiac arrest twenty-four hours after an aortic valve replacement.[96] The pump had an output of 1.8 to 2.5 liters per minute and was connected between the left atrium and the descending aorta by way of a left thoracotomy incision. After four days of assisted circulation the patient's heart improved and mechanical support was discontinued, but the patient had sustained severe brain injury and did not recover. Three years later the device was used again on a similar postoperative patient, and after ten days of support the device was removed, and the patient made a complete recovery. Both of these procedures were done at the Methodist Hospital in Houston. Liotta had also been working on a total artificial heart, but the use of this device in calves was not dependable enough for DeBakey to recommend its use in a clinical trial.

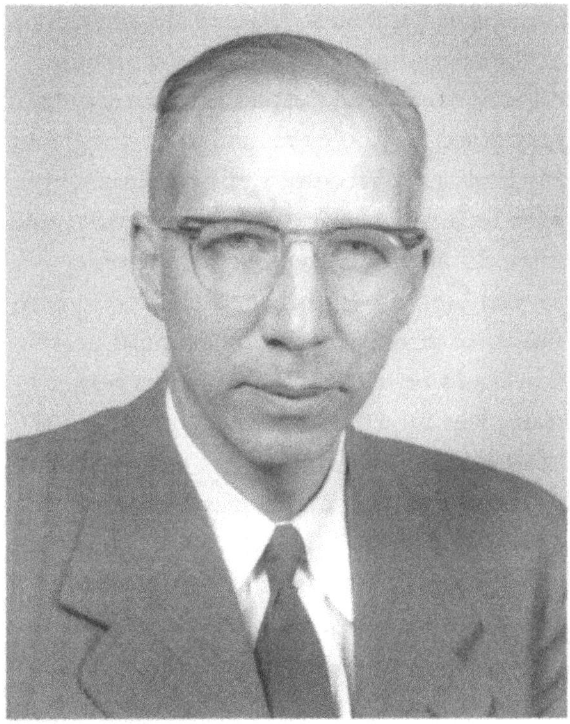

Willem J. Kolff

In 1962 Denton Cooley, Dr. DeBakey's colleague, had moved his practice from Methodist Hospital to nearby St. Luke's Hospital and had formed the Texas Heart Institute. He had moved from Methodist Hospital because Dr. DeBakey, as the senior surgeon at Methodist, utilized the majority of the operating rooms, making scheduling difficult for Cooley's expanding cardiac surgery practice. Cooley remained on the Baylor Medical School faculty, but his relationship with DeBakey became more competitive and more distant. In December 1968 Cooley invited Liotta to his office to discuss the possibility of developing a total artificial heart that could be used temporarily as a bridge to transplant for a dying patient until a donor heart became available. Liotta was enthusiastic about this plan and began working with Dr. Cooley in the evenings and on weekends at the Texas Heart Institute, but he did not resign from his position with Dr. DeBakey. They developed a total artificial heart similar to the one developed for DeBakey, but used the newly developed Wada valves and a new console that was built in the garage of one of the Baylor engineers during his off-duty hours.

On April 3, 1969, Dr. Cooley was asked to see a patient with heart failure secondary to a large left ventricular aneurysm that had resulted from a heart attack. The patient's name was Haskell Karp. The possible need for a heart transplant was discussed, but Karp preferred having the aneurysm removed in spite of the probable high risk. It was agreed that the artificial heart would be used only if his cardiac function at the end of the operation was insufficient for survival. The following day the left ventricular aneurysm was removed. His postoperative cardiac function was inadequate, so Cooley removed Karp's heart and replaced it with the Liotta total artificial heart, with plans to do a heart transplant as soon as a donor could be found. An appeal was immediately made for a donor so that a heart transplant could replace the artificial heart. After two days of circulatory support using the artificial heart, a donor heart became available and the artificial heart was replaced. Unfortunately, Karp developed renal failure followed by an overwhelming pulmonary infection and lived only two more days. This was the first time that a total artificial heart had been used in a clinical setting.[97]

All of this, once again, brought on a media frenzy, and, in addition, it brought onto Denton Cooley the wrath of Michael DeBakey, plus investigations by the National Heart Institute, the Baylor Medical School Institutional Review Board, the American College of Surgeons, and the Harris County Medical Society.

DeBakey was furious that Cooley had used an artificial heart that was very similar to the one developed by Liotta while working in DeBakey's laboratory and funded from a grant controlled by DeBakey.[98] The Baylor Institutional Review Board was distressed that they had not been asked to review the process since it was an experimental device used on a patient. When the smoke cleared, Dr. Cooley resigned from the faculty of Baylor Medical School and from that time worked at St. Luke's Hospital and the Texas Heart Institute, both of which are just a stone's throw from Methodist Hospital.

The American College of Surgeons censured Cooley, as did the Harris County Medical Society of Houston. Both were concerned about the issue of publicity and the use of a device that appeared similar to the one developed with funds from the National Heart Institute. Ironically, the program committee of the American College of Surgeons invited Dr. Cooley to discuss the use of the artificial heart at the same meeting in October 1969 at which the Board of Regents of the College voted that he should be censured. On the same day that he was censured by the Harris County Medical Society, he was chosen by the Seigler Foundation of New York as the recipient of their Humanitarian Award.[99]

Although these events were painful for Dr. Cooley, his reputation was such that his professional life went on much as before. The Texas Heart Institute continued to expand, he was later elected president of the Society of Thoracic Surgeons, and he continued to be a leader and an important influence in the evolution of cardiac surgery and surgical education. Although he made several attempts to reestablish a relationship with Dr. DeBakey, his calls were never returned. Today, Methodist Hospital is no longer affiliated with Baylor Medical School. The primary teaching hospital for Baylor is now St. Luke's Hospital, the location of the Texas Heart Institute, where Dr. Cooley still maintains a major leadership position as president and surgeon-in-chief.

In 1968 Willem Kolff had moved from the Cleveland Clinic to the University of Utah, where he continued his efforts to develop a total artificial heart. He was joined there by Robert Jarvik, an engineer as well as a medical school graduate, and later by a Duke-trained cardiac surgeon, William DeVries. In December 1982 DeVries replaced the heart of a patient, Barney Clark, with a total artificial heart, the Jarvik 7. Mr. Clark had a number of postoperative complications but survived a total of 112 days. He was maintained on an anticoagulation regimen (Coumadin) but had bleeding episodes and embolic strokes. He eventually died of an infection.[100] The power source for the Jarvik 7 was contained in a console, and the compressed air that drove the heart was transmitted through two fairly large tubes that entered his body just below the rib cage. These transcutaneous tubes could have been the source of the bacterial infection. Because of the expense and commitment of hospital resources required for the care of Clark, the University of Utah Hospital decided not to continue additional artificial heart operations until appropriate financing was available. DeVries then accepted an offer by the Humana Corporation to underwrite additional operations at the Audubon Hospital in Louisville, Kentucky, and after moving there he did three additional total artificial heart operations. Although one patient lived for two years, each patient had problems similar to Barney Clark. The National Heart Institute withdrew its support and approval for the use of the Jarvik 7 in patients because of these less than impressive results and because of some difficulties with timely reports from the clinical investigators. The Jarvik 7 is now approved for bridge-to-transplant procedures, but not for long-term total heart replacement.

In 2001 the FDA approved the use of the AbioCor Implantable Replacement Heart for five patients, not as a bridge to transplant but as permanent treatment. The AbioCor was the first completely implantable artificial heart, with a power source implanted within the patient, which was driven by a subcutaneous battery recharged continuously through the skin. This arrangement eliminated the problem of bacteria entering the patient by way of the drive tubing, as in the earlier total heart systems in which the power source was an external console.

The first patient was Bob Tools, whose

operation was done by Dr. Laman Gray on July 2, 2001, at the University of Louisville. Tools did very well at first, but four months later had a severe stroke and died three weeks afterward.[101] A second patient with the AbioCor heart also had a stroke, and another patient died of multiple organ failure. A total of seven patients had placement of the device. Each was in severe biventricular cardiac failure with evidence of cardiogenic shock in spite of maximal medical therapy including inotropic agents and intra-aortic balloon pumps. All were judged likely to die within thirty days. There were only two patients who survived and were discharged to home. There were two early deaths and three late deaths. The early deaths were caused by coagulopathy in one patient and a drug reaction in the other. The late deaths were due to a ceribrovascular accident (day 142), multiple system organ failure (day 56), and retroperitoneal bleeding (day 151). In addition, these very sick patients had multiple postoperative problems of renal failure, prolonged intubation, acute cholecystitis, and malignant hyperthermia.

Although this would appear to be a less than satisfactory trial with only two survivors, it showed that the artificial heart itself functioned well and almost all of the problems were related to the fact that these patients were in an advanced state of total body failure. Hopefully the next trial will include some patients who are not so close to death.

The FDA has also approved at least three devices for left ventricular assist to be used as a bridge to transplant, for postcardiotomy support, or for left ventricular dysfunction after a heart attack. They are the Abiomed BVS 5000, the HeartMate ILVAD, and the Novacor LVAS. In contrast to the total artificial heart, the left ventricular assist devices have been much more effective and satisfactory. Over four thousand have been used in the United States and Europe.

At present in the United States and Europe there are at least eighteen different pulsatile left ventricular assist devices under development and an additional twenty-eight axial or rotary continuous-flow devices. There are at least ten different total artificial hearts in various stages of development.

Obviously, the development of various left ventricular assist devices and total artificial hearts is in a state of rapid change, and the final most satisfactory system is far from settled. It is clear that the need is great. There are more than one hundred thousand patients who die of congestive heart failure each year. If and when a simple, safe, and relatively inexpensive device evolves, it will open a whole new area of cardiac surgery.

The story of heart surgery is the story of American medicine after World War II. It was the result of innovation, hard work, perseverance, and a fair bit of luck. While advances in technology—heparin, plastic tubes, defoamers, Dacron grafts, artificial valves, and immunosuppressive drugs—were all important, we can now say that the pioneer cardiac surgeons "pushed the envelope" to a remarkable degree. As Denton Cooley is fond of saying, they had the "courage to fail." As John Ochsner said, "Today if you did that, you'd probably be put in jail."

While these surgeons were intelligent and enormously productive, they were not born into, nor brought up in, some sophisticated elite group, and this makes their accomplishments even more remarkable. They did not all come from big cities or big universities, although four did come from New York and one each from Boston and Baltimore. They also came from Maple Lake, Minnesota; Sapulpa, Oklahoma; Reynolds, Georgia; and Haskell, Texas—places not often mentioned on the evening news. They were sons of the Depression; many of them knew real hardship as children and worked their way through college and medical school. Many of them served in the armed forces, principally during World War II and Korea, and, in fact, some of them, particularly Dr. Spencer and Dr. DeBakey, made lasting contributions during their time in the military.

One of the remarkable facts was that for a short but significant time in the infancy of heart surgery, in the mid-fifties, the only two locations in the world where successful open-heart procedures were being done were not London, Paris, Rome, or New York, but two cities in Minnesota: Minneapolis and Rochester. Someone once suggested, "There must have been something in the water there." Surgeons came there from all over the world, not only to learn the techniques of the Minnesota surgeons, but also to buy plastic tubing, pumps, and oxygenators so that they, too, could try to jump onto the heart surgery bandwagon. Some succeeded, and some failed. We know a fair amount about the good results, but a lot of carnage went unreported, with whispered tales of "eight operations without a survivor" and "ten operative deaths in a row."

Two features of this period are worth noting. Most of these new operations began with an original observation; for instance, a patient with a massive pulmonary embolus would benefit by using an artificial oxygenator, tetralogy children do well as long as the ductus stays open, dye injected directly into the coronary artery does not harm the heart, and so on. Developing these observations into a procedure led to the heart-lung machine, the Blue Baby operation, coronary artery bypass, and many others. Advances in cardiac surgery were frequently accomplished not by a single investigator working alone, but by the combined knowledge and ideas of two people working together, such as Blalock and Taussig, Shumway and Lower, Starr and Edwards, and Lillehei and DeWall. This has been true in numerous other medical discoveries, not just in the field of cardiac surgery.

These interviews with the early pioneer cardiac surgeons describe their professional lives and the various roles they played in the establishment of the specialty of cardiac surgery. It is the history of cardiac surgery as told by its founders.

References

1. Garrison F. *An Introduction to the History of Medicine* (4th Edition). Philadelphia: W. B. Saunders; 1966. 343.
2. Rutkow IJ. *American Surgery: An Illustrated History*. Philadelphia: Lippencott-Raven; 1998. 308.
3. Hill LL. A Report of a Case of Successful Suturing of the Heart and Table of Thirty-seven Other Cases of Suturing by Different Operators with Various Terminations, and the Conclusions Drawn. *Med Rec.* 1902; 846–848.
4. Carrel A, Guthrie CC. The Transplantation of Veins and Organs. Am Med. 1905; 10:1101–1102.
5. Carrel A. Nobel Lecture 1912. *Nobel Lectures, Physiology or Medicine 1901–1921*. Amsterdam: Elsevier; 1967.
6. Rutkow IJ. *American Surgery: An Illustrated History*. Philadelphia: Lippencott-Raven; 1998. 297–298.

7. Carrel A, Lindbergh C. *The Culture of Organs*. New York: P. B. Hoeber; 1938. 219–221.
8. Trendelenburg F. Zur Operation der Embolie der Lungenarter Ien. *Zlb Chir.*1908; 35:92–94.
9. Cutler EC, Levine SA. Cardiotomy and Valvulotomy for Mitral Stenosis: Experimental Observations and Clinical Notes Concerning an Operated Case with Recovery. *Boston Med Surg J.* 1923; 188:1023–1027.
10. Cutler EC, Beck CS. The Present Status of the Surgical Procedures in Chronic Valvular Diseases of the Heart. Final Report of the Surgical Cases. *Arch Surg.* 1929; 18:402–416.
11. Souttar HS. The Surgical Treatment of Mitral Stenosis. *Brit Med J.* 1925; 2:603–606.
12. Grabiel A, Strieder JW, Boyer NH. An Attempt to Obliterate the Patent Ductus in a Patient with Subacute Bacterial Endocarditis. *Am Heart J.* 1938; 15:621–624.
13. Holcomb GW. Personal Communication. August 2006.
14. Blalock A, Park EA. The Surgical Treatment of Experimental Coarctation (Atresia) of the Aorta. *Ann Surg.* 1944; 119:445–456.
15. Bing RJ, Handelswan JC, Campbell JA, Griswold HE, Blalock A. The Surgical Treatment and Physiopathology of Coarctation of the Aorta. *Ann Surg.* 1948; 803–820.
16. Shumacker HB Jr. Use of the Subclavian Artery in the Surgical Treatment of Coarctation of the Aorta. *Surg Gynec Obst.* 1951; 93:491–495.
17. Gross RE, Hufnagel CA. Coarctation of the Aorta: Experimental Studies Regarding its Surgical Correction. *New Engl J Med.* 1945; 233:287–293.
18. Gross RE. Surgical Correction for Coarctation of the Aorta. *Surgery.* 1945; 18:673–678.
19. Gross RE, Bill AE, Pierce EC. Method for Preservation and Transplantation of Arterial Grafts. Observations on Arterial Grafts in Dogs. Report of Transplantation of Preserved Arterial Grafts in 9 Human Cases. *Surg Gynec Obst.* 1949; 88:689–701.
20. Crafoord C, Nylin G. Congenital Coarctation of the Aorta and Its Surgical Treatment. *J Thorac Surg.* 1945; 14:347–361.
21. Fallot EA. Contribution à l'anatomie pathologique de la maladie bleue (cyanose cardiaque). *Marseilles Med.* 1988; 25:418–420.
22. Thomas VT. *Pioneering Research in Surgical Shock and Cardiovascular Surgery.* Philadelphia: University of Pennsylvania Press; 1985. 80–81.
23. Leeds SE. Alfred Blalock at Vanderbilt: Reminiscences of a Research Associate after 32 Years. *J Cardiovasc Surg* (Torino). 1968; 9:518–525.
24. Levy SE, Blalock A. Experimental Observations on the Effects of Connecting by Suture the Left Main Pulmonary Artery to the Systemic Circulation. *J Thorac Surg.* 1939; 8:525–530.
25. Olch PD. Dr. Sanford Leeds Discusses the Vanderbilt Years of Dr. Alfred Blalock. National Library of Medicine, History of Medicine Division, January 29, 1973.
26. Longmire WP. Alfred Blalock: His Life and Times. Private Publication; 1991. 112.
27. Dalton, ML. Blalock and Harrison—A Rare Friendship. *Pharos.* Summer 1998.
28. Ravitch MM. *The Papers of Alfred Blalock.* Baltimore: Johns Hopkins University Press; 1996. 1:xxxii.
29. Blalock A. Effects of an Artificial Ductus Arteriosus on Experimental Cyanosis and Anoxemia. *Arch Surg.* 1946; 52:247–251.

30. Blalock A, Taussig HB. The Surgical Treatment of Malformations of the Heart in which There Is Pulmonary Stenosis or Pulmonary Atresia. *JAMA*. 1945; 128:189–202.
31. Ravitch MM. *The Papers of Alfred Blalock*. 2 vols. Baltimore: Johns Hopkins University Press, 1966. 1:xlviii–xlix. © 1966 The Johns Hopkins University Press. Printed with permission of the Johns Hopkins University Press.
32. Westaby S. *Landmarks in Cardiac Surgery*. Oxford: ISIS Medical Media; 1997. 113.
33. Harken DE. Foreign Bodies in, and in Relation to the Thoracic Blood Vessels and Heart. *Surg Gynec Obst*. 1946; 83:117–125.
34. Bailey CP. Surgical Treatment of Mitral Stenosis (Mitral Commissurotomy). *Dis Chest*. 1949; 15:377–397.
35. Harken DE, Ellis LB, Ware PF, Norman LR. The Surgical Treatment of Mitral Stenosis I. Valvuloplasty. *N Eng J Med*. 1948; 239:801–809.
36. Brock RC. The Surgery and Pathological Anatomy of the Mitral Valve. *Brit Heart J*. 1952; 14:489–513.
37. Logan A, Turner R. Surgical Treatment of Mitral Stenosis with Particular Reference to the Transventricular Approach with a Mechanical Dilator. *Lancet*. 1959; 2:874–880.
38. Gross RE, Pomeranz AA, Watkins E Jr, Goldsmith EI. Surgical Closure of Defects of the Interauricular Septum by the Atrial Well. *N Eng J Med*. 1952; 247:455–460.
39. Lewis FJ, Taufic M. Closure of Atrial Septal Defects with the Aid of Hypothermia. Experimental Accomplishments and the Report of One Successful Case. *Surgery*. 1953; 33:52–59.
40. Hufnagel CA and Proctor HW. The Surgical Correction of Aortic Regurgitation; A Preliminary Report. *Bull Georgetown U. Med Ctr*. 1962; 6:60–61.
41. Gross RE, Watkins E Jr, Pomeranz AA, and Goldsmith EI. A Method for Closure of Interavicular Septal Defects. *Surg Gynec Obst*. 1953; 96:1–23.
42. Hufnagel CA, Harvey WP, Rabil PJ, McDermott TF. Surgical Correction of Aortic Insufficiency. *Surgery*. 1954; 35:673–683.
43. Gibbon JH Jr. Application of a Mechanical Heart and Lung Apparatus to Cardiac Surgery. *Minn Med*. 1954; 37:171–185.
44. Shumacker HB Jr. *A Dream of the Heart: The Life of John H. Gibbon, Jr., Father of the Heart-Lung Machine*. Santa Barbara, CA: Fithian Press; 1999. 23.
45. Gibbon JH Jr. Artificial Maintenance of the Circulation During Experimental Occlusion of the Pulmonary Artery. *Arch Surg*. 1937; 34:1105–1131.
46. Gibbon JH Jr. The Maintenance of Life During Experimental Occlusion of the Pulmonary Artery Followed by Survival. *Surg Gynec Obst*. 1939; 69:602–614.
47. Romaine-Davis ADA. *John Gibbon and His Heart-Lung Machine*. Philadelphia: University of Pennsylvania Press; 1991. 69.
48. Stoney WS. The History of Cardiac Surgery. Video Interview with Bernard Miller, JY Templeton, and John J. McKeown. July 31, 1996. The Annette and Irwin Eskind Biomedical Library, Special Collections, Vanderbilt University Medical School.
49. Kirklin JW. The Middle 1950s and C. Walton Lillehei. *J Thorac Cardiovasc Surg*. 1989; 98:822–824.
50. Miller WG. *King of Hearts: The True Story of the Maverick Who Pioneered Open-Heart Surgery*. New York: Crown; 2000. 14–17.
51. Miller WG. *King of Hearts: The True Story of the Maverick Who Pioneered Open-Heart Surgery*. New York: Crown; 2000. 111–112.
52. Andreasen AT, Watson F. Experimental Cardiovascular Surgery. *Brit J Surg*. 1952; 39:548–551.

53. Warden HE. C Walton Lillehei: Pioneer Cardiac Surgeon. *J Thorac Cardiovasc Surg.* 1989; 98:833–845.
54. Miller WG. *King of Hearts: The True Story of the Maverick Who Pioneered Open-Heart Surgery.* New York: Crown; 2000. 150.
55. Lillehei CW, Varco RL, Cohen M, Warden HE, Patton RN, Moller JF. The First Open-Heart Repairs of Ventricular Septal Defect, Atrioventricular Communis, and Tetralogy of Fallot Using Extracorporeal Circulation by Cross-circulation: A 30-year Follow-up. *Ann Thorac Surg.* 1986; 41:4–21.
56. Stoney WS. The History of Cardiac Surgery. Video Interview with Vincent L. Gott, MD. August 26, 1997. The Annette and Irwin Eskind Biomedical Library, Special Collections, Vanderbilt University Medical School.
57. DeWall RA, Gott VL, Lillehei CW, Read RC, Varco RL, Warden HE. Total Body Perfusion for Open Cardiotomy Utilizing the Bubble Oxygenator. Physiologic Responses in Man. *J Thorac Cardiovasc Surg.* 1956; 32:591–603.
58. Gravlee GP, Davis RF, Utley JR. *Cardiopulmonary Bypass: Principles and Practice.* Philadelphia: Lippincott, Williams, & Wilkins; 2000. 6
59. Björk VO. An Artificial Heart or Cardiopulmonary Machine. Performance in Animals. *Lancet.* 1948; 2:491–493.
60. Cross FS, Berne RM, Hirose Y, Jones RD, Kay EB. Evaluation of a Rotating Disk-type Reservoir Oxygenator. *Proc Soc Exper Biol and Med.* 1956; 93:210–214.
61. Starr A, Edwards L. Mitral Replacement: Clinical Experience with a Ball-Valve Prosthesis. *Ann Surg.* 1961; 154:726–740.
62. Bender HW. Personal Communication. November 2006.
63. Pleuth JR. The Starr Valve Revisited. *Ann Thorac Surg.* 1991; 51:333–334.
64. Mathews AM. The Development of the Starr-Edwards Heart Valve. *Tex Heart Inst J.* 1998; 25:282–293.
65. Davila JC. Second Henry Ford Hospital International Symposium on Cardiac Surgery. New York: Appleton-Century-Crofts. 1977.
66. Hylen JC, Hodam RP, Kloster RE. Changes in Durability of Silicone Rubber in Ball-Valve Prosthesis. *Ann Thorac Surg.* 1972; 13:324–329.
67. McGoon DC, Wallace RB, Danielson GK. The Rastelli Operation: Its Indications and Results. *J Thorac Cardiovasc Surg.* 1973; 65:65–75.
68. Mustard WT. Successful Two-Stage Correction of Transposition of the Great Vessels. *Surgery.* 1964; 55:469–472.
69. Senning A. Surgical Correction of Transposition of the Great Vessels. *Surgery.* 1959; 45:966–980.
70. Fontan F, Baudet E. Surgical Repair of Tricuspid Atresia. *Thorax.* 1971; 26:240–248.
71. Herrick JB. Clinical Features of Sudden Obstruction of the Coronary Arteries. *JAMA.* 1912; 59:2015–2020.
72. Cutler EC. Summary of Experiences Up-to-Date in the Surgical Treatment of Angina Pectoris. *Am J Med Sc.* 1927; 173:613–624.
73. Blumgart HL, Riseman JE, David D, Berlin DD. Therapeutic Effect of Total Ablation of Normal Thyroid on Congestive Failure and Angina Pectoris. III. Early Results in Various Types of Cardiovascular Disease and Coincident Pathologic States without Clinical or Pathologic Evidence of Thyroid Toxicity. *Arch Int Med.* 1933; 52:165–225.
74. Beck CS. Further Data on the Establishment of a New Blood Supply to the Heart by Operation. *J Thorac Surg.* 1936; 5:604–611.
75. Beck CS, Leightninger C. Scientific Basis for the Surgical Treatment of

Coronary Artery Disease. *JAMA*. 1955; 159:1263–1272.

76. Beck CS. Coronary Disease after Twenty-Five Years. *J Thorac Surg*. 1958; 36:329–351.
77. Vineberg AM. Development of an Anastomosis between the Coronary Vessels and a Transplanted Internal Mammary Artery. *Canad MAJ*. 1946; 55:117–119.
78. Vineberg AM, Miller G. Internal Mammary-Coronary Anastomosis in the Surgical Treatment of Coronary Artery Insufficiency. *Canad MAJ*. 1951; 64:204–210.
79. Effler DB, Groves LK, Sones FM Jr., Shirey EK. Increased Myocardial Perfusion by Internal Mammary Artery Implementation: Vineberg's Operation. *Ann Surg*. 1963; 158:526–536.
80. Sones FM, Shirey EK. Cine Coronary Angiography. *Mod Concepts Cardiovasc Dis*. 1962; 31:735–738.
81. Preston TA. *Coronary Artery Surgery: A Critical Review*. New York: Raven Press; 1977.
82. CASS Principal Investigators and Their Associates. Coronary Artery Surgery Study (CASS): A Randomized Trial of Coronary Bypass Surgery. Survival Data. *Circulation*. 1983; 68:939–950.
83. Longmire WP Jr, Cannon JA, Kattus AA. Direct-Vision Coronary Endarterectomy for Angina Pectoris. *New Eng J Med*. 1958; 259:993–99.
84. Kolessov V. Mammary Artery-Coronary Artery Anastomosis as a Method of Treatment for Coronary Artery Disease. *J Thorac Cardiovasc Surg*. 1967; 54:535–544.
85. Garrett EH, Dennis EW, DeBakey ME. Aortocoronary Bypass with Saphenous Vein Grafts. Seven-Year Follow-up. *JAMA*. 1973; 223:792–794.
86. Westaby S. *Landmarks in Cardiac Surgery*. Oxford: ISIS Medical Media; 1997. 196.
87. Favaloro RG. Saphenous Vein Autograft Replacement of Severe Segmental Coronary Artery Occlusion: Operative Technique. *Ann Thorac Surg*. 1968; 5:334–339.
88. Carrel A, Guthrie CC. The Transplantation of Veins and Organs. *Am Med*. 1905; 10:1101–1102.
89. Lower RR, Dong E, Shumway NE. Long-term Survival of Cardiac Homografts. *Surgery*. 1965; 58:110–119.
90. Hardy JD, Chavez CM, Kurrus FD, Neely WA, Eraslam S, Turner D, Fabian LW, Labecki TD. Heart Transplantation in Man: Developmental Studies and Report of a Case. *JAMA*. 1964; 188:1132–1140.
91. Shumway NE. Way Is Clear for Heart Transplant. *JAMA*. 1967; 202:31–32.
92. Barnard CN. A Human Cardiac Transplant: An Interim Report of a Successful Opertion Performed at the Groote Schuur Hospital, Cape Town. *South Afr Med J*. 1967; 41:1271–1274.
93. Kantrowitz A, Haller JD, Joos H, Cerruti MM, Marcial M, Carstensen HE. Transplantation of the Heart in an Infant and an Adult. *Am J Cardiol*. 1968; 22:782–790.
94. Caves PK, Stinson EB, Anthony FG, Billingham M, Grehl TM, Shumway NE. Percutaneous Endomyocardial Biopsy. *JAMA*. 1985; 225:288–291.
95. Liotta D, Taliani T, Giffoniello AH, Sarria Deheza F, Liotta S, Lizarraga R, Tolocka L, Panano J, Bianciotti E. Artificial Heart in the Chest: Preliminary Report. *Trans Am Soc Artif Int Organs*. 1961; 7:318–322.
96. Liotta D, Hall CW, Henly WS, Cooley DA, Crawford ES, DeBakey ME. Prolonged Assisted Circulation during and after Cardiac or Aortic Surgery: Prolonged Partial Left Ventricular Bypass by Means of an Intrathoracic Circulation. *Am J Cardiol*. 1963; 12:399–405.
97. Cooley DA, Liotta D, Hallman GL, Bloodwell RD, Leachman RD, Milam JD. Orthotopic Cardiac Prosthesis for Two-

staged Cardiac Replacement. *Am J Cardiol.* 1969; 24:723–730.
98. Thomas T. The Doctors' Bitter Feud. *Life.* 1970; 68:62B–74B.
99. Minetree H. *Cooley: The Career of a Great Heart Surgeon.* New York: Harper's Magazine Press; 1973. 36–79, 219–244.
100. DeVries WC. The Permanent Artificial Heart. Four Case Reports. *JAMA.* 1988; 259:849–859.
101. Dowling RD, Etoch SW, Stevens K, Butterfield A, Koenig SE, Johnson A, Chiang B, Gray LA Jr. Initial Experience with the AbioCor Implantable Replacement Heart at the University of Louisville. *ASAIO J.* 2000; 46:579–581.

The Early Years

William P. Longmire, MD

(b. 1913)

I took one look at the little patient and thought, "My God, this man isn't going to operate on this patient." The child was very cyanotic with dark blue lips and fingernails and required oxygen. . . . [The next day] I leaned over the ether screen and looked at the child's face and saw the cherry-red color of her lips.

— On the first Blue Baby operation

Interviewed October 20, 1998

I was born in a little town near Tulsa called Sapulpa, Oklahoma, in 1913. Sapulpa is said to be named for an American Indian who opened a trading post after coming from Tennessee on the "Trail of Tears." In the 1880s the St. Louis–San Francisco Railroad Company built a spur line south to Sapulpa to take advantage of a large number of enormous walnut trees, all of which were cut and transported to Europe. Now there isn't a tree in that part of the country larger than a foot in diameter, a sad ecology lesson for us all. In the late 1880s the Glen Pool oil field was discovered nearby—the largest known reservoir of oil at that time—and stimulated even more growth. My maternal grandfather moved to Sapulpa from Missouri when oil was struck, and later became the mayor.

My father was raised on a beautiful farm in East Tennessee, not far from Knoxville. He went to school in Louisville, Kentucky, and graduated in 1903 from one of the five medical schools that were open in Louisville at that time. After graduation he decided to look for an opportunity to practice in Colorado and bought a train ticket to Denver. On the train west he talked to some passengers who advised him to change his ticket and go down into Indian Territory where there was a great new oil field and a booming part of the country. He changed his ticket, ended up in Sapulpa, and opened a family practice. He was particularly interested in surgery and went to larger cities to take postgraduate classes. These were given in a completely unorthodox manner compared to medical education today. He would go to Tulsa and assist surgeons with some formal training, and so he became a kind of on-the-job self-taught surgeon. Late in life, when he was fifty-five years old, he was taken in as a fellow of the American College of Surgeons. This was one of the greatest landmarks of his whole life. At the time I was a medical student at Johns Hopkins. The College meeting was held in Chicago. I flew from Baltimore to Chicago to attend the meeting with him. It was the first commercial flight I had ever taken, and the plane was a Ford Tri-Motor, the Tin Goose.

The meeting was held in a hotel called the Stevens, which is now the Hilton on Michigan Avenue. As soon as I arrived we rushed downstairs and signed up for the wet clinics, which were held in a large amphitheater with two operating tables. We were up so high that we really couldn't see too much of the operation, but the surgeons talked as they were doing the cases, which did provide a certain amount of educational value.

I don't remember when I decided to study medicine. I just grew up with the idea that I

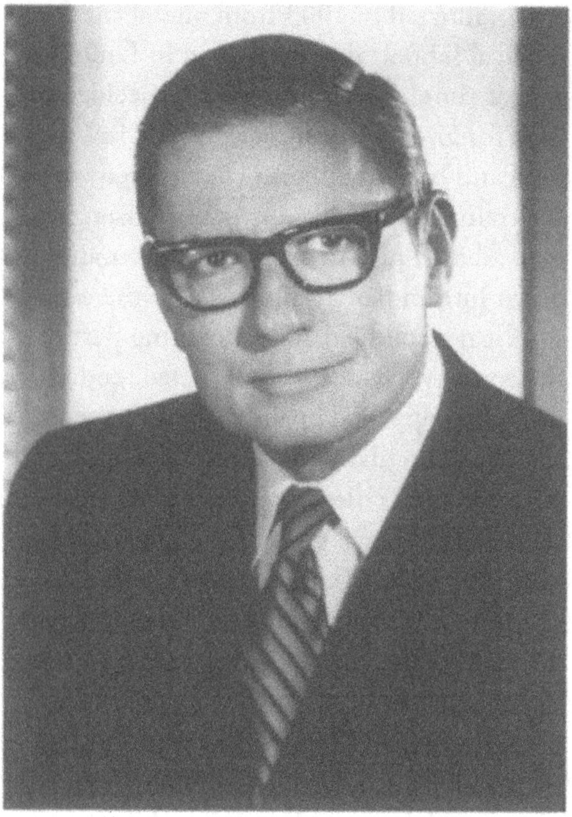

William P. Longmire

wanted to be a doctor. Friends and patients would say, "Oh, you're Dr. Longmire's son, you are going to be a doctor." I planned to practice in Sapulpa when I finished my training, so in planning my education I thought I should go to the University of Oklahoma to become acquainted with people in Oklahoma. My sister had gone to Ward Belmont in Nashville, so I was thinking of Vanderbilt for medical school or possibly Tulane. When I entered the University of Oklahoma in 1930, I enrolled as a premed student with zoology as my major subject. It turned out that my high school education was not as good as I had thought. The premed class had more than two hundred students. After the first meeting they gave us a test and divided us into four groups. I ended up in the "D" class, which I thought was a catastrophe. I thought I would never get into medical school. I went to work and it wasn't long before I was moved up to the "A" group.

The stock market crash of 1929 happened during my sophomore year in college. At that time there were four glass plants and a large oil refinery as well as two brick plants in Sapulpa. Most of these closed, in addition to many of the railroad facilities. My dad had been sending me $60 a month to take care of my expenses. He wrote and said that he would try to keep up these payments, but he was not sure that he could. "I can send you watermelons and tomatoes, but I just don't have much money." I went to the president of my fraternity and said that if he would provide space in the basement I would do all of the laundry for the fraternity members for $1.00 each per week. Most of them mailed their laundry home each week, so it was a little bit cheaper to have it done for $1.00 a week. I hired a laundress to help, collected and sorted the laundry on Sunday night, and delivered it the next Saturday afternoon. With this income I managed to make my way through the rest of the university and eventually with a little help from my father I was able to buy an automobile.

At the end of my third year, the chairman of the zoology department, Dr. Richards, called me into his office to talk to me about medical school. When I told him my plans he shook his head and said, "No, I'm going to send you to Johns Hopkins." I had heard a little about Hopkins and thought it was a good school, but had never really seriously considered it. Dr. Richards arranged for me to go to Fort Worth where there was a physician who was an interviewer for Hopkins. The interviewer said that he enjoyed talking to me and would recommend me. He also said that he recommended everyone that he interviewed. Since then I have thought about being admitted on the basis of one interview and one recommendation, but that was the custom of the times.

I had been to Baltimore once when I was younger. Each summer my father would load us up in a big old Cadillac touring car and we would go to Chicago. It would take three days. We would usually stay a month to get away from the heat and mosquitoes of Oklahoma. He would usually go to one of the Chicago postgraduate courses. One summer we went east to Philadelphia, and as part of that trip drove through Baltimore, as my father wanted to show me Johns Hopkins. We went to the Homewood Campus and my memory of Johns Hopkins was one of beautiful green lawns, trees, and white-columned buildings. Therefore, it was a shock when I arrived in Baltimore on a cold rainy September morning in 1934. As a couple of fraternity members drove me down the street, the first things I noticed were the row houses and no green grass. So I said, "The medical school is located in a different area than this, isn't it?" They said, "It won't be long until we get to the other campus." Soon they pointed up the hill and said, "There's the hospital." I said, "But the medical school is on the other campus, isn't it?" They said, "No, it's just behind the hospital." Well, this was quite a shock coming from Oklahoma. I joined a medical fraternity, which was largely a rooming and boarding house and lived there the rest of my time in medical school.

At the time I thought neurosurgery was evolving most rapidly and that I would become a neurosurgeon. During my first year I would go over to Walter Dandy's operating room on Saturday mornings and watch his operations. I was accustomed to observing in the operating room because my father had taken me into the operating room in Sapulpa on a number of occasions. We had a course in physiology, and I became interested in neurophysiology. Professor Bard was studying the phylogenetic development of the brain, and I worked in his lab on this project. When I went home in the summer I caught a number of lizards and worked out a method of anesthetizing them with a little ether, opening up the brain, and removing part of the brain back to the point where they developed the so-called hopping and jumping reactions. You could touch the front leg and they would either hop or jump. I found you could carry the dissection well down into the hindbrain before it was abolished. As a result of this I wrote my first scientific paper when I got back to Hopkins.

At the end of our first year several of us applied for a job in the Pathology Department to do autopsies. One of the faculty members had a child with a rare form of meningitis, caused by cryptococcus. This child had subsequently died at home on a farm in southern Maryland. Since I was somewhat experienced in doing autopsies, he asked me to go to the home and do a limited autopsy. When I arrived they were having a wake, but they took me into the kitchen and on a table there I took off the top of the deceased child's skull, got some cultures, and took the brain back to Hopkins. We grew the cryptococcus, and subsequently Dr. Goodman and I wrote a paper about torulosis meningitis. This was my second paper.

Near the end of the third year I started substituting as an intern on the surgical service. When the interns planned their vacation, they had to find a student to fill in for them while they were gone. My first opportunity was to substitute on the neurosurgical service, and since I thought that was to be my field I took it. It turned out to be a very tough four weeks, but I did get along well with Dr. Dandy. Later he was very helpful in getting me an internship. I substituted as an intern and continued to substitute during my senior year, possibly more than I should have.

When I became an intern and rotated on the neurosurgical service, I gradually realized that most of the patients that we operated on either had a brain tumor or a lumbar disk. Dandy was one of the leaders in lumbar disk surgery, and he had patients coming in from all over the world. It was a very busy time, and we worked day and night. We would all sit down together as a team on Saturday evening and discuss the week's work. For most of the patients with brain tumors, the operation was only palliative, and we would take out most of the tumor but frequently not all. The mortality rate was also very high. I made the decision that this was not the kind of surgery I would enjoy. I wanted to get to know my patients, to be involved with them, and to help more people than I could in neurosurgery.

At the end of my internship year, along with Rollins Hanlon I applied to spend a year in the surgical research laboratory. I was the Halsted fellow. At that time the research laboratory was run by Dr. Philip Price, who had been born in China where his parents were missionaries. After his medical education he had gone back to China but was driven out by the Japanese invasion. We studied shock, and it was a very profitable year. Dr. Price later became the first chairman of surgery at the University of Utah. During that year I also got married. When I was a student I began to notice a girl who worked as a receptionist and librarian in the Wilmer Eye Institute. I asked one of my friends who was on the ophthalmology service to introduce us, and our friendship developed. It was difficult during our first years since house staff salaries were only $15 each month.

The following year I was scheduled to work in surgical pathology, but my father had a stroke. He understood everything but he couldn't speak. Dr. Firor was then the acting chairman of the department because Dr. Dean Lewis had had a major stroke. I went to see Dr. Firor and explained my father's situation and he said, "Well fine, you go home and get things straightened out and see if your father is going to recover or sell the practice. We will hold your position open for you." That was in 1940.

In 1941 Dr. Alfred Blalock was appointed chairman of the Department of Surgery at Hopkins. Before he moved to Baltimore, I began to get letters and telephone calls from some of the senior residents telling me what a disaster the appointment was and how his proposed changes would completely wreck the residency system. I decided I had better go to Nashville and call on Dr. Blalock and let him know that I was part of his resident team. My grandmother still had a farm in East Tennessee and Jane, my wife, had never visited her, so I said, "This will be our excuse." I didn't want him to think that I was concerned, so I didn't make an appointment. I just stopped by to say "hello" on my way to Knoxville. He was very courteous and gracious. He took me around to see his laboratory even though I was not particularly interested. When we got back to his office the conversation turned serious. He wanted to know how I liked general practice. I told him that it was fine but that I planned to complete my training in surgery at Hopkins. He said, "The training program is too long. For you to finish, it will take eleven years after your graduation from medical school." He said that he was going to have to reduce the number of residents and the only fair way was to cut those at the bottom of the program. After Blalock moved to Baltimore, he wrote and said that he was sorry, but that my leave of absence would have to be extended indefinitely. He also said that he hoped I would be successful in finding another position. Well, I sat down right then and wrote a nasty letter saying that I had been at Hopkins longer than he had, and that I had more friends there than he did, and that he had better be careful about what he was doing. Fortunately, I did have sense enough to put the letter in my desk drawer and let it stay there until I cooled down a little bit. I then wrote him another letter telling him that I was sorry to hear of his decision, and that ended the Hopkins situation for the time being.

Of course in December of that year, the Japanese bombed Pearl Harbor, and I was soon called up by the army to take a physical examination in Oklahoma City. I told the recruiting officer that I would like to join one of the two Johns Hopkins Hospital units that had been formed, but he shook his head and said, "No, you are a healthy young doctor and we need you to follow the troops." However, it turned out that I had a minor physical disability, and they put me in the 4F category but said it was probably temporary. I went back to Sapulpa and began closing my practice, expecting to be called up soon. Our friends began having going-away parties for us. Then to my surprise I received a letter saying that I was deferred from military service. It was not very comfortable to remain in Sapulpa, since I appeared to be perfectly healthy. So I said to Jane, "Let's go to Baltimore and visit your parents, and I will see if I can get into one of the Hopkins units." We drove to Baltimore and the day after we arrived I went to the hospital and walked into the operating rooms. Mark Ravitch was doing an operation and he looked up and said, "Longmire, for God's sake, when can you go to work?" They were very shorthanded and were looking for anybody that could possibly go to work. After he finished the case, we went down to Dr. Blalock's office. At first I didn't think he recognized me as the man he had fired, but Mark Ravitch proposed that I be taken on to help out until I was called up. Dr. Blalock said okay, but then turned to me and said, "Dr. Longmire, we will be glad to have you, but I want you to know that this is not the back door to the Hopkins surgical residency program." That was the beginning of my friendship with Dr. Blalock.

The manpower situation did not improve. The curriculum of the medical school was changed from twelve to nine months, so a new class graduated every nine months. This increased the teaching burden. All of the residency programs were shortened to twenty-seven months, and Dr. Blalock began having two chief residents at the same time, so they would have some major experience prior to leaving for the service. It was during that period of time that Dr. Edwards Park, the chairman of the Department of Pediatrics, asked Dr. Blalock to see a child with coarctation of the aorta. Because of

Helen Taussig's prominence in the field of congenital heart disease, they had attracted a large number of patients with congenital heart abnormalities. Dr. Blalock told Dr. Park of a procedure he had developed at Vanderbilt with Dr. Sanford Leeds. They had tried to produce pulmonary hypertension in dogs by dividing the subclavian artery and then turning it down and anastomosing it to the pulmonary artery. He was disappointed to find that it did not create pulmonary hypertension; perhaps it would have done so if he could have had a longer follow-up. When he was talking with Dr. Park he immediately thought of the idea of turning the subclavian vessel and anastomosing it to the aorta distal to the coarctation, and shortly after, he tried this on a patient. Unfortunately, he divided some of the intercostals to free up the aorta and the patient developed paraplegia, so that was the end of that. In the meantime Clarence Crafoord in Sweden and Robert Gross in Boston developed the technique of excising the coarctation and reanastomosing the aorta, which seemed to be the correct approach. It was during this time that Dr. Park brought up Dr. Taussig's idea of bringing more blood to the pulmonary artery for patients with tetralogy of Fallot. He got Dr. Taussig and Dr. Blalock together to discuss the possibility of an operation to do this. Dr. Blalock always thought you should first go to the laboratory and see how it worked out. He and Vivien Thomas began to try to produce tetralogy of Fallot in a dog. They were never completely successful, but they gained enough experience to conclude that the subclavian artery could be used to direct more blood into the pulmonary artery. It was with this background that Dr. Taussig selected a very sick patient with tetralogy to refer to Dr. Blalock.

By 1944 I had advanced to the position of chief resident. It was the custom then that the chief resident went by Dr. Blalock's office about four o'clock in the afternoon. He would then discuss things with you such as how the residents were doing, what the hospital problems were, and other things far beyond our competence or understanding, but on a very personal basis as if we were equally informed. Then we would leave his office and go around to see the new patients, and if there was a problem of interest, he would select a patient to operate on the next day. The rest of the service we ran as our own private practice.

I went by one afternoon after he had done a couple of rather unusual cases; I can't remember specifically what they were, but they had not turned out well. One had died and the other was having some problems. His face was kind of flushed, and he threw his pencil down on his desk and said, "Bill, I am discouraged. Nothing I do seems to work very well." We then talked about some of the things he was interested in at that time such as the vagus nerve and the pancreas. After he calmed down a little bit, he said he wanted to go over to Harriet Lane, the children's ward, where he had a patient that he was going to operate on the next day. We walked over, went up to the third or fourth floor where there was an infant crib. I took one look at the little patient and thought, "My God, this man isn't going to operate on this patient." The child was very cyanotic with dark blue lips and fingernails and required oxygen. Dr. Blalock briefly described the operation he planned, using an anterior thoracotomy incision on the left. I thought that after this incision and the collapse of the left lung that this child would surely die. At that time the first full-time MD anesthesiologist was on the staff. Hopkins had used only nurse-anesthetists before he came, and some thought because of that we were a little behind the trend. Dr. Austin Lamont must have felt the same concern that I had, because he cancelled the case. However, a day later it was rescheduled, but Dr. Lamont did not give the anesthesia; he had his resident, Merel Harmel, assigned to the operation.

One of the big problems, of course, was anesthesia for a child like this. We did not have endotracheal tubes for a child as small as this patient, so I think the anesthetic was given by mask. Anyway, at the beginning, after the anesthesia was started, the color of the child actually improved, I suppose due to the increase in the oxygen given along with the anesthetic. My next shock was the color of the blood after we made the incision. This thick black blood from the many small vessels looked like purple molasses. I thought to myself that we would never get this under control. Dr. Blalock meticulously set to work and we finally got inside the chest. The lung partially collapsed but things still remained stable. I then took a look at the mediastinum and it looked like a bag of black dilated worms. Again I thought that this was the time to retreat, but instead Dr. Blalock incised the pleura and went right to work and dissected the left pulmonary artery. After this he took a right-angled clamp and stuck it high up in the apex of the mediastinum and shortly pulled down the subclavian artery. Although it was under some tension, it was not injured. The only vascular clamp available was a rubber-shod bulldog clamp, which we placed on the subclavian artery just at its origin from the aortic arch. We tied off the distal end, which gave us as much length as possible. We tied the bulldog clamp with a heavy silk suture and used this as a traction suture. Dr. Blalock passed the traction suture behind the pulmonary artery and then handed it to me and said, "Pull this down." I was concerned that the bulldog clamp might slip off, but it held nicely. He then occluded the left pulmonary artery proximally and distally with bulldog clamps and made a short arteriotomy in the pulmonary artery. During all of this the child was doing all right. We did not have commercial vascular sutures at that time. The night before the operation Vivien Thomas, who was Dr. Blalock's surgical technician in the experimental lab, had prepared a number of very small straight needles with fine silk, which the scrub nurse lubricated with mineral oil just prior to their use. Dr. Blalock then started the posterior row sutures, which was a continuous everting suture placed very loosely. When the posterior row was completed, the opened subclavian artery was brought down to the pulmonary artery and all of the slack was worked out of the suture line. Each end was secured with an everting mattress suture, and the anterior row was finished using interrupted everting mattress sutures.

This was all done with some difficulty but with great skill. Dr. Blalock's surgical skill has been questioned, but if you could have seen him complete one of these difficult operations you would recognize that the skill was there. During the anastomosis he would lean back and speak to Vivien Thomas, standing behind him, and say, "Vivien, do you think that I am doing this right or should I start over there?" Sometimes this was misinterpreted as incompetence or a lack of confidence, but it was one of Dr. Blalock's characteristics to use all of the help and advice of everyone in the operating room. Looking back, it seems to me that part of the difficulty was our lack of proper vascular instruments and sutures.

Then with fear and trepidation, at least on my part, we cut the ligature on the bulldog clamp and slowly removed it, being ready to put it back on the artery if there was too much bleeding. It leaked a little right at first, but almost immediately Merel Harmel, the anesthesiologist, said, "The color is improving." As the anastomosis was opened widely and the circulation in the pulmonary artery resumed he said, "Take a look. Take a look." Dr. Blalock and I leaned over the ether screen and looked at the child's face and saw the cherry-red color of her lips. It was astounding how quickly the child's color improved. It was really quite dramatic. We were all beside ourselves with joy that the operation had worked so well. We put in two chest tubes and closed the chest. The child did fine for the first few hours. The next day she developed a pneumothorax and became quite ill and almost died. However, with constant and skillful care from the nursing staff and the pediatric house staff, she improved. The house staff stayed with her day and night. She eventually went home and did well for a time, but later the cyanosis returned and a second anastomosis was performed. She developed more complications and eventually died, but there had been sufficient improvement to know that the operation would work well for this condition.

It was amazing to me how quickly the word spread across the country without a presentation at a meeting or any publication. It was almost immediate. It was after the first three successful operations that Al and Helen published the results in the *Journal of the American Medical Association*. That really did start an influx of patients to Johns Hopkins from all over the world. Before we knew it we were working night and day. Dr. Taussig made the diagnosis in each child using only her stethoscope and the fluoroscope. As a result, some of the patients selected had more complex problems and did not do well. We needed a more accurate diagnostic method, so Dr. Blalock brought Richard Bing down from New York to establish a heart catheterization laboratory to give additional help with identifying the more complex anomalies. I had the impression that Dr. Taussig never did really accept the value of cardiac catheterization, although most of that happened at the end of my tenure with Dr. Blalock on the heart service. However, some of the things Dr. Bing has said and written would indicate that Dr. Taussig was not enthusiastic about cardiac catheterization. On the other hand, Dr. Blalock felt very definitely that it was an improvement in the preoperative evaluation of the patient. Very soon we had visiting surgeons from everywhere. The operating room had a little stand at one end for visitors, but you could not really see anything in these small children from the stand, so Dr. Blalock, in his courteous manner, tried to oblige them by having them stand on a stool just in back of him, so they could look over his shoulder. Vivien Thomas and Dr. Taussig both came to the operating room for the first half-dozen cases, but it wasn't long before they found other duties, and their places were taken by these visitors who came from everyplace.

All of this made a great story for the newspapers. This all happened in the days of World War II (1944) when there was so much horrible news. It seemed to have great public appeal, because it was about young children who had this bluish discoloration, and it was about the heart. Repair of coarctation of the aorta and closure of a patent ductus had both been done prior to the Blue Baby operation, but neither of these had aroused much public interest. It was the fact that the operation made such a dramatic change from blue babies to pink and red babies that made headlines all across the country in newspapers and magazines. This was at a time when the medical profession did not advertise, or, if one did, it was really frowned upon. There were a few dentists in California that advertised, but no physicians. This led to an episode at the annual meeting of the American Surgical Association. At the business meeting the president criticized Dr. Blalock severely because of all of the newspaper notoriety and publicity. Later the president explained that he meant that Johns Hopkins was using Dr. Blalock to get publicity for the hospital. Al took this as a very personal affront. The following day he got all of his friends together, and they had a weeping and wailing session as to how he had been unjustly criticized. Later the president did kind of rescind his criticism and implied that it was not meant to be so personal. In a way it was a battle that you might say Al came out on top of, but at the same time the president got in a few licks too, so that the controversy did create publicity, and the conflict held on for some time.

In 1947 Dr. Blalock was invited to come to Guy's Hospital in London to demonstrate the Blue Baby operation. He also went to the Hospital Broussais in Paris and to Stockholm. His wife went with him, and he also took Hank Bahnson and his wife, because he planned to do several operations and he wanted Hank Bahnson there as his assistant. I got letters from Hank and a note or two from Dr. Blalock about how they were being received and treated, but I stayed at Hopkins during his trip and did most of the cases and was very busy. While in London he was asked to make a presentation at the Royal College of Surgeons meeting. It was not a scheduled part of the program but was added on for an afternoon toward the end of the meeting. When the time came, the auditorium at the Royal College was filled, and a large crowd was standing in the corridor and outside the auditorium. They arranged a loudspeaker for those outside, but of course they could not see his slides. There was so much interest and acclaim that Dr. Blalock was asked to repeat his presentation for all of those who were standing outside so that they could see the slides and a short movie. He was really an idol of the entire surgical world at that time. Even though the Blue Baby operation was an extracardiac procedure, it does seem to be the stimulus that marks the real beginning of cardiac surgery. The repair of coarctation and closure of a patent ductus were operations that preceded the Blue Baby operation, but these had not caught the interest of the surgical world. I think you could say that the Blue Baby operation was the greatest stimulus to cardiac surgery at that time.

Dr. Blalock really never did have a driving interest in organized medicine. For example, he was made a member of the first Residency Review Committee. He served for a term or two but was not reappointed. Actually, he had a very lackadaisical attitude toward surgical training. This became manifest when he proposed that I become a plastic surgeon. He told me one time, "Bill, these surgical specialties are greatly overrated. You can take any well-trained general surgeon and give him a few months of specialty training, and he can then do it just as well as anybody else." With that he sent me out to visit plastic surgery centers for six months, and then I returned to be the head of plastic surgery at Johns Hopkins.

At about this time the American College of Surgeons was being reorganized and Dr. Blalock was asked to serve on the Board of Regents. That eventually led to his becoming president of the American College of Surgeons and the American Surgical Association. For many years he was the secretary of the Southern Surgical and then eventually the president. He had a great interest in the Southern Surgical Association, perhaps more so than the College of Surgeons, and always took his residents to the meetings. My first presentation was there. His main reason for being interested in organizations was to get a platform where his younger men could present the work they had been doing, and at the same time they could hear what other people were doing, what contributions they were making, and what was in the forefront at that time. This allowed them to go home with their ideas and work on them. This was his primary interest in organizations, and this was why he wanted us to become members of the Southern Surgical and the American Surgical Association as well as others.

Before I really became the head of plastic surgery at Hopkins, I was invited to become the chief of surgery at UCLA in Los Angeles, which was to be the first new medical school established after World War II. Dr. Blalock was ambivalent about my taking the job, and said that I was the only man of thirty-five that he knew who could retire, because I was going to a medical school without a hospital to be the chief of surgery. However, the plan appealed to me, as it was to be a school developed more or less along the Hopkins line, and they seemed to have ample finances to develop a good school and hospital. Harry Muller went to California with me and was able to start a cardiac surgical program, mostly for children, as there was not much adult cardiac surgery at that time.

After I returned from the Air Force there was great interest in peripheral vascular surgery, specifically endarterectomy and endovascular procedures, and Jack Cannon developed a small stripper that we used to do endarterectomies on the proximal coronary arteries. Our first case was very successful, actually the most successful that we did. The patient was a chiropractor. We did an endarterectomy of the right coronary artery, and he lived for six or eight years afterward and was able to return to full activity. The first coronary endarterectomy operations we did without the pump, but then later we did them using the pump. Our major difficulty was that we usually did not get the ostia opened enough, so we never had a good strong blood flow that would have kept the artery from clotting, which a lot of them did. Another problem was with our stripper. If you did not get into the exact right plane, the vessel just disintegrated. This problem ended with us doing the first internal mammary coronary anastomosis. Previously I had used a segment of jejunum to replace the esophagus. When the jejunum turned dusky, I used the internal mammary to revascularize the jejunal artery with success. This was one of the first microvascular procedures performed and was documented in the plastic surgery literature. Having had that experience, I immediately thought of the internal mammary when we found that we had a coronary artery that was damaged by endarterectomy. That patient with a mammary artery–coronary artery anastomosis lived for several years.

The people who had the strongest influence on my life would be first and foremost my father. Second would be Dr. Ott Richards, who was chairman of the Department of Zoology at the University of Oklahoma. Next would be Clint Woolsey of the Department of Physiology at Johns Hopkins. Then it would be Dr. Blalock, of course, who was the most important influence of all on my life. I would add the people that I worked with at UCLA like Harry Muller, Willard Goodwin in urology, and Eugene Stern in neurosurgery, and others who made our department as a whole one of the most outstanding departments in the country.

Note

A portion of this interview is reprinted from W. S. Stoney, "Bill Longmire and the Blue Baby Operation," *Journal of the American College of Surgeons* 198, no. 4: 653–659, © 2004, with permission from The American College of Surgeons.

Bibliography

Longmire WP Jr. The Homologous Transplantation of Tissues; Clinical Aspects. *J Natl Cancer Inst.* 1953; 14:669–681.

Longmire WP Jr, Smith RT, McEachen JA, Adams FA, Yang WW. Interatrial Septal Defects; Review of Thirty-Four Cases and Discussion of Three Current Methods of Closure. *Arch Surg.* 1956; 72:863–870.

Terasaki PI, Cannon JA, Longmire WP Jr. The Specificity of Tolerance to Homografts in the Chicken. *J Immunol.* 1958; 81(3):246–252.

Longmire WP Jr, Cannon JA, Kattus AA. Direct-Vision Coronary Endarterectomy for Angina Pectoris. *N Engl J Med.* 1958; 259:993–999.

Longmire WP Jr. Hepatic Surgery: Trauma, Tumors, and Cysts. *Ann Surg.* 1965; 161:1–14.

Longmire WP Jr. Surgical Treatment of Portal Hypertension: Long-term Results. *Curr Probl Surg.* 1966; Jul:78–88.

Longmire WP Jr. Presidential Address: Some Wise Men in American Surgery. *Ann Surg.* 1968; 168:311–318.

Longmire WP Jr. Loyal Davis' Personal Qualities and Their Influence on American Surgery. *Surg Gynec Obst.* 1983, 157:114–117.

Longmire WP Jr. The Halstedian Influence Goes West: Personal and Historical Remarks. *Pharos Alpha Omega Alpha Honor Med Soc.* 1999; 62:19–24.

Longmire WP Jr. William F. Rienhoff, Jr: A Not-to-Be-Forgotten Mentor. *Surgery.* 2001; 129:110–113.

Viking O. Björk, MD

(b. 1918)

In 1942 I found there was a scholarship available in Italy, at a hospital in Rome with twenty-three hundred beds, where I worked on the tuberculosis wards. I learned that you should wash your hands before you eat, and never kiss a girl with tuberculosis on the mouth.

— On his medical school days

Interviewed June 26, 2001

I was born in Dalecarlia, Sweden, in 1918, where my father ran a sawmill. After my first three years my father realized that I had not made much progress in writing and mathematics. He took me out of school and engaged a well-trained lady to teach me, along with three other students. I was dyslexic and was having a very difficult time. She taught me to read aloud and write at the same time. This solved my problem, and after three years I skipped a grade and returned to school. After I took the first examination I was sent to Uppsala to continue my education. My oldest brother had opened a dental practice in Linköping, and he and his wife had a spare room, so I moved to Linköping for two years and finished my secondary schooling there. I had very good teachers in mathematics and biology, and I developed a special interest in biology and the circulation of blood. I finished school in the summer of 1937 and applied to the engineering school in Stockholm and to the medical schools in Uppsala, Stockholm, and Lund. I had good grades. My family worried that our economy would be all right for four years of engineering but perhaps not for six years of medical school. My brothers thought I should go to engineering school. After a long discussion my mother said, "Don't worry about the expense. Do what you would be happy doing the rest of your life." I said I wanted to be a doctor, and my mother replied, "Then you will be a doctor."

I was accepted to the medical school at Uppsala and finished preclinical studies in 1939. In February 1940 I was one of four students accepted for clinical studies at the University of Lund in Skåne. Also at Lund they had a very good professor of general surgery. He was young and very interested in teaching. By that time the war in Europe had begun.

In 1942 I found that there was a scholarship available in Italy. It was for a hospital in Rome with twenty-three hundred beds. They had developed the technique of treating tuberculosis with pneumothorax. Because of the war, not many students applied for the scholarship, and I was accepted.

I went by air as far as Berlin, but my seat on the next flight to Rome was taken by a German officer. I wandered around the airport for a time and opened a door into a hanger, and there was a Messerschmitt 109. I had my camera, so I took two or three pictures until a soldier came in, pointed his rifle at me, and said his orders would allow him to shoot me, but I looked too silly to be dangerous. He asked me to give him the camera and he took out the film. He then told me to leave, and if I came back he would follow his orders and shoot me.

It took several days and nights to reach Rome by train. I worked on the tuberculosis wards with a Dr. Vincenzo Monaldi. Since I did not know Italian, it was difficult at first. I learned a lot: that you should not be afraid of tuberculosis, that you should wash your hands before you eat, and that you should never kiss a girl on the mouth that had tuberculosis. While in Rome I thought in Swedish, wrote in German, and talked to the patients in Italian. I was there for three and a half months, and when I returned to Sweden I wrote a monograph, *The Treatment of Tuberculous Lung Cavities According to Monaldi.*

I worked with the professor of surgery, Dr. J. P. Strombeck, on why venous thrombosis and pulmonary embolism were more common after abdominal operations. The idea was his, but I carried out the investigations. We injected fluorescein into a vein in the foot and used an ultraviolet light to measure the time it took to reach the mouth. We found that after abdominal operations, patients who were ambulatory immediately had a circulation time that was one-half that of those who stayed in bed for a week. The hospital in Lund was actually the first, in 1943, to institute early ambulation to prevent thromboembolism. Because fluorescein briefly turned the skin and the urine yellow, I was called "the yellow peril" by the nurses.

Since I was interested in lung disease and Clarence Crafoord was doing lung surgery in Stockholm, I spent some time there during my last year in medical school. In October 1944 I happened to be standing on a chair behind him when he did the first repair of a coarctation of the aorta. At times, I was an extra assistant holding a retractor, so he knew who I was.

I was able to get a British Council Scholarship to study in England for a year, and in 1944 Dr. Crafoord helped me arrange a position at the Brompton Hospital with Mr. Tudor Edwards, a leading thoracic surgeon

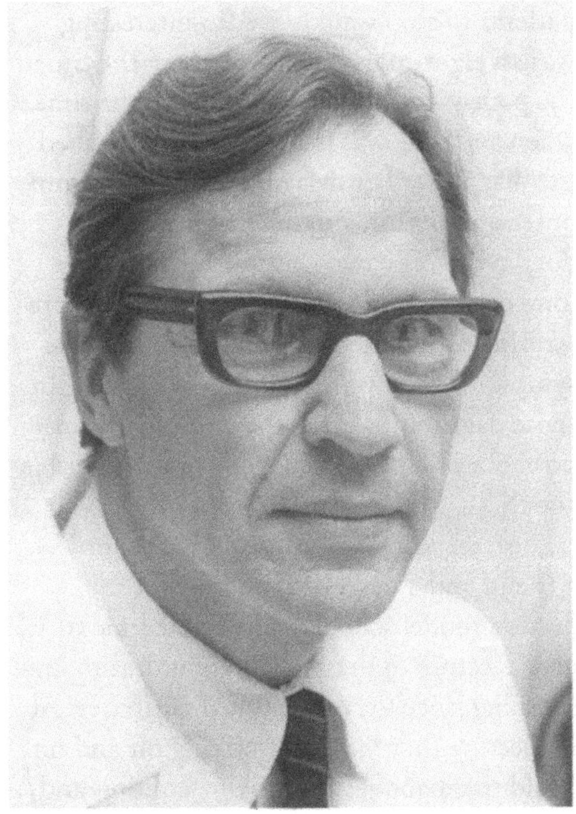

Viking O. Björk

at that time. His assistant was Mr. Clement Price Thomas, who several years later operated on the king. Also working at the Brompton was Mr. Russell Brock, who later became Lord Brock. The other thoracic surgeon at the Brompton was Mr. J. E. H. Roberts, who taught me bronchoscopy and esophagoscopy.

During the war everyone was very busy and no clinical research was being done. I asked Mr. Roberts if I could have permission to review their records of patients with bronchogenic carcinoma. I wrote a book entitled *Bronchogenic Carcinoma*, based on 450 patients. It was clear that if you smoked twenty cigarettes a day for twenty years, there was an 11 percent incidence of carcinoma of the bronchus, and the five-year survival was less that 50 percent, and so I began teaching patients to stop smoking. Also interesting was an eight-month delay between the time the patient first saw his doctor and the time when an X-ray was made which established the diagnosis. The delay by the patient from onset of symptoms to the first visit to the doctor was only two or three months. The long delay was caused by the doctor first prescribing cough medicine and expecting the symptoms to improve. So the main thing in those days was to teach the doctors the importance of an early X-ray for patients with a cough.

Several years later back in Stockholm, a friend and a neighbor was chief of the fashion model school, and he asked me to give a lecture to the models about health and smoking since they all smoked cigarettes. At the lecture they were all smoking off and on. I told them about my study in London and the relationship between smoking and lung cancer, and they listened but kept smoking. I then told them that smoking was not good for blood vessels, caused emphysema, and sometimes duodenal ulcers, and they all kept right on smoking. Then I said that smoking causes deterioration of the subcutaneous muscles in the face, and as these deteriorated you got wrinkles very early. With that they all stopped smoking. That was the only warning that worked—wrinkles.

When I left London, I came back to Stockholm and got a research job at Sabbatsberg Hospital with Dr. Crafoord. He knew about John Gibbon's work on a pump-oxygenator, which could sustain a cat for short periods of time, ten or fifteen minutes. The oxygenator was a large cylinder that rotated. However, as he increased the size of the cylinder to accommodate the larger animals, they were unable to oxygenate the blood efficiently. An engineer working for Crafoord had tried a different type of oxygenator which used multiple discs rotating on a spindle. Blood flowed across the lower edge of each disc, creating a film of blood which was exposed to oxygen. The engineer, Emil Andersson, and I discussed how we should pump the blood. We decided to try the very soft pumps used for milking cows, which do not hurt the cow. We used two milk pumps that alternately compressed the red rubber tubing. With this we began to operate on dogs, supporting the circulation to the brain and other organs and allowing us to isolate and operate on the heart. All eleven dogs survived at first, but they never woke up and all of them died. Crafoord became discouraged and decided to give up the experiments—he decided that the project was impossible.

However, my appointment to work in the experimental laboratory was for a year; therefore I continued. I found a colleague who worked in the blood chemistry laboratory, and together we oxygenated the blood in the machine and took samples. We found, to my astonishment, that during perfusion with our machine, the plasma proteins began to disappear, the platelets all disappeared, and most of the white blood corpuscles disappeared. We found that the rough interior surface of the rubber tubing was the real problem. Our tubing was consuming all of the coagulation products. I had to make an artificial intima, so I spent some time with the chemists of Uddeholm Company and together we developed Siloxan UHB 300. I got a patent for it in 1948. We used this to coat the inside of the rubber tubing, and it solved the problem. Soon after that, silicone rubber became available, and Siloxan fell into disuse.

After that we had six dogs in a row on the pump for ninety minutes, and they all survived. Finally, in October 1947 we clamped both the superior and inferior venae cavae of a dog for thirty-three minutes and that dog survived for several years. I was certain that we had developed a machine that could provide adequate support for clinical use. I published our results in the *Lancet* in 1948. I wanted this project to be the basis for my thesis, but Crafoord would not support me. He told me that one of his principles of leadership was to have his pupils compete against each other so they would not unite against him. Therefore, he chose Ake Senning and did not support my work with the heart-lung machine. However, I wrote a book, *Brain Perfusions in Dogs with Artificially Oxygenated Blood*, and submitted it for my thesis. I was supported by the professor of pharmacology, Goran Liljestrand, who had taken a great interest in the oxygenator. My thesis was accepted, making it possible for me to continue an academic career.

In 1944 Crafoord did the first successful repair of a coarctation. It happened in this way, Crafoord was a very good friend of Clement Price Thomas, a leading young thoracic surgeon in London who had been asked to review Crafoord's academic thesis on the surgical treatment of carcinoma of the lung. They had become very good friends. Price Thomas told Crafoord that he had heard about Robert Gross and his work on coarctation. Gross was trying to produce coarctation in dogs by placing a band around the thoracic aorta just distal to the subclavian artery. He thought that after a year the dogs would develop sufficient collaterals to allow clamping the aorta long enough to excise the coarctation and reanastomose the aorta. Crafoord talked with one of the cardiologists and asked him if he could refer a couple of patients with coarctation to try surgical repair. The first operation was in October 1944, and I happened to be in the operating room that day as an observer. Crafoord was very careful because he had not done such a dissection previously. The operative note that he dictated is very detailed and is five pages long. Gross was very angry that Crafoord had done the first coarctation because it was an operation that he had been planning to do for some time. This was still a sore subject when I visited Boston in 1950. Since I had been one of Crafoord's assistants, Gross did not invite me to come into the operating room, and so I had to go to an observation room above the operating room and, of course, I could not see very much. However, a few years later I again visited Boston and by that time he was using a spinning-disc oxygenator, so I was warmly welcomed and was asked to be in the operating room to observe his cases. We became good friends.

I worked as a general surgeon and also as an assistant to Dr. Crafoord until the fall of 1949 when I received a scholarship for a year of study in the United States. I visited Dr. Chamberlin in New York, Churchill and Gross in Boston, Dr. Blalock in Baltimore, Dr. Graham in St. Louis, Bigelow in Toronto, Ochsner in New Orleans, and Frank Gerbode in San Francisco.

When I returned to Sweden in 1952 I did not have a job. Finally, I was told that if I would like a job working with tuberculosis patients, I could have a position at the Sabbatsberg Hospital in Stockholm. They had built two small TB wards on the grounds of the hospital, one for eight patients and the other for twelve patients. They were happy that I could take over the surgical work for tuberculosis. The operations were done in the hospital so the patients had to be carried on a stretcher outdoors both to and from the operating room, sometimes in snow or rain. I developed a new technique for thoracoplasty for female patients that was not so deforming. I would leave the first rib. After the posterior segments of the next four ribs were removed, the ends of the ribs were anchored to the sixth rib with stainless steel wires. After the operation there was really no external deformity.

The best thing for patients with tuberculosis was to remove the cavity, and then the patient would be sputum negative in a few months. I did a large number of upper lobectomies. It was at this time, while operating on the right lung, that I realized that it would not be difficult to introduce a long needle through the back, straight into the left atrium. At that time cardiologists were having difficulty measuring the gradient across a calcified and stenotic aortic valve. With the right chest open, I tried passing a long needle from the back and found it was very easy to enter the left atrium. I designed a needle eighteen centimeters in length and large enough to pass a small catheter through it. I put the needle over the ninth rib posteriorly directed inward at a forty-five-degree angle until it hit the vertebral body. Then the needle was advanced along the vertebral body and forward right into the left atrium. We could then measure left atrial pressures and could usually get the catheter to cross the mitral valve so that it was possible to inject contrast and obtain both pressures and a ventriculogram. This was in 1952. I was invited to Brazil and Argentina for several weeks, and following that to the World Congress of Cardiology, where I presented our results with this technique for left heart catheterization.

In 1954 I met Henry Swan from Denver, Colorado, who had a lot of experience using hypothermia and inflow occlusion to close atrial septal defects and to relieve pulmonary stenosis. I began operating on patients at the new children's hospital in Stockholm using this technique. The operating rooms were much smaller than the usual, so we had a little trouble getting a bathtub into the operating room. The bathtub was necessary to immerse the anesthetized patient in cold water to reduce the temperature to 30 degrees Celsius preoperatively, and then in warm water at the end of the procedure. We could do intercardiac repair of an atrial septal defect or other procedures that only required five minutes of circulatory arrest.

In 1957 Dr. Crafoord hit his head on the door of his car and developed a subdural hematoma, which was evacuated by a neurosurgeon, Dr. Herbert Olivecrona, my wife's uncle. Dr. Crafoord was away from work for about a year, so they asked me to take over, which included opening the new thoracic surgery department at the Karolinska Hospital. It was then that I first had a heart-lung machine, a Senning-Crafoord model, and we did two or three uncomplicated operations a week. We did not do complicated cases. During that time I also had an accident. I had taken out a lung for tuberculosis and I was putting streptomycin in the chest before it was closed. The glass syringe broke and streptomycin splashed into my eyes. After a few days, I went blind in my left eye with retinal edema, and I was hospitalized for a month. It was thought to be an allergic reaction. I was at home another month before I could see again. I was being considered for the position of chief of thoracic surgery at Uppsala University, and they waited until I was well before appointing me in 1958.

We began a cardiac surgery program right

away at Uppsala, at first using hypothermia and inflow occlusion. We then tried the Drew technique, which used the patients' lungs as an oxygenator and cooled the patient to 8 or 10 degrees centigrade. We then did the operative repair during a period of total circulatory arrest. This method proved to be reasonable for older patients with normal blood viscosity, but patients with tetralogy of Fallot who had high hematocrits developed areas of ischemia and brain injury thought to be due to clotting.

I had visited Jerome Kay in Columbus, Ohio, where they made the Kay-Cross heart-lung machine using a rotating-disc oxygenator. They had the newspaper reporters come and take photos of me as the pioneer developer of the rotating-disc oxygenator, and they promised to send me a machine as soon as I was back in Uppsala. They did finally send me one, but I had to pay for half of it anyway. The Drew techniques took a while to cool the patient, and a very long time to rewarm, usually two or three hours, so the Kay-Cross machine was a big help in saving time. I concluded that the Drew technique did not have a long-term future.

Eventually we built our own disc oxygenator, which incorporated a method of weighing the blood in the reservoir. As the reservoir became lighter, the pump would slow down. If it became too low, the pump would stop so that it was impossible to pump air. We always used a bubble oxygenator for short cases, but we used the rotating-disc oxygenator for long cases, for the first ten or fifteen years.

In the late 1950s and early 1960s a few artificial valves became available. The very first one was a Teflon or nylon leaflet that could be used to replace the aortic valve leaflets. These had been developed by Hank Bahnson. I did a few of these, but they had a tendency to calcify and then fracture between one and two years postoperatively. I had one patient where the leaflet failed in eight months, and so it was not very good.

Next, I tried the aortic valve developed by Charles Hufnagel, a trileaflet with fabric covered by Silastic rubber, but it too failed. Then the Starr valve became available. I had a very good relationship with Al Starr, and I had a lot of patients with aortic valve disease. I used postoperative anticoagulation from the start, and I think I had fewer postop problems because Starr did not use anticoagulation for the first year or so for aortic valves. We did have one Silastic poppet rupture, but they made some changes, so that did not occur again. I thought the Starr valve was very good in the mitral position, but the aortic valve could have a significant postoperative gradient, seventy millimeters in one of our patients. For this reason, I went over to the Kay-Shiley valve. It had a flat disc leaflet and the gradient came down to about thirty millimeters, but that was still not good enough. Don Shiley came over to see me because the Kay-Shiley valve was made to be used in the mitral position only, not as an aortic valve. At first he did not believe that we had used it for aortic valve replacement, but we showed him the X-rays and some of the patients. I told him I would not use it for aortic valve replacement any more, because I had found that the Wada tilting-disc valve made in Japan had a much lower gradient, in the five-millimeter range rather than twenty or thirty millimeters that we had found when there was a small aorta. The Japanese were happy that I started using the Wada valve, but after a few had been implanted we had one fail because of a hinge fracture after only eight months. In Japan they had never had a broken hinge on this valve, I think because the Japanese are much smaller people and have small hearts compared to big Swedes.

This led us to the conclusion that we needed a tilting-disc valve to take advantage of the low gradient, but it shouldn't have a hinge. My engineer and perfusionist was working on a hingeless valve, but when I told Don Shiley, it did not take long for him to send me one, which arrived at Christmas 1968. I spent the holiday evaluating this new valve in the pulse duplicator. I suggested to Shiley that they increase the size of the strut that holds the disc, and then I would use it. We had a very nice cooperative effort in developing the valve. It took some time to understand that the deldrin disc would wear out in large valves over a period of time. We estimated the disc life to be twenty to twenty-five years. Therefore, we changed the tilting disc to pyrolyte, but this is heavy and, later, outflow strut fracture occasionally occurred in the largest valves. The failure rate was not great, but one or two would be too many. Usually if the strut broke, the disc embolized and the patient died. One patient of ours was already in the hospital, and we were able to replace the valve and remove the embolized disc from the abdominal aorta.

The outflow strut was two millimeters in diameter. It was shaped, inserted through drill holes in the valve ring, and welded in place, leading to the possibility of failure at the weld site. The solution was to use a strut and ring all made from a single piece of material without a weld. This mono strut valve was very strong, and I eventually implanted over two thousand of them and we had no strut fractures. However, the strut fracture problem in the original valves was such that eventually the Shiley Company failed and went out of business.

When I had to retire in 1983, I accepted an offer to be the chief of research at the Eisenhower Medical Institute in Rancho Mirage, California, and we built a very nice experimental animal laboratory there. For our experiments we used goats, which were excellent laboratory animals, and eventually I operated on more than one hundred. We were studying valve replacement without anticoagulation, and we had up to five years follow-up with the goats.

The valve that we were investigating had a surface with micropores three to four times the size of a red blood corpuscle, twenty-five to thirty-five microns, and this is the same micropore surface used in one of the artificial heart devices. It allows the body to coat the surface with a very thin layer of tissue that does not increase in thickness and does not interfere with the disc motion. This valve was used in Brazil on ten female patients who were not anticoagulated. There were nine successful pregnancies, and we now have thirteen years follow-up with no embolization. I have tried to get various valve companies interested, but it would require a change from pyrolyte to stainless steel, and none is willing to do that.

I had an especially good relationship with Dr. Kirklin. Several years ago, I had a patient with an aorticopulmonary window. At that time I was visiting in the United States, and I saw a pathological specimen of a patient who had died of this condition. I examined the specimen very carefully, and I immediately saw the best way to repair it. When I went back to Sweden I operated on that patient. We put the patient on bypass

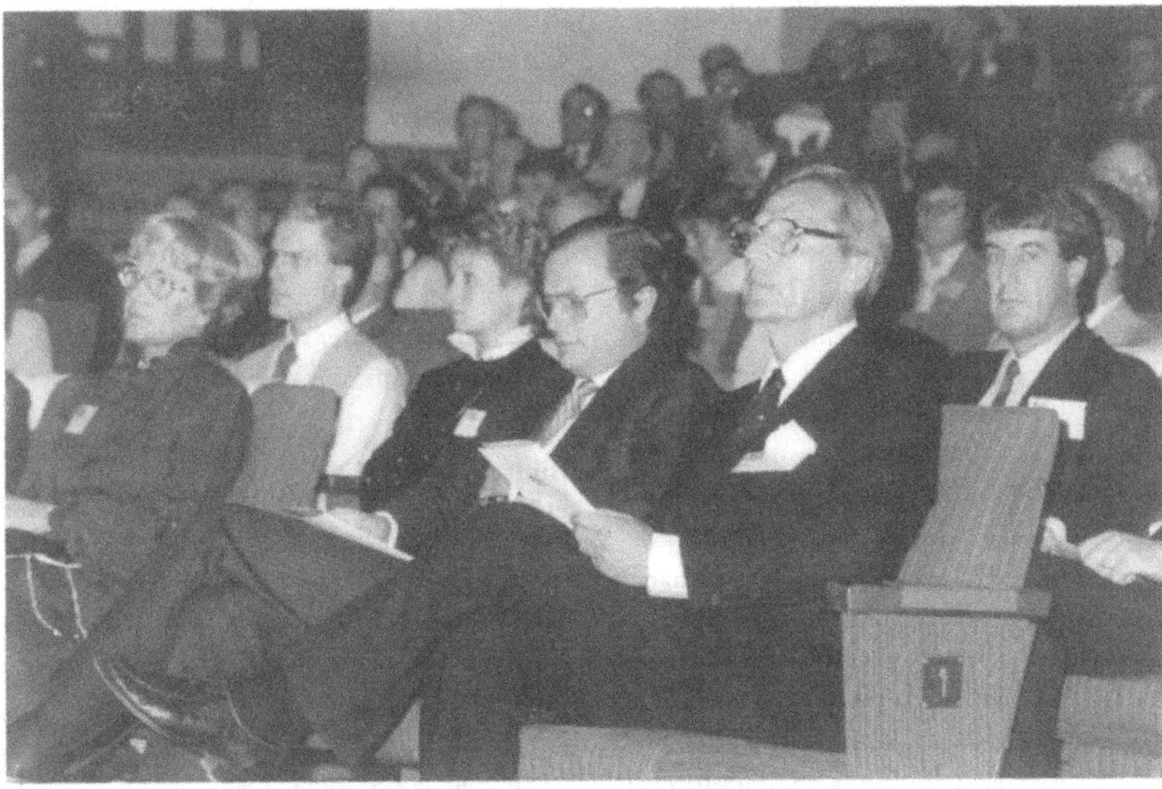

Viking Björk (on the right) seated beside His Majesty King Carl XVI Gustaf of Sweden

and then opened the pulmonary artery and put a patch in the defect just like you would do a VSD. The next time I was in the United States I visited Dr. Kirklin. I was standing behind him, and he was starting to repair a similar defect. I asked him what he planned to do, and he said he planned to dissect the pulmonary artery and the aorta, divide them, and put a patch on each. I told him the technique of repair through an incision in the pulmonary artery, which would be simpler. That is what he did, and after that he was always especially nice to me.

There were many men that had an influence on my career. One of the first was Russell Brock, who was an excellent teacher and spent a lot of time teaching me bronchoscopy. No one could do a thoracoplasty and apicolysis as well as a Clement Price Thomas. When he did a thoracoplasty, it was like a work of art. As an organizer, I think Denton Cooley was the best. His operating rooms could do twenty-five or more heart operations a day. To do that, you have to have a very efficient organization. You could learn a lot about efficiency and organization at the Texas Heart Institute.

I greatly admired Dr. Blalock. When I was there in 1950 he actually offered me a job to stay. He arranged for me to give a talk about the rotating-disc heart-lung machine. After that, whenever we met at a meeting, he would always invite me to sit at his table for lunch or dinner. His assistant, Hank Bahnson, was a very talented surgeon and he seemed to be able to keep Dr. Blalock in balance in the operating room. He and Bahnson visited Sabbatsberg Hospital in Stockholm when I was working on the disc oxygenator. That was when he came to Sweden to demonstrate the Blue Baby operation. When Dr. Blalock came to Sweden, his first visit was to the children's hospital at the University of Lund at the invitation of Philip Sandblom, and he did a Blue Baby operation there. Dr. Crafoord was very upset that Blalock visited Sandblom first before coming to Stockholm.

Dr. Crafoord was able to return to work several months after his operation for a subdural hematoma, but he did not do, or perhaps was not able to do, as much as he had done before. Crafoord wanted his assistant, Johansen, to be his successor at the Karolinska Hospital. Johansen was a very careful surgeon, but he had not done any research. He did most of the operations on Crafoord's private patients. The director of the Karolinska at that time was an ENT surgeon, and I had worked on his service for three months during my training. While there I saw a patient with an unusual problem, and we published a short paper about it. He was the one to choose the new chief of thoracic surgery, and he chose me rather than Johansen. I was at Uppsala at the time, and stayed at Karolinska from 1966 until I retired in 1983.

At Rancho Mirage, I did only research and helped the residents in the operating room, but I did no private patients because of the high cost of malpractice insurance. I was also a visiting professor at UCLA Medical School, where I would go one day a week, lecture from 2:00 P.M. until 3:00 P.M., and then drive home before the rush-hour traffic.

Cardiac surgeons are now doing a lot of new procedures using very small incisions, and the cardiologists are doing more procedures using catheters. This may be good for some special procedures. The preoperative diagnosis is now much better than it was in my time, but there is still the possibility that one may find something unexpected, and in that case one probably needs a larger incision. It may be safer for the patient to have a conventional incision.

Bibliography

Björk VO. Bronchialcancerns Symtomatologi. *Sv Läkartidning*. 1947; 31.

Björk VO. Brain Perfusions in Dogs with Artificially Oxygenated Blood. *Acta Chir Scand*. 1948; Suppl 137.

Björk VO. An Artificial Heart or Cardiopulmonary Machine. *Lancet*. 1948; 25:491–493.

Björk VO, Malmström G, Uggla LG. Left Auricular Pressure Measurements in Man. *Ann Surg*. 1953; 138:718–725.

Björk VO. The Optimal Opening Angle of the Björk-Shiley Tilting Disc Valve Prosthesis. *Scand J Thor Cardiovasc Surg*. 1981; 15:223–227.

Björk VO. Advantages and Long-term Results of the Björk-Shiley Valve. *Cardiovascular Medicine*. 1982; 1:293–304.

Björk VO. Development of an Artificial Heart Valve. Classics in Thoracic Surgery. *Ann Thorac Surg*. 1990; 50: 151–154.

Björk VO, Kaminsky DB. The Five-Year Evaluation of a Mechanical Heart Valve without Anticoagulation in Goats. *J Thorac Cardiovasc Surg*. 1992; 104:22–25.

C. Walton Lillehei, MD, PhD

(b. 1918)

In 1954 you could have quizzed all of the physiologists, surgeons, and cardiologists who were working on this problem and you would have found 100 percent agreement that the one way not to oxygenate the blood was by bubbling.

— On the development of the bubble oxygenator

Interviewed May 4, 1998

My parents were both born and raised in Minnesota. My father graduated from dental school just about the time the United States entered World War I. He went from dental school straight into the army as a dental officer. He and my mother were married, virtually at the train station, and went to Fort Sam Houston in Texas where he was first in training. By the time I was born nine months later, my father was in France. I occasionally tell my Texas friends that I am really part Texan, since by all evidence that was where I was conceived.

When my father returned from the war, he began practicing in Minneapolis and became quite successful. In 1926 when I was eight years old, we moved to a new community outside the city of Minneapolis that was called the Edina Country Club. It was on the edge of the prairie, really, but the developers had put in paved streets and sidewalks. My parents bought one of the lots and built our house there. However, in 1928 the Depression began, sales of lots declined, and very few homes were built during the next ten years. My brothers, our friends, and I had a lot of room for our outdoor activities, much like a huge farm.

When we moved out there I was in the second grade. Our school had only two rooms, but it was very good. It had first through fourth grades in one room, and fifth through eighth in the other. Each row of desks was one grade. When I started, the second row was the second grade, but it was already filled. The teacher gave me a book and said, "See if you can read this." I read it to her satisfaction so she said, "It looks like you can be in the third grade, so sit in the third row." I gained half a year. When we entered high school I was promoted again, so I graduated from high school at age fifteen, almost sixteen. I entered the University of Minnesota before my sixteenth birthday.

While you could enter medical school after two years of undergraduate work, three years were preferred, but I thought that if I needed another year I would rather it be at the end of my education, not the beginning. I spent two years in premed, managed to get into medical school, and also received my undergraduate degree after my second year in medical school. We were scheduled to finish medical school in 1942, but because the war began that year, our graduation was accelerated and part of our last year was turned into the first months of our internship. When I entered the army in June 1942, I had almost finished my internship. My best friend in medical school was John Lewis, and the two of us had signed up, two years before our graduation, for a commission in the Army Medical Corps. We

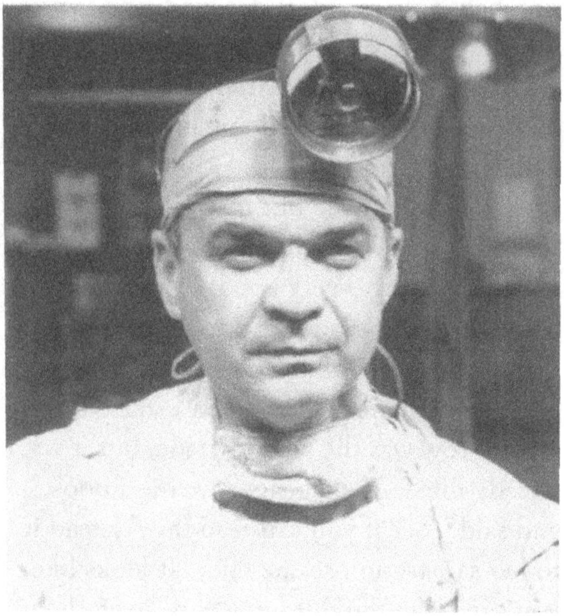

C. Walton Lillehei

were commissioned as first lieutenants and were sent to the West Point of the Medical Corps, Carlisle Barracks in Pennsylvania. We were supposed to be there for an indoctrination course of six months, but it had been shortened to thirty days, which was ample. The instructors spent about half of their time complaining about the shortened course, but they taught us how to salute officers of higher rank, how to police up, pitch tents, and those sorts of things. There were nine hundred of us in that class.

After graduation, I was assigned to go to Fort Devens just outside of Boston. My fiancée, Kaye Lindberg, who was a student nurse at the University of Minnesota Medical School, was then supposed to come to Boston where we planned to be married. However, as soon as I walked into the receiving room at Fort Devens on Monday morning to report for duty, everybody was rushing around packing boxes and shouting, because we were supposed to go overseas at 4:00 A.M. the next day. We had to put off the wedding until after the war. Early the next morning, we went by train to the Brooklyn Navy Yard and were taken on board a British passenger ship converted into a troopship. The next day, we were at sea, headed for England.

We were eventually located in a town of about 150,000 people, located in the midlands of England, called Swindon. Originally it was an industrial town where they made locomotives, but by then they were making tanks. There were no tents or facilities for a military base, so they just put us in the homes of the regular residents. Our unit by that time had eighty officers and about nine hundred enlisted men. Because of this arrangement we were never able, on any given day, to round up all of our men. In October, we were shipped overseas again. Once again we boarded a ship with no idea where we were going. This time we made the landing on D-day in North Africa, and subsequently went through the fighting in North Africa, Algeria, and Tunisia.

When the Germans and Italians in North Africa finally capitulated, we were sent to the invasion of Sicily, which occupied most of the summer of 1943. We were considered to be an amphibious outfit, but of course we never had any training in amphibious techniques. During our first landing in North Africa at Oran, chaos would be the best description of our techniques. We learned fast, and by the time we landed in Italy, and later at Anzio, we were pretty experienced amphibious troops as well as regular soldiers. I was in a clearing company in the beginning, and then we formed the first mobile medical units for the nontransportable wounded, the MASH units, although they were not called that until the Korean War. These mobile medical units became necessary because of the Sahara Desert conditions. The front lines were a fluid area with thirty or forty miles of interchange with German and U.S. troops. The hospitals equipped for major surgery were sometimes as far as one hundred miles behind the area of combat. It could take eight or ten hours for an ambulance to carry the wounded that far back. Many times soldiers wounded in the chest or abdomen would die before they reached the hospital, so it became necessary to have an operating room close to the front lines. We began to steal, beg, and borrow equipment so we could set up an operating room in a tent. Very soon that worked out well. We could take it down and move in about an hour, and set up for surgery in another location in about the same time. This started in North Africa, continued in Sicily, and was perfected in Italy.

The invasion of Italy was stopped by a defensive line the Germans had set up across the country, anchored by a very strong position at Monte Cassino, where the German army was entrenched. Numerous attempts to push through the lines had been made by the British, French, and American troops, all to no avail. Finally the higher-ups decided that if we made a landing at the fishing village of Anzio, about fifty miles northwest of the Monte Cassino line, it would panic the Germans and they would pull back. It didn't work that way; they did not pull back. We could have taken Rome overnight, but General Mark Clark, who was not a very great general, as we now know, thought that advancing quickly to Rome would be a trap. We held back and "established the beachhead" at Anzio. The Germans brought up reserves and contained the Anzio beachhead, and we took an enormous number of casualties both there and at Cassino. We landed at Anzio on January 23, 1944, and did not capture Rome until June 4.

Anzio was a particularly memorable place because ultimately we had two hundred thousand troops (some were British, but most were American) in an area six to eight miles long and only a mile or two inland. The Alban hills were several miles inland and were connected by roads. The Germans overlooked our positions and were able to shell our troops constantly. We all lived underground and there were a lot of casualties.

Our medical unit, the Thirty-third Field Hospital, was set up as a mobile surgical unit. At Anzio, all of the seriously wounded were operated on right there, and then we evacuated them to Naples on barges. The port of Anzio was a little fishing village with an embankment only about as long as a city block and the water was shallow. Large ships could not come in, both because of the geography and because they could be shelled by the German artillery. Each day, we took the wounded out on flat barges to a hospital ship six or eight miles offshore. Part of that job was the responsibility of our outfit, so we had to keep an accurate count of how many wounded were evacuated each day. It was a treacherous business since they shelled the port almost daily, some days almost continuously, and some days they held off. Occasionally they shelled our field hospital, and three of our nurses were killed. We were there for four and a half months until the breakout and the fall of Monte Cassino in May.

After that, we steadily advanced up to the Italian peninsula during the next year. It was a very difficult country for warfare because of the mountains, the many streams and rivers, and the bad weather and rain in winter. It was another twelve months before the war in Europe ended.

Instead of being sent home at the end of the fighting in Italy, we immediately got orders that we were going directly to the Pacific. From May until mid-August we stayed in Italy. Our departure for the Far East was to be in August, and the rumor was that we were going to the Philippines and were going to take part in the invasion of Japan. About a week before our embarkation date, they dropped the bomb on Hiroshima. I knew immediately that we were not going, so I told all of our officers that we should celebrate. Venice was about one hundred miles away, and we all went there and had a great party to celebrate the atomic bomb and the end of the war. I suppose that might upset some people, but the question of whether or not to drop the bomb was never a problem for us at that time. We knew that we were going to be back in combat, and it was estimated that there would have been a half-million soldiers killed in the landing and subsequent fighting in Japan. There was no doubt in my mind that President Truman made the right decision.

We left Italy the first of October, and after landing in the United States in the middle of October, I was immediately discharged. I had had a very good experience in the army, and was a lieutenant colonel and the commanding officer of the Thirty-Third Field Hospital.

I went back home to Minneapolis, and a couple of days later I went to see Dr. Wangensteen, who was chairman of the Department of Surgery. I had known him briefly as a student, but not very well. I had written him a couple of times during the war that I wanted to return for surgical training. He wrote back several times and was very positive and always said, "By all means, do return." I went to the surgery department that day, still in uniform since I had no civilian clothes. His secretary said, "Oh, you are returning for training. You will have to go to see Dr. Varco." He was on the faculty and later became a close friend, but at that time I did not know him very well. My only contact had been as a student. He was very friendly and said that they had organized this wonderful course for returning veterans that was to last for the next nine months. He reeled off a number of lecturers who were going to be imported, as well as some local people. The lectures were to bring us up to date on various subjects that we had perhaps forgotten, and also on the latest developments in medicine. I had a long, unenthusiastic face, I guess, so he said, "What do you think about that?" I said, "I don't see much need for that, Dr. Varco, but I will think it over." I had no real thought of going any other place because of my admiration for Dr. Wangensteen that had developed when I was a student. On my way out of the office, I ran into Miss Jacobson, who had been a secretary in the surgery department for several years. I had known her from my time in medical school, since she had helped me in arranging various surgical rotations and things like that. She said, "How did it go?" I said, "Not very well. He wants me to take this refresher course." She said, "Well, it is a marvelous course, but I'll tell you what. Why don't you stop in to see Dr. Wangensteen? This is Tuesday, but on Thursdays he doesn't operate; he meets with the residents and works on his research and other duties. I will make an appointment for you late in the day, about five o'clock."

I returned on Thursday and he was very friendly. He asked me about some of the other doctors that he knew from Minnesota who had been in the war. After we had talked for about ten minutes he said, "Walt, when do you want to start your residency?" I said, "Right now!" He answered, "Fine." He picked up the phone and called his chief resident and said, "I am going to send over Colonel Lillehei, who is going to join our house staff." That took care of the refresher course. About a week later, my friend John Lewis returned; we had separated in England. He had stayed there and later took part in the D-day landing in Normandy. He told me that he had just talked with Dr. Varco, and he, too, was not very pleased about the course idea. I told him that he should make an appointment the next week to see Dr. Wangensteen. John Lewis had interned at the University of Minnesota Hospital, while I had interned at the Minneapolis City Hospital. The same thing happened with him. Dr. Wangensteen was glad to see him and asked when he wanted to start, so we both got back into training.

There was a strong element of investigation associated with Dr. Wangensteen's training system. It was unique, really, in the United States, or maybe in the world. He had a strong feeling that you learn surgery better by doing research. Even if you didn't accomplish much with research, you learned important lessons of investigation, which could be applied to the understanding and application of good clinical surgery. John Lewis and I both spent a lot of our laboratory time in research aimed at the possibility of open-heart surgery. At that time there was no open-heart surgery. All operations related to the heart, such as closure of a patent ductus or coarctation repair, were extracardiac. That is, they were done outside the heart. The most radical operation at that time was for pulmonary stenosis. It was possible to make a small incision in the right ventricle and advance a knife through the valve so that it had a larger opening and then close the small hole in the ventricle. All of this was done while the heart was beating and filled with blood. Nobody had yet done an open-heart operation. By that I mean stopping the heart, opening it up, and under direct vision repairing whatever defect was present.

John Lewis had been impressed with the work of Wilfred Bigelow in Toronto. We were sitting together at the annual meeting of the American Association for Thoracic Surgery in 1950 when Dr. Bigelow presented his experimental work on hypothermia, lowering the temperature of the body as a possible way of doing open-heart surgery. His work was all done with dogs, not patients. The premise was that if you lower the body temperature 5 to 7 degrees centigrade, you can double the time that the brain can go without oxygen and remain unharmed. The brain is the most sensitive organ in the body to low oxygen levels; normally this time is four minutes. If you lower the body temperature from 37 degrees centigrade to 30 degrees centigrade, it doubles the time to eight minutes. If you lower the temperature another 5 degrees centigrade to 25 degrees centigrade, it doubles the time without circulation to sixteen minutes. You can't go much lower because of the tendency of the heart to fibrillate when the temperature is below 25 degrees centigrade. This was all worked out with a large number of dogs in the experimental laboratory. The limit of operating time with circulatory arrest was about fifteen minutes, which was enough to repair simple problems in the heart such as atrial septal defects. If the patient had an ostium primum defect or ventricular septal defect, all attempts with this technique failed because there was not enough time to complete the repair. Ostium secundum defects could be closed with this technique with a fairly high degree of safety and excellent results. Two other abnormalities that could be dealt with using hypothermia were pulmonary and aortic valvular stenosis. We could visualize the valve, relieve the stenosis, and get things back together in less than fifteen minutes. John Lewis was actually the first person in the world to do a successful open-heart operation. I had the pleasure of assisting him in September 1952. We used hypothermia and inflow occlusion to the right atrium and closed an atrial septal defect. It was a complete success. That experience originating at Minnesota was a powerful stimulus to us at that time. Word spread rapidly around the surgical world that the people at Minnesota were doing successful open-heart surgery on a regular basis. We started out doing three operations a week, but, because of the large backlog of patients, we upped it to one or sometimes two a day. Certainly, the experience with hypothermia was a big success. For some reason Wilfred Bigelow never did any hypothermia operations on patients, even though he had done so much of the experimental work.

That first secundum atrial septal defect closure went incredibly smoothly and only took fifty-five minutes from skin to skin, because it was easier than a similar procedure on a dog. The right atrium was enlarged so there was plenty of room to work, and it was ideal for that technique. The cardiologists were still learning catheterization techniques, and fairly often they were not that accurate —sometimes we found that the defect was an ostium primum or ventricular septal defect. We would try to close these defects in the brief time allowed, but usually we were not successful.

The success rate using hypothermia to close atrial septal defects was about 90 percent, and almost all were later found to remain closed. Most lesions were not that simple, and it was frequently predicted that a heart-lung machine would be necessary to correct complex abnormalities.

The first person, I guess, to really appreciate that was Dr. John Gibbon, because he started working on the development of a heart-lung machine in 1935. In his early experiments he used cats, and gradually progressed to dogs in the late 1940s. The large dog is an excellent animal for research since its heart is almost as large as that of a small person; the anatomy is very similar.

One of the prominent researchers at Minnesota was Clarence Dennis. He was not able to do much research during the war because they were all so busy, but after the war he began to work on the problem of developing a heart-lung machine. He and Dr. Gibbon were good friends, and their machines were similar in some ways, but differed in the mechanism of the oxygenator. The early pioneers of heart-lung machines in the late 1940s and early 1950s were Gibbon in Philadelphia, Dennis in Minneapolis, George Clowes in Cleveland, Ake Senning and Viking Björk in Stockholm, Dennis Melrose in London, Gerard Brom in Brussels, Forest Dodrill in Detroit, and Pogliatti in Italy.

All of these early heart-lung machines were very complex. Gibbon's machine, for example, weighed over two thousand pounds, and it was always a problem getting it to the operating room because it was heavy for the elevator, but it was thought that they should duplicate normal physiology as closely as possible. Initially the trials with dogs were discouraging, but they gradually recognized problems and improved techniques until about 70 percent of the dogs that were on cardiopulmonary bypass for about thirty minutes to an hour would survive.

When the early heart-lung machines were moved to the operating room, there was universal failure at first. The first person to attempt open-heart surgery in a patient was Clarence Dennis at the University of Minnesota. In the spring of 1951 he operated on two patients, and both died in the operating room, due to significant problems with both the heart-lung machine and with the diagnosis. The first patient was thought to have an atrial septal defect, but when the atrium was opened, they found an atrioventricular canal requiring a complex repair of the mitral valve, the ventricular septal defect, the atrial septal defect, and the tricuspid valve. Totally unprepared to deal with this complex lesion, they closed the largest defect, but the heart was not strong enough to come off the heart-lung machine, and she died. The second patient, one month later, did have an atrial septal defect, but during the operation she had an accidental air embolus, and she also died in the operating room.

Dennis and Gibbon both believed that the circulation needed to keep the body alive should approximate normal resting cardiac output; for an adult this would be 100 cubic centimeters per kilogram per minute. However, some experiments from our lab, done by Morley Cohen, suggested that for short periods of time, one hour or less, a flow of only ten cubic centimeters per kilogram per minute was necessary. This conclusion was called the azygos flow principle. If the superior and inferior venae cavae were obstructed so that only the azygos vein remained open, the experimental animals were shown to survive on a very low flow of twenty cubic centimeters per kilogram per minute, as long as it was a limited period of time. We decided to use this low flow for our procedures and selected thirty cubic centimeters per kilogram per minute as our goal. This was important because it made the heart-lung machines simpler. When the heart was opened with the higher flow rates, there was a tremendous influx of blood from the bronchial collaterals, due to most of these patients having been in heart failure for some time. Because of the blood welling up in the heart, it was very difficult to see the anatomy and to carry out the repair. This had been one of the problems for Dennis and Varco during their first two patients.

During the early period, 1951 to 1954, starting with Dennis, not very much progress was made. Thirteen attempts by various surgeons to move into open-heart procedures in humans met with only one success, the one done by John Gibbon in May 1953. That patient had a successful repair of an atrial septal defect, and I think is still alive. That report was, of course, very well received, but it did not engender much enthusiasm for two reasons. One was that others were successful in closing atrial septal defects using hypothermia and inflow occlusion. The second was that Gibbon did four patients and three of them died. Gibbon became discouraged and decided not to do another open-heart operation, but he was considered the guru of heart-lung machines. There was really a small group of people working on this problem, but it was an international group and there was good communication, meetings, and so on. Dr. Dennis left Minnesota to become the chief of surgery at Downstate, New York, and took his heart-lung machine with him.

We were working in the experimental laboratory on another technique called cross-circulation that worked well in dogs. One dog was the donor. With that animal asleep, we would make a small incision over the femoral vessels and advance a catheter into the abdominal aorta. We would then put a second catheter into the saphenous vein and advance it up to the inferior vena cava. These two tubes were then connected to a second dog in the same way. Between the two animals was a Sigmamotor pump, which could pump arterial blood from the donor to the recipient and return venous blood from the recipient back to the donor. We could then occlude the superior and inferior vena cava of the recipient dog and open up the heart while the donor maintained the circulation. With "azygos flow," the heart was not flooded with bronchial venous return, and the visibility was excellent. This simple technique had great promise since the donor animal acted as the oxygenator and also kept everything in balance: liver function, kidney function, and acid-base balance.

All of our early patients were Class IV and were very sick. Part of the problem was that we did not know how to manage heart failure very well, and we were unable to get rapid laboratory results of electrolyte and acid-base balance. With the cross-circulation technique, the donor provided a lot of protection against electrolyte imbalance. It was soon apparent that the dogs on low-flow cross-circulation recovered much more rapidly than those on the high-flow heart-lung machine. My laboratory was in the attic of the physiology building next door to Dr. Dennis's laboratory, so we had an interchange between the residents. The cross-circulation dogs not only recovered more rapidly, but also had a higher survival rate. When the results of open-heart surgery everywhere in the world were so negative and pessimism was so rampant, we felt we should try the cross-circulation technique, especially since other investigators were making no progress.

The first cross-circulation procedures on our patients were highly successful. We were able to correct ventricular septal defects, which had never been done before, as well as atrio-ventricular canals and pulmonary stenosis. The first ventricular septal defect was closed on March 26, 1954, and by August we felt confident enough to do a total correction of a tetralogy of Fallot. Many of the experts, including Blalock and Taussig, had thought that total correction of tetralogy patients would not be possible because the deformities were so severe. Probably part of the reason they thought so was that they had been studying specimens that were formalin fixed. The tissues were like an old shoe that had been left out in the rain. They thought the tissues were too rigid. We were able to repair a tetralogy patient fairly early in our experience, so that was a big breakthrough. Of the first twenty-six patients with a ventricular septal defect that we did with cross-circulation, nineteen left the hospital and actually only two of those patients died in the next thirty years. Good visibility inside the heart was a necessity and made possible what seemed to be a very difficult problem. From March 1954 until July 1955, we operated on forty-five patients using cross-circulation.

Just as we were starting to use cross-circulation on patients, we took on a young resident named Richard DeWall who was very keen and who had a lot of good ideas. I said to him, "Richard, we need a person to run the pump during these open-heart operations." Originally the pump was run by the anesthesiologist, and the operation required four surgeons, two for the patient and two for the donor. Those four were sterile and could not make adjustments to the pump. The anesthesiologist would sometimes go out of the room for coffee and leave the pump unattended, so I asked Dick DeWall to run the pump during these operations.

At that same time we knew that it would be better if we developed a heart-lung machine. Fortunately there was no mortality of a donor during the cross-circulation experience, but we did have one donor who had an injury, and the possibility of a more serious problem was always there. I asked Dick to work on the development of an oxygenator. "The way to do it, I think, is a bubble oxygenator." In 1954 you could have quizzed all of the physiologists, surgeons and cardiologists who were working on this, and you would have found 100 percent agreement that the one way *not* to oxygenate the blood was by bubbling, because, of course, bubbles in the circulation would be a terrible danger to the brain. I was pleased with what he developed in the laboratory. He used a vertical column of polyethylene tubing with a rubber stopper at the bottom. Blood entered the column through a port in the center of the stopper, which also contained a number of 22-gauge needles, each connected to an oxygen source. The vertical column was about two feet long. The blood entering the column was oxygenated very rapidly as it rose to the top and entered a debubbling chamber coated with a silicone defoaming agent from Dow Corning. The real secret of getting rid of the bubbles was a helix of polyethylene tubing about nine or ten feet in length which came down to a reservoir. The bubble-free blood would sink to the bottom as it traversed the nine-foot helix and the blood containing microbubbles would rise to the top until the bubbles dispersed. If the flow was adjusted properly, bubbles did not form in the oxygenated blood, which was then pumped into the patient. Many visitors came to observe our techniques, and we would give them the dimensions and data to make a working bubble oxygenator. This bubble oxygenator had an explosive effect on the growth of open-heart surgery around the world. Cross-circulation was a rather complex procedure, but it showed that the sick human heart could be improved and was not the obstacle that it once was thought to be. The simple, inexpensive, disposable bubble oxygenator was the most important development of that time. It was easy to understand and easy to use. When I left Minnesota in 1966 to go to Cornell as the chairman of the Department of Surgery, we had done over twenty-five hundred open-heart operations using the bubble oxygenator.

One of the important decisions during this early development of open-heart operations was that we realized that we needed some other material for the heart-lung machine rather than glass or rubber; we needed some type of plastic. Just by chance through a conversation, we found a small independent company in Minneapolis called Mayon Plastics. The president turned out to be one of my high school classmates, who had graduated with a degree in chemical engineering at the University of Minnesota and had established a company to make plastic tubing for the milk industry. In separating milk and cream, they needed tubing that could be massaged by an external pump without the pump coming into contact with the milk. The tubing needed to be heat sterilized and cheap enough that it could be discarded after use. This was, of course, ideal for our use. Ray Johnson, the president, was very helpful, and, as it turned out, this became very lucrative for him. As word spread around the United States and the world, he was selling more Mayon plastic to hospitals than he was to the creamery industry. The Dow Corning Antifoam A used in the oxygenator also came from the dairy industry.

The original bubble oxygenator had a vertical oxygenating chamber that was two feet long. The transverse debubbling chamber was larger caliber tubing and was one and a half feet long, coated with Antifoam A that had been baked on in the autoclave. Although it was efficient, it was not enough. It was the descent of the blood through the helix that was the final protection. The pump was a Sigmamotor that was cam operated and massaged the tubing in a progression from the outside. If necessary, we could increase the flow rate by using larger-sized tubing. The pump had eight fingers and was easily calibrated, so we did not need a flow meter.

At first, we used the bubble oxygenator for the simple and shorter cases and continued cross-circulation for the more complex cases, but the bubble oxygenator quickly demonstrated its efficiency, and we stopped cross-circulation completely.

By 1956 Vincent Gott and Dick DeWall had developed a bubble oxygenator which was a double sheet of plastic. It had the same principle as the tubing, but it could be manufactured commercially and could be shipped sterile. The operator could open the package, hang it up, prime it, and in just a few minutes it was ready to go. We patented the design but gave the patent to the medical school. It was licensed to Travenol in Morton Grove, Illinois. These were sold all over the world for seven or eight years. By then a number of other companies realized that they could make a similar design and several more got into the field. I don't think any of them was quite as good as the original sheet oxygenator. The next change in oxygenators was the development of a disposable membrane oxygenator, which also came from Minnesota through the work of a surgeon named Arnold Lande. I guess that all open-heart operations these days are done using a membrane oxygenator, and they have certainly added safety to the operation. The present oxygenators are more expensive than the original bubble oxygenator, but are still relatively cheap as medical devices go.

An important bonus of open-heart surgery in the 1950s was the development, for the first time, of an effective treatment for heart block. Prior to that time the outlook for patients with heart block was not very good. Heart block occurs when the progression of the normal heartbeat from the atria to the ventricles is interrupted. When the conduction tissue is damaged by disease or injury, heart block occurs. This results in a very slow heart rate, usually as slow as thirty or forty beats per minute. That is compatible with life, but those patients are subject to sudden episodes of cardiac arrest and death. In the mid-fifties, heart block was thought to be relatively rare, and no real therapy was developed for its treatment, in part because its importance was not recognized. Since patients with heart block had other cardiac problems such as congestive heart failure and coronary disease, death was attributed to other problems rather than to the heart block.

The main bundle of conduction tissue that carries the signal for each heartbeat travels from the right atrium across the ventricular septum and is in the area where most congenital ventricular septal defects occur. It was predicted by a few that when we began to work inside the heart, particularly placing sutures in and around the ventricular septal defect, we would have 100 percent incidence of heart block. We were concerned about this but hoped for the best. The bad news was that in the first seventy patients that had closure of a ventricular septal defect using cross-circulation or the bubble oxygenator, 10 percent of the patients had permanent complete heart block, and a number of others had heart block that lasted five minutes, ten minutes, or longer, but disappeared by the time the operation was finished. The persistent ones, seven out of seventy patients, all died—not immediately, of course, but within a few days or a week—without leaving the hospital. Our only treatment was epinephrine, which had to be administered by drip. We did not have pumps then and the drips were regulated by a screw clamp, so the heart rates could get out of control, up to two hundred per minute, and then a few minutes later would be down to twenty or thirty per minute. It was very unsatisfactory and we had no survivors. In 1955, we had a new drug, Isuprel, which had to be given by mouth or by rectum, as it was really a drug for asthma. This produced some long-term survivors. Of the next thirteen treated with Isuprel, we had six or seven survivors. Some patients recovered a normal sinus rhythm after a fairly long interval.

We began a very intensive crash program in our experimental laboratory to find a better treatment. Once again the dog was ideal. You could produce complete heart block by a brief period of inflow occlusion, making a short incision in the right atrium and placing a suture in the region of the AV node. This took only a minute or two, and the dog then had complete heart block. We tried a number of drugs, but drugs were not the solution. We knew that Dr. Zoll in Boston had resuscitated a patient with heart block by applying electrodes to the chest wall and stimulating the heart with an electrical current, external cardiac pacing. It required fifty to seventy-five volts, which was very painful for the patients. We tried it, but an electric shock of fifty volts, sixty times a minute, is really intolerable. Blisters developed in the skin at the electrode sites. The problem was solved by several of our researchers in the laboratory, including Dick DeWall. If we applied the electric current directly to the heart, it would respond to a very small electric charge, five to ten milliamps. This would drive the heart at any rate selected, and there was no pain at all for the patient. I was skeptical that this would be a long-term solution, because I didn't think that we could keep a wire attached to a moving organ like the heart, but it turned out that we could. Almost the very next day, we operated on a patient with a large ventricular septal defect who had complete heart block at the end of the operation. I called the laboratory and asked them to bring the pacemaker wires and the pulse generator, which was a device that was used in the physiology lab, called a Grass stimulator. It had two knobs, one for the current, calibrated from zero to one or two volts, and one for the rate. It worked perfectly. The death rate went from 100 percent for our first patients down to 40 percent with the introduction of Isuprel and down to 2 percent using the pacemaker. It would keep the heart rate up, and most of the patients converted to sinus rhythm after a month or so. Those that did not convert were another problem.

It was at that point that I began talking with a young man that we had hired to help with our operating-room equipment. During operations, we used an electrocardiogram and also a Sanborn machine that recorded arterial and venous pressure. Initially we also recorded electroencephalograms, but that turned out not to be very helpful. Our electrical monitors frequently had a lot of sixty-cycle interference. The hospital electricians would not come in the operating room during an operation, because it was not part of their contract, so we hired this fellow named Earl Bakken to be there during heart operations to keep all of our equipment running well. He was a big help. One day I said to Earl, "You know this pulse generator is working pretty well, but it runs on regular wall current. Movement of our patients is limited by the length of the electrical cord, and they can't go down to X-ray or to the lab because we would have to string an electric cord all that way to make it possible." Within three or four months he developed a battery-driven pulse generator, one small enough that the patient could wear it on his belt. This turned out to be the beginning of the Medtronic pacemaker company. He made these first pacemakers in the garage of his home in north Minneapolis in mid-winter of 1958. The first patients to have pacing wires and electrical pacing of the heart started in January 1957. We began presenting this information at meetings and published our results showing that this dreaded complication of heart block could best be treated with pacing wires sutured to the heart and connected to a pulse generator. Many times, the normal sinus rhythm returned and the wires could be pulled out. Earl Bakken started getting orders from all over the country. His company, Medtronic, is now a giant medical company. They have many products, but about half of their income is from pacemakers. Their headquarters is still in north Minneapolis. Their sales last year were about $3.5 billion, and they have something like twenty thousand employees. This is one of the success stories that grew out of the early days of open-heart surgery. There may be as many as five million people in the world today living a normal life with an implanted pacemaker.

The first external unit was made in April 1958, and by 1960 the first implantable pacemakers were being used. Two doctors in Buffalo, William Chardack and Andrew Gage, along with an electrical engineer, Wilson Greatbach, were the developers of the first implantable pacemaker. Greatbach had built about fifty pacemakers in his shop in his backyard. Forty were used in experimental animals and ten in patients. The electronics were embedded in a solid epoxy block.

In 1961 Greatbach and Medtronic began working together after Medtronic bought his patent. The early units were not as reliable as we wanted, particularly the electrodes, but in general they worked well.

Ake Senning in Sweden had been a frequent visitor with us in the early days of open-heart surgery and became a good friend. He was working with a Swedish engineer, Haaken Elmqvist. They developed an implantable pacemaker almost at the same time in 1960. They were using batteries that were charged by radio frequency across the skin, and there were a lot of problems with that approach. Eventually they gave up and relied on conventional batteries.

As word spread that we were doing open-heart surgery every day, we had many visitors. The first group other than ours to begin an open-heart program was led by my good friend John Kirklin at Mayo Clinic, only ninety miles south of Minneapolis. They started doing open-heart procedures on a regular basis in 1955; we had started in 1954. Denton Cooley had come up to visit us with his cardiologist, Dan McNamara, at about that time. I had the honor of showing him the inside of the living heart for the first time. He is a good writer and a good speaker, and later he wrote that "it was like looking through the gates of heaven." He spent a week with us in 1955. I think we used our bubble oxygenator and did one cross-circulation patient. He did not try the cross-circulation, but he went back to Houston and started working in the lab with the bubble oxygenator. His chief, Dr. Michael DeBakey, thought the bubble oxygenator was too simple and pressured him to adopt the Mayo-Gibbon pump, which was very complicated. It also required a large volume of blood to prime it, and some components could not be sterilized by autoclave. It was a difficult machine and was also very expensive. The company licensed to build it estimated a cost of $200,000. Denton Cooley finally prevailed, and in 1956 started his cardiac service using a bubble oxygenator, and was highly successful. When Dr. Kirklin left the Mayo Clinic, his successor, Dwight McGoon, adopted the bubble oxygenator and stopped using the Mayo-Gibbon pump. The bubble oxygenator was simple and inexpensive, a lasting contribution.

During the time from 1952 when John Lewis did the first ASD, through 1956 into 1957, all of the open operations that we did were for various birth defects. The same was true for the Mayo Clinic. By 1956 we had enough confidence in the bubble oxygenator to consider adults for open-heart surgery. Rheumatic heart disease was fairly common, and we thought that we could repair some of it. We started with mitral regurgitation and described an annuloplasty procedure in the journal *Lancet* in 1956. If the valve was leaking and scarred, but still pliable and not calcified, this was an excellent operation. Of the first seven that we did, I think six survived. Of course, for many patients the problem was not that simple, and a lot of patients had valve disease that involved extensive scarring, fibrosis, and calcification. Annuloplasty would not be a satisfactory operation for them, and we began working in the lab to develop an artificial valve, since none was available at that time.

In 1957 we implanted our first successful aortic valve. It was a single leaflet silicone valve shaped like a toilet lid. There were a variety of ideas and a number of people in various places in the world working to develop a useful prosthetic valve. The first really successful and effective artificial valve came from the work of Albert Starr, the caged-ball valve. This original ball valve was very durable and virtually indestructible. The ball occupied a lot of space and that was one of its disadvantages, especially if the patient had a small aorta, but in the mitral area it restored function very well. The valve had a tendency to develop a clot around it, so patients required anticoagulation.

It was at this time that we developed the Lillehei-Kaster valve. It was made with titanium and had a hingeless tilting leaflet that rotated freely. We called it a pivoting-disc or a tilting-disc valve. One of our former residents, Vincent Gott, had gone to the University of Wisconsin after leaving our program and then onto Johns Hopkins. He had been working with an engineer at Gulf Atomic on a new material that they had developed for the space program called pyrolytic carbon. It was an extremely hard and heat-resistant material supposed to be used for the nose cone of the space shuttle. Another material was found that burned and flaked off that was better for that purpose. Pyrolytic carbon was the hardest manmade substance known. The only material harder was a diamond. That attracted Vince Gott, and he and Jack Bokros, the engineer at Gulf Atomic, did a series of animals and found that the durability of pyrolytic carbon was almost infinite. They estimated that a hinged valve could function for over two hundred years. Gott had developed an experimental procedure to evaluate the thrombosis rating of various materials. He would suspend a ring of the material to be tested in the right atrium and then recover it later to determine how quickly it clotted. He found that pyrolytic carbon was resistant to clotting, and as soon as he told us about this material, we incorporated it into the Lillehei-Kaster valve. It was very successful and became the DC-3 of heart valves in those days because it did not wear out. It had better flow characteristics and was less thrombogenic than the caged-ball valve.

By that time our training program in thoracic and cardiac surgery had expanded. We had fifteen residents at first and then twenty; at one time even twenty-five fellows and residents. The basic program for residents was four years, sometimes longer. Those who had already completed their training usually spent a year with us. They were positioned in physiology, electrical engineering, pathology, zoology, and various other things under the guidance of Dr. Wangensteen. He felt that knowledge from other fields was often slow to get back to the surgical world, and this greatly improved the interchange of information. We were able to attract some of the best and brightest young men in the world. They didn't look like it when they came; they were somewhat like John Hunter's residents in surgery three hundred years ago. He said they were "loud, profane, often addicted to spirits and low company, and especially women." They sometimes fit that description, but their later records show that many became world-famous leaders like Norman Shumway, Christiaan Barnard, Christian Cabrol, Donald Ross, Juro Wada, Herbert Warden, Vincent Gott, Dick DeWall, Nazih Zuhdi, Aldo Castaneda, E. D. Zerbini, and B. R. Kalke.

Dr. Kalke was from Bombay and was a cardiac resident from 1964 to 1968. We were walking down the hall one day, and he said he was due to go to the lab for six months and would like to work on a bileaflet valve.

Kalke had observed a similar ancient design of a one-way valve used in the irrigation system in India. So I said, "Why try a bileaflet valve? There are already plenty of valve designs around." He said that no one had worked on a flexible bileaflet valve because there were problems with wear and flow. I said, "The reason no one has worked on it is that it has a fixed hinge which will wear out, and the stasis around the hinge will promote clotting." I had learned by this time that one of the hazards of progress is when a young investigator goes to the professor with a new idea that there is almost a knee-jerk reaction to say, "It won't work. It has been tried before." I caught myself and instead said, "Well, we will authorize some funds, you can have a bileaflet valve made in the machine shop. I think the first thing to do is to test the flow." We had an engineering student working with us named Robert Kaster. He had developed a very sensitive and durable flowmeter, which he called the analog pulse duplicator. I said, "Ask Bob Kaster to measure the flow and see how it compares." Four or five weeks later he came back one day while we were making rounds and showed me the valve and the flow data. The valve was cumbersome with metal leaflets and a metal cage, but the flow studies were better than for the Lillehei-Kaster valve we were using. I said, "I can hardly believe this. I would like to come down to the lab on Saturday and see for myself." Sure enough, the flow studies were superior. We worked on the valve some more and eliminated the cage and refined the structure, and eventually by 1968 had a clinical model. It was titanium with two leaflets that opened to sixty degrees, and a knee-joint type of pivot, which was about half open to promote flow around it. It looked a lot like the present St. Jude valve. I went to see the CEOs of the three largest valve companies in the U.S. and asked, "Can you make it?" That was before the FDA required any review of devices; there was no valve device legislation so there were no hurdles. We had a lot of data on the flow and the use in experimental animals, all of which were favorable, because Dr. Kalke had used this project for his PhD thesis. The CEOs all said the same thing, "It won't work in humans. It will wear out or it will clot," so the valve was put on the shelf. Dr. Kalke got his PhD and went back to India, where he became the chief of surgery in one of the major hospitals. The bileaflet valve remained on the shelf from 1968 until 1976.

The final development of the St. Jude bileaflet valve came about in the following roundabout way. A friend of mine, Manuel Villafaña, worked on the development of the early pacemakers and became an employee of Medtronic. He had become interested in using lithium batteries for implantable pacemakers. Up to that time all pacemakers were powered by mercury batteries, but lithium batteries had the advantage of a much longer battery life, and, unlike mercury batteries, they gave off no gas. Mercury batteries gave off hydrogen and pacemakers had to have a one-way valve to vent the hydrogen. This sometimes led to fluid entering the pacemaker, which could cause trouble. However, the Medtronic Company did not want to try lithium batteries because in the past lithium batteries used by the military had exploded. Manny Villafaña formed his own pacemaker company, Cardiac Pacemakers Incorporated, in nearby St. Paul. Medtronic officials said his company would not last more than a month or two, but it was very successful and very soon all pacemaker companies were scrambling to convert to lithium batteries. Eventually Manny Villafaña sold his pacemaker company to Eli Lily for $136 million, which doesn't sound like much these days, but in the late sixties it was a pretty significant sum. Mr. Villafaña was not the sole owner, but he was the CEO. He then began looking into prospects for starting another company.

A surgeon who had trained with me, Demetre Nicoloff, and a couple of other people advised Mr. Villafaña to consider making a better heart valve just like he had made a better pacemaker. They decided on a bileaflet valve and became interested in the idea of not just coating the valve with pyrolyte but making the valve out of pyrolytic carbon. This was in 1976, and the Lillehei-Kalke valve had been on the shelf for eight years. I sort of forgot about it in a way. The old titanium valve opened to sixty degrees, and in the new design, the leaflets opened to eighty-five degrees. The pivot mechanism was the same, and they added a pivot guard on the inflow side of the valve. Gulf Atomic was the only company that could make pyrolyte and at first they said they could not make the pivot, but with persistence and determination, they eventually solved that problem. In 1976 Mr. Villafaña established his company, St. Jude Medical, and the valve was their only product. The first implant was in October 1977. The valve worked beautifully, but most surgeons were skeptical of the design. It took eight years, until 1985, for the first one hundred thousand to be used. By that time the results were so impressive, with both flow characteristics and diminished clotting, plus no problems of durability, that the valve really took off. We had a twentieth year celebration in 1997 and eight hundred thousand St. Jude valves had been implanted at that point. It is still going strong and there is still some controversy, but the controversy now is how to make tissue valves last longer and better. We know tissue valves are excellent, especially for the older patient, because they do not require anticoagulation, but they do wear out.

The final solution for valve replacement will be in the foreseeable future. In the meantime, the St. Jude valve is the most successful valve that has ever been developed. It is especially interesting that it started out as a valve that violated all of the principles which we held at that time. This is one of the important things that I have tried to teach my fellows. The way to make a contribution is through research. It is hard work, and serendipity (an elegant word for good luck) sometimes helps. The more research and hard work that you do, the more good luck you will have. The third factor is a paradox: Challenge accepted beliefs. All through this story we have had breakthroughs that went against the accepted beliefs. Examples are the azygos flow, the bubble oxygenator, total correction of tetralogy of Fallot, and the bileaflet valve; all were at first said to be wrong. It is a valid concept: hard work, research, and paradox. I have always said, "What you dream, if you are willing to work, science and technology can achieve it."

One thing seems to me to be clear. There is no monopoly on creativity. Young people have creativity whether they are in our medical school here or elsewhere in the United States, Europe, or Asia. If you give them an opportunity to work, and provide some material assistance and stimulation, great advances will occur.

Bibliography

Cohen M, Lillehei CW. A Quantitative Study of the Azygos Factor during Vena Caval Occlusion in the Dog. *Surg Gynec Obst.* 1954; 98:225–232.

Warden HE, Cohen M, Read RC, Lillehei CW. Controlled Cross Circulation for Open Intracardic Surgery: Physiologic Studies and Results of Creation and Closure of Ventricular Septal Defects. *J Thorac Surg.* 1954; 28:331–341.

Lillehei CW, DeWall RA, Read RC, Warden HE, Varco RL. Direct Vision Intracardiac Surgery in Man Using a Simple, Disposable Artificial Oxygenator. *Dis Chest.* 1956; 29:1–8.

Weirich WL, Gott VL, Lillehei CW. The Treatment of Complete Heart Block by the Combined Use of a Myocardial Electrode and an Artificial Pacemaker. *Surg Forum.* 1957; 8:360–363.

Lillehei CW, Gott VL, DeWall RA, Varco RL. Surgical Correction of Pure Mitral Insufficciency by Annuloplasty under Direct Vision. *Lancet.* 1957; 77:446–449.

Lillehei CW, Levy MJ, Bonnabeau RC Jr. Mitral Valve Replacement with Preservation of Papillary Muscles and Chordae Tendineae. *J Thorac Cardiovasc Surg.* 1964; 47:532–543.

Kalke BR, Carlson RG, Lillehei CW. Hingeless Double-Leaflet Prosthetic Heart Valve for Aortic, Mitral, or Triscuspid Positions. *Biomed Sci Instrum.* 1968; 4:190–196.

Lillehei CW. A Personalized History of Extracorporeal Circulation. *Trans Am Soc Artif Intern Organs.* 1982; 28:5–16.

Lillehei CW. St. Jude Valve. *Ann Thorac Surg.* 1983; 35:475–476.

Lillehei CW, Varco RL, Cohen M, Warden HE, Patton C, Moller JH. The First Open-Heart Repairs of Ventricular Septal Defect, Atrioventricular Communis, and Tetralogy of Fallot Using Extracorporeal Circulation by Cross-Circulation: A 30-Year Follow-up. *Ann Thorac Surg.* 1986; 41:4–21.

Richard A. DeWall, MD

(b. 1926)

My device was a kind of Rube Goldberg affair with a bunch of tubes gathered in a heap and on a stand, but every curve and bend and piece had a purpose. A lot of people would think, "I can do better than that," and have it changed by the time they got on the plane to go home. Of course, they had disasters.

— On the evolution
of the bubble oxygenator

Interviewed May 3, 2003

I grew up on the western prairies of Minnesota, in a little country town 150 miles west of Minneapolis. I had a brother who was thirteen years older than me and two sisters, nine and ten years older. I grew up virtually as an only child, because my brothers and sisters were gone by the time I had grown to any extent. I had a very happy childhood and a good education. The major event in my life, though, was the death of my father when I was fourteen. He had an adhesive obstruction of the small intestine. He was operated on by a country general practitioner surgeon, who opened him up, didn't know what he saw, sewed him back up, put him to bed, and let him die. Of course his death bothered me greatly, but later I was even more disturbed when I came to realize that Dr. Wangensteen at the University of Minnesota had developed an international reputation for the use of nasogastric tubes, the Wangensteen suction system, to relieve bowel obstruction. He was world famous for the treatment of bowel obstruction. I had a great deal of animosity toward that local GP who had allowed my father to die at the age of fifty-three.

The unnecessary death of my father put thoughts of medicine in my mind at an early age. At first I was more interested in orthopedic surgery and the more mechanical aspects of medicine. When I graduated from high school, World War II had begun, but I was only seventeen and too young to go immediately into the service. I went down to the University of Minnesota because it was quick and easy. After a year there, I turned eighteen and had to go into the service. I was in the navy for a little less than a year, and then the war was over. I immediately came back to Minnesota and started at the university again in January 1946.

As an undergraduate I took pre-engineering and premedical courses. As time went on, I realized that I was just not that strong a student in mathematics and engineering, but the biologic sciences came easy to me, and I was interested in biology. I started out as a bacteriology major, slid off into premed courses, and ended up in medical school at the University of Minnesota.

The Korean War was in progress during the last two years that I was in medical school. At that time, if you had not been in World War II for at least two years, you were subject to recall for the Korean War. Since I had been in World War II for a little less than a year, I knew for sure that I was going to be called up. I had been in the navy before, and so I ended up in the United States Public Health Service, which took care of the Coast Guard, some of the merchant marines, the naval patrol, and so on. I was sent to Staten Island Hospital in New York City.

One of my patients there made an indelible impression on me. He was a teenage boy who was literally dying of rheumatic heart disease, with mitral insufficiency and heart failure. I was partially responsible for caring for him. It began to occur to me that the heart is a pump, and in this boy the pump had a defective valve. Well, I thought, why don't we just open up the pump and replace the valve as people have been doing with pumps for two thousand years? You opened it up, and you fixed it. But, of course, at that time it was not possible to fix a heart valve like that.

I finished my internship in the Public Health Service, and I went back to Minnesota because that was where my roots were, and I really didn't have any other place to go. I found a situation in a suburb of Minneapolis, in family practice, but in the evenings when I had some spare time, that young lad who had been my patient preyed on my mind. I started carving a mitral valve prosthesis out of plaster of Paris. Obviously it was nonfunctioning; it was just a prototype to get some ideas and concepts started about mitral valve prostheses.

It was a standard flutter valve, but there were some internal reinforcements, so it didn't have to have chordae on it. Of course, I didn't really know what I was doing. I didn't really have much idea of what the internal anatomy of the heart was; I had just been an ordinary medical student. Anyway, I fashioned this prototype valve and thought I would talk to Dr. Richard Varco, who was the chief of cardiac surgery at the university. He had been one of my teachers when I was a student, so I was acquainted with him. I talked to his secretary, and I asked if I could make an appointment to see him. She said, "He's up in the operating room right now. Why don't you just go up there and talk to him?" Back in those days, they weren't so compulsive about sterile techniques. So I went up to the operating room and walked into the operating suite in my street clothes. There were other people there in street clothes; nobody thought anything about it. I remember sitting on a litter outside Dr. Varco's operating room, waiting for him to come out. He came out in his scrub suit and was very pleasant. Why he was so patient with a total stranger walking into his operating suite off the street, I can't imagine. Anyway, I had the plaster valve in my hand. We sat on the litter outside of the operating room until he

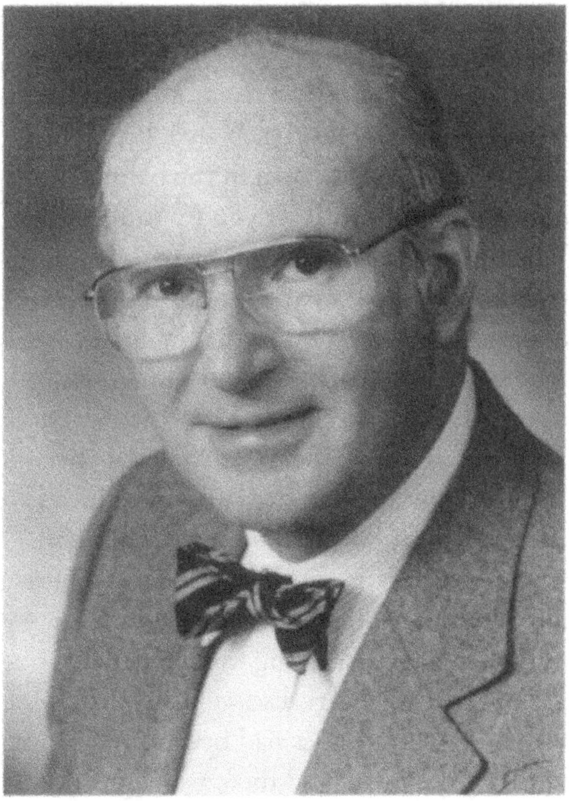

Richard A. DeWall

had to go back in, talking over my thoughts about the valve. He said, "Well, if you're interested in that sort of thing, I think that one of my colleagues, Dr. Walt Lillehei, has a heart research lab down in the basement, and if you wish I will set you up to meet Dr. Lillehei and see what we can work out." I was not interested at all in inquiring about a surgical residency, but rather laboratory medicine. I was curious about mechanics, heart-valve mechanics to be specific. So Dick Varco arranged for me to see Walt Lillehei.

Walt took me to his lab and introduced me to Herbert Warden, who was a resident doing his research year in Dr. Lillehei's laboratory. For a while there had been interest at the university in trying to help patients with congenital heart disease. This was an era when German measles had been rampant for twenty years or so, and there was a great deal of congenital heart disease, as well as other congenital defects. Clarence Dennis had really helped initiate the interest in congenital heart disease and heart surgery in the late 1940s. He and his team had developed a rotating-disc oxygenator. They had used it in the laboratory where it worked pretty well, and so they took it up to the operating room. He did his first patient in 1951, and unfortunately, for a variety of reasons, that patient died. The procedure was probably basically successful, but the patient died for reasons that I won't go into. As a result of this tragedy, Clarence Dennis stopped operating and later went to Stonybrook University on Long Island as the professor of surgery.

The pediatric cardiologists at the University of Minnesota had clinics that were literally flooded with patients with congenital heart disease, because the university saw patients from several states with these difficult problems. Dick Varco took over after Clarence Dennis left, but he was not very interested in laboratory work. The baton was passed on to C. Walton Lillehei, who had come back from World War II after a very meritorious career as a military surgeon in North Africa. Walt finished his residency at the university under the influence of Dick Varco. Of course, I can't leave out Dr. Owen Wangensteen, who was the chief of surgery. He was a marvelous mentor who encouraged all of his residents and students in the disciplines of physiology and surgical research. You couldn't complete your residency program unless you spent a year in surgical research and preferably an additional year in physiology. Everybody had a good grounding of two years in research and physiology before they completed their residency program. At that time I was interested in laboratory medicine.

Dr. Lillehei introduced me to Dr. Herb Warden, who was running the lab. Dr. Warden and his colleague, Dr. Cohen, had developed the idea of cross-circulation. He and Dr. Warden were working on ideas about how one could operate inside the interior of the heart to take care of congenital heart disease problems. Dr. Cohen had initiated the idea of an autologous lobe oxygenator. The autologous lobe system was as follows: First cannulate the azygous vein and the pulmonary artery of the upper lobe of the lung. These were connected with plastic tubing so that the azygous venous blood could be pumped into the pulmonary artery of the upper lobe. A second circuit was set up with a cannula in the right pulmonary vein to pick up oxygenated blood, which was then pumped into the femoral artery. When all was ready, the superior and inferior venae cavae were clamped and the dog could be maintained by this system for thirty minutes, long enough for many open-heart operations. The oxygenator was the dog's own upper lobe and the blood was pumped by a Sigmamotor finger pump. It worked very well, but as you can well imagine, it was a very difficult cannulation, because anytime a cannula was kinked, or drainage was impeded coming out of the lung, the lung would go into pulmonary edema. A number of these animal experiments were successful, but some of them did not work. Fortunately, this system was never used for a patient.

After Cohen developed this procedure, Warden took over running Lillehei's lab, and that was when I came into the scene. Warden took me on essentially as a student. He taught me all the perfusion physiology, but his main goal was to understand and work on the pathophysiology of controlled cross-circulation. The way they became interested in it was as follows: Cohen and Warden were talking one night after their day's work and about the fact that Cohen's wife was pregnant, and that here was an ideal example of a donor-patient relationship—the mother supplies oxygenated blood to the fetus, which is totally dependent. So the thought emerged, "Why don't we take a big donor animal and connect it to a small animal and perfuse the small patient from the donor animal?"

Warden and Cohen then took a donor dog and connected it with a cannula through its femoral artery and vein into the blood vessels of the recipient dog. They perfused the recipient dog at a low-flow rate for a short period of time, but long enough to operate inside the heart. These experiments were the origin of controlled cross-circulation.

Of course, the circulation from the donor animal to the recipient animal, as well as the return circulation, went through a calibrated pump so that the inflow and the outflow were adjusted to keep things in balance. Warden's main responsibility was to study the pathophysiology of controlled cross-circulation. He had a chemistry laboratory set up with a couple of technicians, so a great deal of effort was spent in studying both the donor and the recipient's biochemical response. Of course, sham operations were performed on the recipient heart, by opening the heart, reviewing the inside, making sham ventricular defects, and repairing them. It proved to be a feasible project. Once the project was well under way, the whole concept was then brought to a faculty committee of the university to see if they would approve of moving the procedure to the operating room and using it on patients. There was a great deal of controversy about taking a normal individual, giving him or her a general anesthetic and using his or her blood to support another patient. These, of course, were usually parents and their children, so there was no problem getting the parents to agree to it. The blood types were generally the same so it usually did not present a problem.

The parent functioned as the oxygenator. We used a pump in between the two patients, and the flow rate was calibrated at about 20 percent of the normal cardiac output of the patient. We would be operating on infants, or children up to thirty pounds, so their total cardiac output was not great. The idea with other perfusion systems at that time had been that you had to pump a normal cardiac output to a patient. But to pump the total normal cardiac output of the patient, or five times the volume that we were pumping, escalated the problems exponentially. The reduced volume really simplified the operation. We did not use hypothermia; we used normothermia. The first controlled cross-circulation operation was in March 1954.

Dr. Lillehei and I were aware of Dr. Gibbon's patients and his device, but it had not been very well publicized yet, and his heart-lung machine seemed enormously complex and expensive. Dr. Gibbon's device and his early operations with it were not a big event like the Blue Baby operation or heart transplant. Dr. Gibbon was a very modest and humble man, and a very fine scientist, but he did not publicize his procedure widely. I think his first paper on his operation came out in 1954 in *Minnesota Medicine*. Simultaneously, the Mayo Clinic, under John Kirklin, took the Gibbon concept and modified the Gibbon machine for their hospital. Earl Wood, an outstanding physiologist, and Jesse Edwards, a world-renowned pathologist, helped put this together. Not many institutions could afford either the mechanical equipment or the high-caliber staff to do such a thing. Their first operation with the Mayo-Gibbon machine was in March 1955. By that time we were already doing cross-circulation.

My main role in the laboratory was to run the pump between the donor animal and the recipient. Eventually I became the perfusionist when the whole procedure went to the operating room, but Dr. Warden ran the pump for the first couple of patients, and then I took over. The pump that we used was the Sigmamotor Model T-6S finger pump originally used in the milk industry. This one was an old laboratory pump that Dr. Lillehei took from the physiology laboratory one dark night. It wasn't a great pump, but it worked. It was noisy, but you could control it very well and very precisely.

After they had done several cases, I became involved in the operating room running the pump. I had never been in an operating room before, and I had no knowledge of hearts or surgery, so I wasn't interested in getting up and watching what was going on. My role was to pay attention to the pump, which I did. I was the first full-time perfusionist in the business of open-heart surgery.

People began coming to find out about cross-circulation right away. Somehow the news got out, and it became a worldwide sensation. People came from all over the world, visiting the laboratory and the operating room. The operating room had a large glass dome over it, and it could seat twenty people or more. It was not unusual for the whole dome to be crowded with people.

Dr. Lillehei did about forty-five cross-circulation operations over an eighteen-month period. A few other people tried it, but not very successfully. Others thought this was a pretty simple thing; you just take one individual, plug him into the other, turn on the pump, and go to work. They didn't understand the physiology of it, didn't understand the perfusion techniques, and they didn't understand the postoperative care. So, unfortunately, there were a number of disasters. I heard about them through the grapevine. They were never really publicized because people were very reluctant to admit what had happened. If you looked at the literature, you would think that nobody else did any cross-circulation operations. They did, but the outcome was tragic more often than not. It was like the early heart transplants in that way.

We had several good people working together on this at the University of Minnesota. Herb Warden went on to be the chief of cardiac surgery at the new medical school in Morgantown, West Virginia. Norm Shumway was working in a lab adjacent to mine, and he too went on to develop a reputation of his own. There was a core of people there who later went on to make significant contributions to heart surgery.

The way we got started on developing the bubble oxygenator was interesting. After an operation using cross-circulation one day, I was talking to Walt Lillehei, and he was saying that it was obvious that we need a replacement for the donor. The cross-circulation couldn't go on indefinitely, because we would eventually have to work on larger patients. We couldn't take a full-sized adult and tie them up to a full-sized patient. We would have to develop a substitute technique. He said that a very good project would be to work on developing a pump-oxygenator system. He said, "Now if that interests you, that would be a good project for you to work on in the lab." I was always very grateful to him that he didn't say, "You have to go down and work in the lab." He gave it to me as an option. That was Walt's generosity. He didn't force anything on anybody, and neither did Dr. Wangensteen. I thought it was a good project for me. And was interested in it because it drew on the laboratory and medical experience that I already had, and it would expand my knowledge in those areas as well.

As you would expect, I went through a number of false starts. You don't start out with a success right off the bat on any complex project. Dr. Lillehei had a couple of admonitions for me. He said, "If you're going to work on this project, I suggest that you consider two things. First of all, do not go to bubble oxygenator systems because they have a very poor history of success. Second, avoid libraries and avoid literature searches, because I want you to keep an open mind and not be prejudiced by the mistakes of others." This was a unique approach, but it suited me fine. I was glad to do whatever he said because I greatly admired him. I just went ahead and used my own mechanical ability to approach the project.

After these false starts, I was advised by Dr. Lillehei to contact a friend of his who was in the food-processing business. He made polyvinyl tubing to transfer beer, mayonnaise, and other food substances from one place to another. It was called the Mayon Tubing Company. Fortunately, the polyvinyl tubing was very blood-compatible. I didn't know this at the time, but a lot of oxygenator systems had used glass vessels. There had been some papers demonstrating that raw glass had a very negative effect on blood. It would activate thromboplastin and destroy the clotting mechanism of blood. A lot of experiments using glass systems ended up with uncontrollable bleeding problems because of the loss of thrombin. But serendipitously, because of Walt's suggestion to use polyvinyl tubes, we didn't have to go through all that.

It occurred to me while working on this that there had not been any efforts at hyperbaric oxygenation. We knew that three atmospheres of pressure would drive enough oxygen into the blood to equalize the entire arterial-venous difference. You would not even need red cells. You would get all the oxygen you need in the plasma alone. There are a number of variables, of course, that you have to consider, and one of these is the time of exposure of your film of blood. Whether it's the film surrounding a bubble or a film spread over a sheet, either way it is still a film. The oxygenation speed depends on how oxygen will penetrate through the plasma. The oxygen-hemoglobin reaction is virtually instantaneous, but the delay is the time it takes for the gas to go through the plasma to get to the red blood cell. I knew that we were supposed to avoid bubbles, and that I could film blood down a long plastic tube. I could control the rate of flow by the tilt of the tube, and I could manage the thickness of the film by the input and the angle of incline. In other words, you could manipulate the variables fairly easily just by taking a six-foot-long tube and tilting it one way or the other. I devised a system in which the lower part of the tube served as a reservoir, and the upper two-thirds of the tube was an oxygenator. Venous blood was put into the top of the tube and would run down the incline plane of the tilted tube. There was an insert near the top of the reservoir for oxygen input, and I would tie it to a tank of oxygen so that I could really pump up the pressure as high as I wanted. Of course, I would hold the pressure in the tube by a release valve. By controlling the release valve I could control the pressure, and I had it gauged, so I could measure the pressure. I didn't know whether the polyvinyl tube would hold three atmospheres of pressure or if it would blow up in my face. Being naïve, I just took the chance that it would hold, and it did. That is how I developed a hyperbaric oxygenator.

A problem arose, though. What happens to hyperbaric blood when you decompress it to normospheric pressure? Caisson's disease. Bubbles would come out of the blood, and of course you would end up with bubbles in the system. I noticed that on this long inclined tube, the bubbles that came out of the system would be trapped in the upper layer of blood. The heavier blood would slide down, and the lighter blood containing the bubbles would rise to the top and be trapped. So the tube was an excellent bubble trap. You could really prevent any bubbles from moving on. Having a long inclined tube was cumbersome, so the obvious solution for me was to wrap it around a stand. You could still control the incline to whatever degree you wanted if you wrapped it around the stand, and that is how the helix developed in the reservoir system.

However, I was still getting bubbles on decompression, and I realized that I couldn't avoid bubbles and might as well learn to live with them. The reservoir was a good bubble trap, but I wanted to make a bubble dispersion system. I took another piece of plastic hose, and I got a black rubber cork. I put eighteen number-22 needles through the bottom of it and enclosed that in the chamber as the bubble dispersion system. Of course, I put a venous input into the base of it also. This was a tube about three feet long. I could put the venous blood in the base of this tube around this nest of hypodermic needles, and it would introduce multiple small bubbles into the system.

Bubble size was an important variable. Carbon dioxide is about twenty times more soluble in water or blood than oxygen, so that with a very tiny bubble, or with foam, you had carbon dioxide retention. It would be hard to get all the carbon dioxide out because of the much greater surface area represented in the tiny bubbles. The larger bubbles that could be produced by the number-22 needles were able to maintain a level of carbon dioxide retention that would be compatible with physiology. I pumped this up to the top of the vertical tube, and then tilted it over so that it entered the helical reservoir. There was always a volume of blood in the reservoir, so the blood would fall into that. In this way, the polyvinyl tubing by itself served as a debubbler.

Also at that time silicone was used to line glass blood bottles in blood banks. Silicone had recently entered the market as a useful blood interface. There was also a silicone defoaming agent called Antifoam A, made by Dow Corning, which had been developed in the aerospace industry for the jet fighters that were coming out at the time. These jets ascended very rapidly to high altitudes, and as they came down again, they were having trouble with bubble formation in the jet fuel and the bubbles would jam up the system. As I understood it, Antifoam A was invented to disperse the bubbles in jet aircraft, and it helped in my bubble oxygenator, with debubbling and with the coalescing of the bubbles. I found the maximum flow rate that I could use, but I didn't tell Walt what I was doing until I had done ten perfusions on dogs using this system. Every dog survived, and none of them had any physical disability, they all looked good. I finally told Walt about it. He came down and took all the dogs out of their cages. I remember walking them out in the field in front of the grassy meadow by the research lab. We were just walking the dogs around and analyzing them and checking them over. There was no apparent damage to them. It was then that Walt decided that we would try this in the operating room.

We did have some funding for this research, both from the Life Insurance Medical Research Fund, which provided some money, and from the American Heart Association. This was before the government was involved in this kind of research. Dr. Wangensteen ran his laboratory in such a way that each staff man had his own laboratory, and it was his responsibility to get it funded. Some people funded their research with income from private practice, which was permitted at that time. They would also raise some money in the community. We didn't have a lot of funding, so we had to be careful, and my project was worthwhile as it could be done very inexpensively.

The first case that we did in the operating room was in May 1955. From my experiences in the animal lab, I knew that I could safely oxygenate an animal up to fifteen pounds with the system I had designed. Walt said, "I've got a patient that weighs twenty-five pounds. Do you think you can do that?" I told him no because this hadn't been tested in the lab. I asked him to give me a couple of weeks. I upsized the system, increased its dimensions, and got an inch-and-a-quarter-diameter tubing and made various other adaptations. I found that the system could perfuse a twenty-five-pound patient. That's how we gradually moved the system to an adult size. But it came to the point that the polyvinyl tubing was not available in the size that I needed. To get around that, I developed my own blow-molding technique. I took a four-inch diameter brass tube, put a piece of polyvinyl tubing in the tube, corked it at both ends, and put it in the autoclave to heat it up. After it got hot, I would bring it out of the autoclave and then put a bit of pressure into it. The pressure would blow that tube up to four inches in diameter, allowing me to blow-mold my own parts. In this way I upgraded the system for larger patients.

Once we had a disposable oxygenator, we really started having a lot of visitors. All of the pioneer cardiac surgeons came: Denton Cooley from Texas, Charles Dubost from Paris, Russell Brock from London, Clarence Crafoord from Stockholm, and people from Russia, India, and South America. They would write down the exact measurements in order to copy my device. Actually, I published a paper with diagrams and measurements. My device was a kind of Rube Goldberg affair with a bunch of tubes gathered in a heap and on a stand, but every curve and bend and piece had a purpose. A lot of people would look at it and think, "This is stupid. I can do better than that." They would have it changed by the time they got on the plane to go home, and, of course, they had disasters in their laboratories. There was a paper given at the American Surgical Association written by a surgeon who had tried it in the laboratory and had had disaster after disaster. He obviously didn't know what he was doing. He presented this at a national meeting of very distinguished people condemning my work, which was rather hurtful in its own way. There were comments at the end of the paper, and Denton Cooley responded and said, "I went to Minnesota, and I studied what they did there. I took it home to Texas, and now I have 125 patients that have done well with it." That was the end of the discussion. Denton was a great supporter of mine, and I became very fond of him.

After I served my time in the laboratory, Dr. Lillehei suggested that I go through the surgery residency program. I hadn't really considered that before, but I thought, well, I'm mechanically inclined, it's very interesting, and I would like to do that. When I left the laboratory, Vince Gott came in and took over my role directing the laboratory. Obviously, the idea of taking a few coils of plastic hose and making your own oxygenator was causing some disasters when people did not understand what they were doing, so the idea of commercializing it became desirable. A company called Travenol became involved and they worked with Vince Gott. They developed the sheet oxygenator, in which two sheets of polyvinyl plastic were fused together, creating a similar-type oxygenator to the one I had had with the helical system. This turned out to be a huge success. I think Denton Cooley helped a bit in the development of it, and the University of Minnesota patented it. That was one way that they developed some funding for research. It didn't occur to me to patent it. They provided me with an excellent education, and if I could give something back to them, so much the better.

I finished my residency in 1960 or 1961 and stayed on for a year as a faculty member in charge of one of the surgery divisions. My colleague was Richard Lillehei, who was C. Walton's younger brother. Richard and I were good friends for many years, living close to each other, and going through parallel stages of residency together.

When I left Minnesota, I went to the Chicago Medical School as chairman of the Department of Surgery. At that time I had become acquainted with Jim Bentley, who was an engineer working with Lowell Edwards in the Starr-Edwards valve company. Jim wanted to start his own company, and we talked about building our own oxygenator based on some new ideas that I had. I wanted to develop a system with a built-in

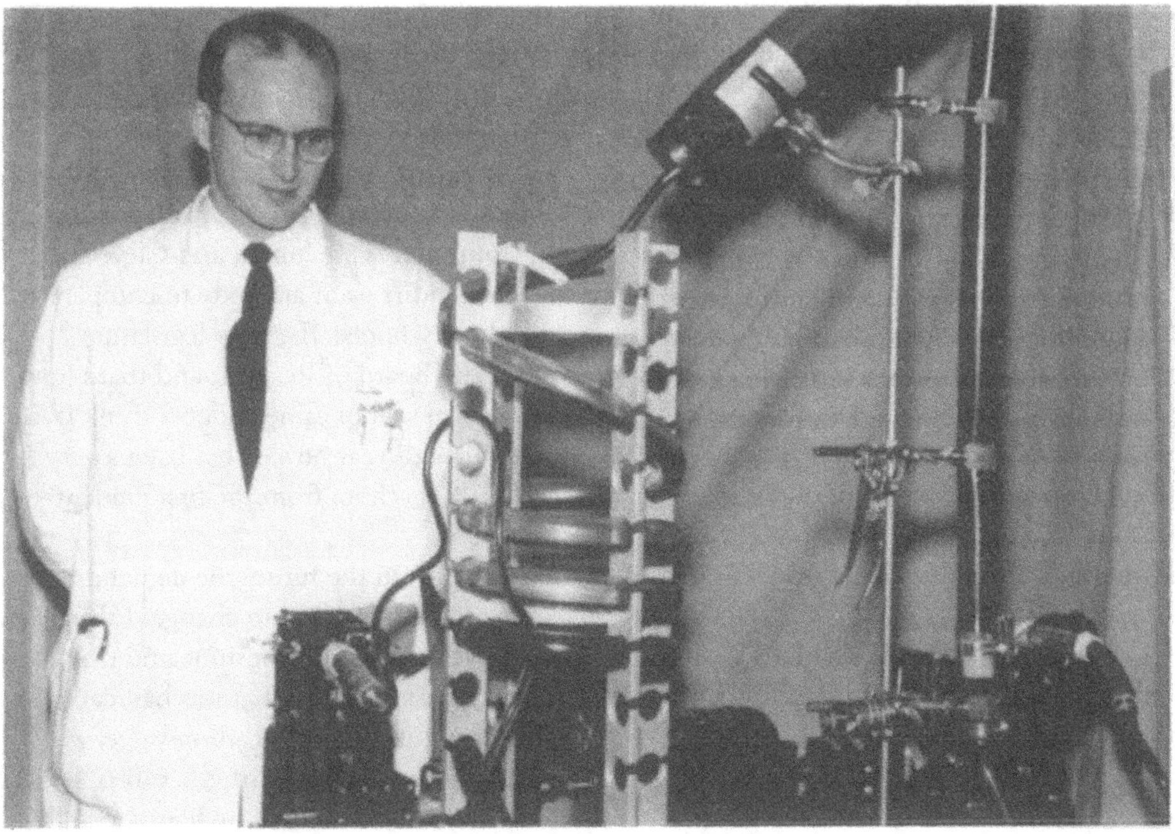

Dick DeWall and an early bubble oxygenator, 1956

control for cooling and warming. This developed into the Temptrol oxygenator. It was a rigid plastic body with a built-in canister for the heat exchanger. The blood would run down over it on an inclined path, which served as the debubbler. It incorporated a lot of my ideas. That device became moderately successful for a period of time.

While I was still at Minnesota, I started thinking that to duplicate the normal lung was the way to go. I made some prototypes of a capillary membrane oxygenator using silicone rubber tubing. It was very attractive and interesting, but I left that project behind in Minnesota. It was ultimately taken over by Dow Corning and later used in the hollow-fiber artificial kidney. Later some other companies developed a hollow-fiber oxygenator, which is used today in most cardiac surgery operations.

Walt Lillehei was a very good friend and supporter. During his senior residency he developed what was probably a follicular lymphoblastoma of the parotid gland, and he had to have an extensive operation, excision of the paratoid, and a radical neck dissection. At Dr. Wangensteen's insistence, they even split his sternum and did an internal mammary artery node dissection. He went through a lot at that time, and I think this changed his attitude. He decided to live for the present, one day at a time, because he didn't know if he was really cured. After that, he always had great compassion for other people. Because he had radiation for the tumor in his neck, later in his life he developed cataracts and had problems with his vision. He gave up surgery and came back to Minnesota. He became a medical advisor to St Jude Medical for the next twenty years until he died. In spite of all his health problems he lived a pretty full life until his eighty-first birthday.

As I said, I went to Chicago Medical School when I left Minnesota, and I was there for three or four years. After the third year I decided that administrative work was not my calling. I was not mentally suited to sit at a desk, and my surgical program was not well supported, so I thought I should get out of the role as the chairman of surgery.

At that time I was a consultant for the artificial heart program at the NIH. I went to one of the meetings in Washington and mentioned to a doctor at the meeting that I was amenable to transferring out of academia. At the time Dayton had a new hospital called the Cox Heart Hospital. They invited me to come down there as a surgeon. It was an opportunity to start a cardiac program.

When I got to Dayton, I found that the hospitals there had very fine residency training programs. The city fathers had started a state university there, Wright State University, named after the Wright brothers. The university developed very nicely, but it did not have a medical school at the time. When I got to Dayton and saw the residency programs and the academic programs that were already there, I thought they should have a medical school attached to the state university. The idea of a new medical school had fallen into disfavor because people thought that a new medical school would require a $120-million hospital to support it. I began to draw up a program. It took me three years to put together a proposal to create a medical school there using local hospitals.

The Board of Regents of the state of Ohio was against it. They were all sponsoring Columbus, Cincinnati, and Cleveland, and they didn't want anybody to compete with those schools. The state legislature vetoed the Board of Regents, and that's how the medical school came about. I think it is in its thirtieth year now. It has been a very fine medical school from the first graduating class.

Certainly, in the future the demand for cardiac surgery is going to change. I think that valve surgery will continue and maybe even increase. I foresee that mechanical valves, such as the omni-carbon valve, will eventually replace bioprosthesic valves, because they have an indefinite lifespan, and we are now titrating down the amount of coumadin that is necessary for these valves. I have had to take out some bioprosthetic valves only a couple of years after their implant. Bioprostheses are better now, and many of them may last for ten years. But if you put a bioprosthesis in a person at the age of seventy, and then you have to replace it when they are eighty years old, that is a formidable procedure. However, if you put in a good mechanical valve, that's it; you don't have to go back and do it again.

Looking back on my life, there have been many people who have influenced me. Certainly Herb Warden would be in that group, and also Dr. Wangensteen and Dr. Lillehei. I had several outstanding high school teachers, but I can't remember their names. I went to the university right after World War II, when it was flooded with students, and my classes were very large. We didn't really develop a relationship with any professors at that time. I did have some influential teachers in medical school, like Dick Varco in the surgery department. He made you think. Of course, Owen Wangensteen was a wonderful man, just outstanding. Walt was very supportive to me, and Herb Warden was a very close personal friend for many years, as were Vince Gott and Rich Lillehei, Walt's younger brother.

I am proud of my work on the bubble oxygenator. It certainly created a great deal of interest at the time. Many people worldwide used it because it was easy and simple. It had the advantage of a small priming volume. By contrast, the Gibbon system might require ten to fifteen bottles of blood. At that time there was also the Kay-Cross disc oxygenator. Crafoord and Anderson in Stockholm originally designed this, and it was subsequently taken over by Viking Björk. They did some updating and called it the Björk oxygenator. Then Fred Cross and Jerome Kay in Cleveland took that design and turned it into a very useful machine that became quite popular. It presented some real maintenance problems as it had fifty discs that you had to take apart and clean. The priming volume was large, but the rotating-disc oxygenator had certain adherents. It was reliable and could be used without a large staff, unlike the Gibbon screen oxygenator, which never achieved much popularity because of its complexity.

The bubble oxygenator ultimately did influence the early days of cardiac surgery. It was truly the can opener for the cardiac surgery picnic.

Bibliography

DeWall RA, Warden HE, Read RC, Gott VL, Ziegler, NR, Varco, RL, Lillehei CW. A Simple Expendable, Artificial Oxygenator for Open Heart Surgery. *Surg Clin N Amer.* 1956; Aug;1025–1034.

DeWall RA, Warden HE, Lillehei CW. The Helix Reservoir Bubble Oxygenator and Its Clinical Application. *Extracorporeal Circulation.* Springfield, Illinois: Charles C. Thomas; 1958. 41–56.

DeWall RA, Grage TB, McFee AS, Chiechi MA. Theme and Variations on Blood Oxygenators. I. Bubble Oxygenators. *Surgery.* 1961; 50:931–932.

Gott VL, Sellers RD, DeWall RA, Varco RL, Lillehei CW. A Disposable Unitized Plastic Sheet Oxygenator for Open Heart Surgery. *Dis Chest.* 1957; 32:615–625.

DeWall RA, Lillehei RC, Sellers RD. Hemodilution Perfusions for Open Heart Surgery. Use of Five Percent Dextrose in Water for the Priming Volume. *New Eng J Med.* 1962; 266:1078–1084.

DeWall RA, Najafi H, Roden T. A Hard-Shell Temperature-Controlling Disposable Blood Oxygenator. Use in Clinical Open Heart Surgery. *JAMA.* 1966; 197:1065–1068.

DeWall RA, Pelletier LC, Panebianco A, Hicks G, Schuster B, Bonan R, Martineau J-P, Yip L. Five Year Clinical Experience with the Omniscience Cardiac Valve. *Ann of Thorac Surg.* 1984; 38:275–280.

DeWall RA. The Evolution of the Helical Reservoir Pump-Oxygenator System at the University of Minnesota. *Ann Thorac Surg.* 2003; 76:2210–2215.

William H. Muller, MD

(b. 1919)

I arrived in Baltimore in December 1943, and for the first three or four months I literally did not set foot outside the building. The work schedule was so heavy that one outstanding intern rolled the gurney from the operating room back to the ward, and then just walked out of the institution. He later wrote to Dr. Blalock that the work was more than he could tolerate.

— On the surgical training program at Johns Hopkins

Interviewed October 20, 1998

I was born in 1919 in Dillon, South Carolina, and I grew up there. My father was an attorney and had a fairly successful law firm with his brother-in-law, who was a politician and was speaker of the House of Representatives in South Carolina.

My father had married a woman from a large, old family in South Carolina. They had originally traveled from Mississippi through Georgia about the time of the Civil War. Food and places to stay were difficult to come by on the trip, but a family in Marietta, Georgia, took them in and was very kind to them. My grandmother was born while they were there, and they named her Marietta Georgia Buffet. The family moved up near Dillon, South Carolina, and eventually owned a large farm. My grandfather died around 1895, but my grandmother, a rather stately, matriarchal woman, lived until about 1955. She apparently had some means, and lived in a large house. She had five daughters and two sons, and, interestingly enough, all of the daughters went to college, which was a little unusual in the South at that time.

Dillon was a town of about seven thousand people, and it was a wonderful place to grow up. My father had a great influence on me, as did my mother, but I think my father had the greater influence. Although I was making good grades, he realized that I was learning very little at Dillon High School, so he sent me to McCallie for one year. I went there in 1935, in the middle of the Depression; he could only scrape together enough tuition money for that one year. I thought it was the best educational year of my life. After McCallie, I thought of what I wanted to do, and I thought of medicine. Times were tough then, so I also thought about the armed services and about going to one of the military academies. My father was a good friend of Senator Burnet Maybank of South Carolina, and he asked the senator if he would give me a principal appointment to West Point, which he did. I had a year to wait, though, so I went to the Citadel in the meantime. During my first year at the Citadel, I decided that instead of majoring in physics and going on to West Point, I would try to study medicine. I had a wonderful experience there. There was not the hazing there then that we hear about today. It was a good educational experience, and one that instilled some discipline in me, which I probably needed and which has served me to this day.

When I finished at the Citadel, I applied to Duke University Medical School.

I only applied to that one school, and they accepted me. I went to Duke in 1940, and it was indeed a wonderful experience. The medical school had only been open for ten years. Most of the faculty had come from Johns Hopkins and were very interested in the students and in teaching. Elizabeth, the wife of the anatomy professor, Dr. Sweat, was sort of the majordomo on the anatomy floor. She recognized every student except two out of my class of sixty-five or seventy as they walked in the door. That gives you some idea of the interest and attention given to medical students at Duke.

The teaching was excellent and the environment was simply great. At about that time, in 1941, World War II began, and there was considerable emphasis on tropical medicine, but we had superb instruction in everything else as well. During the last part of my junior year and during all of my senior year, I substituted as an intern, since the number of interns and residents had been significantly reduced because of the war. I performed surgical operations as a senior student, appendectomies and so on, and by the time I started my internship, I already had quite a bit of clinical experience.

When I was thinking about where to do my internship, I talked to some of my instructors, many of whom were from Hopkins, including the chief of surgery, Deryl Hart, and a surgeon named Joseph Beard from Vanderbilt, with whom I had worked in the research laboratory as a senior student. Although Dr. Hart very kindly and graciously offered me a position there at Duke, they encouraged me to go to Hopkins. Joe Beard said, "You should go look at Hopkins, and I think you will like it," and so a friend of mine, Ray Ramage, and I decided to go by train to Baltimore in April 1943. It happened Dr. Tinsley Harrison was the AOA lecturer in the afternoon of the day that we were to leave to go to Baltimore. He had been Dr. Blalock's roommate in medical school. I was invited with some others to Dean Davidson's home for a little reception for Dr. Harrison. I chatted with Tinsley Harrison, who was a very interesting and charismatic individual. He said, "I would like to go to the train station and put you on the train to see that you get well ensconced for your trip to Baltimore." I said, "Well, that's very kind of you, Dr. Harrison." When we got to the station, I told Dr. Harrison that I would see Dr. Blalock and that I would give him his regards. Dr. Harrison pulled me aside and said, "Son, do you really want an internship at Johns Hopkins?" I said, "Yes, Dr. Harrison, I would like that very much." He said,

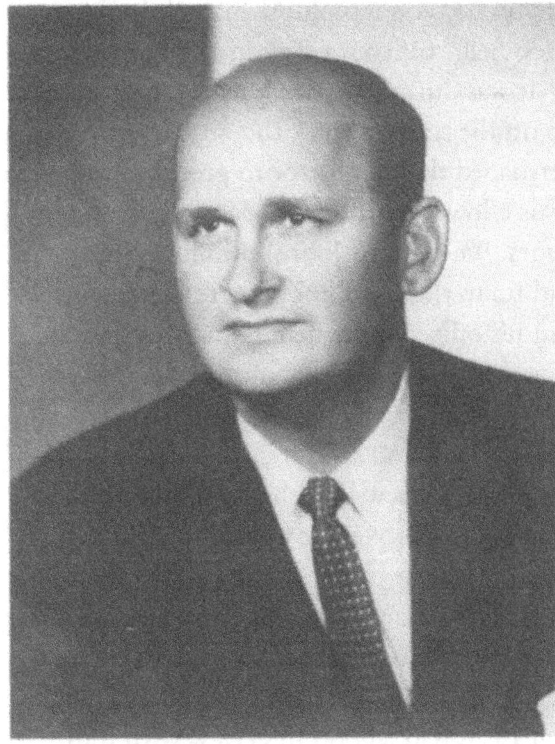

William H. Muller

"If you do, you tell old Al Blalock I said to go to hell." Of course I didn't.

It was during World War II and we stood up on the train most of the way. I finally persuaded the conductor to give the two of us a lower berth for the last two or three hours. We went to Johns Hopkins Hospital, and up to the sixth floor where Dr. Blalock had his office, and where Francis Grebel, his secretary, presided. In about ten minutes, a very young man in a tweed sports coat, a little ruffled, and saddle shoes came out of the office. I knew that that could not be Dr. Blalock, so I looked down and continued reading, but he came over and said, "I am Alfred Blalock." I was a little startled, but he very graciously took me into his office and treated me very kindly. After I left, I thought that I had had a good interview with him, although I was somewhat worried about one thing I had said. I was talking to Dr. Blalock about an experiment I was working on in Dr. Beard's laboratory with the Shope papilloma virus, and I said that cortisone increased capillary permeability. Dr. Blalock said, "No, I think it decreases capillary permeability." I really didn't argue with him, and I wondered if that might have an influence on my being given an internship, but in about three or four weeks, I received a letter offering me the position.

After we left Dr. Blalock's office, we went to the Chi Phi house (a medical school fraternity), which was across the street from the hospital. They offered to let my friend and me stay there for the evening. They had a sleeping porch with screen wire on the sides and over the top, and they offered us a bed there; we gladly accepted. We had left Durham the afternoon before, and it had been a beautiful day, with the gardens in bloom and everything lush. That night it snowed five inches in Baltimore. The Duke facilities were relatively new and shiny, but the Baltimore facilities had a lot of coal dust and other industrial sediment on them. I said to myself, "Well, I will never go to Hopkins."

I returned to Durham, and I spoke to Keith Grimson, who had come to Duke while I was a student. I also spoke to Joe Beard about going to Hopkins for an internship. I remember that he said, "If you have an opportunity to go there, you do it. Alfred Blalock will never forget you." He was absolutely right; Dr. Blalock never forgot me, and I think he felt that way about many of his trainees.

I decided to go to Hopkins, and it certainly was one of the best decisions I ever made. I arrived in Baltimore in the latter part of December 1943. When I got there, I learned that the number of internships at Johns Hopkins had been reduced from about twenty to about twelve or thirteen. For the first three or four months, I literally did not set foot outside of the institution, or even outside of the building. We worked very hard, on duty every night. It was just continuous work. We covered the emergency room and it was very busy. In East Baltimore they had a lot of stab wounds, industrial accidents, and all sorts of the usual emergency problems such as perforated ulcers, acute gallbladders, and so on. We had a very busy schedule in the operating room.

There were two chief residents on the surgical service. One was Herb Sloan, who became very successful and head of thoracic surgery at Michigan. The other was George Duncan, who was very bright and interested in research, and who had come from Vanderbilt with Dr. Blalock.

As I said, we had a very busy surgical schedule. It was a great opportunity because I was able to be the operating physician in cases where I might not have been otherwise. The work schedule was very heavy, so heavy that one outstanding intern from Columbia rolled the gurney from the operating room back to the ward and then just walked out of the institution. We understood that he later wrote to Dr. Blalock that the work was just more than he could tolerate. Although the workload was great, we were very focused, and it was a wonderful learning experience.

It was a twenty-seven-month program, divided into three segments of nine months each. Three interns out of our original group were kept on after the first nine months, and I was fortunate enough to be one of the three selected. I began to do a moderate amount of surgery, something that Mark Ravitch had waited eight or nine years to do. When he returned from the service, he could not believe that I was doing all of these major procedures that had taken him so long to reach.

In 1944 we learned that Dr. Blalock was going to perform an operation on a blue baby. I hardly knew what a blue baby was, so I began talking to some of the pediatric cardiologists and the pediatricians. There weren't many pediatric cardiologists except for Helen Taussig and one or two of her assistants. Dr. Blalock asked the then chief of anesthesiology, Austin Lamont, if he would provide the anesthetic, and Austin, an aristocratic man from a very prominent and wealthy New York family, said that he would not do it. Merel Harmel, the second in command, said he would do it. He later became the chief of anesthesiology at Chicago and at Duke. The patient was an eighteen-month-old child who was given open-drop ether for a thoracotomy.

During the operation, Dr. Blalock's laboratory assistant, Vivien Thomas, came to the operating room and stood behind Dr. Blalock to make sure that Dr. Blalock did it properly. Vivien Thomas had been performing the pulmonary subclavian shunts in the animal laboratory, the old Hunterian laboratory. At least, we were led to believe that Vivien was to tell Dr. Blalock what to do. We knew Dr. Blalock knew exactly what to do, but he was a very generous man, and he would turn to Vivien and say, "Well, now, Vivien, shall I put this stitch in here?" He completed the operation and the patient survived, but she died about a year later. Some other Blue Baby operations were attempted some time later, and these were successful. Blalock and Taussig published a paper within the next year on the early tetralogy of Fallot operations. Dr. Blalock continued to do these procedures, and he also performed patent ductus procedures, as well as other operations. At that time, though, he did not do any operations for coarctation of the aorta.

I was elected as the final one to stay on for the last nine months, and it was a great privilege to do so. Bill Longmire had stepped aside for two other residents to be chief residents for six months, and he then became a chief resident and stayed on for more than eighteen months. The opportunity to work with Bill Longmire was really something special. We had a kind of chemistry, and he was very good to me. He trusted me and was very helpful. Bill Longmire helped Dr. Blalock a great deal with these operations, so much so that if Dr. Blalock did not want to do an operation, he would ask Bill to do it, whether it was GI or plastic surgery or anything. After

Bill had stayed on as a resident for eighteen months, he became a member of the faculty. Dr. Blalock asked him if he would become the first full-time plastic surgeon at Johns Hopkins, and Bill made a trip around the country to plastic surgery centers, returned, and became the head of plastic surgery.

In late 1945 some of the men began returning from the armed services, such as Mark Ravitch and Bill Gross. Bill Scott had come down from the Brigham as a resident during my last nine months. Although he was senior to me and had completed a residency in neurological surgery with Frank Ingram, Dr. Blalock gave me the more senior position.

As we stayed on at Hopkins and things relaxed a little bit, Dr. Blalock became much more approachable, and I got to know him a little better. He was a simply wonderful man and had a lot of charisma. I asked surgeons who visited Hopkins to tell me what this man had, and none of them could really explain it, but he had a great influence on the people who were there. His personality was not ebullient. He wasn't like William Rienhoff, who became one of his closest friends, but he had a very pleasing personality, and he had something that attracted people to him.

He had a Christmas party every year. Once he made me feel so good at that party. Ogden Nash was there, and at that time he was a very popular author of ditties and such. Dr. Blalock grabbed me by the shoulder and said, "Ogden, I want you to meet my star assistant resident." I felt just about as good as I have ever felt. Not only that, but I had asked a lovely nurse there if she would marry me, and she said she would, and she was with me at the party.

In 1946 I was called up for military service, and we were married en route to San Antonio, Texas, where the Officers Field Service School for Medicine was located. It had been moved there from Valley Forge, Pennsylvania. We were married in Roanoke, and we went down to New Orleans to spend a few days for a honeymoon. We went on to San Antonio, and then I received word that I would be sent overseas to Berlin, Germany. I had hoped that I would not be sent overseas, because I was just married.

It was a great opportunity. I was supposed to be the chief of surgery in the 271st Station Hospital in Berlin, but there were a couple of other surgeons who had been there for a while, and since I was a lot younger than one of them, he became the chief of surgery, and I was made chief of proctology. I accepted that, and I did some hemorrhoids and things like that.

I became quite ill in Berlin, with a very thick membrane in my throat, and was thought to have diphtheria. A number of GIs who had had the vaccine, as I had, came down with diphtheria. They decided to give me the diphtheria antitoxin, even though I was allergic to the horse serum. I received it in divided, increasing doses, and nine days later, I had the worst serum sickness imaginable. I ended up with a bilateral brachial plexus paralysis and was sent home.

We were sent to Coral Gables, Florida, to Pratt General Hospital. It had formerly been the Miami Biltmore Hotel, with three eighteen-hole golf courses that surrounded it, and beautiful pools. It was great to be there, and we made a lot of friends there, people with whom we are still in touch.

My father was dying at that time of coronary disease, and we went to South Carolina for the better part of a year to take care of him. My brother had stayed out of Duke for a quarter to care for my father and had to go back to medical school. I had separated from the service by then, and I decided to go into practice in my hometown in South Carolina. A small new Catholic hospital had been built, and there was no surgeon. I made some inquiries, and they welcomed me with open arms. Within three weeks, I had all the surgery I could do. I did a lot of gynecological surgery, in which I had no prior experience. I also did everything from hernias to thyroids to nephrectomies, you name it. I did fifteen caesarean sections in the nine months I was there.

Then I received a letter from Bill Longmire, who invited me to return to Hopkins and work with him. When I had asked Alfred Blalock, he had not given me any assurance that I could return. He had said, "Well, you know, a lot of people are coming back, and I just can't tell you." The letter from Bill Longmire, though, said, "You're probably in the best situation you could be in, and maybe it would be wrong for you to return to Hopkins, but if you do want to come, please let us know." I learned that Dr. Blalock had asked him to write to me. I got all of my operative records together and took the train to Baltimore. When I presented Dr. Blalock with a stack of about three hundred operative records, I will never forget what he said. He looked at them and said, "Fifteen caesarian sections? Well, you can come back."

That was in March 1948, and I returned the following July. I was a little aghast to find out that I was to be the chief resident. I thought I could handle the surgery, but I did not know if I could handle the administration of the service, which had become much, much larger by that time. They assured me

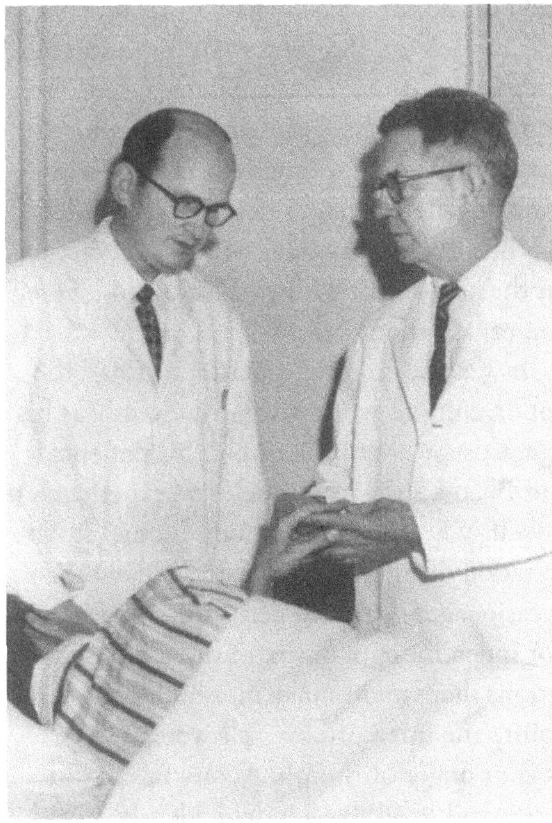

Harry Muller and Alfred Blalock

that I could handle it, and, as it turned out, I did. My co-resident was Richard Clay from Miami, Florida. He was very bright and had returned from the service. He was a wonderful speaker, which I wasn't, but I think that technically I was a significantly better operating surgeon.

I went through the six months, and in about the fifth month Dr. Blalock said, "Well, I think you have had enough training." I learned later that Dr. Blalock did not believe that one needed long periods of technical training, such as had been the case when Dean Lewis had been the chief at Hopkins. Dr. Blalock thought you could spend two, three, or four years training, and that was all you needed. Part of the reason for this could have been that his resident experience had been so limited. He had a year of ENT, a year of urology, and then went to Vanderbilt with Barney Brooks. At any rate, I said, "You know, Dr. Blalock, I thought I was going to have more training." He said, "You've had enough general surgery now. What would you like to do?" I said, "I would like to come on the heart team with you." He said, "Fine, you can do that."

It was a wonderful experience. I had the opportunity to work with him directly as his first assistant. We took care of his patients, and I had a significant operative experience myself. We were doing patent ductus, coarctation of the aorta, tetralogy of Fallot, an occasional constrictive pericarditis, but really not much more than that. I did adult coarctations that would make me shudder at this point. The intercostal vessels were as large as your finger or thumb. At any rate, I did those, and I did them independently. I could call on someone if I needed help. I was busy most of the time with patients on the heart service. Bill Longmire did very few of these patients; he was head of plastic surgery, and he was also the professor of difficult surgery. If Dr. Blalock had a difficult problem, Bill often did it.

I had returned to Hopkins with the thought that I was going to work with Bill Longmire in plastic surgery. When I returned, though, Bill was not there; he had gone to Los Angeles for a week. He was being considered as the first chairman of the Department of Surgery at UCLA. He was offered that position, and when he came back, he said to me, "I would like for you to come out there with me if you wish." A little later, Dr. Blalock offered me the position that Bill was vacating; I was to go to St. Louis or New York and spend a few months in plastic surgery and then return and become the full-time head of plastic surgery at Hopkins. When Dr. Blalock made me this offer, I said, "Dr. Blalock, I have been offered a position with Bill. Will you give me some time to consider your offer?" He said, "Yes, we are going to Gibson Island on vacation for a month. Bill Longmire and Jane are going with us, and when you make your decision, will you come down and tell me?" The next two weeks was a very trying time for me, because Hopkins was well established, and there were a lot of prominent surgeons there that I had come to know and like, such as Bill Reinhoff, Warfield Firor, George Finney, Ridgeway Trimble, and of course Dr. Blalock. I also knew the plastic surgeons, Ed Hannahan and John Stage Davis, so I thought I might like to stay there. The more we thought about it, the more we decided that it would be a great opportunity to go to Los Angeles with this first group to start the new UCLA medical school. I went down to Gibson Island one evening to tell Dr. Blalock, and what I said was, "I think I will stay in general surgery." I didn't say I would go with Bill Longmire, but he knew what I meant. He said, "Let's play a game of ping-pong," and he beat me. He was a real competitor and a great sports enthusiast, so much so that he used to take his vacations up in Cooperstown where the Baseball Hall of Fame is located.

Bill Longmire went to Los Angeles in November 1948, and then we followed him to Los Angeles in early June 1949. The UCLA medical school facility consisted of one small metal Quonset hut. The new dean was Stafford Warren, who had been the chief medical officer during World War II for those developing the atomic bomb.

The chief of medicine was John Lawrence. Charles Carpenter was in infectious disease, Andy Dowdy was in radiology, and Bill was surgery. They were the original four department chairmen. I wasn't quite sure what I was to do. Bill said, "You will be the chief at the Harbor General Hospital." This had been a port of embarkation hospital for Los Angeles, and the state had bought it for about five cents on the dollar.

Being the new man on the block, and with UCLA just beginning, I had a real honeymoon. I was accepted very well, and we started doing surgery at the Harbor General Hospital and the VA hospital. We made a lot of equipment lists and designs for operating rooms and that sort of thing. I was interested in getting a cardiac surgery program going. A man named John Jones, a prominent thoracic surgeon who had been trained at Michigan, was doing patent ductus and Blalock-Taussig procedures, but somehow or other he kept everyone else from doing it.

Eventually a thoracic surgeon named Artie Goldman invited me to his home to give a talk about congenital heart disease. He had invited the chief cardiologist from the county hospital and a number of others. At the end of my talk, I was pulled aside by the chief from the county hospital, and he said, "I have got about a hundred catheterized patients with tetralogy and other things. Will you operate on them at the Harbor Hospital?" I said, "Sure." I began to operate on tetralogy patients at the Harbor Hospital. The next thing I knew, John Jones had acquired an associate and placed him at the county hospital, and my supply of patients diminished somewhat. By that time it had become known that we were doing cardiac surgery.

When I was at Hopkins, Dr. Charles Bailey came for a week as a visiting professor. At Dr. Blalock's request I brought a crock of preserved hearts with valvular disease from the pathology department so that Dr. Bailey could demonstrate how he was performing the splitting operations for the stenosed mitral valve, which he had been doing for the past year or so. I felt that this was a very viable operation and that it should not have a great deal of risk associated with it. I began doing them at the Harbor General Hospital in Los Angeles. The next thing we knew, we had more surgery than we could do.

About that time (1952), Bill Longmire, who had not yet been in the service, decided that he wanted to enlist. He really had a great experience in the European theater. He became the chief surgeon for the European theater, and he made many contacts and friends. Bill returned after two years, but during his absence, we further developed vascular and cardiac surgery. I did an aneurysm of the aorta about 1953, the first one at the Santa Monica hospital. It was one of the largest abdominal aneurysms I had ever seen. I called one of the fellows in the little laboratory that we had set up at UCLA, to please bring me a homograft. We had prepared some homografts, thinking that we might have this opportunity. At any rate, we resected the aneurysm, and I was very fortunate that the patient survived and seemed to do well.

After that I did many aneurysms in the Veterans Administration Hospital where there was a ready supply of them. I did a good deal of cardiac surgery in the St. John's Hospital, which was a private hospital. This was the hospital where most of the movie crowd went for their medical care. They went there and also to the Sinai Hospital, which was not quite as prominent then as it is now. The nuns very kindly gave me three operating days at the St. John's Hospital.

I had asked Frank Dammann, who had been with Helen Taussig at Hopkins as a fellow, to join us. When he came out, the program became viable because he was very good at cardiac catheterization, having worked closely with Richard Bing at Hopkins. We developed a catheterization program and had more cardiac operations than we could do, plus many vascular operations.

About 1951 or 1952 Charles Bailey began to perform aortic valvulotomies with a tribladed instrument. He slipped it in through an incision in the left ventricle and split the valve. About the same time, I made a somewhat similar instrument. We had a wonderful shop associated with our little UCLA school because of the atomic energy program there. We had really good metal mechanics that could make any instrument that we wanted. We began to do valvulotomies, and I did ten without a fatality and reported them in the *Annals of Surgery*.

In the meantime, I had been asked to come to the University of Virginia to be interviewed for the position of chairman of the department. I had visited several other places but had not been offered a position. At the meeting of the Society for Vascular Surgery in San Francisco, which occurred just a few weeks later, I looked out in the audience and there was the dean from the University of Virginia. He invited me to have lunch with him, and at lunch he said, "We want you to come." I said, "Well, you know, really I am so happy at UCLA that I am not sure I want to move to Virginia." During the first two years we were in Los Angeles, I had said to myself, "This will never be home." After that I thought, "We'll never leave." I was undecided, and I called Alfred Blalock, Mike DeBakey, and several other people for advice. When I called Alfred Blalock, he said, "You've got to accept it; you've got to return and be my neighbor." That wasn't the deciding factor, but my wife and I thought that Charlottesville would be a nice place to live and rear the three children that we had by that time. It also seemed as if the medical center in Charlottesville was at very low ebb and could go nowhere but up. We decided to return to the East Coast, and I'm glad we did.

I told Tom Hunter, the dean, that we would like to set up a department called surgical cardiology, and I asked him if he could get Frank Dammann an appointment as a member of the Department of Surgery rather than medicine or pediatrics. We cleared it with the chiefs of cardiology and pediatrics, and they said it would be fine. Frank returned, and we set up a very modest cardiac catheterization lab. George Minor, a Michigan-trained thoracic surgeon, had already done a few ductus closures and one or two mitrals. Almost from the beginning we began to perform cardiac surgery, a lot of mitrals, and operations for atherosclerotic disease of the lower extremities and of the aorta.

I especially began to pursue my interest in valvular heart disease. While we were in LA we saw a child with a single ventricle who had equal pulmonary artery and aortic pressures. We thought that putting a band on the pulmonary artery might protect the lungs and might allow the patient to survive. This idea was not original with us. As a matter of fact, it was first suggested by a cardiologist at the Mayo Clinic, and Dr. Blalock had tried the procedure once, but it had failed. I went to the laboratory and developed a procedure that would allow us to reduce the size of the pulmonary artery small enough to maintain flow but also to reduce the pressure. We did that procedure on a very small eighteen-month-old infant who weighed something like eight or nine pounds. The child began to flourish, and the sisters at the hospital kept the child there for months on end.

At the same time I had begun experiments in the laboratory to see what caused the vascular changes in the lungs of the patients who had equal pressures in the pulmonary and aortic systems. For the first time we produced, in laboratory animals, the medial hypertrophy and intimal necrosis in the pulmonary vasculature, and I reported this at the Society of University Surgeons. A short time later I reported this one case of pulmonary banding at the American Surgical Association, and we began to see many of those types of patients.

Dr. John Gibbon of Philadelphia had developed a heart-lung machine. I had visited him in 1952 and seen the screen oxygenator that he was using in the lab. I wanted to do open-heart surgery, but we did not have the resources nor was such a device available to us at that time. I began to use what we had used in California for interatrial septal defects: hypothermia and venous inflow occlusion. We began to try to open stenotic aortic valves that same way. We had about five minutes during which we could have the circulation arrested, and within that time we could easily make an incision in the aorta, put a partial occlusion clamp on it, and then restart the circulation. We then began to see patients with aortic insufficiency. We began to open them in a similar manner, and we would make compressed Ivalon sponge leaflet extensions and suture them on one or more of the aortic valve leaflets. Some of these operations were amazingly successful, but we did not do a great many.

We learned that a man at the Yellow Springs Institute, a company in Ohio near Cleveland, had developed a heart-lung machine with a bubble oxygenator. I can't tell you exactly how it worked, but it seemed as if it would blow the air through in pulses. Frank Dammann went to visit the manufacturer, and when he came back he said that it was great and we ought to get one, so we did. The man who devised it visited us, and when he ran the pump, the patient came off, woke up, and did well. However, we could never make it work correctly.

In 1958 I went to a meeting of the Society of University Surgeons in Boston. Bob Gross had a small heart-lung machine with a Kay-Cross oxygenator on the top and with the DeBakey-type roller pumps on it, and it was just wonderful. His machinist was there in the operating room, and I asked him how long it would take him to make one for me. He said, "Oh, more than a year." I said that I couldn't wait that long. I returned to Charlottesville and found out that there was a wonderful company in Cleveland that made the Kay-Cross oxygenator, in which the oxygen flowed over a series of stainless-steel discs rotating in the pool of blood. I went to see William Cotelles, who was the head of that company. I drew a diagram of what I wanted. Within a month he had delivered it in a station wagon, and I had it in my operating room. The first procedure I performed on it was a ventricular septal defect closure, and the operation went beautifully. After that, everything just worked very well. With the stainless-steel oxygenator one had to be sure that it was cleaned completely in order to remove any foreign protein. From time to time a patient would wake up with a high fever, and we attributed that to retained foreign protein in the pump-oxygenator.

One of the early operations we did after we received that machine was the partial replacement of an aortic valve. In those days we saw, not infrequently, patients who had holes in the aortic valve secondary to subacute bacterial endocarditis, and I had operated on some of those under venous inflow occlusion and hypothermia and closed the defect with sutures. Two or three patients seemed to do fairly well. We opened one patient up on the pump-oxygenator, and she had a leaflet that had been virtually destroyed. Having nothing else, we made a compressed Ivalon sponge leaflet and sutured it in. That patient recovered and seemed to do well for about six weeks, but then she developed aortic insufficiency again. With the pump-oxygenator we explored her again and found that the apposition of the leaflets against the Ivalon sponge had apparently destroyed them enough to cause severe insufficiency. We sewed in one more leaflet, giving her a bicuspid valve, and she did well and lived for a number of years. This may have been the first complete replacement of an aortic valve. Larry Michaelis, who was the chief at Northwestern and who was then at the NIH, made a documentary movie that indicated that ours was the first one, but someone at the NIH indicated that Walt Lillehei had done one already. His operation was a single leaflet that closed over a calcified valve, and they called it the "toilet seat operation" in Minnesota.

Priority wasn't that important. We gained confidence, and I began to fashion some trileaflet valves out of nylon and suture them in, and they seemed to work fairly well. Then I learned that a company in Glens Falls, New York, could knit these valves. I went up to see them, and they showed us how they knitted the valves. They started manufacturing the valves for us, and we put in about seventy-five of them. Most of them lasted from two to ten years. We replaced many of them, and I'm sure that other people did too. We replaced them with the Starr-Edwards valve, or the Magovern valve, the one you did not have to suture. The Magovern valve was a mechanical valve that had fingers that grasped the annulus of the aorta. I put in a number of those. Later on we used the Starr-Edwards more than any other design.

At any rate, we developed a rather vigorous program in cardiac surgery at the University of Virginia. I headed it until about 1970. In 1968 I had brought one of my former residents, Dr. Stanton Nolan, back from the National Institutes of Health, and I told him that if he returned, he could head the program in two years. In 1970 he became the head of it, and he did a very good job. He gave it up about six years ago, and Irvin Kron is now head of that service. We now have five cardiac surgeons and it is a very viable program.

When I first came to the University of Virginia, we had virtually no house staff, and about a month before I arrived the Joint Commission or the Resident Review Committee had disapproved the program. I had one very poor intern, and I later learned that he was really working part-time in construction and during his internship was building three houses in the community. He has since become a very wealthy, very prominent real estate and construction man. We had two or three residents in whom I was very interested. A number of residents that had had one year at various other institutions, some very fine people, came to me and said that they would like to become general surgical residents. I did a good deal of general surgery at that time as well as cardiac surgery. Gradually, we developed a residency program, and we turned out some very good residents. At least they have been very successful, both in practice and in academic medicine.

I think the training of residents has changed a lot. When I was a resident, we had great independence as we continued through the residency toward our senior years. We did a lot of independent operating, really without necessarily notifying one of the attending staff. We just handled whatever came in. I think that with the advent of Medicare, all of that has changed, because in order to collect Medicare bills, one has to have the attending physician sign that he has supervised or assisted in this procedure or in the care of the patient. This is one of the factors that has changed residency the most. I think it is for the better in terms of the patients' care, because the residents are much more closely supervised than when I came through. Of course, that was during the war, but even when I became chief of surgery at Virginia, our residents worked much more independently than they do now.

The advent of Medicare did drive up the cost of medical care astronomically, because all of the ward patients or service patients paid a very small amount when I was in medical school. When I came back to Virginia, they paid four dollars a day for their hospital care. Even later on, in the early 1970s before Medicare, they didn't pay very much. The cost of medical care began to rise at that time. I think this increased cost of health care brought on much of the managed care that we see today.

I became involved in many surgical and parasurgical organizations. I worked with the American Board of Surgery and the Board of Thoracic Surgery, the Forum Committee of the College, the Southern Surgical Association, the American College of Surgeons, and the American Surgical Association. I really did not have as much time to devote to operative surgery as I had earlier, although I continued to do a good deal of surgery. In 1976 a situation developed at my institution that required a committee to assess the senior administration of the medical center. The committee advised the president to make some changes. They also advised that I be made the chief administrator of the medical center. At any rate, the president asked me if I would become the vice-president for health affairs and director of the medical center. I had never thought about it or coveted that position. I thought that being the chief of surgery and chairman of the department was the best job in the institution. But I said, "I'll let you know in a week."

I returned to him and said, "I will do it for one year if you will let me retain the position as chairman of the Department of Surgery." He said that that was fine; I held both jobs. The first thing that landed in my lap when I became vice-president was the committee report assessing the need for more in-patient facilities, a new hospital. Initially we thought of a wing on the present hospital, but as we moved along, we realized that we needed a new university hospital. I talked with the finance people and the president, and they said that the most we could spend would be $30 million, which in 1976 would not purchase much of a university hospital. To make a long story short, we obtained consultants and architects, and we ended up building a $260-million hospital, which was completed in 1988. I gave up the chairmanship after I had been president of the American College of Surgeons, in order to devote all of my time to building that hospital. We received funding from private sources; we got some from the state, from our faculty (not much, but they were as generous as they could be), and we floated a $150-million revenue bond issue. Goldman Sachs did it for us, and we built a really lovely, state-of-the-art hospital. It made all the difference in the world to our institution, at least among our personnel, including the faculty, the nurses, the attendants, and all the people who worked in the hospital. It elevated their morale tremendously.

It's important for anyone, but especially for people in professions such as this, to have mentors and teachers who provide guidance and influence, and there were several important people in my life. The first was my mother, of course, and also my father, who was a self-made man. He came from a farm in South Carolina, worked his way through the University of South Carolina, graduated in 1905 as salutatorian of his class, and was determined that we would all be educated and that we would make something of ourselves. He was a great influence. Duke was a great influence on me, but I can't pick out any individual people as I can at Hopkins. At Hopkins there was Alfred Blalock, who was a remarkable man whom I admired very much, who later became my friend after I returned to Virginia, and who was a great influence and motivator in my life. Bill Longmire was also a great influence, and I rank him right up there with Alfred Blalock. He invited me to California and was very helpful to me, but at the same time he gave me a lot of independence. He was always there, as was Alfred Blalock, pushing me along and helping me. I thank them.

Bibliography

Muller WH Jr., Longmire WP Jr. The Surgical Treatment of Pure Pulmonic Stenosis: A Description of an Expansible Valvulotomy. *Surgery.* 1951; 30:275–282.

Muller WH Jr. The Surgical Treatment of Mitral Stenosis. *Calif Med.* 1951; 75:285–289.

Muller WH Jr. The Surgical Treatment of Pulmonic Valvular Stenosis. *Dis Chest.* 1952; 22:152–158.

Muller WH Jr, Hyman M. Valvulotomy for the Surgical Relief of Aortic Stenosis. *Surg Gynec Obst.* 1954; 99:587–594.

Muller WH Jr, Warren WD, Blanton FS Jr. A Method for Resection of Aortic Arch Aneurysms. *Ann Surg.* 1960; 151:225–230.

Muller WH Jr, Dammann JF Jr, Warren WD. Surgical Correction of Cardiovascular Deformities in Marfan's Syndrome. *Ann Surg.* 1960; 152:506–517.

Muller WH Jr. New Valves for Old. *Surg Gynec Obstet.* 1962; 115:233–234.

Muller WH Jr. Presidential Address: Societies, Surgeons, and Surgery. *Ann Surg.* 1976; 183:449–462.

Muller WH Jr. The John H. Gibbon, Jr. Lecture: The Evolution and Current Status of Surgery of the Aortic Valve. *Bull Am Coll Surg.* 1977; 62:20–31.

Harris B. Shumacker Jr., MD

(b. 1908)

I have no doubt that the best elective operation we ever did was the coronary artery bypass graft.
— On cardiac surgery of the 1970s and 1980s

Interviewed December 3, 1996

I was born in 1908 in Laurel, Mississippi. I was not supposed to be born there, because all of the Shumackers lived in the northern part of Mississippi in Holly Springs, and that is where Shumackers are supposed to be born. My father was buying cotton and managing the cotton compress down in Laurel when I was born. Laurel is in Jones County, which has an interesting history. It was covered with pine woods, and the soil was not good for cotton. Most of the gentlemen in the South were only interested in growing cotton, so people from the upper Midwest came down, cut down the trees and built lumber mills, and made fortunes. That is how the town evolved and really got going. It was a nice place, I think, but I really do not remember it because I was only three years old when we left. I went back for the first time in 1975, and it was just the way my father had described it.

We then moved to the northern part of Mississippi, to Holly Springs, for a few years, and I started public school there. When I was seven, we moved over to the delta region of Arkansas, which was about like Mississippi. We lived in a small country town called Marianna, where I thoroughly enjoyed my years as a child and teenager. There was not a thing in town, no tennis courts, golf course, nor swimming pools, and yet we never lacked in the way of fun. One really good but perhaps a little unusual thing that we did in the hot summer months was to listen to our neighbor, Miss Effie, read aloud to all the children in the neighborhood from Dickens and Thackeray and all the great novelists of that period. Miss Effie was the wife of a country doctor whom I admired very much. We sat there starry-eyed, listening to every word that Miss Effie read. I think it probably instilled the love of good literature in all of us; certainly it helped in my case. In those days books were really the only entertainment in a little town of that sort, except for the things that boys would do, like digging caves in the hills and scrounging around, making boats and putting them in the river. We had a good time. I do not regret the lack of anything, because our days were full.

I was a good student, and I enjoyed studying and learning. I was accepted at Harvard for college, and that is where I had planned to go, but then I got a letter from a cousin and a close friend in Chattanooga, who asked me if I would give up my plans to go to Harvard and come to school at the University of Chattanooga instead. His father was having such bad financial problems that if he went to college at all, he would have to go there, so I did. I had a very good education, but I think if I were living my life over again, I would have said, "I am sorry, but I am going to Harvard." However, I have never felt handicapped from attending the University of Chattanooga.

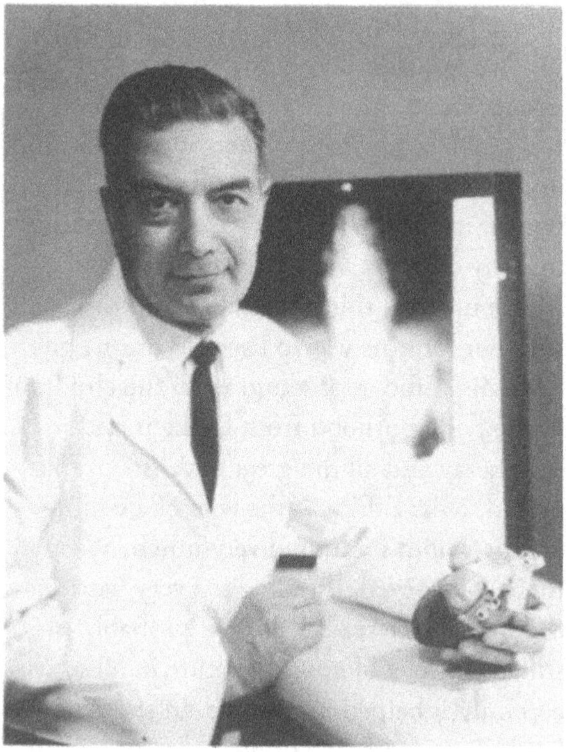

Harris B. Shumacker

I do not know why children aim in certain directions, but even as a small boy I did not want to be a fireman, a horseback rider, a circus performer, or anything else. I just wanted to be a doctor, but I have no idea why. One of my father's brothers was a physician, a very good one, but that was certainly not the reason I was interested in medicine. I just never wanted to be anything except a doctor. The role models in Marianna were country doctors. They did a wonderful job with scanty preparation. I had great admiration, and as the years passed and I could assess what they were really doing, my admiration of them grew more and more.

I finished college very early, in two years instead of four. The reason I finished early was that a wonderful person, the head of the schools in Marianna, said to me, "When you go off to college, you must promise me that you will go to the dean's office and ask them to let you take the maximum amount of work." He said, "I am going to tell you what will happen. You are going to get As, and then I want you to go back at the end of the semester and say, 'That was easy, and I want to take more.'" He said, "If you do not do that, you are going to get in trouble." I am not sure I know exactly what he meant by that, but I have an idea. At any rate, that is precisely what I did. At the end of each semester, I would go to the dean's office, say that I had made As and it was not enough work for me, and that I would like to take more hours. That is why I only spent two years in college.

I was admitted to Johns Hopkins medical school, but before I went there, I spent an extra undergraduate year at Vanderbilt, because I had the impression that chemistry was terribly important. I got this idea from a friend who had graduated from Yale, was a good student, but was having trouble with chemistry at Johns Hopkins. The new professor of chemistry at Johns Hopkins, Mansfield Clark, was no longer teaching chemistry the way most medical schools were teaching it, which was cookbook chemistry, and he was deeply into really modern chemistry. I think now that it may have been a mistake to spend that year at Vanderbilt, but I learned a great deal. I learned how to work hard, how to organize a research program, how to prosecute it, how to look up the literature thoroughly, and how to write a proper thesis. My Vanderbilt year was good, but I doubt I would do it over if I were living my life again.

I went to Baltimore in the fall of 1928, and graduated in 1932. I had hardly been there any time before I decided I would like to be a surgeon. I did not meet any of the clinical people in the first year, but in the second year we had a bit of clinical experience. Dr. Dean Lewis, the chief of surgery, had a clinic every week, designed for the third- and fourth-year students, but the house staff and all of the faculty members also attended. He had a clinic for second-year students, and it was very clever the way he structured it. He would bring in patients with some disorder that a young medical student would be interested in from the standpoint of physiology or anatomy. He held these clinics in the amphitheater, would sit in the pit, and the nurses would bring in the patients. He would look up in the stands and say, "You, come down here," and the very first clinic I went to, I was the "you." A lady had been brought in by the nurse and was draped so that one could only see her shoulders, neck, and head. Dr. Lewis said to me, "Take a look at this lady, and tell me what you see." Well, I saw a rather nice-looking African American, but I did not see anything else. I said, "I am sorry, I don't see anything unusual." He said, "Well, walk around and look again." I walked around and looked at her back, and she had atrophy of the supraspinatus and infraspinatus muscles. When I told him what I saw, he said, "Do you know anything about Erb's palsy?" I said, "No, sir." "Klumpke's palsy?" I again said, "No, sir." He said, "Well, do you read German?" We had to have a reading knowledge of Latin, French, and German to apply for medical school at Hopkins. I said, "Yes, sir, I can struggle through it." He said, "Well, struggle through this," and he handed me a book. He said, "This book has the best chapter on brachial and cervical palsies that has ever been written." It was written by a man named Levendofsky. He said, "I will ask you about that some time." I took the book. The chapter was seventy-eight pages long, and the print was fine. The German was very difficult, and I practically had to quit school to read those seventy-eight pages. I expected him to ask me about it, but he did not mention it the rest of that year or the next. In my fourth year, or maybe even when I was an intern, he pointed to me and said, "Shumacker, come down here. Did you read that chapter by Levendofsky?" I said, "Yes, sir, I did." He said, "Then tell me what you learned." That was my first patient, a case of Erb's palsy.

I stayed on at Johns Hopkins as an intern. The internships were hard to get. Dr. Lewis took almost all of his interns from the Hopkins senior class, but you had to be in the upper fifteen of the class or you did not have a chance. I think they appointed six interns, so I was really quite fortunate. It was a good internship, and I enjoyed it. We did not consider it work, but thought it was a real opportunity. We were on call from the first of September of that year until the first of September the next year. There were only two ways an intern could get out of the hospital. One way was to ask a fellow intern to take your calls. You could say, "I have been in this place now for two months, night and day, and I would like to go out tonight. Would you take my calls?" If the other intern said yes, you could call the telephone operator and tell her your fellow intern was going to take your calls. The other way was to visit a friend who lived within five minutes of the hospital. You could call the operator and tell her that you would take calls there, but you could not do that if the friend lived any distance away.

It was great fun. I have difficulty understanding why interns are concerned about the hours or nights that they work, because we thought Saturday nights were one of the best times to be around the hospital. There was a lot going on in the emergency room, and we liked being involved. Dr. Lewis kept two of the six interns after the internship, one for the whole residency, which would be a total of seven years in training including the intern year. The other would be appointed a research fellow and spend a year in the Hunterian Laboratory, and then that person's time at Johns Hopkins was over. That is what he did with me.

I worked in the Hunterian with Dr. Firor, and one of the things we worked on was tetanus. The retired professor of pharmacology was president of the American Association for the Advancement of Science, and in his presidential address he talked about poisons. He was fascinated with the fact that a tiny bit of a really bad poison could do a lot of damage to a lot of people, and that is how he got interested in tetanus. He asked Dr. Firor and me if we would try to find something about the real cause of death in tetanus. When the new Society of University Surgeons was started, the first paper I gave was on tetanus. At that time, almost everybody at Johns Hopkins was interested in the endocrine glands because nobody knew anything about them. Dr. Firor and I investigated the effects of removing adrenals and pituitary glands in various animals, and the first paper I gave at a national meeting was to the endocrinology section of the American Medical Association meeting in Cleveland, on the interrelationship of the pituitary and adrenal glands. I had published a previous paper when I was a first-year medical student.

At the end of that year we were getting along with our research, and Dr. Firor persuaded me to stay at least part of another year. We were also looking around for an appointment for me to continue my surgical training, and he would not let me accept any resident position that he did not consider to be top-notch, which meant a place where the residency training program was modeled on the one at Johns Hopkins. There were only a few like that: Vanderbilt, Yale, Rochester in New York, Washington University, and Duke, and he would not let me apply to any other. I was thinking maybe I would go into neurosurgery. One day Dr. Wilder Penfield at the Montreal Neurological Institute sent me a telegram saying that I could come up there. On that same day, within an hour of my receiving his telegram, I was called back to the front desk at Hopkins for another telegram. This time it was from Yale, saying that I had an appointment there for the next year. I decided I would go to Montreal to the Neurological Institute for several months until it was time to start at Yale, and I was an assistant resident in neurosurgery for the rest of that year. Dr. Penfield was very nice and said that if I ever wanted to come back, I could complete my training in neurosurgery, but when I got to Yale and started back into general surgery, I knew that that was what I wanted to do.

I was lucky, and it was a wonderful program at Yale. It is difficult to understand how I got into the business of cardiovascular surgery, but it happened in this way. Once I had completed my surgical training, I was offered a number of jobs. One of them was to go back to Johns Hopkins, and another was to stay on at Yale. I asked Dr. Harvey, "If I stay here at Yale, what would you like me to do?" He said, "I would like for you to establish a real cardiovascular surgical unit." I went back to Johns Hopkins, where the person who had been in charge of the almost nonexistent section of cardiovascular surgery had just left. The professor, Dean Lewis, called me to his office and asked me to take charge of it.

I accepted his offer, moved back to Baltimore in 1938, and ended up in cardiovascular surgery. I was still interested in every phase of surgery. I might have had an entirely different career except for the forces that pushed me into cardiovascular surgery. During my training period, the only cardiac operations that were done were pericardiectomies for constrictive pericarditis, but they were rarely done and then not very well. Surgeons were afraid of the heart, and they did piddling little operations like resecting a little bit of the pericardium and then redoing it six months later. That was one operation. The other one was just repairing stab wounds of the heart. There were not any others. Of course, after 1938, when Gross successfully ligated a patent ductus, the congenital heart problems came into prominence as surgically treatable diseases and made cardiac surgery a viable specialty.

In 1941, after I had been on the faculty for a few years, Dr. Blalock arrived at Hopkins, and we were happy to see him. We knew what he had accomplished, and that he was interested in investigative work and new ideas. It was a good appointment, but some of the people at Hopkins who had wanted a local person to get the chairmanship were not happy. We had a custom at Hopkins that whenever a vacancy occurred in the chairmanship, those of us who had positions in the department wrote a nice letter offering to resign, and we put those letters on the chairman's desk. When Blalock came, all of those resignations were on his desk, and he accepted all of them except for mine and maybe one other person's. All the rest of them had to get positions in other universities, go into practice, or they could keep a part-time affiliation. Blalock was very fortunate in that respect, and I thought it was a mighty good custom not to confront the new professor with a lot of positions filled in a way that he did not like.

Blalock came in July 1941, just before the beginning of World War II. Like many other university hospitals, we had organized an army reserve hospital unit, because the war was obviously going to involve our country. Many of us were looking forward to our entry into the war. We thought it was inevitable and the right thing to do, so we were all commissioned as army reserve officers in 1941 prior to Blalock's arrival at Hopkins. Dr. Blalock knew this, and when our unit was activated he called me into his office. Blalock was very close to Fred Rankin, the surgical consultant to the surgeon general. Dr. Rankin was from Lexington, Kentucky, and had trained at the Mayo Clinic. Blalock and Rankin frequently talked by telephone, and I think Fred shared some secrets with Al, because Al seemed to know everything that was going on about the war. He called me to his office and said that he did not want me to go into the army, and that he wanted me to stay at Hopkins. He said that each university professor had been assured that he could keep one man who would be declared essential and would not ever be called for military service. He said, "I would like for you to be that man, my associate." Well, that was a very nice thing, and I was appreciative. I said, "May I have a day or so to think it over and talk with my wife, Myrtie, about it?" I thought it over, and I knew that to stay at Johns Hopkins presented me with an unusual career-building opportunity, but I had the feeling that I really ought to put on a uniform. I guess I wanted to be a soldier. I went back to see him and said, "Thank you very much, Al, but I have to go to the war." He said, "You are a goddamned fool, but if that is what you are, you can not help it." However, I kept my appointment at Johns Hopkins so that when the war was over, I could go back.

I went into the army, and after a very pleasant thirteen or fourteen days in a camp up in New England, we were put on a train. We did not know where we were going, because everything was secret, as it should have been, but the train kept going so we were obviously crossing the country. When we got to San Francisco, we boarded a ship, and again we did not know where we were going, but when we landed we found we were in Australia. When the war started we had organized a one-thousand-bed general hospital, but the surgeon general's office did not have enough hospitals, so they asked us to split it into two units. We made two one-thousand-bed hospitals, and then they picked the senior officers and split us up. I happened to go with the hospital that was lucky to be busy, and the other one was not busy at all.

My hospital was located on the outskirts of Sydney, one of the most wonderful cities in the world. I was busy and happy there, but at the end of May or first of June 1943, a surgical consultant came and talked with us. We should have had a surgical consultant long before, but qualified people were scarce during the war. The consultant was Barkley Parsons, and he had been a prominent member of the surgical faculty of Columbia Presbyterian before the war. He came to our hospital and said that the previous arrangements with the surgeon general's office were such that we had been assured that we would never be transferred out of our Johns Hopkins organization, but, he said, "I need people to head surgical services in other hospitals. I am going to have to take some of you, and the only way I can do it is if you volunteer to go." Two of us volunteered: I did and also a wonderful fellow who had gone through the residency at Johns Hopkins the same year I finished at Yale. The very next day, Barkley Parsons appointed me the head of the surgical service of a very busy hospital in Sydney, and I was very happy there. It gave me a chance to help some young men, and, I thought, this was not a bad move at all.

Very soon we got orders to go somewhere else, but they were written so that you could not understand them. We had a commanding officer whom I did not like, and maybe he did not like me either, but he called me to his office and he said, "I have just received some orders to move this hospital, and I am appointing you to be the officer in charge of the movement." I said, "There is not any such position in the table of organization." He said, "Well, there is now, and you are it." At first I was mad at him, but it turned out that this job was interesting, and I had a good time doing it. It gave me the opportunity to do an unusual bit of maneuvering. The orders simply said that this station hospital would be transferred via (and there was a code name) to (and there was a code name), so I did not know where we were going or by what means. The only way you could move out in the Pacific was by ship. So I went down to the harbor, and I found the hospital ship. It turned out that I knew the commanding officer, and he told me his ship had the same code number. The next problem was that my orders said to put our hospital on it for the move, but there was no way in the world they could take the whole hospital on that little ship. I did not follow the orders, and it was not the last time I did either. I finally got the hospital moved on thirteen separate ships, a little bit here, and a little bit there.

We went to New Guinea, which was not the most pleasant part of the world. The temperature was about 120 degrees, and it rained all the time. When we got there, it turned out that there was a very peculiar disease that we had not observed before. This disorder was the sudden onset of an isolated nerve paralysis. I do not think anybody had any idea about this disorder other than that it was perhaps some type of viral infection, but it was a peculiar thing. The patient would go to bed perfectly healthy, get up the next morning, go to the latrine to shave, and find that he could not pick up his arm. He had axillary paralysis. He could be walking and suddenly fall, and that is what happened to me. It always rained and the paths were muddy. I got out of my tent to go to breakfast, and I fell down. The path was slippery, so I got up and brushed the mud off, and soon the rain had me clean again. I took a few steps and fell again. Then I examined myself and found that I had a peroneal nerve paralysis. I knew then that I could not go forward with that unit. The other Hopkins man who had volunteered was in the same area in New Guinea, and I went over to see him. He confirmed the diagnosis, and I was sent down to Sydney, then sent home. We did not have much of anything in the Pacific, certainly no leg braces, and I had to come home with my leg in a cast. When I got to a hospital here, they fitted me with a brace. Then I was much more mobile and was anxious to go back to work. I think I wore that brace for about five years, and my leg gradually got a little stronger after a couple of years. I still have some weakness in my right leg, but it is not really a handicap.

I got back home about April or May 1944. Then I had really good luck, and I suppose Al Blalock had something to do with it. When I got to San Francisco, there were orders waiting for me saying that I was to appear at the surgeon general's office within ten days. When I got to his office, I found that the orders were to establish the third and last military vascular surgery center. This was a great opportunity for me, and it was a very wise thing to gather the patients with disorders of a given sort in special military installations. During the Civil War, we had one on Christian Street in Philadelphia, where only nerve injuries and neurological disease patients were treated. That is where Weir Mitchell observed patients with major causalgia, which he reported: the first paper on causalgia in this country.

When I left the military, I went back to Johns Hopkins and had every intention of staying there. I was Blalock's senior associate, and he was very good to me. Within a week or two, I got a call from Yale, asking me to come up there and start a cardiac surgical program. I had a good job at Hopkins, but I felt I would like to take the job at Yale, because I wanted to give myself a chance to work in a place where I was totally in charge. When I accepted the Yale job, Blalock again thought I was stark raving mad, and he told me so quite emphatically. He said, "You have the best job of any university surgeon in the

United States! The hospital is filled with children with congenital heart defects, you can operate all day long every day, and you do not have any other responsibilities. Nobody could ask for anything better. Is it a problem with your title? Because if it is, I could promote you, and if it is money, I could see that you get more money." We were paid something like five or six thousand dollars a year. I said, "No, it is not that." I did leave, and fortunately Al Blalock and I remained very close, good friends over the years.

I enjoyed being back at Yale and starting that heart service. It was good fun. It was a long time, though, before we were doing any open hearts. We did not even have a heart-lung machine. We were operating on patent ductus arteriosus patients, coarctation of the aorta, pulmonary stenosis, and other congenital abnormalities, all of which could be treated with the heart beating, performing its normal function. We also had patients with cardiac constriction from pericarditis. Since there had not been any prior treatment, there was a backlog of children with congenital heart difficulties, and I was just as busy in New Haven as I had been in Baltimore. There were not many surgical centers that were doing surgery of this sort, certainly none in Connecticut, western Massachusetts, or the eastern part of New York state. We had a very busy and active service.

I only stayed at Yale for two years, because I was then offered the position of chairman of surgery at Indiana. That year, in 1948, there were three chairmanships to be filled, and the same people were considered for each of them. Bill Longmire went to UCLA, which had no hospital at the time, but that job turned out to be a great appointment for him. Mike DeBakey went down to Houston where everybody was opposed to the whole business of cardiac surgery. He had a struggle, but it turned out well for him. I went to Indiana, where I had many happy years. I was chairman of the Department of Surgery and had a house staff that did general surgery as well as thoracic and cardiac surgery. Since I was training surgeons, I thought that I personally should keep my hand in general surgical procedures as well as in cardiovascular procedures. Most of the patients who were referred to me, and there were gobs of them, had cardiovascular problems, such as cardiac and peripheral vascular disease, aneurysms, and things of that sort. In addition, a lot of doctors referred general surgical patients to me. I would always ask them whether it was all right if I had one of my associates take over, and the doctors always said yes, but every week I would do two or three cases, a colon resection, a cholecystectomy, or something of that sort. I think it was the right thing to do, because that way my house staff knew that I could operate well on other things besides the heart and blood vessels and could make sure they learned techniques properly.

The heart-lung machine that John Gibbon developed was very expensive, and it was not commercially available. Gibbon demonstrated on May 6, 1953, that the heart-lung machine could take over the function of the heart and lungs successfully while you opened the heart and did what you needed to do. Shortly after that, various people began working madly to develop other kinds of heart-lung machines that would be easier to acquire and less expensive. Walt Lillehei and Richard DeWall in Minnesota were really responsible for developing the bubble oxygenator. Lillehei showed that you could use it as a substitute for the function of the heart and lungs for a short period, and he began to operate on patients, making some very significant contributions of a technical nature. We owe a great deal to him.

I did not try to get a machine like the Gibbon machine, even though John Gibbon and I were good friends. I did not have the money. DeWall and Lillehei were successful with the bubble oxygenator, so I went that route. We made our own bubble oxygenators at first, but then they became available commercially. Denton Cooley, for example, devised one that had a base of steel, and it was manufactured and sold commercially. Soon that technology spread all over the world because anybody could make or acquire a bubble oxygenator, and they were inexpensive. They worked well for short procedures, and so they became popular everywhere. We used the bubble oxygenator for a while, until eventually we began to work with the better disc oxygenators.

We had a wonderful lady working with us who was a nurse, and I put her in charge of the experimental surgical laboratory. When we first started using an oxygenator on patients, she would come to the OR and operate the bubble oxygenator. Her name was Ms. Brumbaugh, and she was a self-trained perfusionist. We soon started using a disc oxygenator that we purchased. They were not terribly expensive. Kay and Cross developed one, and there were a number of others available. They were a nuisance to clean, wash, sterilize, and get together again, but they worked, and they were safer and better than the bubble oxygenator.

We began by doing a mixture of congenital and adult-acquired patients. We were fortunate in Indiana in that we had the largest university children's hospital in the country, and we had many, many children that needed operations, but we also began to attract a lot of adult patients. This was the late 1950s and early 1960s, and at the beginning we made some mistakes. The operations on the mitral valve carried some risk, and at first the total repair of tetralogy of Fallot was very complex. When we first began putting patches in the ventricular septum in cases of ventricular septal defect, we did not understand where the conduction mechanism was located, and we produced some cases of total heart block.

The pacemakers at that time were also pretty poor. The problem with the pacemakers then was that they were not as reliable as they are now, and the batteries did not last as long. At the beginning the principal trouble was with the electrodes. They would fatigue and break. The patient would have to come back, and you would have to mend the electrodes or replace them. We were putting pacemakers in at one time below the costal margin, and I put one in a lady who was fat and had been much fatter. She lost a lot of weight, and she would play with this pacemaker, turning it all around beneath the skin. She did that until she broke the wires. Eventually somebody was smart enough to say, "The wires in a watch or clock last for years and years and they do not break. There must be something good about those wires." So that technology helped to solve the problem of broken electrodes.

Although we were not doing coronary artery bypass operations, we were doing everything we could think of to try to increase myocardial circulation in patients who had coronary disease, hoping that creating pericardial adhesions would do some good. We were struggling, and we knew it was questionable whether we were getting anywhere, but there was nothing else to do. I will tell a story about an incident that gave me great respect for people who are careful in reaching conclusions about clinical work. I had a patient, a big husky man, who lived down in southern Indiana or over in Kentucky, and he was sent to me because he had severe angina and was taking an average of a hundred nitroglycerin tablets a day. His angina would occur at rest, or any time. At that time we were using various indirect methods, hoping that they would help the myocardial circulation. As he was being anaesthetized, he developed ventricular fibrillation, and I started external cardiac massage. Fortunately, the anesthesiologist could ventilate him. I was compressing his heart rhythmically, but nothing was happening. I told one of the people in the operating room to go down and tell his family that we were having difficulty, and that I doubted that he would survive. The person came back and said that the family could not be found, that they were in the chapel. I thought that was a good place for them. Anyway, I kept compressing his heart and applying electrical shocks, and long after I thought it possible, the heart started beating vigorously. He woke up and I cancelled the operation. I was not going to operate on him after all that. I went to see him that evening, and he was very alert and had taken no nitroglycerin. He said, "I have not had any angina. Whatever you did was good." The next day he did not have any angina and did not take any nitroglycerin. He did not take any for the few days that he remained in the hospital. The last time I saw him was six or seven years later when he told me he told me he was free of angina. The day before he had been rabbit hunting and had walked five or six miles. The day after I operated on him he said, "Doctor, did something go wrong with the electrical system while I was in the operating room? I thought I felt a shock, and it was the damnedest shock you can imagine." I said, "You felt plenty of them," and I told him what had happened. If we had done the operation and created pericardial adhesions we would have thought it was a great procedure when, in fact, he may not have had coronary artery disease at all.

By the time cardiac bypass procedures came along, I was ready to turn over my operative work to my associates. The first coronary bypass operation done by Mike DeBakey was an extraordinary thing. Mike DeBakey has a mind that is appreciative of new things, and yet he did a vein bypass operation in 1964 that was successful and was still successful seven years later. The graft was patent, and yet during those seven years Mike did not do a single other coronary bypass operation. I am sure that others have passed over opportunities like that. The interesting thing is that they did that operation off the pump. They had the pump ready, but they did it without going on bypass, and now we have circled back around to that method today. In the early 1950s Bill Longmire was trying to remove obstructing atheroma from coronary arteries on the beating heart out in Los Angeles, the so-called thromboendarterectomy, which is pretty difficult to do with the heart beating. The outcome of those operations was not that favorable.

When I gave up my chairmanship at Indiana, they appointed a chairman that I did not particularly like. I stayed around there for a year or two and had an office that I suppose I could have kept for the rest of my life at the university. I was still getting a small university salary, and I was operating and had a good practice of referred patients. One of the residents that I had trained was a very popular general surgeon in Indianapolis, and he was the chief of the surgical service at St. Vincent's Hospital. He asked me to come over to St. Vincent's and start a cardiac surgical program there. I was very impressed with the sister who was in charge of the hospital, and I had nothing to lose and everything to gain. I went across town to St. Vincent's. It was affiliated with the university, but at St. Vincent's I not only had patients who were referred from other places, but for the first time I had patients from Indianapolis. Before that my patients were mostly from out of town. We were just overwhelmed with cardiac cases, and I got a bright young fellow, John Isch, to come to work with me just after he finished his residency. He was an excellent surgeon, and the two of us worked ourselves to death that first year, night and day, because the volume was too much for two people. John and I had to have some help, so we got first one surgeon and then another to join us, and things were going well. I did that for seven years. It was essentially a private practice, and it enabled me to make some money for the first time in my life. After that, one of my friends who is head of the surgical service of the Uniformed Services University in Bethesda said, "Why not come and help me?" By that time things were going well at St. Vincent's and I was not needed there any more. I thought I might as well do something different, so I went to Bethesda, Maryland, and helped him acquire a staff and get his department going.

The last operation I did was a Bentall procedure. The man had wide-open aortic insufficiency and a big ascending aortic aneurysm. The operation went nicely, and the patient did well. I put in a valve, a conduit, and reimplanted the coronary arteries. I was interested in the conduits because I had worked in the experimental laboratory on plastic materials as vascular substitutes in the early days of vascular surgery. I heard that my friend Arthur Blakemore was working on them too, and that he had operated on a patient and had inserted an aortic graft made of nylon. In 1953 I had a patient who had a large abdominal aneurysm with a retroperitoneal leak. We did not have a suitable homograft. We were putting plastic grafts in animals but not patients. I called Arthur and asked him if he had really put a nylon graft in a patient. He said, "Yes, I did, a couple of weeks ago, and the patient has done well." I told the patient what I was going to do, and I operated on him. We put in a nylon graft, and that was the second time a plastic graft was used in a human, in July of 1953.

Mike DeBakey was using homografts, but once I used the nylon graft, I thought, "There is no sense in using homografts; these are better." It turned out to be true, and we did a pile of them. I started out using nylon, which was stronger in the beginning than Orlon or Dacron. I did not know that after four or five years it would begin to wear out, and I had to get the patients back and do them over. I was not going to allow any of them to have an expanding aneurysm again, so I reoperated on all except one. He lived in Ohio or Pennsylvania, and I wrote him a letter and told him I thought it was important. My letter was not returned, so I know he got it.

As I said, I left Indiana and went to the Uniformed Services University in Bethesda.

After I got there, I wrote a biography of Leo Eloesser, and it was published in 1979. Then I wrote *The Evolution of Cardiac Surgery*, on which I had actually been working off and on for about ten years, but I finished it in Bethesda. I think it is a useful book, and for that sort of book it has done well. Recently I finished writing a biography of John Gibbon, and now I must find somebody who is willing to publish and promote it. It is not that I want to make money from it, I just want people to know about him. I imagine that I could get it published by the Indiana University Press, which did such a beautiful job with *The Evolution of Cardiac Surgery*, or by some other university press.

If I were advising a young person who is thinking about a medical career now, I would say to go ahead and do it. It is a wonderful opportunity for a person to spend his life doing something that is worthwhile and really interesting. There have been a lot of changes in hospitals and in the business of medicine with managed care, but I still think medicine is tops. If I were living my life over again I would hope that I could become a doctor, and that if I became a doctor I would hope that I could then become a surgeon.

It is great fun to think back over all these times. Those of us who have been in this particular area of work have been lucky, because it has been so rewarding. To have been there from the beginning was a rare opportunity. I have been fortunate to know people like Alfred Blalock, Walt Lillehei, and Jack Gibbon. Bill Bigelow made a great contribution because of his devoted interest in the possibility of using cold to stop the heart for a moment and not have the patient harmed by the lack of circulation. In the area of valve surgery, you would have to include my English friend, Dennis Melrose, who did some of the first important work on the use of potassium to stop the heart. You would also have to include Donald Ross, at the National Heart Hospital in London, who transplanted the pulmonary valve to replace the diseased aortic valve.

Geoffrey Wooler was one of the first doctors to use pericardial pig valves and to constrict the mitral valve annulus. They worked very well. When I first learned that Donald Ross, Ake Senning, and Geoffrey Wooler were taking the patient's own fascia lata and making that into valves, I thought, "This is the answer. It is autogenous and has a good strong structure." So I hopped on a plane and went to London to see Ross, to Zurich to see Senning, and to Leeds to see Geoffrey Wooler. When I came home I put in a great many fascia lata valves, but they began to go bad pretty soon. We had a conference up in Toronto on fascia lata valves, and unfortunately I had operated on more patients using that technique than anybody in North America. Most of them had done ten or fifteen, or at most a couple of dozen. I had operated on seventy-three. To my dismay, they did not do well. It has been a long struggle, and it is not over yet. Somebody will improve the valves, I am sure. The perfect valve is not available yet by any means.

The oxygenators have come a long way, though. Just think of that cumbersome Gibbon screen oxygenator that required exposing a film of blood over many square inches of surface. Now a little membrane oxygenator can do the job. I think you would have to include George Clowes among the great contributors, because he really stuck with the membrane oxygenator concept when most people thought it was too cumbersome. His membrane oxygenators *were* cumbersome, difficult to make, and hard to assemble and use, but I would include him as an important contributor.

I have no doubt that the best elective operation we ever did was the coronary artery bypass graft. If you remove a gallbladder, the patient is relieved of his symptoms, and perhaps in a rare case some disaster is prevented. With the bypass operation, you give new life to a person. There are patients living long lives in families where none of the men ever lived past the age of forty. Many people in their seventies are out playing tennis as a result of that operation. It was a hard struggle coming up, and those of us who are old enough to have tried those various indirect methods long ago can hardly believe what has happened. We had to wait for the technology to develop. Arthur Vineberg and René Favaloro would be surprised to see what has occurred.

Bibliography

Shumacker HB Jr. Use of the Subclavian Artery in the Surgical Treatment of Coarctation of the Aorta. *Surg Gynec Obstet.* 1951; 93:491–495.

Shumacker HB Jr. Surgical Repair of Atrial Septal Defects. *Ann Surg.* 1953; 138:404–414.

Shumacker HB Jr. Plastic Grafts for Aortic Substitution in Man. *Arch Surg.* 1957; 75:413–422.

Shumacker HB Jr, Lurie PR. Patent Ductus Arteriosus with Pulmonary Hypertension. *Arch Surg.* 1958; 76:179–192.

Shumacker HB Jr. The Surgical Volumes of the History of the United States Army Medical Department in World War II. Vascular Surgery. *Arch Surg.* 1960; 80:379–383.

Burns WH, Shumacker HB Jr. Implantable Mechanical Cardiac Substitute. *J Cardiovasc Surg* (Torino). 1968; 9:17–21.

Shumacker HB Jr, Barnes DL, King H. Ruptured Abdominal Aortic Aneurysms. *Ann Surg.* 1973; 177:772–779.

Shumacker HB Jr. The Value of Accurate Observations and Clear Clinical Reports: A Tribute to Harvey W. Cushing. *Surgery.* 1975; 78:269–272.

Shumacker HB Jr. A History of Modern Treatment of Aortic Aneurysms. *World J Surg.* 1980; 4:503–509.

Shumacker HB Jr. Reminiscences of John H. Gibbon, Jr., MD. *Ann Thorac Surg.* 2003; 76:S2195–S2196

Geoffrey Wooler, FRCS

(b. 1911)

In London, a thoracic surgeon makes an incision in the chest, and he is confined to the chest. In Leeds, an operation may start in the chest, but the incision can be extended the full length of the body if necessary. I have seen the fundus of the bladder taken out through a chest incision. He [Vernon Thompson] just looked at me and said, "How frightful!"

— On surgery at the
General Infirmary at Leeds

Interviewed June 10, 1997

My family has lived in Leeds for over 250 years. We have a marriage certificate between Hannah Wainwright and John Wooler dated December 22, 1778. We have a collection of certificates from that date until today: marriage certificates, baptisms, and all that nonsense.

My father was a successful businessman, and he stabilized the finances of the family. My mother, unfortunately, was blind. She had picked up an infection when my brother, the first child, was born, and she lost her sight the following year. It was seven years before they decided to have another child. In 1911 I was the next child to arrive, and my sister came a year after I was born. I went to a private kindergarten school run by four spinsters, the Misses Newman. I had to be looked after by a nursemaid because of my mother's disability, a maid called Winnie. Winnie taught me to sew, crochet, and knit at a very early age, and I would like to think that her tuition at that time had something to do with my success later in life as a surgeon. At nine years of age, I went to Leeds Grammar School, and then after that, at age thirteen I went to Giggleswick School. The headmaster, a Mr. Douglas, was a devout Christian, and we had prayers two or three times a day. I managed to get eleven credits in the school certificate, which was sufficient for me to be exempted from the Cambridge entrance examination. I still lacked a credit in Latin, so I had to take the exam again and managed to pass. I obtained a place at Selwyn College, Cambridge, but I had not made up my mind which subject to read. My brother had just become a lawyer in Leeds, and I thought I might be able to follow his example, so I put myself down for law. I was horrified to discover when you are reading law at Cambridge, you had to learn Roman law in Latin for the first two years. It was a subject that I hated, but our tutors said they wished us to be "cultured lawyers," not just lawyers.

It was during my third term, after I had been there for nearly a year, that I decided to change. One of my friends, John McKeller, had been at Giggleswick with me and afterwards at Selwyn College. One day he took me around the dissecting room and showed me the human body with all the dissected muscles. I thought this was fascinating, and I decided to give up law and change to medicine.

I passed the second MB examination at Cambridge at the end of my third year and obtained a BA degree at the same time. In 1930 I went to the London Hospital to do my clinical work. My first dressership was to a Mr. Russell Howard, who would not change things unless he was really forced to. In the operating theatre, he still retained large cisterns of carbolic acid used in the Listerian period for irrigating wounds. He never changed clothes to do an operation, and in the operating theatre he wore a stiff collar, a waistcoat with a gold Albert pocketwatch and boots. He was also a farmer, so presumably that is why he liked to wear boots. All he did was to put on a large rubber apron to protect his clothing, his mask merely covering his chin, and then he would start scrubbing up. He was actually the senior surgeon at the London Hospital, was a great teacher, and taught me a lot about surgery. He used to say, "Surgery is anatomy, common sense, and nothing more."

The other surgeons at the London Hospital were really quite an eminent crowd. There was Sir Henry Souttar, who later flew out to India to operate on an Indian princess who had carcinoma of the tongue; Hugh Cairns, who became the Nuffield Professor at Oxford; and Sir James Walton, who was the surgeon to the royal household. He was very fast and a very good technician. Finally there was Tudor Edwards, who was one of the leading thoracic surgeons during the 1930s. I had no difficulty passing the final examinations and qualified in 1937. My first house surgical appointment that I had was with Norman Patterson, the ear, nose, and throat consultant, who was a fantastically good surgeon, but he was also completely absentminded, and I had to make sure that he did the right operation on each patient. This was especially difficult because he always had a long list of operations to do. On one occasion he removed the tonsils inadvertently, but the patient seemed quite pleased when he was told about it.

After my appointment with Norman Patterson I joined Tudor Edwards in 1937. He was one of the pioneers of thoracic surgery in England, and while I was with him, he had his first heart attack. He had been to Grenoble University to receive an honorary degree and was taken ill on the way home. After that I was house surgeon to Russell Howard, the general surgeon for whom I had been a dresser.

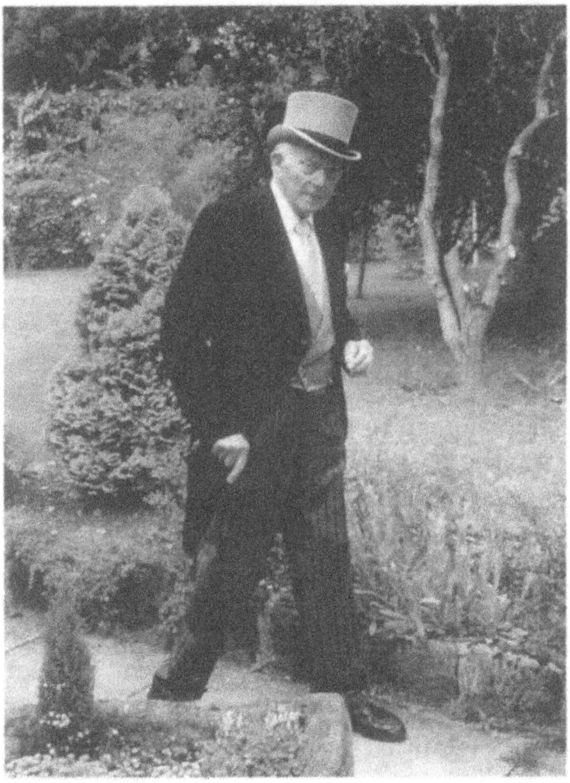

Geoffrey Wooler

In 1937 I joined the Territorial Army, and in August of 1939 I was called up for duty. I had not taken my final fellowship exam, and Russell Howard wanted me to stay and pass the exams before going into the services. I was the medical officer to the Second Battalion of the Queen's Westminsters, and as I knew everybody in the battalion, I agreed to stay with them.

After about a year I was getting a bit tired

of it, and Tudor Edwards asked me to have dinner with him. He said, "You are wasting your time here. I want you to go to South Wales to look after the chest casualties. The Germans are bombing the ports and airfields, and there is nobody in South Wales to do the thoracic surgery." I was loaned, although still in the army, to the Emergency Medical Service to deal with chest casualties. While I was there I was able to take and pass the final fellowship, and I stayed there for about a year until the work quieted down.

I was then sent to the Seventieth General Hospital in Oxford. This was an interesting time when penicillin had just been introduced. Mrs. Florey, the wife of Howard W. Florey of penicillin fame, used to come down to see us, asking if she could be of help. One day we admitted a young officer who was seriously ill. He had been married for two to three weeks. He and his bride had gone to the Lake District on their honeymoon. While there, he had developed a boil on his nose, squeezed it, soon developed a severe headache, and went into a coma with a cavernous sinus thrombosis. We fed him by tube, and he remained unconscious for at least ten days. Mrs. Florey gave all the penicillin she could spare for him, but it had no effect. One day she said, "One of my cases has completely recovered, and I can let you have much more. Tomorrow I will send triple the dose." She would come every day and bring the penicillin in her handbag and then take the patient's urine back in the same handbag, because they could extract the penicillin from it. We were all worried that this young man would never regain consciousness or would never be able to speak properly. After he received the triple dose, he woke up within a few hours. The nurse in charge was taking his pulse, and he looked at her and said, "Come, come, nurse, my days of frolicking are over. I am a married man," so we knew that he had no brain damage.

In November of 1942 I went with the First Army to North Africa, landed at Algiers in the third convoy. I was still with the Seventieth General Hospital. One day I was asked to go up to the front to a place called Sejename, where a factory had been converted to a hospital, to help a surgeon who was dealing with a lot of casualties. The third day I was there, we were dive-bombed. It was very noisy and rather dangerous for a short time. The Stuka dive-bombers came in suddenly out of the sun so we couldn't see them. The bombs and bullets came through the roof of the tobacco factory, the wood stove that was in our bedroom disappeared through the open door, and all patients in the adjoining room were killed. At the time I was not frightened, but I had an awful reaction afterwards.

Several months later I was again at the front with the French Army, and one day our senior surgeon arrived with an American colonel called Ed Churchill. He looked around the ward and asked to see our operating room and instruments. He picked up a Doyen lung forceps and asked if I had ever used it. He did not know that I had worked for Tudor Edwards. I said, "Quite honestly, no." Then I looked at him and asked, "Are you interested in lung surgery?" It turned out he was the senior thoracic surgeon of the American Army, and prior to the war had been professor of surgery and dean of Harvard Medical School.

Our largest number of casualties occurred in the last stand of the German Army at Cape Bon in North Africa. We were mass-ing all of our troops for a final attack, but the Germans must have been alerted and attacked first. In my unit, we took 580 casualties in one day. We obviously couldn't operate on such a large number of people, and started with the ones that we thought had a chance of survival, but it was some hours, about half a day, before other surgical teams arrived to help us. I did an enormous number of operations during the war.

In July of 1943 I was ordered to join the invasion force for the island of Pantelleria, which was the first part of Europe to be taken by the Allies. We went over on LCIs (Landing Craft Infantry). The Americans had built LCIs and LCTs (Landing Craft Tanks), and were trying them out prior to the invasion of Sicily and later Normandy. We were fired on by the Germans as we landed. The local inhabitants had been using a large gallery dug into a hillside as an air-raid shelter, and it was there that we set up our hospital. The place had previously been used to store petrol for submarines, and the floor was raised on duck boarding. It was infested with fleas; indeed, we could see them jumping at us. The whole place was full of fleas, flies, and feces, and we had to operate under those conditions. I de-fleaed myself twice a day. Gradually my clothing became spotted with my own blood from fleabites. I eventually discarded my clothes, and when we left I reported back to duty in Italian Navy fatigue kit.

We went on through the invasions of Sicily and Italy and eventually were involved with the battle for Monte Cassino. There were so many dead at Cassino that the smell was terrible, and it took us ten days to bury the bodies and to clear the area assigned to us. I took a camera case from a dead German that I still use today. The German dugouts at Cassino had been lined with furniture taken from the local houses, and they looked very comfortable. I worked in a field surgical unit, to which most assignments were for about a year because it was so physically and mentally exhausting.

I served in that unit for fourteen months, and during that period I operated on fifteen hundred patients. They were all serious cases, and I operated on abdominal injuries, compound fractures, chest injuries, and any other "priority one" injuries. I was finally demobilized in February of 1946, after nearly seven years in the army.

When I got back to London there were many opportunities. Several people approached me offering me a job. For instance, I was offered a consultant job in ear, nose, and throat surgery at the London Hospital where I had trained. I was offered an assistant professorial appointment in Newcastle, and I was offered a consultant post in Cape Town, but I had quite definitely decided to continue with thoracic surgery. I really enjoyed working as surgical first assistant for Tudor Edwards, who was an extremely good technician. I joined him in February of 1946, but he died of a heart attack in August of that year. The London Hospital was not the same without him.

I was then approached by John Lachmore, who was a consulting surgeon on the staff at the General Infirmary in Leeds. He came to see me in London and said, "Phillip Allison wants someone in Leeds to be his assistant. Would you be interested?" I said I would think it over. I asked Vernon Thompson what he thought about this, and he said, "I will release you for a year. You won't like it. It's terrible in Yorkshire; they speak another language. If you don't like it you can come back and join me." I rang up John Latchmore and said that I would like to join Phillip Allison. I had been away from home since I was thirteen, and I could not think of anything better than going back to Leeds. Six months later, Vernon Thompson invited me to have dinner with him in London. He said, "How are you getting on?" I told him that I was enjoying it immensely. He asked me why. I said, "In London a thoracic surgeon makes an incision in the chest and he is confined to the chest. In Leeds an operation may start in the chest, but the incision can be extended the full length of the body if necessary. I have seen the fundus of the bladder taken out through a chest incision, which would be unheard of in London." He just looked at me and said, "How frightful!"

I stayed in Leeds and the following year became a consultant on the staff of the Leeds General Infirmary. We were operating on a lot of patients with tuberculosis, doing lung resections and thoracoplasties. I don't know how many ribs I have taken out. There was a surgeon at Killingbeck Hospital, a Polish man, Dr. Roscyski, and he used to take ribs out like teeth. I have never seen ribs come out so fast. We never thought tuberculosis would disappear like it did. Drugs were the cure, not surgery.

I became interested in portocaval shunts. Glenn Morrow came over from Bethesda to spend a year with us, and he showed me how to do the operation. I was fascinated with it. Glenn did the first case in Leeds, and I continued the good work doing a "side-to-side" shunt. Dr. Sheila Sherlock from the Hammersmith Hospital began sending me patients from London. I would, from time to time, go back to London to see how the patients were progressing. On one of these visits, I was introduced to Dennis Melrose, who was working on a prototype heart-lung machine. I was most interested in what he was doing and his prototype machine. I collect clocks and thought having something like that working in the operating room was wonderful. I kept writing to Dennis asking if we could buy one. He eventually persuaded a firm in London, New Electronic Products, to build three pumps. The first one went to Hammersmith, the second to Moscow, and the third came to Leeds. They were the first heart-lung machines built in this country. That was in 1956. Two benefactors helped us with the purchase, the Bernard Cayzer Trust Fund and the Nuffield Foundation.

We were told that we could only have the machine on the condition that we would work closely with the Department of Physiology in their laboratory. We wanted to use the pump on dogs to train a team to do the surgery so that everybody would know what was expected of them. The Department of Physiology at Leeds helped us and provided facilities in their animal operating theatre. I found out that there was a dog dealer at Thirsk in North Yorkshire where we could buy stray dogs for three pounds each. I bought a van and our technician, Leslie Catchpole, and I would drive up there and collect them as needed.

The original Melrose machines had bar pumps, but they produced an unacceptable amount of haemolysis. I asked Dennis Melrose if my research fellow, Peter Nixon, could join him at Hammersmith for a while. Together they removed the bar pumps and replaced them with the so-called DeBakey roller pumps. They also altered some of the tubing connections, and these changes reduced the haemolysis to a minimum. The first plastic tubing that we obtained was too rough. Glenn Morrow brought a whole lot of tubing from America as well as some connectors and cannulae, which were most helpful.

After six months in the lab, our morale improved as more of the dogs survived being on the pump, and we thought it was time to move our equipment to the General Infirmary and to begin a clinical service. The cardiologists were happy to send us a number of patients, most of whom had liver and kidney disease and were in the last stage of heart failure. The chest X-rays would show an enormous heart filling the chest with only the upper lobes of the lungs visible. At a meeting I remember Lord Brock saying he was surprised that we accepted such advanced cases for surgery.

Almost all of our early patients had mitral insufficiency. Our first successful mitral valve repair was in 1957. In those early days, the operative mortality was at least 50 percent, but the patients were all high risk and the mortality of those on the waiting list was almost as high. Reviewing those patient's records later, we realized that many should not have been accepted for surgery. At that time there was no artificial valve available, so the valve (either mitral or aortic) had to be improved a lot for the patient to survive. This was frequently achieved, but some of the patients died a few days later because of the lack of modern postoperative care. We did not have an intensive care unit, no ventilator, and no haemodynamic monitoring. I remember a time we stayed in the hospital five days and nights taking turns to ventilate a patient by squeezing the bag on the anesthetic machine in three- or four-hour shifts.

I first got the idea of mitral valve repair when I was in Munich visiting Professor Zenker. His young German assistant had been working on the anatomy of the heart, and he showed me several dissected specimens that clearly demonstrated the aortic annulus, the mitral annulus, and the tricuspid annulus. After looking at them I remember saying to him that the aortic annulus is a very tough structure and that we should be able to suspend the mitral annulus from the tissue of the aortic annulus.

The incompetence caused by the dilatation of the mitral annulus with minimal disease of the cusps and chordae is the easiest to repair. The incompetence is usually through the center of the valve, apparently due to laxity of the mural cusp, so it must be elevated and tightened by deep sutures which are inserted across each commissure but not tied immediately. These sutures act as "stay sutures," and when they are pulled upon, it can be seen if they would deform the cusps when tied. Frequently they do, so the offending suture is held while a second suture is inserted. If it produces no deformity, it is tied and the offending first suture removed. This method also prevents damage to an aortic cusp. Mixed lesions are dealt with by mobilizing the cusps as much as possible without increasing the incompetence. Adherent commissures are opened up with scissors, adherent cordae separated, and the valve dealt with as I have already described, except the deep sutures must be further out so as not to diminish the lumen when the valve is open. Sometimes only one commissure requires a deep suture.

It was not really possible to work out how

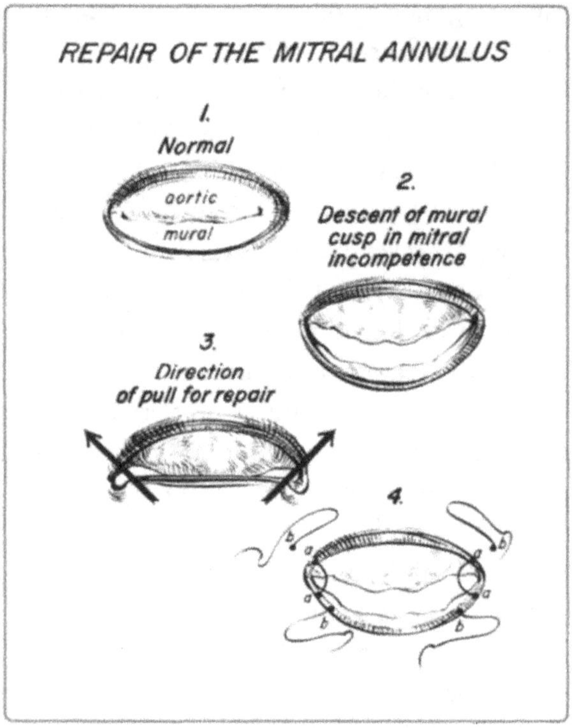

Illustration of Mr. Wooler's operation for mitral insufficiency

to repair a diseased valve in the experimental animal using healthy dogs. It was necessary to work out the technique on humans, and I think this is why most American surgeons concentrated on developing a mechanical valve rather than a technique for repair.

Sometime during that period, at a meeting of the European Cardiological Society in Naples, I was asked to chair a panel to discuss various methods of valve repair. Donald Ross was there as well as Lord Brock and surgeons from the whole of Europe, each claiming he had a lesser mortality than the previous speaker. The last man to speak claimed a mortality of 5 percent, which I thought was pretty ridiculous. At the end of the session, I had to get up and summarize what had been said and talk about our work at Leeds. I stood up and said, "I am one of those people who believe that our life on earth is really just a part of our continuous existence. Under these conditions I have no operative mortality." A report in the Naples newspaper the next day stated, "Professor Wooler believes in eternity so he has had no operative mortality."

In 1958 our cardiac surgery unit was working nicely, and we were having reasonable success. Toward the end of that year, I noticed a swelling on the right side of my chest, which gradually got larger. Professor Goligher aspirated it twice, but nothing was proved about the diagnosis. I thought I had better have something done about it and went to Hammersmith to see my friend there, Bill Cleland. He operated on me and removed a tuberculous abscess from the side of my chest beneath the pectoral muscle. I also had a right apical infiltrate, and so was put on drugs which I did not like. This all happened just before my first visit to America. I did not tell anyone about it, but when I went over I had not really recovered; the wound had hardly healed. I was the visiting professor at the University of Virginia and two other medical centers and was there for three weeks. I flew back on the British Airways' airplane called the Comet, which was later removed from service after two crashes caused by metal fatigue.

The Hammersmith surgeons recommended that I should give up heart surgery altogether, so I put David Watson on the staff. He was a young cardiac surgeon who had trained at the London Hospital and had an interest in congenital heart problems. After about a year I was in reasonable shape again, so I came back and started doing more open-heart operations.

In 1964 the Medical University of Istanbul asked me to bring my whole team there for a week to help them. They were in the process of developing an open-heart programme and various members of their operating room and anesthesia staff had previously visited Leeds for several weeks, observing our staff and procedures. It was about three months before we could clear up our schedule to go, and in the meantime there was a revolution in Turkey. The army deposed the older professors at the medical school who had invited us to come and replaced them with a group of younger men. The day before we arrived, the old professors were let out of the university compound where they had been detained, presumably because the army thought it would create a bad impression if we saw our hosts all locked up. When we arrived at the Istanbul airport, a fleet of Mercedes cars met us, took us across the Bosporus to Scutari, past the Florence Nightingale Hospital, to a sanitarium up in the snow-covered hills, and there we were kept. The young professors had kidnapped us, determined that we should not share any of our surgical secrets with their elderly rivals, and we were kept in this isolated spot for a week. Living conditions there were primitive, as indeed was the operating theatre.

Their heart-lung machine, if I remember correctly, was a Wolff machine with a bubble oxygenator. It was still in a packing case and no doubt had been taken from the university before the old professors were released. I told them I was not prepared to operate on a patient until I was sure that their equipment would work and asked that we be allowed to perform some trials on dogs. In Turkey they use goats instead of dogs for experimental work. I noticed that every time we did a goat experiment, we had goat for lunch the following day. When I questioned them about this, they answered that it would be a pity to waste such excellent meat!

There was a lot of local publicity about our work, and several reporters were milling about in the theatre each day. After a few days we had everything working, more or less successfully, and I thought before we left, it would please and satisfy them for us to do two simple operations. I chose two patients whom I knew we could do at a normal temperature with just inflow occlusion, if necessary; a pulmonary valve stenosis and a straightforward atrial septal defect. Both patients recovered, and we were hailed as a great success in the local press.

One day, one of my surgical friends in Paris, Philip Daumet, rang and said, "Geoff, I've got a first-class surgeon here who has escaped from Romania. We don't really have a place for him, but I don't think you could find anyone better." I flew over to Paris and watched him operate, and I decided to get him and his wife to come to Leeds. His name was Marion Ionescu. Prior to his escape, he had been dealing almost entirely with congenital heart conditions when he was the chief of cardiac surgery in Bucharest.

I persuaded him and his wife to come to Leeds and asked him to concentrate on mitral and aortic valve problems, because we had such a long waiting list. For valves unsuitable for repair, we first tried pig valves mounted on a cloth-covered frame, but they were not too successful—probably the sterilization process was at fault. Next we tried constructing a valve from the patients own fascia lata taken from the thigh. This was an improvement, but the fascia lata varies in

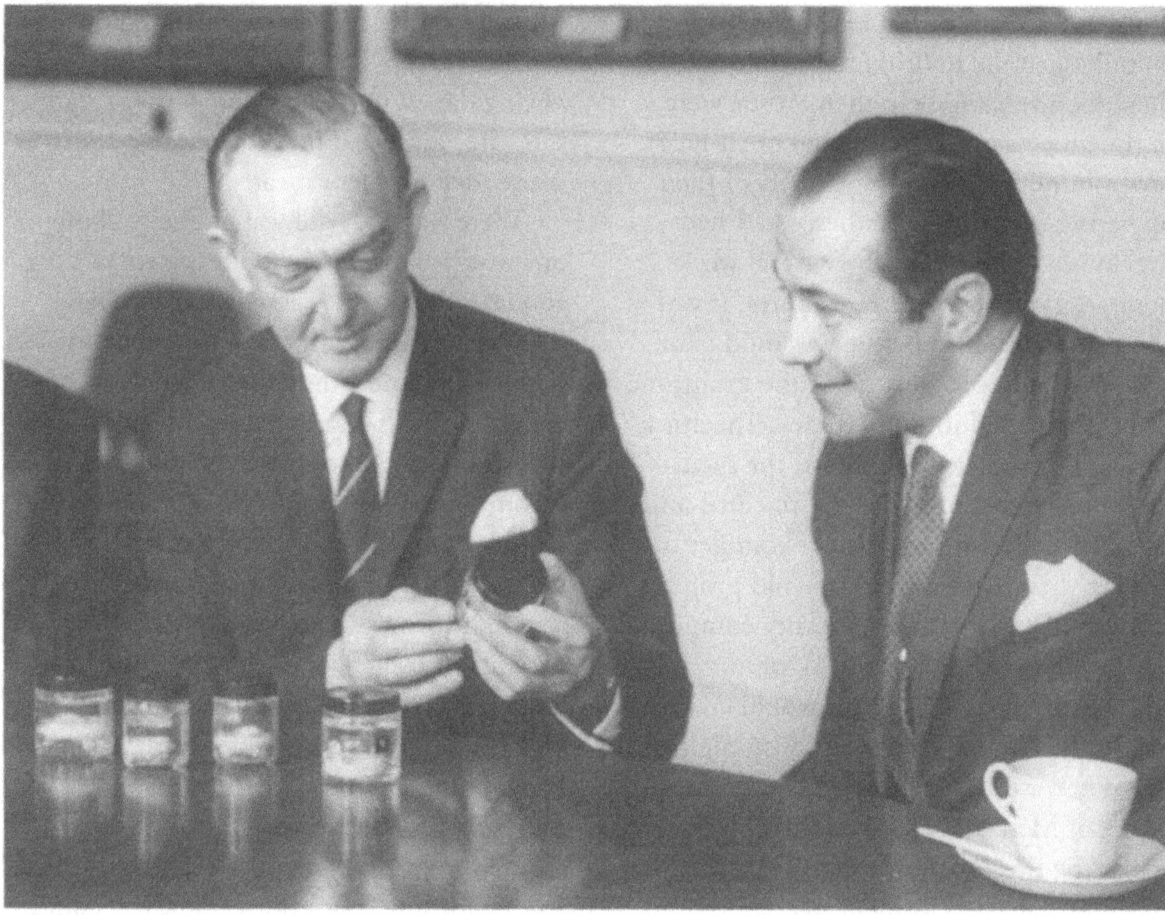

Geoffrey Wooler and Marion Ionescu inspecting porcine valves

thickness and texture and these valves did not last very long. Lastly, we began to use bovine pericardium fixed in gluteraldehyde, and some of these did extremely well. They lasted ten years or more, which is not bad for a biological valve.

While we had been busy developing cardiac surgery, we had observed other changes in the wider world of thoracic surgery. Tuberculosis had been eradicated. Patients with operable lung cancer were diminishing in number, and cancer of the stomach and oesophagus was being dealt with by the general surgeons. Coronary artery surgery had come into fashion with a flood of patients so that there was little time to do anything else. The daily repetition of similar operations did not interest me, so I retired to the Yorkshire Dales. I have been retired now for twenty-three years, almost as long as I was on the staff of the General Infirmary.

I have a country house in West Burton in Wensleydale, and I began spending a lot of time there. The local vicar came to see me, looked at me very seriously, and said that I was in for a very difficult time. He said I would become bored and depressed and when that happened I should come to see him for counseling. I said, "Look here old man, I have been waiting for this moment for years. I have so many things that I want to do, I just hope that I will have time to do them all."

I would like to thank Geoffrey Bunch, one of my former registrars, who has helped me to edit this article based on material published previously in my autobiography.

Would anybody like to help me with the garden?

Bibliography

Wooler GH. Subphrenic Abscess. *Thorax*. 1956; 11:211–222.

Allison PR, Wooler GH, Gunning AJ. Esophagojejunogastrostomy. *J Thorac Surg*. 1957; 33:738–748.

Austen WG, Wooler GH. Surgical Treatment of Mitral Stenosis by the Transventricular Approach with a Mechanical Dilator. *N Engl J Med.* 1960; 263:661–665.

Wooler GH, Nixon PG, Grimshaw VA, Watson DA. Experiences with the Repair of the Mitral Valve in Mitral Incompetence. *Thorax*. 1962; 17:49–57.

Ionescu MI, Wooler GH, Smith DR, Grimshaw VA. Mitral Valve Replacement with Aortic Heterografts in Humans. *Thorax*. 1967; 22:305–313.

Wooler GH. Experiences in Mitral Valve Surgery. *Anglo Ger Med Rev*. 1967; 4:39–41.

Wooler GH, Mashhour YA, Garcia JB, Holden MP, Ionescu MI. Pectus Excavatum. *Thorax*. 1969; 24:557–562.

Ionescu MI, Ross DN, Deac R, Grimshaw VA, Taylor SH, Whitaker W, Wooler GH. Autologous Fascia Lata for Heart Valve Replacement. *Thorax*. 1970; 25:46–56.

Holden MP, Wooler GH. Tracheo-oesophageal Fistula and Oesophageal Atresia: Results of 30 Years Experience. *Thorax*. 1970; 25:406–412.

Donnelly RJ, Smith DR, Ionescu MI, Wooler GH. Mitral Valve Repair; Results at 5 and 10 years. *Br Heart J*. 1972; 34:207.

Michael E. DeBakey, MD

(b. 1908)

I went downtown to get nylon shirt material, and when I got there, the clerk said, "We are fresh out of nylon, but we have a new material called Dacron."

— On the first prosthetic grafts for aortic aneurysm repair

Interview December 14, 1998

I was born in a small town in Louisiana called Lake Charles in 1908. My father was a pharmacist and ran two drug stores, where I worked as a boy, particularly in the summertime. In those days, the drug store was a hangout for doctors, especially in a small town, because they would come in to get their drugs. There wasn't a great deal of surgery; most of them were general practitioners. I think they influenced me; I know that I liked and admired them. I think that was the reason I wanted to go into medicine. As far back as I can remember, I wanted to be a doctor.

I did my undergraduate work at Tulane. After two years of college, I had enough credits to go into medical school, but also I wanted to get my bachelor's degree. I went around to some of my professors and asked them if I could take the rest of my college courses while I was in medical school. They were a little skeptical at first. Because I was a student instructor in zoology, the professor of zoology was a good friend of mine, and he helped me persuade the rest of the professors to approve my plan. When I finished my sophomore year in medical school, I graduated with my original college class and got my bachelor's and MD degrees in six years.

As a senior medical student, I met Dr. Alton Ochsner, who was the professor of surgery at Tulane. He was looking for some students to act as technicians in his lab. I volunteered, and he liked the work I was doing. He said to me, "You know, you ought to be a surgeon. I would like for you to come on my service when you graduate." After that I came under his influence and worked very closely with him. I did my internship and residency under Dr. Ochsner.

I went abroad for two years: one year with Dr. René Leriche at the University of Strasbourg, and one year with Dr. Kirschner at the University of Heidelberg. At that time Dr. Leriche was doing lumbar sympathectomies. He would resect a part of an artery with the idea of dilating it. He had a curious philosophy about that. He was a philosopher as well as a scientist, and he had all kinds of ideas, many of them very innovative. For example, he described the Leriche syndrome absolutely perfectly, without an aortogram. He even indicated what the surgical treatment ought to be. He said it wasn't possible yet, but said what it should be. Later a French surgeon in Paris, Dubost, did the first bypass for the Leriche syndrome, using a homograft, just as Leriche in his 1926 article had predicted it should be done. Leriche never did the procedure himself, he only did sympathectomies.

After two years in Europe, I came back to Tulane, and I was made an assistant professor. Dr. Ochsner had started the Ochsner Clinic, and I worked there for a while.

Dr. Ochsner had fallen out with the governor of Louisiana, Huey Long. I knew Dr. Vidrine, who had operated on the governor after he was shot. He was not really a surgeon; he was a general practitioner and only dabbled in surgery. A good surgeon wouldn't have missed the bleeding problem that was the cause of Long's death.

I went into the Army Medical Corps in 1942. Fred Rankin was the chief surgical consultant in Washington. He called Dr. Ochsner when he found out that I was going into the service and said that he wanted me to come up there. I immediately went into that department and was stationed in Washington, in the surgeon general's office. I wrote every surgical order for the surgeon general, and from time to time I would have to go to the surgeon general's library. Since it was a wonderful library, I came to believe that it should become the National Library of Medicine, and I began working to make that happen. Of course you can imagine the objections to my proposal, because the army didn't want to give it up. But they couldn't take care of it. They had been waiting to get a new building for over thirty years. They hadn't been able to get it, because a new library was a much lower priority than new military equipment. That's when I realized it didn't belong with the army.

I had the good fortune to write the medical task force report for the Hoover Commission in Washington after the war, and recommended that the army's medical library should become the National Library of Medicine. There were about twenty recommendations in that report, and when I briefed Mr. Hoover on it, he said, "You know, I have over fifty task forces, and if everybody comes in with some twenty recommendations, who is going to read those reports?" He said he wanted the single recommendation that I thought was most important, so I said it was the library, and that's what went into the report. John Kennedy in the House and Senator Hill in the Senate picked it up, and I worked with Senator Hill's staff to develop the legislation for it. Everything went smoothly until just before the Democratic Convention, which was to be held in Chicago. That was the convention that nominated Adlai Stevenson. A little quarrel developed between the congressmen in Chicago and others about the location of the library. The congressmen in Chicago were being pressured by the AMA to put it in Chicago. We didn't want it there; we wanted it at the NIH in Washington. The speaker of the House, a fellow named Sam Rayburn from Texas, tabled it. Senator Hill called me and told me what had happened. He said,

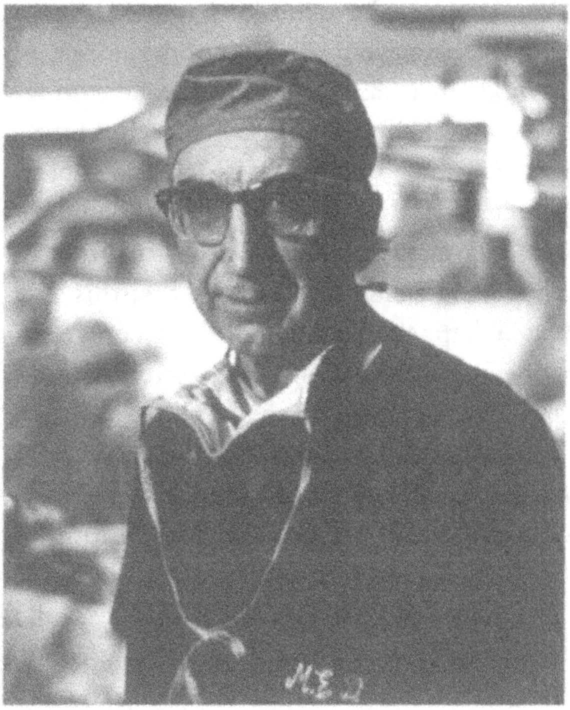

Michael E. DeBakey

"You know, we have the votes to pass it if we can just get Rayburn to let it come up. Does anybody in Texas have any influence with this fellow?" Well, I had only been in Houston for a short time, and I didn't know many people there, and the people I did know didn't have any influence with Rayburn. But when Senator Hill told me that this had all happened because of the Democratic Convention, it suddenly came into my mind that I had operated on the husband of the secretary of the National Democratic Party. I had done an abdominal aneurysm resection on him. The secretary's name was Dorothy Fredenberg, and I called her and asked if she could influence Sam Rayburn. She said, "Mike, I'll let you know." The next morning she called and said that he was going to let it come up for a vote, and that's how we got the library. The library is now part of the NIH, but it has its own budget.

In 1948 I went to Houston to be the chairman of the Department of Surgery at Baylor. At that time it was a very small department, not at all what it is today. I turned the job down twice before I decided to accept. I wasn't at all proud that I had a letter of invitation from Baylor University College of Medicine because I thought it was a pretty third-rate school. I had already turned down three jobs in the East from good schools. I was also surprised when I saw the letterhead stating that it was in Houston, as I thought it was in Dallas; it had moved during the war. But Dr. Ochsner, who was my chief, was a consultant to the Texas Medical Center, and he told me that I should look into it, because they had great plans. I came down to look into it, and I found that they didn't have a real teaching service, and they were teaching students through doctors at the various hospitals in town. Most of them were not really surgeons. As a matter of fact, when I moved here I was the only board-certified surgeon in Houston.

I turned down the job, telling them I couldn't have a residency program if I had no service. They came back a second time, and I told them the same thing. When they asked the third time, they had a promise of a twenty-bed surgical service at Hermann Hospital, which was right next door. I agreed to come on that basis, but after I had been here for two months, nothing had happened with Hermann Hospital. I went to the dean and told him that I was getting a little anxious about this, and if they weren't going to give me a service, I was going back to New Orleans. They had an emergency meeting. The chief of staff of Hermann Hospital came to see me and said, "We just had a meeting and unanimously voted you to be professor of the teaching service." There was something about that title that I didn't like. I said, "Who is in charge of the service?" They said, "Oh, the doctors that are there." I said, "Well, that's not going to work. Suppose I come in there with some students and I tell them that the operation that was done was not the right operation, or that it shouldn't have been done?" They said, "Well, you know, that would be rare." I said, "Not from what I've seen around here. It would be very common." You see how I endeared myself to them. I told them that I was leaving.

However, fate intervened. When I was in Washington writing the Hoover Commission report, I had pointed out that the Veterans' Administration was about to build a hospital right next door to the old Navy Hospital here in Houston. The old Navy Hospital was supposed to serve as a veterans' hospital at the end of the war, according to a memo that I had unearthed signed by Franklin Roosevelt. But the navy brass didn't want to turn it over to the VA. I spotlighted the construction of the new VA hospital as a complete waste of money. That hit the papers around the time that I was negotiating with Baylor. Truman ordered the navy to turn it over to the VA the week before I was getting ready to leave Houston. I got a call from the VA stating that Truman had ordered them to take over the hospital, and the VA director said, "You know, we don't have any personnel to take over the hospital. Can you organize the personnel to take it over?" I just moved in and suddenly had a teaching hospital of my own in Houston. Within a few weeks I was able to convince the chairman of the Board of Trustees that the local county hospital should be affiliated with us, and so I had two teaching hospitals right away. That is what kept me in Houston. As soon as I moved into the VA I started scouting around the country to get new faculty members. I got some pretty good young people from Pennsylvania and Boston. I had friends who were professors, and they helped me find some good people. We got a residency program approved right away, because I was on the board at the time. I got it approved verbally at first, and then they came down and checked us later.

At that time Baylor University College of Medicine had no teaching hospital, no service, and no NIH grants. It was getting along from day to day financially with very poor management. In fact, in 1968 they had a financial crisis and almost had to close the place down. That was when they asked me to be the dean. I ended up separating the medical school from Baylor University. Baylor is a Baptist school, and they have a rule that all of the trustees must be Baptist; all of the trustees of our medical school were Baptists. I said, "You know, I don't have anything against Baptists, but they are long on prayer and short on money." It was quite an unusual thing for a medical school to separate from its parent university, but I separated it, and it's still separate today. We got a charter from the state that it's a separate institution with its own board of trustees. I reorganized the board and got the best people I could find in Houston, particularly those with money. We immediately went out for a campaign of $30 million, and we got $35 million. We have had several campaigns since then and are now in the midst of a campaign for $500 million. We have never been in a deficit since we separated from Baylor University. We are now among the top seventeen schools in the country for NIH grants. We went from nothing to the top seventeen.

In 1952 we did our first abdominal aortic aneurysm. We didn't know that Charles Dubost had done one in Paris a few months before us. We thought ours was the first, and afterwards we found out about Dubost, who hadn't published it at that time. The interesting thing was that he never did anything more. Once I did the abdominal aneurysm, I thought that it could be applied to the thoracic aorta also. It wasn't long before I had a good thoracic aneurysm case, and I did it. We used fresh homografts, taken in the autopsy room. I took them out myself. I had a great opportunity because the coroner in Houston became a good friend, but he was a very lazy fellow. Most of these trauma emergencies happened at night, and he didn't want to come out to perform the autopsies. Back then there was a lot of violence in Houston, knife wounds and gunshot wounds, and the victims were usually young people. So I would come out in the middle of the night and do the autopsies and collect the grafts. I had a little team to prep and scrub and help me take out the fresh homografts.

We stored them in the refrigerator, in antibiotic solution, for up to several weeks. Later on we used freeze-dried grafts, but by the 1960s I had pretty much given up on homografts completely. I had developed the Dacron graft. I put the first Dacron graft in a human being in 1954, and it was two sheets of Dacron that I sewed together. I bought the fabric that was shirt material. It came on a bolt from a department store in Houston. I went down there to get nylon, and when I got there the store clerk said they were fresh out of nylon, but they had a new material called Dacron. Eventually I did get some nylon and did some experimental work with it, but Dacron proved to be better. Later on, I was able to work with a fellow at the Franklin Institute in Philadelphia, Pennsylvania, which was a textile institute. He built the first machine to knit the Dacron grafts, and all of the machines today are derivatives of that first machinery.

The first Dacron grafts did have some porosity, and they would bleed. We preclotted them the best we could, and even after preclotting they would bleed a little, but we sort of squeezed the aorta a bit to reduce the flow. We could slow down the flow intermittently like that until the clotting was pretty good. They were durable and lasted a long time. I have patients walking around now with Dacron grafts I put in thirty years ago.

When I was a junior medical student, there was a faculty member who was interested in the pulse-wave. I worked in his lab as a technician, and one day he said, "Do you suppose you could find me a pump?" I asked what kind of pump he wanted, and he said he wanted one that would pump fluid. Being naïve, I thought, "There are all kinds of pumps and I won't have any trouble finding a pump." But I found out it was a real problem. I went to the medical library and looked up pumps and couldn't find much. I called one of my classmates, a close friend from undergraduate school, who had gone into engineering. I said, "I am trying to find out something about pumps and went to the medical library but didn't find much." He said, "Well, you went to the wrong library. You should go to the engineering library; there's plenty of information available there on pumps." I went uptown to the Tulane engineering school and found that he was right. There were all kinds of pumps dating back over two thousand years. Archimedes developed a pump for irrigation purposes that is still used in some developing countries. I learned a lot about pumps.

I discovered that in the mid-nineteenth century, rubber tubing was developed for the first time, and that is what gave me the idea to develop the roller pump. When I became a resident, blood transfusions were rather rare because we didn't have a blood bank, therefore they would transfuse blood directly from the donor. I used my roller pump to pump blood from the donor to the patient. I would put the donor next to the patient, and I would take my pump, and I would pump the blood from the donor into the patient's arm. The pump was calibrated. I became an expert on blood transfusions. I used to go all around town giving blood transfusions. We didn't use any anticoagulant, because there was none in those days. That came along in World War II.

The roller pump later became part of most heart-lung machines. John Gibbon was working on his heart-lung machine, and he invited me to his lab. He showed it to me, and he said that the oxygenator was doing pretty well, but that the pump was not good. He had what is called a Sigmamotor pump. I said, "Let me send you a sample of my pump." I told him about it, sent it to him, and in a subsequent article he described the whole episode of getting the pump from me. He adapted it to the heart-lung machine, and from that point on everybody adopted the roller pump, even to this day.

We made our own first pump-oxygenator here ourselves shortly after the first Gibbon case. He did his first case in May 1953, and we did ours in September 1953. We began working in the lab building on our own machine, like everybody else. You couldn't buy them because there was nobody making them. We had a machine shop in the lab to build it. Of course, we already had the roller pump, and we used a bubble oxygenator that was based on the Lillehei-DeWall oxygenator. We used it for atrial septal defects, ventricular septal defects, valve replacements, and thoracic aneurysms.

We did the first thoracic aneurysm before the pump was available, in 1952. The patient was a fellow from Arkansas. I remember him very well. He had a huge aneurysm of the descending thoracic aorta, eroding the vertebral bodies, so I thought it was syphilitic in origin. He was having a lot of pain in his back. I told him, "I have done these in the abdomen, but I haven't done these in the chest and nobody else has, but I think the same technique will apply." Fortunately, it was in the lower part of the descending thoracic aorta. We didn't have any experience at that time with the possibility of ischemic damage to the spinal cord, so I never said anything to him about that. Of course, he didn't have any damage anyway and came through the surgery beautifully. That was a very satisfying experience for us to have it work so well. He lived for about thirteen or fourteen years and came back for a check-up. The homograft was fine, even after such a long time. I did an aortogram on him, but he had a lesion on his lung that turned out to be cancer, and I did a lobectomy on him. Two years later he died of metastasis to the brain. He was the first patient to have a descending thoracic aneurysm removed. Later we had several more successful cases, but then we had a patient that developed some weakness in his legs because of damage to the spinal cord. That is when I developed the technique of atrial femoral bypass. That procedure didn't stop the problem, but it was somewhat reduced. Even today you can get 4 to 5 percent ischemic damage to the spinal cord no matter what you do. I started going up the aorta, went up to the upper thoracic aorta, and then to the ascending and the aortic arch. By 1954 I had done all of it, the whole thing, including acute dissecting aneurysms.

We were still using homografts. I used my first Dacron graft in 1954 in an abdominal aorta. Then by 1955 and 1956 I began using Dacron grafts for the thoracic aorta. By 1958 I had quit using homografts and was using Dacron entirely. In fact, I was going around telling people to throw away their homograft banks. I went out to Los Angeles, California, where they were trying to build a multi-institutional homograft bank. They had asked me to come and consult with them about their organization, and I told them to throw away all the homografts.

By about 1958 or 1959 the Dacron graft was commercially available, and anyone could get one. In the meantime, I was making them and sending them to my friends. Actually, a fellow in Philadelphia was making them for me. They were crimped. We put them on a stent, wrapped nylon around them, put accordion pleats in them, and then baked them. They are still made using virtually the same process.

In 1953 I did my first endarterectomy procedure on the carotid artery. I had been reading some interesting articles in the *New England Journal of Medicine* by a couple of neurologists at Massachusetts General Hospital, who had prepared a study on patients with strokes. They found that in patients who had died of strokes, there was a fairly high incidence of carotid disease. One of the neurologists suggested that strokes might be preventable if you could remove the carotid lesion. He wasn't talking about endarterectomy; he was just talking about resecting it. That sounded very reasonable to me. I thought there must be some patients who would benefit from that.

Then all of a sudden I got a patient just like that. He was a school bus driver and was having intermittent attacks of little strokes. All of a sudden his leg and arm would be paralyzed, and his speech would be slurred. They had to stop him from driving the bus, because it was dangerous. He couldn't tell when the little strokes were going to happen. When he came in and I examined him, I remembered the syndrome described by the neurologists in the *New England Journal of Medicine.* It was very similar to the bus driver's symptoms, so I studied him. We did an arteriogram, and we found that he did have a lesion in the carotid artery. I told him what I thought should be done. I told him that nobody had ever done an endarterectomy on the carotid artery, only on the femoral artery, but that it was the same thing. He was from Lake Charles, my hometown, so he knew my family and me, and I think he sort of trusted me. He agreed to let me do it. I didn't use a patch with this first patient, but in later endarterectomies, I used a vein patch. Later I switched to Dacron patches.

The endarterectomy is very successful in the carotid artery, although endarterectomy is not used much elsewhere. It could be successful elsewhere, but the problem is that other arteries are not as easily exposed as the carotid artery. For example, the renal arteries are not easily exposed, and it is a difficult procedure to perform. Usually a bypass procedure is used on the renal arteries. I have done endarterectomies in the renal arteries. In fact, the first coronary revascularization was an endarterectomy. But the bypass became a much simpler procedure where exposure is a problem, and that's why endarterectomy is not used much in places other than the carotid.

I used some early prosthetic heart valves. Other people had been working on these prosthetic valves before we did. The only contribution I made to prosthetic valves was the addition of pyrolytic carbon. Ball valves were clinically successful and had been developed by Starr and others preceding me. I had learned about pyrolytic carbon from Jack Bokros in California. I had the idea of putting pyrolytic carbon on the valve in order to reduce the chance of clotting and started putting it on my valves. That ultimately led to pyrolytic carbon being put on all the valves, and that was my contribution to the valves.

In 1961 I began working on an artificial heart, and I finally forced NIH to dedicate some funds by persuading Senator Hill that we needed NIH money for development of an artificial heart. They didn't want it at the NIH. The director at NIH at that time, Jim Shannon, thought that the science wasn't good, that it was soft science. He may have been right, too, but I thought we needed some money to get started and work on it. As time went on, I became more and more convinced that the total artificial heart was too complicated, and that it was much simpler to work on an LVAD, a left ventricular assist device, because it involved just the one ventricle. I used it for the first time clinically in 1966, and it was successful, which confirmed my bias in favor of the LVAD. I continued to stress that the LVAD was more practical than the artificial heart. About fifteen years ago I did a heart transplant on a NASA engineer who became interested in our work. Through him I was able to contact some NASA hydraulic engineers, who worked with us on the LVAD. Through their cooperation we developed an axial flow pump that is very small and have now put it in four patients in Europe for a clinical trial. The pump moves blood from the apex of the left ventricle to the ascending aorta. Because of its small size, it is very easily implanted without displacing anything and uses only eight watts of power. The battery is worn on a little belt and can last about eight hours before recharging the two batteries. The four patients have done extremely well.

Left ventricular assist devices will eventually become as common as pacemakers or defibrillators. We know that the technology exists to be able to make these small enough that the battery can be put under the skin and recharged through the skin. The controller can be the size of a pacemaker so that it can be inside the body. Everything is inside, which means you don't have to remove the heart. The great majority of patients that we thought needed a heart transplant actually will not need a transplant. They could have a right or left ventricular assist device, or both. This is a great advantage because we have around five thousand patients annually awaiting heart transplants in this country. Only about twenty-three hundred to twenty-four hundred transplants are performed because of the lack of donors, resulting in a large number of patients never receiving the necessary transplant.

In the early years of heart transplant surgery, 1968 through 1970, many people thought that the artificial heart would eventually become available and that, by the early twenty-first century, heart transplantation would be a thing of the past. I didn't feel that way. I wrote an article in 1977 in which I concluded that the artificial heart was not worth experimenting with any more. I reviewed the whole literature about it, and I examined our own experience operating on seventy-seven calves. I concluded that it was very disheartening to take a very healthy calf and put an artificial heart in him and kill him. They often died on the table because the hemorrhage couldn't be controlled. If they did survive the operation, you had hemolysis, thrombosis, and infections. We never had a single animal to survive more than forty-eight hours; not a single one. I said in that article that I was giving up doing any more artificial heart research, and that I would concentrate on left ventricular bypass.

I don't think the heart transplant program is wrong; it's just that there aren't enough donors, and the donor pool is shrinking. Secondly, we still haven't solved the problem of coronary occlusive lesions developing in some of these hearts, causing deaths in seven to twelve years, no matter what you do.

In 1973 Ed Garrett and I reported a coronary artery bypass patient who was still doing well, having been operated on seven years previously. That was our first vein coronary artery bypass operation. In the early sixties there were twelve or fourteen laboratories in this country doing coronary artery bypass on animals, and we were one of them. In 1964 I wrote a paper summarizing our experience up to that time in animals, in which I said, in conclusion, that we had had about a 50 percent success rate at the end of six months. This was very encouraging, and I thought that it indicated that we had a feasible procedure (vein grafts), but I said I didn't think we were quite ready for human use. I didn't ask for the approval from our hospital committee. In 1965 David Sabiston did a coronary artery bypass operation on a patient, but the patient died three days later of a stroke. In 1966 we had a patient who had been scheduled for a coronary endarterectomy, which was what we were still doing at that time. We usually did this operation off the pump, but for this patient we had to go on the pump. When I got in, we tried to do the endarterectomy, but, as it sometimes happens, the lesion was so intimately adhered that by the time we got through, we had virtually destroyed the artery. We were desperate. We weren't going to get the patient off the table unless I did something else, so I decided to do what we had been doing in dogs and did a vein bypass. It was successful, and after seven years we did a follow-up coronary arteriogram, and it was still functioning well. This illustrates how luck can sometimes play a role in the development of new procedures.

There are many people who have had a significant influence on me and my life. Dr. Ochsner was the most significant, I would say. René Leriche had some influence on me, and so did Dr. Rudolph Matas. I didn't work with Dr. Matas, but I had a close relationship with him before he died. Before the war, a lot of the scientific and medical literature was in foreign journals, which I read because I could translate French and German. I did translations of these articles for professors while I was a student at Tulane. Dr. Matas had the best foreign journal library in town other than the medical library. I would go to the medical library to get articles that the professors wanted me to translate, and the librarian would have to go over to Dr. Matas's library to get the ones that the medical library didn't have. One day the librarian told me that Dr. Matas wanted me to come get the journals myself, because he wanted to meet the fellow who was reading all of his journals. I went over to his house, and he met me at the door. He was a nice, heavy gentleman, and he invited me in and offered me a glass of port. He found it fascinating that I was translating these articles, and he wanted to know who I was and all about my family. I got to know him after that, and he was very kind to me. He invited me to his home and told me to come get the books myself, rather than sending for them, because he would like to see me. Because he lived on St. Charles Avenue, every year when the Mardi Gras parade went by, the King of Mardi Gras always toasted Dr. Matas. He always invited me to be there when that happened. I had a great respect for him. He was a wonderful, very scholarly man.

I had the good fortune of getting to know quite a few people like Fred Rankin, Nick Carter, Pete Churchill, and Isadore Ravdin at Pennsylvania, who were all very kind to me. They had an influence on me, and I respect them highly.

Sometimes I run into some of my residents who are retired now, and I say, "My goodness, you can't be retired. You just got through here." They will say, "Dr. DeBakey, that was thirty years ago." I have been lucky in that the great majority of the people I have trained have been very fine individuals and have turned out very well. People like Ed Garrett, George Morris, Bob Wallace, and Bill Blaisdell have become leaders in vascular surgery in this country. Bill Blaisdell just won the DeBakey Award in the society. The people I trained formed an organization called the Michael DeBakey Society, and they put on a good meeting in Lisbon recently. I was there for it, and it was nice to see them. They usually invite me. I run into them at other meetings too and find that some of them are retired. Here I am working, and they are retired! But one of the most gratifying aspects of my career is the success of people who have trained with me, because they are such wonderful people and they carry on. You try to impart some of the values in surgery to them, and it is nice to see that they have accepted those values and are imparting them to their own trainees. That is very gratifying.

I think medicine as a profession and as a science is very strong and very good right now. Surgery is excellent. What is unfortunate about medicine today is the third-party payment system and the fact that third parties control the payment and therefore control also, to some extent, the way in which medicine can be practiced. I don't think this is going to last, though, because I don't think the American people are going to stand for it. They are beginning to rise up in arms already, and in time they will demand a change. The so-called HMOs are making tremendous amounts of money out of this third-party payment system, and yet they deny people care. I think that people will demand a change and will not allow this. The HMOs are almost fraudulent. The name itself, health maintenance organization, gives a misleading idea of what they want to do. They are not interested in health maintenance; they are interested in financial maintenance. To hell with your health. That is the lowest priority in their book. You see, the great majority of their insurees are among the middle section of the population, between the ages of eighteen and fifty, and the health of those people is pretty good, so the HMOs can get by with allowing them a minimum amount of care. It's the people younger and older that are getting the short end of the stick, but they constitute a smaller percentage of the population, so the HMOs get away with denying them the care they need. This minority group is beginning to cry out and make themselves heard. They are applying political pressure, and I think in time they are going to make a change. We are going through a transition, but you've got to remember one thing, medicine is needed in a society, no matter what else the society needs, and if society needs medicine, it will be supported.

Despite the fact that all of these things are taking place in the clinical area, there is also a great deal of research going on that is pouring out new knowledge. This new research will ultimately affect the clinical work and make it better. There is more good research going on now than ever before, and this is true not only in the medical professional area and in institutions of higher learning, but also in the private area, in pharmaceutical companies. The future of medicine is very bright and very good. The way medicine is organized in practice and the way it is organized for the financial support of insurance companies is bad right now, but I think that is going to be corrected. I think you can look forward to a great future for medicine because the people need it.

Bibliography

Kilduffe RA, DeBakey ME. *The Blood Bank and the Technique and Therapeutics of Transfusions.* St. Louis: C. V. Mosby; 1942.

DeBakey ME, Beebe GW. *Battle Casualties: Incidence, Mortality, and Logistic Considerations.* Springfield, IL: Charles C. Thomas; 1952.

DeBakey ME, Cooley DA. Successful Resection of Aneurysm of Thoracic Aorta and Replacement by Graft. *JAMA.* 1953; 152:673–676.

Elkin DC, DeBakey ME (Editors). Vascular Surgery in World War II. Washington, DC, Office of the Surgeon General, Department of the Army, 1955.

DeBakey ME, Cooley DA, Crawford ES, Morris GC. Clinical Application of a New Flexible Knitted Dacron Arterial Substitute. *Arch Surg.* 1958; 74:713–724.

Liotta D, Hall WC, Henly WC, Cooley DA, Crawford ES, DeBakey ME. Prolonged Assisted Circulation during and after Cardiac or Aortic Surgery. Prolonged Partial Left Ventricular Bypass by Means of Intracorporeal Circulation. *Am J Cardiol.* 1963; 12:399–405.

DeBakey ME (Chairman). The President's Commission on Heart Disease, Cancer, and Stroke: A Report to the President: A National Program to Conquer Heart Disease, Cancer, and Stroke, Volume I. Washington, DC, 1964.

DeBakey ME. Left Ventricular Bypass Pump for Cardiac Assistance. Clinical Experience. *Am J Cardiol.* 1971; 27:3–11.

Garrett HE, Dennis EW, DeBakey ME. Aortocoronary Bypass with Saphenous Vein Graft. Seven-Year Follow-up. *JAMA.* 1973; 223:792–794.

DeBakey ME. John Gibbon and the Heart-lung Machine: A Personal Encounter and His Import for Cardiovascular Surgery. *Ann Thorac Surg.* 2003; 76:2188–2194.

DeBakey ME. Development of Mechanical Heart Devices. *Ann Thorac Surg.* 2005; 79:2228–2231.

C. Rollins Hanlon, MD

(b. 1915)

Dr. Taussig had an immense reservoir of knowledge about cardiac malformations. Clearly she said to Dr. Blalock, "What we need is to improve the blood flow to the lungs of these babies." She didn't say, "I think you ought to do a subclavian-pulmonary shunt."
— On the origin of the Blue Baby operation

Interview October 26, 2000

I grew up in Baltimore when it was a rather sleepy town of 750,000 people. It was the seventh largest city in the country, but it rapidly lost that distinction to a lot of newer and more active cities. It had a Southern ambiance. I went to a parochial school, just a few blocks from my home. My father never went to college. He was a salesman, and a very good one, for a firm that made straw hats, so-called Panama hats, which were actually Ecuadorian. In those days most men wore hats.

Although my father never went to college, he was a prolific reader. He had a large room in the front of our house that was covered on all sides with books, except for the one side that looked out. There were bookcases filled with books. Things like the eleventh edition of the Britannica, an India paper edition, which I still have. He was interested in philosophy and history. My mother used to express a not-so-polite surprise and amazement when he would bring home more books. I think my brothers, sisters, and I inherited a love of reading from him early on, and an interest and curiosity about many things. He used to have clubs, as he would call them. "You're the head of the tool-chest club," he would tell me, and that meant that I took care of his tool chest. I still have a big saw that he had years ago. I was also the head of the poetry club, and I would have to memorize great long poems like *Gunga Din* and *Hiawatha*. I would be given some small pittance for recalling those. Memorizing these poems instilled in me a love of memorization, and a capacity for memorizing things, both to please him and to please myself.

My mother also didn't go to college, but she was a great homemaker. There were seven children, and I was the sixth child. My younger sister and I are the only survivors of those seven. One sister died in the great flu pandemic of 1918, and the others lived to a pretty old age, as did my mother and father. My mother was just short of eighty when she died. She was a small, wiry woman, never over a hundred pounds maximum. She was interested in supporting schools, both my grade school and high school. She put on fundraising card parties and things like that. She was a very religious woman; she said her rosary every morning while she was getting us ready for school. She grew up in Port Royal, Virginia, and was a Baptist before she married my father and converted to Catholicism. My family was a very settled, simple, middle-class Irish-Catholic family. All of my siblings went to college, and some to universities, as I did. I think that was a great accomplishment for my parents. They had a reasonable income, because my father was a crackerjack salesman. In 1915, when I was

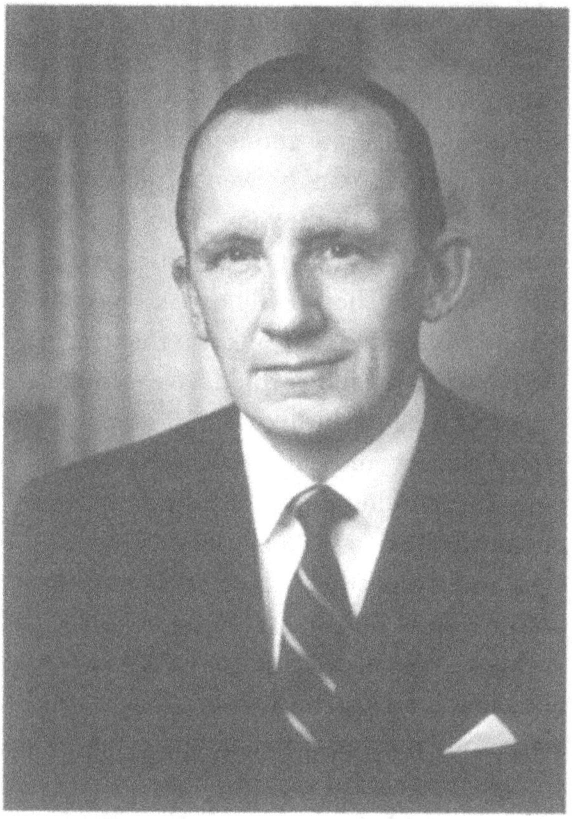

C. Rollins Hanlon

born, the income tax was not much of a factor, so if you made $15,000 a year, you could do quite a bit with it.

I went to Loyola College and graduated in 1934. I was interested in science and in learning about nature. During my sophomore year in college, I decided that I was going to medical school. I had worked the summer before my sophomore year with a distinguished Jesuit biologist who was a world-class authority on the paramecium, the single-cell organism. I had spent that summer working on and publishing my first scientific paper. I think that was indicative of the fact that I was interested in learning about nature. There were only forty people in my graduating class, and the total student body of Loyola College, which was not a boarding school, was about two hundred students. My older brother was in the class ahead of me. In my sophomore year when I decided that I was going to go to medical school, the dean adjusted things so that I could do the science courses during the Christmas holidays. I could do all the laboratory tests and run through all the exercises for physics by working with the fellow who ran the physics lab, who was kind enough to accommodate me. I think I was pretty relaxed about school in my first year of college, but by the second year I knew where I was going.

Johns Hopkins was always a large presence in Baltimore. My father was keenly interested in Hopkins and its accomplishments, and he had a very high opinion of it. I didn't grow up literally in the shadow of the dome of Johns Hopkins, but I was very conscious of its role in the city. When I was in my latter years of college I used to go over on Saturday and slip into the operating rooms to watch operations all day. There was no such thing as security in those days. If you knew where to go you could just put on a blue gown and go down to the gallery and watch the surgeons. I used to watch Walter Dandy every Saturday. He was a world-famous neurological surgeon. I would see in the paper that a child was being flown in from Texas with hydrocephalus, and the next day I would be over in the gallery watching that operation. I was a part of Hopkins. A student who graduated ahead of me at Loyola College showed me the ropes, and from then on I just went from operating room to operating room. I knew I was going to be a surgeon right from the start. I don't know if they kept statistics the way they do now about the number of applicants and whether they accepted one out of two or one out of twenty applicants, but I applied to Johns Hopkins and was accepted.

After college, but before I went to medical school, I went to Europe. I worked my way over there on a ship. In those days there wasn't much union activity on the docks, so I went as a work-away. I got a penny a trip and worked as an ordinary seaman. I got to travel through the ports wherever the ship docked. As soon as it docked, I was free to go about my business. I didn't have to work on the ship when it was in dock; I just had to be back before they raised the hook to go on to the next place. I would have done that again, but that process was abolished after 1934.

I graduated from Hopkins in 1938 and then stayed on as an intern. They took eight interns in those days, and one of my fellow interns was Bill Longmire. After our second year in medical school, Bill and I worked in pathology during the summer under W. G. McCallum, who was the professor of pathology, and under Arnold Rich, who became the professor. We did autopsies and attended all the conferences. It was good discipline, and we learned a lot. I also did some work in physiology, as did Dr. Longmire. We were both kept on for a second year to be fellows in the experimental laboratory.

Being an intern at Johns Hopkins in those days was a serious commitment compared to today's internships. No interns were married. Our life was in the hospital. The professor of surgery, Dean Dewitt Lewis, was a surgeon of the old school, literally a railroad surgeon, and had been president of the AMA. He was trained by Arthur Dean Bevan, who was a quick and masterful surgeon. With Dean Lewis, the way to become one of his interns was to sit down in front in his clinics and answer all of the questions. You made yourself available and vulnerable, and if you knew all the answers, then he invited you to become an intern. One day I was going into the elevator as he was coming out. He said, "Do you want an internship in surgery?" I said, "Yes, sir." He said, "See Ms. Baker." She was his secretary, and that was the end of it.

He forbade marriage, and it was understood that if you got married during your internship, you were automatically out. That would be a violation of civil rights now, and it was then, but that is how it was. There was no smoking. Smoking was forbidden. They gave us six white suits and our room and board, and that was all we got. No pay. You were paid by what you were learning, and we were very glad to do it. We thought that if we had to be paid to do it, we must not be having a very high-class experience.

We were on call all the time, unless we got someone to take our place. Of course, we worked very hard, as we had in medical school. When we were students it had been customary, at least for me, to go into the emergency room before leaving the hospital, and open the screen door and see what was going on there. If it was something interesting, somebody setting a fracture or something, we learned a little bit about that process. It made us late getting home, but you went home to study anyway, so it didn't make any difference.

I stayed on as a Halsted fellow. Out of the original eight interns, Bill Longmire and I were the two selected to stay. We worked on shock. Philip Price was our professor, a very interesting man who had spent twelve years in China as a medical missionary. He was the most meticulous researcher I have ever known. He did a study in China on degerming the hands by using a certain percentage of alcohol, comparing that to scrubbing. He had a glacier-like speed of operation. He worked on that study for twelve years and was in no haste to publish anything.

Shock was an unsolved problem then and later. In those days the concept of shock was that it had a toxic element. Around that time Blalock demonstrated beautifully that it was a matter of fluid loss, and we knew about that, but there were a lot of conflicting theories about it. Bill Longmire was injecting a T1824 solution, a blue dye, to determine what the blood volume was, and then putting the dog into shock by various ways. He would then see what the physiological activities of the dog were at that time and what the blood volume was. It was a very complicated process because you had to draw disappearance curves, the sort of thing that you can do in five minutes now with a computer, but then you had to do it by trial and error. I was working on a variety of methods of producing shock, such as causing constriction of the heart by putting pressure in the pericardial sac. With the output and the blood pressure low, the animal would go into shock. We were studying the performance and physiology of the animals, and the experiments were long, some of them taking twenty-four hours. We considered that this was just good discipline, and we would start again the next day. This was all done in the old Hunterian laboratory, where the conditions were pretty primitive and there were a lot of cockroaches.

We measured cardiac output the same way people do now. We would do studies of the blood gases, oxygen, hemoglobin, and hematocrit. As the shock went on, the hematocrit rose, of course, and as the blood level and circulating volume diminished, the blood counts would go up. There were a lot of things we didn't know about, like ejection fractions and stroke volume, things I worked on later in the cardiac lab in St. Louis. We used to say that if you worked on shock it was like working on pulmonary physiology. One of the cardiologists at Hopkins, E. Cowles Andrus, used to say that when you finished the year, you would have a laboratory full of equipment, but you wouldn't have very much information.

After my Halsted Fellowship at Hopkins, I went to Cincinnati as an assistant resident at Cincinnati General Hospital. Cincinnati General, at that time, was under Mont Reid, who had also been a Halsted resident. Indeed, he and George Heuer, who had also gone to Cincinnati, came back to Hopkins to operate on Halsted during his terminal illness in 1922. It was a diversified program at a municipal university in a city hospital. Cincinnati General Hospital was a huge hospital with pavilions: A, B, C, D, continuing on up to K and L. The surgical wards were open with thirty-four-bed wards, seventeen beds down each side. The surgical program there was widespread, and we did everything, including neurological surgery, urology, and fractures. We did the whole spectrum of surgery, so general surgery to us meant surgery in general, plus every specialty. We didn't do ophthalmology in its present sense, but we shared all the other areas of surgery. We didn't do definitive orthopedics such as fixation of the back and that sort of thing, but we shared the fractures with the orthopedists.

When the war began, I was on a fellowship in California, because Cincinnati had an exchange program with the University of California. A man from the University of

California program would come to Cincinnati General Hospital, and his counterpart from Cincinnati would go out to San Francisco to work six months of the year in neurological surgery with Dr. Howard Naffziger and six months in general surgery with H. Glenn Bell. The day after Pearl Harbor, I tried to join the navy. The lieutenant commander thought I had flat feet. I also had an enlarged inguinal ring and a varicocele and had a history of sinusitis, which I have to this day. He said, "You won't do." I went back home, and somebody suggested that I have a little incision made and closed up so that I could say that I had had my hernia fixed. That didn't appeal to me particularly, although it might have worked, but it wouldn't have fixed the other things. I applied to the Hopkins unit that was forming, but they were all filled up. I completed my fellowship in San Francisco and went back to Cincinnati.

I was accepted into the navy later in 1944. My first duty station was in Memphis, and I got orders that I could volunteer for detached and dangerous duty. I showed this letter to all the old hands around there, but they didn't know what it meant. I knew it wasn't the Fleet Marines. I thought it was some intelligence group. They flew me to Washington, and there I got an idea of what it was. It was an organization called Sino-American Cooperative Organization (SACO) that really worked with the guerrillas in China. I was assigned to the Fourteenth Air Force with General Clair Chenault. SACO also ran an intelligence outfit that was monitoring the Japanese codes that had been broken. That was a highly guarded secret, and I didn't understand it. In the interior of China we had a radio unit that was getting Japanese signals and decoding them and then sending those instructions to our navy. Bull Halsey was the head of the Seventh China Fleet, and the intelligence people gave him some information that permitted him to have some very effective strikes. I knew it was top secret, and I knew that Chenault's Fourteenth Air Force was running sorties here and there. I worked with the people in the counterintelligence agency, most of whom were sons and daughters of old China missionaries. They spoke Chinese. I didn't know whether they were colonels or privates; they had no pips on them. I would do physical exams on them and take care of them for other things. I had some of Stilwell's people who had come up from Burma working with me, corpsmen and others, and I worked there until they dropped the bomb.

Then I went up to Shanghai and was lucky to get on a hospital ship. As soon as I got on the hospital ship, it was like being stateside. I had a surgical assignment on the hospital ship. The chief of surgery on the ship, a lieutenant commander, was a great fellow, but I was better trained than he was. I became the de facto chief of surgery, and we worked up and down the coast. There were fifty-seven thousand marines in north China at that time, and we would take care of their problems. I was on that ship until I came back to the states.

When I came back, like a lot of other people, I didn't have a job or any prospects. I stopped at a couple of places, John Alexander's place in Michigan, Frank Berry's in New York, and then I went down to Baltimore. Bill Longmire was nominally the chief of plastic surgery at Hopkins, but he was really what they called the chief of difficult surgery. They just gave him an assignment, and he did it. He did marvelous things, like total gastrectomies, with remarkably low mortalities. He did some remarkable operations like transplanting loops of bowel and sewing the internal mammary arteries into the jejunal arteries to vitalize the loop. He was an extremely skilled and innovative surgeon. Bill and I had been friends for a long time, and he suggested that I might stay there at Hopkins. He spoke with Dr. Blalock, and Dr. Blalock spoke with John Alexander. I had a sort of tentative commitment with John, but I wasn't very happy about it. Dr. Blalock called him and said, "John, I need this fellow more than you do." So I was lucky and got on as a resident under Blalock, and then I stayed on and ran the experimental laboratory, the Hunterian laboratory.

That was at the peak of Dr. Blalock's Blue Baby career. When I came back, they were in about the three hundredth Blue Baby operation. People came from all over the world to see it. I was working on comparable things in the laboratory, doing venous transpositions and trying to ameliorate various cardiac conditions without, of course, having a heart-lung machine. We also did clinical work, but it was pretty limited. We did Blue Baby operations, ductus, and coarctations; that was pretty much the repertoire of what we did in those days. It wasn't a very extensive thing. Then, of course, a few years later in the fifties, Jack Gibbon invented the heart-lung machine and brought that to fruition.

The Blue Baby operation caught the fancy of both the professionals and the public. It was so dramatic. Dr. Longmire was in on the first one of those operations, and my future wife was a pediatrician working with Dr. Taussig at the time. We were married in 1949. We went to Italy on our honeymoon where, with the Rome surgeon Pietro Valdoni, I did a Blue Baby operation. Dr. Blalock was not very pleased about that; he thought it was a poor idea. I had more enthusiasm than good sense, but it went all right.

Dr. Blalock had come to Hopkins while I was in Cincinnati, and I had reports on his arrival from Dr. Ravitch. When Dr. Blalock arrived, there was an entrenched system of residency in place at Hopkins, with residents who stayed on a long time, were very skillful, and had a great deal of authority. He called them in one by one and told them what they were going to do. He dismissed some of them, and he told others that they could stay on provisionally. He made some quick decisions that seemed to many people to be autocratic, and they attempted an abortive resistance. According to Dr. Blalock's secretary, the "revolt" made him extremely angry; he fired some people. This seemed unfair to some.

He was actually a very low-key, relaxed Southern gentleman who knew exactly what he wanted and how to get it. He really wasn't autocratic; as a matter of fact, he was very receptive to ideas both before and during an operation. He would get a little tense sometimes. People would mimic the rather high, querulous voice that he had when he would get in a tight spot. Overall, he had an abiding interest in the careers of his residents and in seeing that the men he picked were successful later in life. I say men, because he picked very few women. He told Rowena Spencer, who was quite a spunky little person, that she wasn't going to make it through the residency. He knew that research and discipline were important, and he knew that his main interest was in training a group of people who would become administrators and high-level surgeons. They were his legacy. In effect, he was like a latter-day John Hunter who founded a school of surgery.

His residents were fiercely loyal to him. They recognized certain characteristics that he had, but they admired and respected him. There was an interesting interplay between him and the pediatricians, who were of course vital in the whole Blue Baby procedure. My wife was a pediatric cardiologist. Our first date was a fairly extensive one, starting with a football game, going through dinner and a party, and one of the animated topics of conversation that evening was the relationship between Dr. Blalock and Dr. Taussig. We, the house officers, would be in the operating room, and the pediatricians would make rounds on our patients. The pediatricians would sometimes change the medication orders, and we would tolerate that for a while, but then we would complain to the professor, and the professor would speak to Dr. Taussig. It wasn't violent, but there was the usual question of turf and privileges when it came to who was running the postoperative care.

I had known Dr. Taussig as a sophomore student in medical school, because between our first and second year we worked in pathology, and whenever we had an abortion or a miscarriage or a damaged baby at term, Dr. Taussig had to see that baby. We were not particularly interested in doing autopsies on these children, many of whom had cardiac disease. It was difficult because we had to wait until she came; she supervised and directed the autopsy and took the heart. She was following up on the researches of Maude Abbott, who wrote the classic monograph on congenital heart disease. Dr. Taussig was storing away all these defects, and she was classifying and codifying them until she put them in her two books on congenital heart disease. I knew that Dr. Taussig had a great volume of pathological information, which she correlated with clinical information, as did some of her fellows, like Mary Allen Engle and my wife. Margaret Hammond was my wife's maiden name, which led to interesting confusion over the public address system. I would get her calls and she would get my calls.

I think that Dr. Taussig and Dr. Blalock maintained a very cordial relationship, at least superficially, although at times the various members of the house staff would have disagreements, and they had to adjudicate this. Dr. Taussig was obviously a woman of immense capacity. She was quite deaf, so she used an electronic stethoscope, which in those days was a rather large box. Also, because of her deafness she had a high-pitched undulating voice, as deaf people sometimes do, and when she became excited her voice would rise very high. Her fellows would come and sit in her office, and when she came back from whatever she was doing, she would say, "May I please have my office?" in her high-pitched voice, and they would mimic the way she said that, just as the surgeons used to mimic the annoying voice that Dr. Blalock had when he got upset in the operating room.

Dr. Blalock and Dr. Taussig had an interesting and productive relationship. There has been much debate about whose idea it was to do the bypass of the obstruction at the outflow of the right ventricle for patients with tetralogy of Fallot. It is sufficient to say that the technicality of the operation was worked out long before with Sanford Leeds and Dr.

Blalock while at Vanderbilt, so it was simply a matter of adapting that procedure. Robert Gross and Clarence Crafoord in Sweden did the first coarctation by resecting the narrow segment and putting the ends together, but Dr. Blalock also used the turndown of the subclavian artery beyond the narrowed place. The concept of bypassing either the outflow tract of the right ventricle or the obstruction by the coarctation in the aorta was adapted from his early work. Dr. Blalock used to say that he was adding one defect to correct another.

Dr. Blalock had hoped, with Sanford Leeds, that if you increased the blood flow into the lungs a lot, then the blood pressure in the lung would go up and you would have pulmonary hypertension, but that didn't occur. The reason it did not happen is that the lungs are immensely adaptable to increased flow. In essence, he failed to do what he set out to do, but he did succeed in increasing the blood flow to the lungs. The fundamental problem in tetralogy of Fallot is that the blood flow to the lungs is inadequate. The operation was a simple way to increase the blood flow, and the results were spectacular, even though the operation did not correct the basic malformation.

The Blue Baby operation could not have happened anywhere else but right there, because of those two people. Dr. Taussig had the expertise in pathology. She had an immense reservoir of knowledge about all the different malformations: the coarctations, the pulmonary obstructions, the interventricular and atrial septal defects, and the transpositions that we subsequently worked on. All of those things were cataloged in her mind, based both on Maude Abbott's previous work and on her own expertise from immense experience with pathological specimens. Clearly, she said to Edwards Park and Dr. Blalock, "What we need to do is to improve the blood flow to the lungs of these babies." She didn't say, "What I think you ought to do is a subclavian pulmonary shunt." That may seem like a subtle distinction, but I think that is about the sum and substance of how the operation came about.

Dr. Blalock had a technician working for him, Vivien Thomas, a most agreeable, soft-spoken man. Vivien had had an interest in going on to medical school. He was such a superb technician that when Dr. Blalock conceptualized a procedure, he would give it to Vivien, and Vivien would carry out the details. Dr. Blalock would come over to the lab periodically to see how the procedures were going. When he came to Baltimore from Nashville, he brought Vivien with him and put him in charge of the laboratory. Vivien ran the laboratory with a few assistants, who took care of the animals and so forth. Vivien, by virtue of working alone, became a very skilled operator. When he was working by himself, he would take blood vessels and put loops around them and hang clamps on them, so instead of having an assistant to do that for him, he was in effect his own assistant. Also, from working with Dr. Blalock he had learned the physiology, the technicalities of doing the anastomoses, how you pulled up the back row of sutures, and so forth. He did that day after day. When the fellows of the surgical department went to work for a year in the laboratory, he was their mentor and taught them the technical aspects. A number of people, including myself, learned a great deal from Vivien. When the first operations were done, he was standing behind Dr. Blalock, not telling him what to do, but giving him pointers. Dr. Blalock would ask Vivien what to do next. During operations he would often say, "Now, can I have suggestions? I want wise ideas." He didn't want people interfering and telling him how to do it, but he would ask for advice and follow it. He knew that Vivien had done a lot of these in the laboratory, so he was not above asking for Vivien's advice, and he got it. Some people have confused Dr. Blalock's request for advice with the idea that he did not know what he was doing, but that was not so.

Vivien himself was a most agreeable person. In those days, if Dr. Blalock had the house staff out to his house, Vivien would act as the bartender. Nowadays this would seem to be demeaning to have a technician with excellent skills and capacity working with you in the laboratory, and then use him as a bartender. In the politically correct environment in the year 2000, that would be unthinkable. I got along extremely well with Vivien and read the citation when he got his honorary degree.

Vivien would tease us a little bit if he thought we were not giving him due credit. He was the coauthor on one of my papers. On at least one occasion, he said that he should have been on some paper that he hadn't been listed as an author, but the relationship between Vivien Thomas and Dr. Blalock was one of collaboration and of co-worker. At the same time, they were in different social spheres; it was a different time. They came from a Southern town to Baltimore, which was also a Southern town. Baltimore was not just technically south of the Mason-Dixon line, but was Southern in its social persuasions, which were wrong but at that time were not perceived as wrong.

In 1950 I became the chief of surgery at St. Louis University, the first full-time professor of anything in the clinical departments. Ordinarily, you would expect that they would bring in a full-time professor of medicine and then expand from there. But in this case, the dean, Mel Casberg, came to Hopkins and talked to Dr. Blalock. He suggested me for the job, and I went out there. It was basically a school that did not have a research background. It was oriented toward producing general practitioners. What we were attempting to do was not to make it into a Harvard or a Johns Hopkins or a Vanderbilt, but to upgrade the research aspects of the department. We wanted to publish some papers, which would give us a national presence. We developed the cardiac research laboratory, and we expanded to other departments. We were able to bring a more academic environment to what had previously been a strictly clinical medical and surgical faculty.

By 1950 surgery had come a long way technically, but we still did not have the heart-lung machine. In St. Louis, we were doing the same cardiac cases that we had done at Hopkins. Jack Gibbon had worked on his heart-lung machine for twenty years with support from IBM and Thomas Watson. This has recently been written about in Harry Shumacker's book on Jack Gibbon, *A Dream of the Heart*. The book doesn't go into all the technical details. It's more about the personality of John Gibbon and his wife, who was his collaborator, and his relationships with his children. He came from a long, distinguished line of physicians who had also been military physicians, and he wanted to continue that tradition. When World War II began, he left his wife and children, and his research, to go into the military in the South Pacific.

We were making homemade heart-lung machines that were based on the DeWall model, in which you just took two sheets of plastic—we used to call them window shades—and you put blood in a film and bubbled oxygen in at the bottom in small bubbles. The bubbles went up and oxygenated the blood, which then ran down into a container, and you debubbled it by running it through a metal sponge and then down a slope to a reservoir. From there it could be pumped to the patient. It was pretty crude, but in the early days it was reasonably effective for what we were doing. Our first heart-lung machine was a disposable bubble oxygenator, and that was about 1952 or 1953, after the first successful ones had been made. They were very active in Minnesota, of course, and the innovators were not only DeWall, who was the inventor of that basic oxygenator, but also Clarence Dennis, who invented another type of oxygenator, which spun the blood into a film on a screen and thereby exposed the blood to oxygen. The people in Minnesota were also using a live donor—a parent of the patient—to oxygenate the blood. That was pretty precarious because you ran the risk of losing more than one person when you were doing the operation.

Most of our cases were congenital heart defects. After 1948 when Charlie Bailey and Harken began to crack the mitral valves and do finger fractures for mitral stenosis, we began to do that as well. Those were closed procedures in those days, and then we evolved into doing them open, using the pump.

In 1969 I decided to go to Chicago, to be the director of the American College of Surgeons. Two years before that, to my surprise, I had been elected to the Board of Regents of the American College of Surgeons, the nineteen people who are the senior administrators, or the decision makers of the College. From 1967 to 1969 I went to Chicago, or wherever the regents met, three times a year and worked as a regent of the College. Before I finished the first year of a three-year term (you could have a maximum of three three-year terms), the previous director announced his intention to resign. A committee asked me whether I would be interested in being the director of the College. I had never thought about it. I was fifty-four at the time, and I had expected that I would go on being a professor of surgery for another five or ten years where I was, and that would be it. But I had become interested in the College because of my work as a regent, and I was interested in the possibility of not retiring but of doing something at the college. Somewhat regretfully I gave up clinical surgery and went into full-time administration.

The American College of Surgeons is unique in many ways. It was founded by a farm boy from Wisconsin, Franklin Martin. He was very hard-nosed and knew exactly what he wanted to do. In 1905 he formed a journal called *Surgery, Gynecology, and Obstetrics*. It was a scientific journal that would be authored and supervised by practicing surgeons, of which he was one, with an emphasis on gynecology. He had a friend, Donnelly, who could publish it in a high-class way. The Donnelly Printing Company afterwards became a mammoth organization. He started that journal, and in 1910 it occurred to him that he should bring people in to see the leading surgeons of the day operate in Chicago. John B. Murphy was one of those surgeons. They called these events clinical or bedside conferences. They gave these clinics, and they gave people tickets to come. At the first one, hundreds of people fought to get in, and instead of a couple of hundred people, twelve hundred people came. They gave a clinic again the next year, and by the third year, 1912, it became apparent that some organization should be formed to coordinate the work of the Clinical College of Surgeons of North America. Martin's idea was that he would form an organization comparable to the Royal Colleges of Edinburgh, Glasgow, and London. He went to Britain to visit them, and then in 1913 he brought some of the fellows over to the United States, with all the ceremonies of those colleges. He made several of them honorary fellows of the American College, and he took on the pomp and ceremony of the British organizations. He was strongly ridiculed for that, and the idea of an American College was strongly resisted by much of organized medicine, including the AMA. The AMA had resisted the American Surgical Association being formed thirty-five years earlier.

For a couple of years the Clinical College of Surgeons of North America and the American College of Surgeons were separate entities, then they fused. The journal started the clinical series of demonstrations and clinics, and then one organization followed and absorbed the two previous organizations. From 1913 on, the College became an organization with a structure that was carefully worked out. It had a board of regents, which made decisions about the College, and it had a board of governors that acted as the liaison between the fellows and the regents.

Today, the College is educational, and it's also interested in managed care and other issues. The original bylaws of the college state that it was formed for scientific research, for educational purposes, and for the ethical and competent practice of the art. That is in the original charter of the College. That was a departure, because in many surgical organizations, and in the AMA, the question of a person's ethics was not a determinant of whether the person got in or not. At the time the College was started, one of the plagues of the surgical profession was the practice of fee splitting. A general practitioner would refer a case to the surgeon who would give him the biggest kickback. It was determined that that practice should be forbidden and was explicitly condemned in the charter of the American College of Surgeons. To have a criterion of ethical behavior as well as competence was a really new departure.

Itinerant surgery was common in the 1930s and was still common in some areas as late as the early 1970s. At one time it was so bad in Iowa that all admissions to the College from Iowa were interdicted and nobody was allowed to join from Iowa. We just quarantined Iowa. This was before my time. Of course the AMA and its subsidiary organizations fought against this, because the AMA from the start has basically been a local organization with state and county medical societies, and its backbone has been general practitioners. They didn't have a problem with itinerant surgery. The main problem with itinerant surgery is not that you go somewhere and operate, it is the fact that you leave the patient in the care of somebody who has no surgical knowledge. The idea that practitioners with no surgical background are capable of detecting and taking care of complications is simply not valid. That concept is a hard sell because it has important political and economic components to it. Itinerant surgery has been a very comfortable arrangement for some people. A surgeon would go out in the morning, operate on a patient that he had never seen before and would never see again, and leave the patient in the hands of general practitioners who were absolutely not competent to supervise the patient's postoperative care. As a result, there were a number of deaths and other complications that were smoothed over. We resolved that we were going to fight this through even though it was troublesome and expensive, and we made our point.

The College is dealing now with issues such as managed care and malpractice insurance. Managed care is getting a lot of very bad press at the present time. This is because it isn't so much "managed care" that is occurring, but what is happening is "managed costs." The administrators shrink services and make it difficult to get things done. One of the simplest ways, clearly, to cut costs is to shut down medical care. The ultimate economy would be if you didn't have any medical practice, then it wouldn't cost anything. I think the concept of managed care is not in itself inherently wrong. Everybody admits that there is a great deal of waste in the system. The idea that managed care can both eliminate waste and improve care is a nice visionary thought, but it hasn't worked out that way. The main reason that managed care is not saving as much money as we hoped is that managers are drawing very large salaries, with chief executive officers getting multi-million-dollar annual recompense. That has to come from somewhere, and it comes out of the system. Some aspects of managed care, such as having a protocol for doing things, are not inherently bad ideas, as long as the decision making is in the hands of the people who have the medical expertise rather than in the hands of managerial personnel.

There is no question that a single-payer system is simpler and easier to administer. But where it has been put in place, such as in Britain or Canada, you see gradual evolution toward private practice. Margaret Thatcher introduced and fostered that in Britain. I think that there are creaks and groans also in the Canadian system. The main advantage of the single-payer system is that it cuts costs because the overhead is less. It is a bit misleading, though, to compare the 14 percent of the GDP that is being devoted to health care to the amounts being spent on other sectors of the economy, such as education. Health care is not just about spending money on illness; it is also about employing a huge number of people. Health care is an industry that has its own merits.

I can't say what the future will be, but if past performance is any indication of the future, and the Congress works the way it has done for a long time, we will have incremental change bit by bit, rather than a wrenching change into a completely new system. The Clinton attempt to change managed care suffered not just from the work of the insurance companies to abort it but from the fact that it was done in a surreptitious and illegal manner. They were fined $200,000 for violating some of the premises under which they were supposed to be operating. That was clearly an emotional response to an attempt to do it the wrong way.

The fact that there are some forty million people who don't have insurance is a huge problem, there's no question about that. This is not equivalent to not having care, because some people who don't have insurance nevertheless have care. Equating insurance with care is a mistake. There are a lot of people who are outside the safety net, and we need to do something about that. One of the reasons that we're in the fix we're in now is that many of us did charity care for many years before Medicare and Medicaid came in, and then charity care was immediately abolished. People began to be paid for what they had previously done as a charitable operation. They did very well by getting paid for what had previously been a charitable commitment. We're going to have a hard time reversing this trend and going back to doing this work as charity. We have small areas where people are treating groups of patients, under various auspices, on a voluntary basis, but to get forty million people into the safety net is going to take more than a few voluntary areas of care without pay.

Malpractice insurance is another issue that the College has looked at. I don't think we will ever have a no-fault system as we have done with automobile accidents, because the trial lawyers are so powerful and so rich. I worked for years with Jeffrey O'Connell, the main apostle of the no-fault system. That system makes logical sense, it is a superb idea, and it would cut costs. But the people who are arrayed against the idea, the entire legal profession on both sides, are so strong that the idea that we will ever get to a no-fault system seems to be only a happy dream, not something that will come to pass. I hate to admit this because I worked so diligently on it, and I have seen people work on it since I dropped out of active involvement with the College. I'm afraid it isn't within the realm of possibility to push through a strong bill or set of bills to implement a no-fault system.

Cardiac surgery continues to evolve. First there was the idea that we should make the operation as open as we could, with the heart quiet. We began to do smaller incisions, and we began to work with the heart on bypass. We began to work with the beating heart compressed by instruments, working through a small opening. We then began to do things like genetic manipulations and laser boring of holes through the myocardium to increase the blood supply. Now there is the technique of doing a bypass operation where you push down on the heart so that it moves only a millimeter or two. It is not dead quiet, but quiet enough that you can do the operation. Is that going to be the answer, or is that an unsatisfactory way to do things? Is there something better? There will be some kind of evolution, both technical and philosophical. There has to be, because there's no question that when you put somebody my age or even younger on bypass for forty-five minutes, all sorts of things happen to the neurological system. It's not anything gross, such as an inability to do serial sevens backwards. We don't know if it's fat or bubbles, but whatever it is, people sometimes come out of that operation not exactly the same person that they were before. It's becoming increasingly apparent that the idea that cardiopulmonary bypass is a benign procedure, either to the heart or to the head, is false. It is not benign.

People ask me what the secret is of my vigor and health at my age. I don't have a secret. My parents lived to be eighty, and I have beaten them by a little bit. Anybody that gets old and starts giving recipes for other people about how to get old is foolish, I think.

Bibliography

Blalock A, Hanlon CR. The Surgical Treatment of Complete Transposition of the Aorta and the Pulmonary Artery. *Surg Gynec Obstet.* 1950; 90:1–15.

Hanlon CR. Surgery of Heart Disease. *Postgrad Med.* 1952; 12:228–232.

Hanlon CR. Surgery for Congenital Heart Disease. *Postgrad Med.* 1955; 18:207–211.

Hanlon CR. Surgical Treatment of Funnel Chest (Pectus Excavatum). *Am Surg.* 1956; 22:408–414.

Hanlon CR, Danis RK. Superior Vena Caval Obstruction: Indications for Diagnostic Thoracotomy. *Ann Surg.* 1965; 161:771–777.

Hanlon CR, Kaiser GC, Mudd JG, Willman VL. Closed Mitral Commissurotomy for Mitral Stenosis. *Ann Surg.* 1968; 167:796–800.

Hanlon CR. Advantages and Disadvantages of a Program for Basic Surgical Education. *Ann Surg.* 1968; 168:579–581.

Hanlon CR. Shattuck Lecture—The Physician and Organized Medicine. *N Engl J Med.* 1971; 284:1131–1134.

Hanlon CR. Presidential Address: The Surgical Presidency. *Ann Surg.* 1982; 196:233–238.

Hanlon CR. Quality Assessment and Tracking Results of Cardiac Surgery. *Ann Thorac Surg.* 1997; 64:1569–1573.

Frank C. Spencer, MD

(b. 1925)

I saw a nineteen-year-old Marine with a gangrenous leg from a small wound of the superficial femoral artery. I asked why the femoral artery had not been repaired, and the answer was that repair was contrary to orders. I said, "What the hell do you mean, orders?" I suggested an experimental program on arterial repair. We still couldn't get permission. An advisor said, "Why don't you go ahead and do it anyhow?" If it worked, I would get a decoration, and if it didn't, I could well get a court martial. We did one hundred patients with a 90 percent success rate.

— On the use of homografts for wartime arterial injuries

Interviewed April 19, 1999

I was born seven miles north of Haskell, Texas, which had a population of thirty-five hundred. This was a farming and ranching region, and that has always been a part of my background. The nearest house to our home was about a half-mile away so it was a sparsely populated area. The advantage of that was that we learned self-reliance very early because if we had a problem there was no one to help and no one was coming. We learned about problem solving from the cradle up. This background gave me a sense of self-reliance and a capacity for hard work. Because of the economy, everybody worked, not because we were told to, but because we felt embarrassed if we were not working. In a typical rural area children worked in the cotton fields with the adults.

My education began in a two-room country schoolhouse. When the Texas Panhandle was settled in 1880 and 1890, two-room schoolhouses were built every six miles along the main roads. The wisdom was that no child would be more than three miles from a source of education. If the roads were impassable in wintertime, the children could walk three miles to school. They built hundreds of these two-room country schoolhouses, and they built teachers' colleges to supply the teachers. My grade-school education was in a two-room country schoolhouse, and it has been surprising to me that during my professional career I have been associated with people who have had the best education that money could buy, and my education was just as good as anybody's, with the exception of music. It was all reading, writing, spelling, and mathematics. I owe it all to the dedication of the two teachers who taught those grades, and the key to my professional success was access to a good public education. I was the first child in my family, and my mother began to teach me to read and write at a very early age. When I was ready to start school, I could do multiplication tables, write, and spell. My mother timidly suggested that I might be ready for the second grade rather than the first. This was not greeted very warmly by the schoolteacher. They said they would let me try it for a week. After a week, I was put in the third grade rather than the second. That had an effect on my career later on.

I rode a school bus to Haskell for my high-school education and graduated when I was fifteen. I then entered North

Texas State College. This was a marvelous school with an excellent faculty. Pearl Harbor occurred during my freshman year, so thereafter we went summer and winter. Because of this, I finished college in two and a half years. I liked both chemistry and mathematics and considered a career in mathematics, but finally decided to apply to medical school. Being a very loyal Texan, I applied to both of the Texas medical schools. With the confidence of youth, I thought I would apply to both and then decide which one I would go to. I had no advisors. Early in World War II, if you were accepted in medical school you were inducted into the army or navy and given a commission. The military then paid your tuition and also a salary. It was an enormous financial advantage. It was one of the darkest days of my life when in the spring of 1943 I was rejected by both schools on the same day. Both sent me a note stating that my grades were fine, but they thought seventeen was too young and would consider accepting me a year later. A year from then I would be eighteen and draftable and probably be in the South Pacific. There was an urgency for me to find a medical school. Someone in my chemistry class was planning to go to a place called Vanderbilt. I asked where that was, and they said Tennessee. I said, "I never heard of it, is it any good?" They said it was a great school. I mailed my application and my grades, and three weeks later received a note that said, "Congratulations, you have been accepted and there is a $50.00 deposit required." This made me a lifelong Vanderbilt enthusiast. There was no interview and no comment about my age. I traveled to Nashville and entered medical school just before my eighteenth birthday. It was the first time I had ever been in that part of the world.

Our class began in late December of 1943. We had a small class, about forty-five students. We had a standard curriculum but went to class winter and summer. Many members of the faculty were away in military service. There was a very warm relationship between teachers and students, and I became personal friends with the legendary professor of anatomy, Sam Clark, who was brilliant but very modest. Billy Orr taught us psychiatry and was a close friend. The professor of surgery was the well-known Barney Brooks, who taught by terror, but he was a brilliant teacher and decades later I can still remember his lectures. When we had bedside rounds he sat at the patient's bedside and the students stood at attention around the bed and made notes standing. I have never seen another personality quite like his.

During that time I met my wife Connie, who was an undergraduate student at Vanderbilt. We were married between her junior and senior years. She was a Southern belle from Manchester, Tennessee. Her family was concerned that she married an impoverished medical student and that she needed to go to work right after her graduation. Her maiden name was Ewell, and there has been a Ewell practicing law in Coffee County for more than one hundred years. My brother-in-law is a circuit judge there, and his son is an attorney there, just like his father and grandfather.

In my third year, when it came time to apply for internships, we all got a letter from the dean. "Dear Mr. Spencer, you have expressed an interest in surgery so you have been assigned Dr. Cobb Pilcher as your advisor. You have an appointment to be in his office next Tuesday at 4:15 P.M." Dr. Pilcher was an outstanding neurosurgeon. In his office the next week he looked at me and said, "You must be Spencer." I replied, "Yes, sir." "Well, come in. I'm looking at your grades, they are fine. I understand you are interested in surgery. Where do you want to train?" I was nineteen years old, a little frightened, and replied, "I would like to train somewhere in the East. I have heard that there are some good places, and I have never been east of Nashville." I remember the conversation almost verbatim because it was a turning point in my career. He smiled and said, "Well, Spencer, you are right, there are some good places in the East. Where do you want to go?" I replied, "I don't know. I thought you would know better than I would." He said that I was probably right and told me to apply to Johns Hopkins, Yale, and Rochester. He added, "They probably will have a place for you at Hopkins," and he told me not to accept any of them until I talked to him. The interview was less than fifteen minutes, but it was pivotal for the remainder of my career as I was accepted at Johns Hopkins. Dr. Pilcher and Dr. Blalock had been good friends during the fifteen years that Blalock was on the faculty at Vanderbilt.

I arrived in Baltimore in the summer of 1947. Connie and I were married but had no money, so Connie stayed with her parents until I could find an apartment. The idea of my finding an apartment turned out to be a myth. The interns were on call seven days a week, twenty-four hours a day. If we wanted to go to a movie, we had to sign out to another intern. The hours were brutal, but nobody thought a thing about it. We could either live in the hospital or live close by. After being there ten days, I had not been

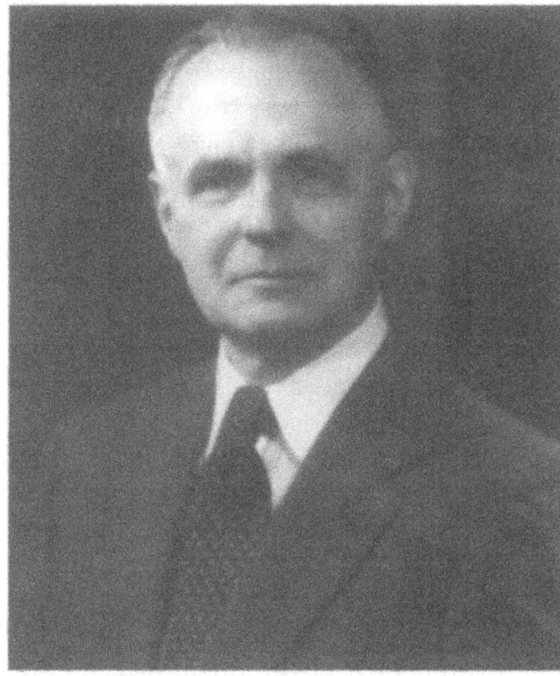

Frank C. Spencer

out of the building. I was making rounds with the chief resident one evening when he turned to me and said, "Spencer, aren't you married?" I told him I was; only two in the group of ten interns were married. He said, "Where is your wife?" I told him she was in Tennessee until I could find an apartment. He said, "That is crazy. You will never get out of the hospital. When we finish rounds I will call my wife. We have an extra room. You call your wife and she can come to Baltimore, stay with us, and look for an apartment." The house staff was very close and much like a family. If we were having trouble, the others would always help out. Connie came to Baltimore and found an apartment near the hospital.

The house staff at Hopkins had an unusual number of very talented people, although at the time we were not really aware of this. The intern group included David Sabiston and Jim Maloney, and they became my lifelong friends. Hank Bahnson was a junior resident as was Glenn Morrow. Rollins Hanlon was the chief resident. During that year, Denton Cooley and Harry Muller came back from the army as senior assistant residents, and the junior faculty members were Bill Longmire, Mark Ravitch, and Bill Scott. I had told my wife that my fellow residents were some of the smartest people I had ever seen, but I had no idea that so many were destined to become chairmen of surgical departments and national leaders of surgery. The workplace was intense but collegial.

What was not collegial was the rather brutal pyramid system of promotion. They brought in ten interns each year and in a highly competitive environment picked only two to go through residency training. The other eight had to move to another training program or enter practice. They couldn't decide what to do with Jim Maloney and me. We were both parked in the experimental surgery laboratory for a year. Jim went to Boston the following year, and I worked in the cardiac catheterization laboratory. This turned out to be an invaluable experience and led to a publication in the *Journal of Physiology* in 1949. As that year went on I was uncertain if I would be asked to stay for another year since my fellowship would end in June. Bill Longmire was leaving to go to UCLA so I asked him if I could go with him, and he was delighted. I liked the people at Hopkins, but I had some anger about the pyramid system, so I left with perfectly good intentions of never coming back.

Life is certainly not always a success story; it has ups and downs. When I have advised younger people, I often point out that it is not always your achievements but how you handle your failures that determine a lot of things in the future. When I had come to Hopkins, life never looked better. I had a young bride, had graduated first in my class, was awarded the Founders Medal, and was appointed an intern at Hopkins. The next five years saw a series of failures, one right after another.

We arrived in California to work in a new medical school, but construction of the hospital had not even started. We all went to work at Wadsworth Veterans Hospital, which turned out to be superb, and I was there for eighteen months. They had moved the faculty and house staff there because they had fallen behind, actually five years behind, on opening the hospital. The surgical training was good and I was an assistant resident, but we had no interns, so essentially I repeated my intern year. Longmire got together some research money and proposed that I drop out of the residency program, work in the research lab, and then be his chief resident in the new hospital, so Harry Muller and I started a cardiac research laboratory on the UCLA campus in a war-surplus wood-frame hut. Six months later, the Korean War broke out. Since I had a military commission in the navy but had never been called up, I was promptly sent to the Oakland Naval Base. The hospital there was filling with patients evacuated from Korea. Because of a letter of recommendation by Dr. Longmire, I was assigned a ward for patients with vascular injuries. In advising young residents about work and career, I have often said, "Don't pay a lot of attention to your long-term plan. Do whatever you are doing the very best that you can. Those observing you will make doors open for you." That was the case at Oakland. Dr. Longmire's letter made it possible for me to be assigned to a busy surgical ward rather than the outpatient dermatology clinic.

The chief of surgery at Oakland wanted new ideas. Jack Wiley in San Francisco had started doing a few aortograms, so we were able to begin aortography by injecting dye into the aorta through long needles. That was in 1951. Also, since I had worked in a cath lab, they asked me to set up a cath lab at Oakland. We ordered about $200,000 worth of equipment.

I asked the chief of surgery about our spending money on a cath lab. I said, "The normal tour of duty in the navy now is a year in a hospital and then a year with the Marine Corps or on a ship." I felt guilty about spending money for a cath lab if I was not going to be there to use it. He replied, "Well, Spencer, you are going to stay here for two years. After getting all this started you are not going anywhere." That seemed fine with me. A few weeks later, after being out of town for temporary duty, my wife told me I had this official-looking letter. The letter stated that I was hereby detached to report for training with the Marine Corps at Camp Pendleton. They gave me a thirty-day leave; my wife was pregnant with our second child. All that talk about staying at Oakland had gone out the window. Being very disappointed and upset, I went to the admiral to see if I could stay at Oakland. I was given about two and a half minutes. "Come in Frank, my boy. This is a great opportunity for you to see the world. Goodbye and good luck," and I was out the door.

During this time it became apparent that the Marine Corps needed more trained surgeons in Korea, but there was a problem with the division surgeon. He believed that regardless of background, every surgeon sent to Korea should spend the first four to five months in a battalion aid station starting IVs and holding sick call. He had board-certified surgeons in the front lines instead of in the mobile hospitals where they were needed.

So I'm packing and moaning and complaining. They needed surgeons in Korea, but I'm going to a battalion aid station. Nobody here will be able to use all this expensive equipment I have ordered. What can I do about it? Well, there is a principle of military service that you can always write a letter to the secretary of the navy or army. The letter always goes through, but must go up the chain of command. Through that chain, each person can add whatever comment seems appropriate. The letter eventually resides in your permanent record. I wrote a five-page letter, keeping it as neutral as possible. I did not complain about going to Korea, but I did complain about not being used as a surgeon, especially since the need for surgeons in Korea was so pressing. Twenty-four hours after submitting the letter I got a phone call that said, "Lieutenant Spencer, the admiral wants to see you right now." I explained that he told me good-bye two days ago. The answer was to come down now. I walked in and got this warm greeting, "Come in, Frank my boy, have a cigar. You don't need to write any letters. I just talked to so and so in Honolulu and you are going to be chief of surgery in the EZ Medical Company in Korea. You can operate all you want, and you won't need to send any letters." I arrived in Korea in the summer of '52. They were negotiating peace terms and the lines were frozen around Panmunjon. EZ Medical Company was one of three or four medical companies that covered the first Marine division on the line, as well as one Korean division. The truce teams negotiated in a five-mile no-fire circle. Every day there was machine gun and mortar fire. EZ Medical Company was two miles behind the battle lines, and had two Quonset huts, tents with space for sixty cots, and eight or ten medical officers.

Shortly after I arrived, a nineteen-year-old marine who had a gangrenous leg was scheduled for an amputation. His injury was a small mortar wound that had involved the superficial femoral artery. All of the marines wore armored vests, so we saw very few chest or abdominal injuries. Most injuries were from mortar or grenades. A 50-caliber machine gun could penetrate an armored vest, so most of these were fatal. I asked why the femoral artery had not been repaired and the answer was that repair was contrary to orders. I said, "What the hell do you mean, orders?" They showed me this large manual about how each type of injury should be handled. This was a perfectly sound conclusion from the studies of vascular injuries in World War II by Dr. DeBakey and Simione, because at that time evacuation to a hospital was eight hours or more, causing extensive ischemic damage. Vascular repair at that stage had a high probability of myoglobinemia and renal failure, so ligation of the artery was the policy. In Korea for the first time they had rapid helicopter evacuation, and the marines were very aggressive in going out and bringing in wounded comrades. We were just behind the lines, so we had these people arriving very early after injury being treated by an old policy that required ligation of injured arteries rather than repair. I knew how to repair arteries, having had a lot of experience in the experimental laboratory, but we were unable to get permission. It was suggested that if we did not follow orders on this, we would risk court martial. I suggested an experimental program on arterial repair. We still couldn't get permission. Finally, after a couple of weeks, we talked to an advisor for our group and he said, "Frank, you will never get permission, why don't you go ahead and do it anyhow?" He thought that command structures were more flexible this close to the front line. That was the only encouragement I needed. There were concerns, however. We did not have vascular instruments, only bulldog clamps; I was not board certified; and my rank was only Lieutenant (JG). If it worked I would get a decoration, and if it didn't, I could well get a court martial.

We set up an arterial tissue bank. If a patient tragically arrived dead, we would remove both femoral arteries under sterile conditions and store them in plasma under refrigeration. No one thought about informed consent. We used the protocol developed at Bethesda for bone grafts, and it worked like gangbusters. Our patients were young, healthy marines operated on within two hours of injury. Our only problem was infection since all of the wounds were contaminated. We always did a radical debridement, covered the vascular graft with fascia, and delayed closure of the wound for four or five days. Our infection rate was about 5 percent. If we were unable to completely cover the graft, there was the risk of rupture of the graft. Most of the grafts did not go beyond the knee joint. Blast injuries around the knee joint were our biggest problem, since frequently there was not enough viable tissue to cover the graft. We needed a free graft of muscle or something. We did one hundred patients with a 90 percent success rate. We did not do carotids, as the neurosurgeons thought that ligation would be safer, so we did only extremities. Word spread rapidly over the division, and our operating tent was frequently filled with visitors. The navy was very pleased. One day my commanding officer called and said, "Spencer, they have an arterial injury patient at Inchon Harbor. A helicopter will be here in twenty minutes to pick you up, go fix it." I was dispatched with my carbine and a bottle of grafts from our bank. Our only equipment was bulldog clamps, 4–0 silk sutures, and homografts. This was the same equipment Dr. Blalock had used ten years before for the Blue Baby operation. We did end-to-end interposition grafts. I don't recall how long our grafts could be stored before use, but we had a fairly rapid turnover. The longest graft that we used was about fifteen centimeters.

We were able to restore arterial flow to almost all limbs with only two or three failures due to technical errors. One problem was popliteal vein occlusion, where we had massive swelling and sometimes a compartment syndrome leading to gangrene. Also we had a long delay getting Potts clamps. The military had requested Potts clamps from their instrument company, but they said they were committed to other orders and we would have to wait nine months. Someone high up told the instrument company to deliver six pairs of Potts clamps in two weeks or lose their contract. Five sets went to John Howard who was setting up a research team for a vascular surgical unit for Korea and the sixth pair was for Lt. J.G. Spencer. They were delivered by Colonel Carl Hughes one afternoon six months after I arrived in Korea.

One afternoon a reporter came by and said that he had heard we were doing some interesting work. It was a time when there was a lull in the combat, so we sat around and talked about the vascular surgery that was being done. I thought that the reporter and I were just having a conversation, but to my astonishment the stories we told him went out over three wire services and appeared in the newspapers at home. I was very embarrassed and angry because it didn't give any credit to my colleagues or the corpsmen and nurses, and it made me out as a boy hero. It did capture national interest in the concept of arterial repair, and it also changed my career, because I was sent back to present our results at a meeting of the American Medical Association. It was published in the *Annals of Surgery* in 1955.

I had left Johns Hopkins with the intention of not ever going back and had planned to continue my training with Dr. Longmire at UCLA. My last duty station for a few weeks prior to discharge from the navy was Bethesda, and while there I received word that Dr. Blalock wanted to see me, so I went up to Baltimore to see him. He asked me to come back on the house staff as a senior resident and promised that I would be the chief resident in about six months. This was a tremendous opportunity. Because of my commitment, I tried to reach Dr. Longmire, but he was in the air force in Europe. The professor said correctly that the UCLA hospital was still not built and that I might be an old man by the time it was finished. After three weeks of deliberation, I decided to return to Hopkins. I felt badly about UCLA, but as it turned out it was another two years before the hospital was completed. Jim Maloney had returned and we were co-residents. After I finished my residency, I joined the faculty and stayed at Hopkins from 1955 to 1961, being primarily involved in developing a vascular surgical service.

Dr. Blalock had a unique personality, and I have never met anyone quite equal to him. His main interest was developing his faculty and helping them obtain positions of national prominence. At the same time he kept himself in the background. To a remarkable degree he tried to avoid having his name appear in the newspapers. He gave us big opportunities and then stayed behind us with a pitchfork to be sure we were working hard. In the operating room he was good but not a brilliant technician. Throughout his life he would do only one operation a day, very seldom two, because in the afternoon he always went to the laboratory. If we did more than two operations a day he would criticize us. He said you can't do two or three operations and still get to the lab. He was not interested in developing a large clinical series. His health was somewhat frail. He had spent two years in a tuberculosis sanatorium and had only one kidney. He did not have a lot of stamina, although he and Tinsley Harrison had been star tennis players at Vanderbilt. He grew up in a generation where the sight of blood in the operative field made one very uncomfortable since blood transfusions were not always available. Blood loss was often the sign of impending disaster. He never recovered from that instinctive anxiety over the sight of bleeding. When I was on the faculty, either Hank Bahnson or I always stayed in our office one floor below the operating room where he was operating. If he had a problem he would call one of us. Hank was away one day and Dr. Blalock's secretary called and said he wanted me in the OR. He had a room full of prominent visiting surgeons. He introduced me to them and then said, "I have these guests and I am demonstrating a subclavian-pulmonary anastomosis. I have a lot of bleeding and I am making a mess of it. I want you to get it under control, and I have a clinic at 11:30, so I want to finish here as soon as possible." He then asked the nurse for a towel, wrapped it over his gloves, and sat down on a stool in the corner. I quietly scrubbed and began working and after about five minutes he said, "Have you got it fixed?" I said, "No, sir, still working." He said, "See if you can hurry it up. I have patients at 11:30 and I don't want to be late." A few minutes later things were under control. He came up and said, "That will be all right, you can leave now. If I need you I will call." Then he went on with the demonstration. He was a great leader and he had great confidence in young people. We took orders and felt they were for our benefit, not his. He molded our careers with his leadership.

At that time we wanted to begin doing mitral valve surgery, open commissurotomy, and valve repair using the pump-oxygenator, but we could not get anyone to do a left heart catheterization. I read some articles by Bill Blakemore about catheterizing the left atrium by introducing a long percutaneous needle through the back. At first I did these procedures myself until the cardiologists began the trans-septal technique, which, to my relief, put me out of business. We would leave a catheter in the heart at the end of an operation, and could then measure mixed venous oxygen levels as well as left atrial oxygen and pick up low cardiac output. With those early patients, I would often sleep in the recovery room in an adjacent bed, and the nurse would wake me every three hours or so to look at the patient.

For the most part we were doing open mitral commissurotomy. There were also some primitive techniques for annuloplasty.

If the patient had mitral stenosis we could fix that, but if the patient had mitral insufficiency, it often failed and the patient died. To measure the gradient across the aortic valve we put a needle into the chest to enter the apex of the left ventricle. Fairly often we got a pneumothorax. I wouldn't dare do that now.

We used a roller pump and a bubble oxygenator for a time, but we gradually moved away from the early bubblers because the patient frequently did not wake up if he had been on bypass more than thirty to forty minutes. We tried a disc oxygenator developed by Viking Björk and eventually used a version of the screen oxygenator. Jerry Kay had been at the NIH with Glenn Morrow, and he and Bob Gaertner built a modified Gibbon screen oxygenator that was called the Kay-Gaertner. The bulk of patients were children until prosthetic valves became available.

Ben Eiseman was appointed chairman of the Department of Surgery at Kentucky, and he had a very persuasive personality that could sell a refrigerator to an Eskimo. He wanted me to come down and join him, especially to develop cardiac surgery. I told him I was not interested in moving, that I was having a good time at Hopkins. He said please just come and look. I finally told him I would come for twenty-four hours and that I was not sure where Lexington was. As soon as I saw how beautifully the hospital was built, I told Dr. Blalock, and he said you are going to have trouble turning that down. When I finally arrived in Lexington, the hospital was completed, but there were no patients, no nurses, no staff, no nothing. We began to recruit everything. Because of the shortage of nurses we could only open a small wing at a time. We first opened forty beds. It was hard work because we had no house staff. First we had to find patients and then recruit house staff. Lexington at that time had a population of about seventy thousand and had a lot of good physicians and surgeons. They really did not need another hospital, but they were very supportive. To find patients I became the busiest circuit rider in Kentucky. If six doctors were meeting in a café, I would be there and show them my slides. If they called about a patient, I always asked them to send the patient to the hospital. In time we filled the hospital and had a good time doing it.

I was interested in the mammary artery, so I made that my research project for the next two to three years. I tried different concepts and in 1964 published an article about mammary-to-coronary anastomosis in a group of dogs. These were done with 4–0 silk sutures and no magnification. Everybody assured me that the artery was too small to be much good.

In 1966 I went to New York as chairman of the Department of Surgery at NYU. They did not have a thoracic surgery training program. Columbia had a thoracic program at Bellevue that had once been famous for tuberculosis, but NYU was not part of it and was not especially welcomed. At that time you could start a thoracic residency program by decree. The board would allow you to start, and if the residents were not adequately trained, they would not be accepted for examination, and if they were trained, they would be accepted. It was that casual in the sixties. I started a thoracic training program and recruited a faculty. I was told that there was a young resident named George Green who was in the lab working with the mammary artery using a dissecting microscope.

That pricked up my ears, and he became one of our first thoracic residents. Dr. Blalock always said that you should train people and let them make their own decisions. If you disagree with their research, you should first look at your own because you may be wrong. This was true of George Green and the mammary artery. He had continued his research, and when he completed his training, I put him on the faculty. I wanted to see what could be done with the mammary artery. About four months later he had a patient at the VA Hospital with David Tice, and he wanted permission to do a mammary-coronary anastomosis. I said, "Well, if you think it is safe, go ahead. I think it is too small but I hope I am wrong." That was the first use of the mammary as a coronary artery graft in the U.S.

My contribution was giving him permission to do it, even though I thought that it was probably a waste of time. We did not realize the true value of the mammary artery, and it was not until the mid-eighties that the long-term value of the mammary artery became clear. Early in my tenure in New York I was interested in using the mammary artery for the Vineberg procedure, and with the usual Texas reasoning, I said if a small artery is good maybe a large artery will be better. I mobilized the splenic artery and tunneled it into the myocardium of a patient. It made a heck of a hematoma.

My father discouraged me from becoming a rancher, and of course there were other people who had a big influence in my life. At North Texas State Teachers College, Dr. Carico was the chairman of chemistry department. I was fifteen years old, scared, and homesick, and he treated me with interest and friendship. He was in his thirties and was a brilliant teacher and a great outdoorsman. He picked out several of us from the freshman class to have a job to help run the laboratory, and paid us something like $30 a month. I worked for him for two years, and this $30 a month paid most of my expenses. He treated his students as if they were part of his family. He would take us quail hunting on Saturday afternoons or take us to a baseball game. He had the spark of intellectual excitement, was the epitome of the ideal teacher, and I have quoted him many times. Since then I have tried to make the students comfortable with the professor, because the most effective atmosphere for teaching is the excitement of learning. If you are scared of the professor it is difficult to experience the fun of learning.

When I was a teenager in college, I took a course in abnormal psychology from a teacher who could absolutely mesmerize the students. He had excitement, enthusiasm, and clarity. He was like a magician. I decided I wanted to be a psychiatrist, and when I went to Vanderbilt, I told them I was interested in psychiatry. They asked if I knew any psychiatrists. No. Ever seen a psychiatric patient? No. But you are going to be a psychiatrist? Yep. When I was a third-year student I had a psychiatric rotation. All of the patients were in an institution. The chairman of psychiatry was a brilliant man, but he would put you to sleep talking to him. In the state mental hospital my first patient was a catatonic schizophrenic who had been there for fifteen years. I thought, "My God, is this what I have been talking about?" That was when I became a surgeon.

When I got to New York, I had never been in a courtroom in my life. I thought a tort was something that you bought in a bakery store. I had been there two or three years when I got this subpoena. I wound up in a malpractice trial over a child who had a crippling injury, but we never knew the cause of the injury. It was finally settled for an annuity. After it was over the plaintiffs' attorney said that he admired Dr. Spencer's courage and tenacity, but doesn't he know that he couldn't win a case that involved a brain-injured child? One of the problems of cardiac surgery is that the most complicated and sickest patients are the biggest challenge, and the more complicated the patient, the bigger the likelihood of an imperfect result and the chance of litigation. As time went on, I had two or three malpractice cases that were not malpractice but were complications of complex surgical procedures. I began to look at it as blackmail, not malpractice, so I decided to say, "Go to hell, I will see you in court," when urged to settle. I have been through six jury trials as a defendant and won five of them because there was actually no malpractice; it was just a form of blackmail. Many physicians are vulnerable to the tactics of a skilled plaintiffs' attorney who will insult the physician with insinuation until he is angry, which suggests to the jury that there is something to hide. The plan is to distort the facts to achieve a big award. Because of this experience, I went on to promote a committee of the College of Surgeons to develop guidelines for physicians who find themselves facing malpractice litigation.

What will be the future of cardiac surgery? Of course it is impossible to judge. Gene therapy will probably change things. There are no more obvious frontiers now that coronary artery surgery has evolved. Initially when cardiac surgery first started it involved congenital heart abnormalities. Later we had prosthetic heart valves. We developed procedures for complex congenital problems and, later, coronary bypass techniques. Probably there will be new developments in cardiac transplantation, and certainly there will be progress with left ventricular assist devices. It is important to remember that none of the operations that I have done for the past twenty years existed when I finished my training. Not one. When I was a house officer, I heard that Tom Starzl was trying to do something with a wire to start the heart. Everybody was laughing to think you could run the heart with an electric battery like an automobile, so you can't always tell. Dr. Blalock always told me that it was important to keep your interest in a broad selection of problems. He advised that I do other procedures and not just heart surgery, because he thought that most major developments came from those people with a broad background. When you are working on a problem and nothing that you have tried has worked, don't quit. You can't always solve every problem, but you can always learn something in the process. Persistence is important.

Bibliography

Spencer FC, Grewe RV. The Management of Arterial Injuries in Battle Casualties. *Ann Surg.* 1955; 141:304–313.

Spencer FC, Bahnson HT. Intracardiac Surgery Employing Hypothermia and Coronary Perfusion Performed on 100 Patients. *Surgery.* 1959; 46:987–995.

Green GE, Spencer FC, Tice DA, Stertzer SH. Arterial and Venous Microsurgical Bypass Grafts for Coronary Artery Disease. *J Thorac Cardiovasc Surg.* 1970; 60:491–503.

Spencer FC, Reemtsma K, Ebert PA. The

Surgical Residency: Length and Quality. *Surgery*. 1973; 74:791–793.

Spencer FC. The Gibbon Lecture—Competence and Compassion: Two Qualities of Surgical Excellence. *Bull Am Coll Surg*. 1979; 64:15–22.

Spencer FC. Presidential Address. Intellectual Creativity in Thoracic Surgeons. *J Thorac Cardiovasc Surg*. 1983; 86:163–179.

Spencer FC, Colvin SB, Culliford AT, Isom OW. Experiences with the Carpentier Techniques of Mitral Valve Reconstruction in 103 Patients (1980–1985). *J Thorac Cardiovasc Surg*. 1985; 90:341–350.

Spencer FC. The Internal Mammary Artery: The Ideal Coronary Bypass Graft? *N Engl J Med*. 1986; 314:50–51.

Spencer FC. The Development of Valvular Heart Surgery over the Past 50 Years (1947–1997): Personal Recollections. *Ann Thorac Surg*. 1997; 64:1549–1554.

Spencer FC, Guice KS. The Expert Medical Witness: Concerns, Limits, and Remedies. *Bull Am Coll Surg*. 2000; 85:22–23.

Henry T. Bahnson, MD

(b. 1920)

The allocation of organs from donors is controversial as to whether the donated organ should be offered to the closest transplant team or should be offered first to the sickest patient on the National Registry. I think that organs should go to the sickest patient first.
— On allocation of donor hearts

Interviewed August 3, 1999

I grew up in Winston-Salem, North Carolina, in a Moravian church community. When I was a boy, the opinion of other people in your community and service to the community were very important. Early in life, it was one of my goals to find a way to serve my community. I was sent to a boys' camp outside Winston-Salem—Camp Haines—and one of the camp activities was to go next door to the Covington farm and pick tobacco. It turned out that my grandfather had delivered all of the babies at that farm, which made a big impression on me. It seemed very noble, and it made me want to go into medicine.

I went to Davidson College for my undergraduate work, and because I did pretty well I was accepted at Harvard Medical School. When I came home after the first summer at Harvard, the war was on. I looked for some research to do and got in touch with Dr. Tinsley Harrison, who at that time was a newcomer to Winston-Salem. I told him I wanted to do some research, and he lined me up with a project involving hemorrhage and vascular grafts. Dr. Harrison was not much on technical things, and so I did all the technical work. This honed my skills a bit, and I worked pretty hard and earned the approval of Dr. Harrison. I ended up with material for a paper, which was subsequently published. Later, when I was getting ready to apply for an internship, Dr. Harrison told me that he would only approve three places for me to go, and one of those was Johns Hopkins. A number of my friends had been there, so I applied in the usual manner. Dr. Blalock at Hopkins normally asked for interviews, but I was excused from that because of Dr. Harrison's recommendation. Dr. Blalock said that if I was good enough for Dr. Harrison, that was good enough.

It was a very good time to be at Johns Hopkins. It was wartime in 1944, and there were only eight interns. There were four residents, and the chief resident was Bill Longmire, who, of course, was a tremendous leader, surgeon, advisor, and head of the surgical service. I got involved in research on hypertension, one aspect of which was working on coarctation of the aorta. We tried to create a stenosis by first dividing the subclavian artery and turning it down and anastomosing it to the distal aorta. We would then divide the aorta between the subclavian and the distal anastomosis so that all of the aortic flow had to go through the subclavian artery. This produced a constriction to the flow similar to a coarctation. This was my own project. Vivien Thomas was there, and he was a tremendous help. He showed me how to anesthetize dogs and anastomose arteries. He taught me a lot of other techniques as well.

Nothing really came of this except some

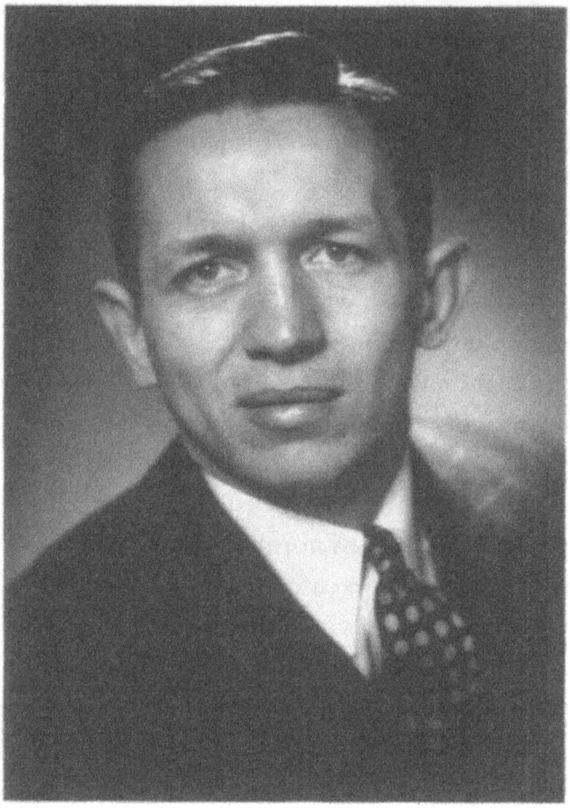

Henry T. Bahnson

improved technical skills on my part, but I think it had something to do with my staying on at Hopkins. The number of assistant residents was cut from eight to three during the war. I was drafted for one year, and when I came home from the war, I stopped by to see Dr. Harrison, who at that time was in Dallas. He urged me to go back to Hopkins, so I did.

In late November 1944 Dr. Blalock did the first Blue Baby operation on Eileen Saxon. I believe that Denton Cooley was the intern. The operation was done in late November just before changing services, and I rotated onto the service as Denton rotated off. My job was to take care of Eileen. A lot of people, mainly Dr. Blalock and Dr. Taussig, were hovering over her. She didn't seem to be less blue than she had been before the operation, but Eileen got better over the next few days. It is interesting how little treatment we had to give back then. There wasn't really much you could do except put a child in an oxygen tent, which increased the oxygen from 20 percent to 28 percent, obviously not much help. We did not have chest tubes, no intubation during general anesthesia, and none of the other things that are commonly done at the present time. Her operation had been done without an endotracheal tube, only with a mask. Ms. Berger, the nurse-anesthetist, did the procedure. I think other anesthesiologists did not want to do it. Ms. Berger was a devoted nurse-anesthetist and always did a beautiful job.

It became more of a landmark procedure than it really deserved to be, I think. Loads of people came to Hopkins to see it done. Dr. Blalock was very receptive and welcomed people. The idea for that sort of shunt had been around for a while. It had been mentioned at a pathology session at Harvard during my second year. The pathologist was talking about patent ductus and congenital heart disease, and he mentioned that you might get a benefit from creating a ductus in patients with tetralogy. The idea may have come from Dr. Taussig's visit to the Boston Children's Hospital, or it may have predated her visit, I am not sure. She often did claim credit for the idea, but regardless of who invented it, it was a nice technical feat. Of course, Dr. Blalock had previously done this operation in the experimental lab at Vanderbilt. They did a subclavian pulmonary anastomosis while trying to produce pulmonary hypertension, so he had the operation ready and available.

One characteristic of Dr. Blalock was his

whiny voice. He was always saying, "Won't somebody help me?" when things weren't going right. He was demanding, and he didn't always recognize that he had to settle down and do the job. On at least one occasion he apologized to me about being whiny, saying that he thought he did better work when he complained a bit. He was not a brilliant surgical technician, but he was good. He was a very thoughtful surgeon, which was the key to his success, I think. Also, he was a good speaker and had a homey way of talking. He was just a friendly, nice guy. He made friends easily, and he maintained his friendships. It was not put on; it was his natural attitude.

I helped him with a large number of Blue Baby operations, probably as many as two hundred. I also went with him when he was invited to go to Guy's Hospital in London. Guy's Hospital had extended an invitation to some of the faculty at Hopkins for a visit for several months. Most people were not willing to take the time away, and Dr. Blalock didn't want to go either, but they urged him and he agreed. He was apprehensive about it. Dr. Ridge Trimble suggested that he take someone with him. I had been working on nothing but tetralogies, coarctations, and patent ductus, so Dr. Blalock asked me if I would like to go with him. It was one of the best experiences of my life, I guess.

A number of interesting things happened on that trip. When we got there, we had to go through customs, and while Dr. Blalock was still trying to get through, I just went straight through because I had a letter from him. I just showed the letter and went straight through, but it took Dr. Blalock an hour or so to get through. He didn't have any identification, and they held him up to explain all the instruments and medicines he had brought. While I was waiting for Dr. Blalock, a friend came down to customs and asked how much bourbon and scotch Dr. Blalock wanted. Dr. Blalock was accustomed to having a drink every day after work was done. I never knew him to drink other than at the end of the day. He rarely drank much, but he regularly drank something each night. Not many drinks though. That was his drinking habit, which so far as I know never affected his ability to function. He used his friends in London to get a case of one of the whiskeys. He entertained frequently.

In London we stayed at the Norfolk Hotel. I don't know where it is in relation to anything other than Guy's Hospital. We worked every day at the hospital. I think we did thirteen cases in four weeks. Then, we all went to Paris: his wife Mary, my wife Louise, Dr. Blalock, and myself. We did seven cases in Paris. Dr. Blalock didn't do all the cases himself. He was getting tired after being away from home almost six weeks. They had a ductus that needed to be done, and he asked me if I would do it. That was the first ductus that had ever been operated on in France. He didn't even go to the hospital the morning I did it. He was out in the gardens touring around. The operating room and the French technical staff were fine, but there were a bunch of Frenchmen in the room crawling all over my back, and it was quite an experience for a young resident.

Hedley Adkins had been our host at Guy's Hospital in London. Guy's Hospital was a general surgical hospital, but at that point there was not much of a distinction between thoracic and general surgery either in England or the United States. There were no boards until about that time. Dr. Blalock gave two talks on that trip to London that drew a lot of attention. He even had a movie to go with the tetralogy operation talk. His lectures were given at the Royal College of Surgeons. There was a series of talks going on, with leaders from the American College of Surgeons, such as Evarts Graham and people of like stature. Dr. Blalock's talk had not been scheduled as part of that series, but a bigger crowd turned out than for the regularly scheduled speakers. The lecture hall filled and there was standing room only, and so he offered to give another lecture afterwards, which he did. They cleared the hall, and he gave another lecture, on coarctation of the aorta. Neither one of these lectures was announced prior to that time except to a small group, but word got around. It was a stimulating experience going to Europe as an instrument carrier of this great man.

After that trip I went back to Baltimore and continued as a resident and then as chief resident. I joined the faculty in 1951 as an assistant professor. By that time I had published a number of articles on abdominal and thoracic aneurysm surgery. For that procedure we were using homografts from the morgue. We had our own system of freeze-drying them, and then we would put them up in a sealed glass container. The main limitation was that it was sometimes difficult to procure them or to get permission to use them, and there was concern about the freeze-drying and reconstituting processes. We used ethylene oxide to sterilize them. I worked with Jim Maloney on developing a sealed vacuum glass container.

About that time, Jack Gibbon first successfully used a heart-lung machine. He was a good friend of Dr. Blalock, and Dr. Blalock asked if we could visit him with several of our residents and junior faculty. Dr. Gibbon got Tom Watson at IBM interested in the heart-lung machine; they developed several models. When we went to visit, we realized it was the best machine going at the time, although it was very expensive. In 1953, I think, Gibbon did his first open-heart procedure on a patient with an atrial septal defect. He was very open about helping to get the information out about what was going on. I had been to Minnesota earlier to see Clarence Dennis's rotating disc, and it was obviously not very good at that time. I worked with him though, and got to know the people in Minneapolis. Later I went there with Tom Starzl to watch them do one of their cross-circulation procedures. Unfortunately, the case we saw was the one in which the patient had air pumped into her system, and she suffered badly from it. We never used the cross-circulation procedure at Johns Hopkins.

The cross-circulation concept was successful in Minnesota, but I don't think it was ever used at other institutions. The Gibbon machine came out so quickly that people waited for that, and then the bubble oxygenator took over. I think they did only about forty cases with cross-circulation.

The first machine that we used at Hopkins was a disc oxygenator. I am not sure how much clinical use that got. Then we used a hanging screen, which was modeled after a Gibbon screen oxygenator. It was designed by Bob Gaertner, who was one of the residents in the lab at Hopkins.

I had an interest in cusp replacement for aortic and mitral valve operations. It was plastic, made of woven Teflon. We had worked a lot with the anatomy of the aortic valve, working out some of the finer points about the shape and mathematical configuration of the leaflets. We made them with a New York company, because they had developed fabrics of Teflon. In developing that, we had initially just gone to the Hudson's department store and bought fabric off the shelf to try to model the shape of the leaflets. The valves worked, but we had a little trouble getting patients off the pump, and it was obvious that this was not going to be successful.

About that time, 1961, I published a paper about closed-chest resuscitation. Before that time, resuscitation of cardiac arrest was usually done with a thoracotomy and manual massage of the heart. It seems hard to believe now that closed-chest resuscitation was developed as recently as 1961, but it was developed at Johns Hopkins. I remember several of those patients. One of them was having trouble, and we had opened his chest and were massaging his heart. At first he was talking to us, but then he couldn't talk any more and he somehow indicated to us, with a very anxious look, to continue it. That was the standard treatment at the time.

I had watched Dr. W. B. Kouwenhoven work in the surgical lab. He was a former chairman of engineering, and he had became interested in defibrillating linemen who got shocked while working on electrical lines. Dr. Blalock turned over part of the lab to Dr. Kouwenhoven, and he was very diligent and hardworking. I had seen him work with dogs, and you could easily get increased blood pressure in the dog by chest compressions. He had suggested that we do this with patients. I did the first closed-chest resuscitation on a patient with a congenital heart lesion. I don't remember the condition other than he arrested during the postop period. We did closed-chest massage and he survived.

This technique spread pretty quickly after that and became the standard for cardiac arrest. It was very commonly done in the hospital, on people who were dying of pneumonia and other things. I remember going to a meeting of the American College of Surgeons in San Francisco, and there was an exhibit on how to do closed-chest resuscitation. Then shortly thereafter I went to see La Boheme and saw Mimi stretched out on the couch singing her last aria, and nobody was there beating on her chest. I thought it was much better to die peacefully like that than to be resuscitated through heart massage, but it was done on virtually everyone who died in the hospital before guidelines were developed.

I moved to Pittsburgh in 1963 to be the chairman of the Department of Surgery at the University of Pittsburgh. The oxygenator that we used there was a screen, and you had to spread the blood over the screen. It had a roller pump on each side of the screen to fill it with blood. It was made by the Edwards Company in Virginia. We didn't use the bubble oxygenator until later. One of the reasons we were having postoperative problems at that time was the screen oxygenator; we weren't cleaning the screens adequately. The screen oxygenator was reusable, in contrast to the bubble oxygenator, which was disposable. We subsequently found out that there were protein deposits on the screen, most of which were probably coming from bacteria and E. coli. When we started really cleaning the screens the results became much better. I don't think we ever got a dog to survive using the screen oxygenator. Denton Cooley commented that we had to use very short pump times, but most of us weren't able to do that at first. Once we learned to clean the screen properly, the machine was a pretty good one. Later we went to the bubble oxygenator like everybody else, and then finally the disposable membrane oxygenator.

Around that time I wrote a paper about the EKG changes with heart transplants. We had started doing heart transplants very quickly after Christiaan Barnard did the first one in late 1967. We did three. It was technically possible to do heart transplants, but taking care of the patients afterwards was the problem.

In 1962 I invited Tom Starzl to come to Pittsburgh, but at first he didn't want to leave his job in Denver. When he finally came, he not only started a liver transplant program, but he also stimulated the cardiac transplantation program. He had gotten the wrinkles out of kidney transplantation, and he continued to do those. The urologists were unhappy about that and wanted to take over, but neither Tom nor I would accept that, so we agreed to divide the kidney transplant patients fifty-fifty. Tom very quickly got a better procurement system going and began getting better results, and so it worked out.

His recruitment to the University of Pittsburgh had been opposed very vigorously by the medical service, so we had to get another recommendation. I got one from the chairman of the Nobel committee and one from a Nobel Prize winner. I found out by talking with friends who had worked with him that he was not easy to work with, but he was straightforward, hardworking, and he came strongly recommended. It seemed to me that he would add a lot to our environment. It was difficult at first, for he didn't stand for idleness. He worked hard and hoped others would work with him, but if they didn't, he simply did their work too. Sometimes that involved taking over patients, and that didn't fit our pattern entirely. It was not easy at first.

Tom brought cyclosporine to our program. It had been tried by Roy Calne in England, but in England they thought it was too toxic and set it aside. Tom thought it might work after all, and he started doing his own experiments with it. He found out that if it was properly handled, it was as good as, or better than, Imuran. Initially cyclosporine was used as a substitute for Imuran when it caused trouble or complications. Later cyclosporine was used for almost all transplant patients.

In 1982 we revived the heart transplant program and began to get very good results, similar to those that Shumway was getting. A few months after Tom arrived he got us going more vigorously with his organ procurement organization and with the use of cyclosporine.

The allocation of organs from donors is controversial as to whether the donated organ should be offered first to the closest transplant team or should be offered first to the sickest patient on the national registry. I think that organs should go to the sickest patient first. Since we have a very large transplant service at the University of Pittsburgh, we naturally have a lot of very sick patients. If that were the case, we would be allocated a large share of donated organs, and fewer organs would go to smaller, local transplant teams. Probably this would lead to better outcomes, but there is also the argument that a family that donates would prefer that it benefit someone in their community. The sickest patient is not always in the same area.

Ten or fifteen years ago, I would have predicted that the mechanical heart would be the solution to end-state heart disease, but this has not turned out to be the case. I am not sure that we will ever be able to get a mechanical heart to last fifteen to twenty years, much less five, or even one to two years. There are some things that are worse than dying. I think we have a long way to go before we develop an implantable, long-lasting artificial heart. It does seem that it can be used for a temporary period of time. We are working on it, trying to improve the pumps and so forth, and they may eventually last for several years, but not much longer than that. It may work for bridging the transition from heart failure to a transplanted heart. Maybe the American public will become more generous in making organs available for donation. The artificial heart may be like the screen oxygenator or the bubble oxygenator. The early oxygenators were worlds apart from the refinement of our machines today. I think the same sort of improvement will happen with the mechanical heart for bridging to transplant, but not for long-term replacement.

I have had a long life and a long career in medicine, and there have been many people who have had a profound influence on my life and medical career. The first were my parents. I was raised in a good Moravian Christian family with four brothers. My parents taught us about honesty and integrity, which, I think, are the prime virtues. I was brought up in a Christian environment.

When I worked at Camp Sequoia, teaching horseback riding, I met a guy named Clovis Alexander, who was a fun-loving bachelor. He was as interested in horses as I was, and he had a joy of life that I think I have never seen in anyone else. I had a couple of influential professors at Davidson College, and then the group at Hopkins, Dr. Blalock leading them, along with Bill Longmire, who was my resident. You always think your resident is the best, and I always think my resident was the best, but there were other people who have come along and done equally well, for example Bill Scott. I was four years behind him at Harvard. He was a resident there when I was a fourth-year student, and he became the chief resident when I came back after the navy. Some of my other influences have been Rollins Hanlon, Harry Muller, and Frank Spencer because we worked together. Dr. Blalock commissioned Frank and me to build the heart-lung machine and establish the open-heart program at Hopkins. Most of the good things that I got credit for were really Frank's work; he was a tremendously hard worker. Denton Cooley was a fellow intern and has always been a good friend.

Vivien Thomas was an important colleague of Dr. Blalock, and they worked very well as a team. Dr. Blalock taught Vivien a lot, but Vivien also discovered a lot of new techniques himself and taught them to Dr. Blalock. I was going to say that Vivien would have gotten nowhere without Dr. Blalock and that Dr. Blalock would have gotten somewhere without Vivien because there were others around that could have done what Vivien did. But Vivien thought of a number of ways to do things, and Dr. Blalock realized this and gave Vivien a lot of credit. The race issue was quite a concern, as you know, and Vivien was slow to get credit. He got a fair amount, but perhaps he should have gotten more credit earlier. He was given an honorary degree at Hopkins, and I think that was laudable and appropriate. Vivien certainly taught me easy ways of doing a lot of things and improved my technical skills and my work with Dr. Blalock. He was one reason I was on the heart service for eight months. I had picked up a lot of my skills from Vivien, who was a nice guy and a positive influence on me. He was also a good role model for many blacks at that time.

One of the other things I did when I was a student was to watch Dr. Gross do a ductus. It made a big impression on me. The operating room at Children's Hospital was small. I had an elective there for a month in pediatric surgery. That time at Children's Hospital was part of the reason I was invited to come to Pittsburgh. The resident in orthopedics offered to help me do a circumcision, and I did mine so well that I impressed him. Later he was one of the people who was instrumental in my coming to Pittsburgh. I am indebted to a lot of people at Children's and the Brigham; they were just nice places to work. Mass General was a little more businesslike and bigger, and so it had a different atmosphere.

Anyway, doing the ductus back then was a pretty stressful procedure because of the instruments and anesthesia that were available at the time. When I was Dr. Gross's student, he was ligating them. Dividing them came later. He got into an argument with Dr. Blalock about that fairly early. Dr. Blalock thought that ligating them was good enough, and I still believe it is all right and satisfactory. Dividing them is a better procedure, and in later years almost all of them were divided. That one I did in France wasn't divided, though. I had those Frenchmen crawling all over me. In fact, it bled when I tried to get around it, but it worked out all right. A ductus had never been done in France until that time.

Looking back on my career, I can see that every surgical procedure I did in my last year of practice was a procedure that did not exist when I was a student. I would be a fool to say anything other than that the same thing could happen again. I am not sure where we are going, but you can be very sure it will be different.

When I retired, I started playing the harmonica. I had played it as a kid, never very well, and never for a long time. I used it on horseback riding trips when I worked on a ranch in Wyoming for a couple of summers. When I retired, I wanted to learn how to play it better, so I went to a folk festival in Elkins, West Virginia, and I took a course on harmonica playing. When you play a harmonica, there are a number of notes that are straightforward: You just blow on them or draw on them to get a tone. You also need to bend notes by changing the reeds. It is a lot harder to explain than to do, although it is not that easy to do. People remember where they were when JFK was shot, but harmonica players remember where they were when they managed to bend a note on the harmonica. Well, I remember exactly where I was and what I was doing. At the camp, our instructor had taken the cover off the harmonica, and we looked at the reeds. He said, "Can't you see it bending?" Well, I couldn't see them bending. I could see that the thing was vibrating and moving, but I couldn't see what I thought would be curling or bending. I knew that we had the tools at home that would let us visualize that. We came back home and used some of the engineering equipment, various scopes and things, to see the reed, see how it functioned, and what made the sound. It took forever to get all the wrinkles out, but I ended up with a publication about it. The same month I got a patent on a type of harmonica, a four-inch thing, hoping to sell some of them. We sold a couple of hundred of them, but that is all we ever got around to, because they were so expensive to make. You have to make them in large numbers, and I haven't been able to do that yet. What we did was modify a Horner harmonica, first using shops and machinists around town. Finally, the Horner Company made them for us. I wish I had one of them to play right now.

Bibliography

Bahnson, HT. Definitive Treatment of Saccular Aneurysms of the Aorta with Excision of Sac and Aortic Suture. *Surg Gynec Obst.* 1953; 96:383–402.

Waldhausen JA, Webb RC, Spencer FC, Bahnson HT. Study of Canine Lung as an Oxygenator of Human and Canine Blood in Extracorporeal Circulation. *Surgery.* 1957; 42:726–733.

Spencer FC, Bahnson HT. Intracardiac Surgery Employing Hypothermia and Coronary Perfusion Performed on 100 Patients. *Surgery.* 1959; 46:987–995.

Bahnson HT, Spencer FC, Busse EFG, Davis FW Jr. Cusp Replacement and Coronary Artery Perfusion in Open Operations on the Aortic Valve. *Ann Surg.* 1960; 152:494–503.

Bahnson HT. Closed-Chest Cardiac Resuscitation. *Surg Gynec Obstet.* 1961; 112:622–623.

Bahnson HT, Spencer FC, Landtman B, Wolf MD, Neill CA, Taussig HB. Surgical Treatment and Follow-up of 147 cases of Tetralogy of Fallot Treated by Correction. *J Thorac Cardiovasc Surg.* 1962; 44:419–432.

Scheuer J, Shaver JA, Harris BC, Leonard JJ, Bahnson HT. Electrocardiographic Findings in Cardiac Transplantation. *Circulation.* 1969; 40:289–296.

Shaver JA, Leon DF, Gray S III, Leonard JJ, Bahnson HT. Hemodynamic Observations after Cardiac Transplantation. *N Engl J Med.* 1969; 281:822–827.

Bahnson HT. Substitute Hearts. *Bull Am Coll Surg.* 1987; 72:4–10.

Bahnson HT, Antaki JF, Beery QC. Acoustical Physical Dynamics of the Diatonic Harmonica. *J Acoust Soc Am.* 1998; 103:2134–2144.

Congenital Heart Surgery

Judson G. Randolph, MD

(b. 1927)

When Dr. Ladd left to go on vacation he said to Dr. Gross, "Whatever you do, don't operate on that little girl with a patent ductus."

— On the first closure
of a patent ductus

Interviewed February 4, 2004

I was born in Georgia in 1927, and I went to school in Nashville, Tennessee. I graduated from Vanderbilt University and then went to medical school at Vanderbilt, graduating in 1953. I did my internship at the University of Rochester, and then I came back to Vanderbilt briefly while I was waiting for a position to be available for me at the Boston Children's Hospital. I went to the Boston Children's Hospital as an assistant resident, and then as a resident at Massachusetts General Hospital. Ultimately, I was chief resident at the Boston Children's Hospital in 1960 and 1961. I stayed on the faculty there, and during that time I worked with Dr. Robert Gross. Dr. Gross is a great hero of mine, and he was my close associate while I was working in Boston. He was my teacher and was almost like a father figure to me. So first I'd like to talk about Dr. Gross and how he got started in medicine, and about his various interests and contributions.

Robert Gross was born in Baltimore on July 2, 1905. He was the son of a piano maker, and his father hoped that Robert would come into the piano-making business when he grew up. When Robert was in high school, his father had him work after school in piano construction, for two reasons. One reason was his hope that Robert would come into the business, but the other concerned Robert's eye problem. He had trouble with one of his eyes, and his father hoped that working with the fine tools and movements of piano construction would help him learn to adapt to the partial loss of vision in one eye. From that experience Robert Gross became a mechanic. In the second half of the twentieth century, most surgical contributions have been physiological, but Dr. Gross's contributions were mechanical.

He graduated from Harvard Medical School AOA but couldn't get the surgical internship he wanted, so he went into pathology with Dr. Bert Wolbach. He was a pathology resident at the Brigham and at Children's Hospital, and ultimately he was the chief resident in pathology at the Brigham, but at the same time he was appointed to the surgical house staff of Elliott Cutler at Harvard and at the Brigham. When he was doing his work in pathology, he kept seeing little children who had died because they had acute bacterial endocarditis involving the ductus arteriosus. He kept looking at the ductus, and the mechanic in him said, "You know, we ought to be able to shut that thing off." He went to the dog lab and devised a method to divide the ductus. This was in the mid-1930s, and you must remember that we didn't have endotracheal anesthesia or antibiotics. The heart was a big heaving thing that everybody avoided because they couldn't get to it or do anything with it. But Dr. Gross worked out a method. It was a bit

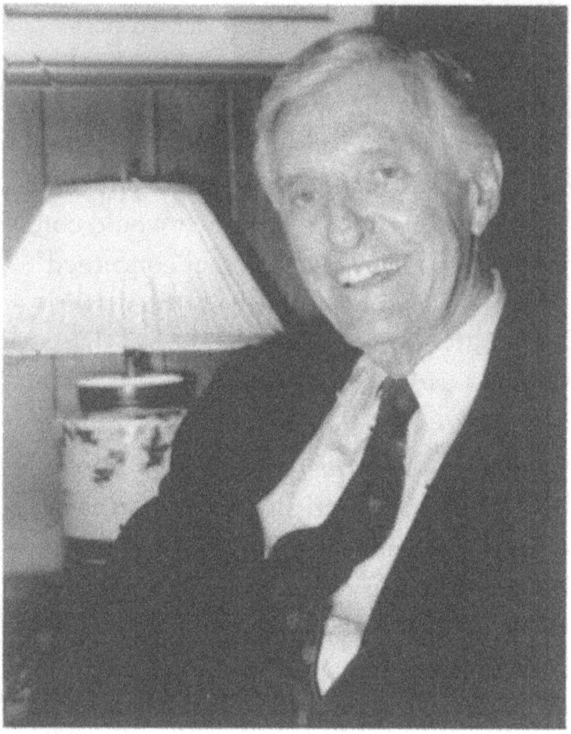

Judson G. Randolph

primitive. He put four hemostats across the ductus, and he put rubber bands around the handles of the hemostats so they wouldn't spring open, causing unexpected blood loss. It was that primitive. We were still using the rubber bands when I was his resident. Once the four hemostats were on, he would take the two inner hemostats off and transect the ductus. Then he insisted on silk sutures to close the ductus, not just to tie it off. He wanted silk sutures to close the end of the ductus, and that's how he really began his inquiries into various extracardiac mechanical problems and operations.

He discussed this research with Dr. Ladd, his chief at the Children's Hospital. He thought that maybe this ductus work could go forward clinically, but Dr. Ladd told him that he should stay in the lab, that they weren't ready to do such a procedure on a patient. Dr. Ladd always took a month off in August for his vacation. While he was gone, Dr. Gross, who at that time was a thirty-three-year-old assistant resident, mind you, not even a chief resident, lined up two children with patent ductus arteriosus, to operate on. He was so sure that this was the right thing to do that he planned to do the second child if he lost the first one. But he didn't have to do the second child that day. The first operation went very well. Actually, he ligated the ductus, as it was too short to be divided. This trial was hailed around the world as an inroad into cardiac surgery. The operation was done on August 26, 1938. When Dr. Ladd left for his vacation, he had said to Dr. Gross, "Whatever you do, don't operate on that little girl with the patent ductus." Of course, Dr. Gross did the operation anyway. Dr. Ladd came back from his vacation a few days later, and he asked Dr. Gross, "Well, is anything new?" and Dr. Gross said, "Nope, not much, nothing new." He didn't want to tell him, even though it was a success.

His lab work progressed and he became interested in two other problems. Back then, there were a lot of children born with a constricting vascular ring around their esophagus or their trachea, and that was another mechanical problem. He gradually distinguished the different patterns of this problem and developed different surgical approaches to each. While he was working on that, he realized that there were also a lot of children who had coarctation of the aorta. Dr. Gross believed that the coarctation could be excised and that a direct union could be brought about, eliminating the narrow area of the aorta. Clarence Crafoord did the coarctation operation just before Gross did, but loyalists of Dr. Gross believe that Crafoord knew of the work Gross had done in the lab, and this led him to go ahead with an operation on a patient. Then, of course, Gross repaired a coarctation also, and was given a lot of credit for working out the details and some of the difficulties with the long-gap coarctation. The situation was analogous to that of Christiaan Barnard and Norman Shumway, when Barnard visited Shumway's colleague, Richard Lower, in Richmond and then went home and did a heart transplant before Shumway did one.

In the late forties, Dr. Gross also became interested in arterial homografts. This interest was related to the coarctation of the aorta. I think he might well be lionized for that contribution alone, because in a way he opened up the whole field of vascular surgery. The homograft research came about because he was seeing patients with a long aortic coarctation. If he resected enough to eliminate the narrow place, he might not be able to get the two ends together. He went through a series of experiments in the lab to see if they could put an aortic sleeve around the thoracic artery. What would happen to it? What would happen to a dog that had an aortic sleeve for a year? Would the sleeve calcify? Would it become necrotic? Nobody knew. He worked out a whole process where you could use homografts as aortic sleeves. All of us on the house staff used to be required to go to the autopsy room and resect segments of the aorta. We would then put them in packages, and they would be freeze-dried, radiated, and refrigerated. When Dr. Gross needed to put a sleeve in, he would have somebody go to the freezer and get one and reconstitute it, and he would sew it in place. You see, that was the first real progress in vascular grafting, and it opened up the whole field of vascular surgery. This by itself is a major contribution. Dr. Gross wrote his first paper on the use of aortic homografts in 1948.

In the early 1950s, surgeons started using Dacron woven grafts. I think Dr. DeBakey had a lot to do with that development. At that time there was an explosion of vascular surgery procedures involving aortas and aneurysms, and surgeons started using various plastic and woven materials. It was Sterling Edwards who put the crinkle in the vascular grafts. We used to have trouble with the Dacron grafts. They would get kinked under a vessel, or they would get kinked going around an organ. Sterling was home with the flu one time, and his wife kept bringing him fluids with those new straws that had the little crinkle so they would bend and not kink. Sterling kept looking at that crinkle. He went back to the lab and put the crinkles in the vascular grafts so they would not kink. All the grafts are that way now.

Before he built his own pump, Dr. Gross used an atrial well to close atrial septal defects. We were still using it in the lab when I worked there. That was another Gross mechanical concept. The question was, since we don't have a pump-oxygenator, how can we get our fingers inside the heart? Elton Watkins was working in the lab, and he was also very mechanically gifted, so the two of them took a big rubber cone with a smaller bottom to it, and they sewed the small end onto the side of the atrial appendage in a laboratory animal. Then they opened up the atrium through the bottom of the cone or well and the atrial pressure would fill the well to about twenty millimeters of mercury. Dr. Gross could put his finger inside this big well and reach in and feel, for example, an atrial septal defect. They would put sutures in from the outside of the atrial wall and guide the needle with the finger down to the defect, or they could actually put the sutures in through this well of blood and sew up the atrial defect. They did that on a number of patients. This was quite an ingenious approach before there was such a thing as an open-heart or pump-oxygenator procedure, because it enabled them to operate on a beating heart. Dr. Gross was a mechanic and a very successful one.

In the early forties Helen Taussig came to Boston to talk to Dr. Gross about the Blue Baby operation. You see, Dr. Blalock had just arrived at Hopkins, and she wasn't used to working with him, but she knew what Dr. Gross had done with the ductus and coarctation. She came to Boston and she just laid it out for Dr. Gross; she gave it to him. She said, "Dr. Gross, in these blue babies, if you could just put an artery into the pulmonary artery, and if we could perfuse blood that way into the lung system, we would save a lot of children's lives." Dr. Gross didn't get it. I will never understand why, with his facile mind and his mechanical sense, he didn't get that, but he said to Dr. Taussig, "You know, I spent years trying to develop a way to divide the ductus, and now you want me to make one." Helen Taussig went home and gave the problem to Blalock, and the rest is history. For years Dr. Gross used to kick himself for not grasping that opportunity. Of course, if he had followed Dr. Taussig's suggestion, he would have held all the cards in the congenital heart surgical game. This situation took place a couple of years before Dr. Blalock did the first Blue Baby operation in 1944.

John Gibbon did the first open-heart procedure in 1953 in Philadelphia. This came about after he worked in Churchill's lab in Boston in the 1930s. After the war he had the idea that a machine could take over for the heart so that surgeons could operate inside the heart, and he finally demonstrated the practicality of that with the repair of an atrial septal defect patient in 1953. Dr. Gross really jumped on that. He thought, "This is the future for cardiac surgery in children." He had a very bright resident, Lester Sauvage, working in the lab and on the clinical service with him at that time. Lester had been a student of Henry Harken's in Seattle and had come to work with Dr. Gross. Dr. Gross sent Lester around the country to see the different kinds of heart-lung devices that were being used. Of course, he spent time in Minnesota and Philadelphia and other places, and when he came back, he and Dr. Gross developed their own pump-oxygenator, a disc oxygenator. It was Dr. Gross who figured out that you needed to raise the OR table to put the patient up high above the floor and then put the pump down low so you could get gravity flow for the venous drainage. He was good at little mechanical things like that. He started doing more and more open-heart surgery, and that happened to be the time that I was in Boston at Children's Hospital. It was a very exciting and wonderful time.

Dr. Gross had a toolbox that he kept in the operating room. He had it there because he liked to fool with the pump, the plumbing, and the scrub sink, even the door if it was squeaking. He didn't like it when it squeaked on opening. He really worked with his tools. After he retired, I visited him up in Vermont, in Brattleboro, where he had his home. In his basement he had a splendid array of tools carefully hanging in all the right places. He was a mechanic until the day he died, but he never went back to making pianos.

He had a strained relationship with Dr. Ladd. Dr. Ladd was concluding his time in Boston in 1945 or 1946, and he wanted Dr. Orvar Swenson to succeed him there. Of course, Dr. Swenson had done wonderful work on Hirschsprung's disease, and he had written a very fundamental paper on esophageal atresia in 1948. But Harvard chose Gross to succeed Dr. Ladd, instead of Swenson. Dr. Gross was basically very shy. He was quite good in a professional setting when he gave a paper or commented on a paper, but in a social gathering he was quite shy.

I could have said a lot more about Dr. Gross. He loved pretty girls. George Holcomb and I used to say that the reason for our success at Boston Children's was that we were married to such pretty girls. Alice, George's wife, was Miss Vanderbilt. My wife, Comfort, was awfully pretty, and Dr. Gross thought that they were two lovely ladies. Comfort knew him well enough to call him Bob, and he gloried in that, but he said, "What are we going to do about Jud?" Comfort said, "Bob, he's going to call you Dr. Gross until one of you dies," and that was true. I could never call him Bob.

I had not always planned to be a surgeon. When I was growing up thinking about medical school, I thought I wanted to be a pediatrician, because I had been in Boy Scouts. I liked working with and teaching younger boys, and pediatrics seemed to be the right medical field for me. At the same time, going through high school, I had a little trouble with my knee, so I never amounted to much on the football field. I played a little basketball and baseball, but I never was a hot stick like I wished I could be.

I got to Vanderbilt medical school, and in my third year I had surgery as my first rotation. Man, I got in the OR, and after I had been there two or three days, I looked around and said to myself, "These people have uniforms, a locker room, an arena, and a team. This is for me. You can be as good as you want, and it doesn't matter how much you weigh." I just found the OR to be something I was pleased to be a part of. It was my briar patch. This was during a transitional time at Vanderbilt, after Barney Brooks retired. Rollin Daniel was the acting chief of surgery, and soon thereafter Dr. Scott came.

I went to Rochester, New York, for my internship. While I was there, Dr. Gross's book came out. It cost $18, but I had no money. I bought that book anyway and took it home to my wife. I said, "Look, you can do it all. You can be a surgeon, and you can work with children. I'm going to write a letter to this fellow Gross." She said, "No, you're not," and I thought, "She doesn't want me to go for the extra training." Then she said something that only a wife could say: "No, you're not going to write to him. We're going to find the money for an air ticket, and you're going to Boston to meet him because you're a lot better in person than you are on paper."

I went to Boston, and Dr. Gross and I hit it off. He got out a great big roll of paper with years marked on it, in two-month intervals. He had slots for junior residents, senior residents, and a chief resident. He wrote me down for a slot as a junior resident. Dr. Gross took a new junior resident every two months so that there wouldn't be a big transition in July when nobody knew where they were going. He penciled me in for March

1955. I said to him, "Dr. Gross, what should I do during this interval of eight months?" He said, "Well, you've got that great pathologist, Ernest Goodpasture, there at Vanderbilt. Why don't you go down there and work with him? I think it will help you." He told me that when he couldn't get the surgical internship that he wanted, he went into pathology for a while. That's what I did. I went to Vanderbilt to work for Dr. Goodpasture and Dr. John Shapiro, and that was a very productive time.

Dr. Shapiro was a great friend of mine. If you looked up the word "integrity" in the dictionary, you ought to find his picture next to it. He terrified us students during the six months of his pathology course; he would look down his nose and say, "Mr. Randolph, do you know anything at all about rheumatoid arthritis?" We would just freeze up, paralyzed. He instilled a lot of fear in the students. The message was, "Work hard, and no funny business." He never called the students by their first names, and he treated everybody exactly the same throughout the course, but the day after you got out of that course and you weren't under his thumb any more, you might be walking down the hall and he would look over at you and say, "Hello, Jud." Then you felt like somebody had said, "I knight thee." He was a most warm, affable person to work for as a house staff member, a magnificent man and leader. Because he thought so much of Dr. Shapiro's judgment, Dr. Harvey Branscomb, chancellor of Vanderbilt University, used to call and talk to him about the university as a whole, not just the medical school.

Dr. Shapiro had an ankylosed knee from an injury he got during World War II in Italy working in a front-line hospital, and he walked with a stiff-legged gait. He was hit, and Dr. Jimmy Kirtley of the Vanderbilt Hospital in Italy wanted to take his leg off, but he begged Jimmy not to do that. There was some brand new stuff called sulfanilimide, and they put it in his wound. They managed to save his leg, but the knee joint became ankylosed. John Shapiro came home and was given a 50 percent disability. Before the war he had had two years of surgical training at Western Reserve, and he had wanted to be a surgeon, but when he tried to go back, he found that he couldn't stand in the operating room. So he went into pathology, came home to Vanderbilt, and worked with Dr. Goodpasture, and in 1948 he finished his residency. Then Dr. Goodpasture asked him to stay on the full-time staff as an instructor. By this time Dr. Shapiro was married to Elizabeth, whom he had met in Cleveland. Of course, he was making very little money as an instructor in pathology. John Shapiro then wrote to the VA and said, "I am no longer disabled from my profession. You can stop sending my 50 percent disability check." I am sure they didn't know where to file that letter, because they had never received another one like it from anybody.

During the summer after our sophomore year, Bill Edwards and I were working in the pathology lab, and we did an autopsy together. We were doing the organ recital later, and we couldn't figure out what had caused the death. Dr. Goodpasture came in, and he was like a little terrier, small and intense. He leaned over and looked at the slices of the liver, and I had the feeling that he was looking into it as if it were under a microscope, because he was right down on it. He said, "I believe that you will find that there is fibrosis around the veins. . . ." He just laid it all out for us. Then he turned around and walked out. Shapiro looked at Edwards and me and said, "Boys, there's no substitute for brains."

I was telling this story at home the next Sunday during dinner. My brother, Somers, was there, and he was a wonderful baseball player. At that time he was playing for John Shapiro's brother, Joe Shapiro—a legendary coach—in the summer leagues. We were always trying to get Somers, my brother, to study, so I was telling that story where Dr. Shapiro says, "Boys, there's no substitute for brains," and my brother said, "That's not what his brother says. His brother says there's no substitute for team hustle." Dr. Shapiro loved that story. He was later elected to be chairman of the pathology department for fifteen or twenty years at Vanderbilt until 1971. He was a fine one and a rock on the faculty during those years.

After eight months at Vanderbilt with Dr. Goodpasture and Dr. Shapiro, I went to Boston to start my residency with Dr. Gross. Back in those days, we were having trouble getting enough blood to prime the pump-oxygenator. Sometimes we needed five, six, or even seven units of blood. But if you could get two patients whose blood type matched, there was no reason not to clamp all of the tubing after the first case, save the blood, and use that blood to prime the pump for the second case. As a matter of fact, the second pump run was probably better because the first patient's own fresh blood and clotting factors were warm and ready to go. Two pumps, one after another, was really an ingenious idea, and it worked well. I don't believe there were ever any dire consequences. It was a unique concept and was not done any other place except possibly in Memphis, because Bobby Allen, who was the cardiac resident at that time in Boston, liked it, and he later went to Memphis to start a cardiac surgery program there.

We had a disc oxygenator, and the discs chewed up blood cells. Then Teflon was invented, and they started using Teflon to coat the discs. The blood slipped off the Teflon and wasn't damaged as much. Later I told my wife about that and she said, "If you had had a brain in your head, you would have figured out that you could put that stuff on the bottom of a cooking pan, and we would have been millionaires!" I never did make that conceptual leap.

My job with Dr. Gross was really just for one year. After that, I had the great good fortune to meet Dr. Churchill, and he invited me to come over to Massachusetts General after I finished my year at the Children's Hospital. My job with Dr. Gross was a junior resident's position. People were knocking down the doors to get that junior job, and then they would go out and do either pediatric surgery or cardiac surgery. We had people with thoracic boards coming just to do that junior job. The senior residency at Boston Children's was four six-month units, including six months as a cardiac resident. Once in a while Dr. Gross would select somebody to be the chief resident. That person didn't do any cardiac surgery, but took care of the ward service and did all the noncardiac general surgery in newborns and children of all ages. That was the job that propelled so many young people into academic jobs around the country in the fifties and sixties as chiefs of pediatric surgery, since those were the days that the specialty of pediatric surgery was just taking off.

I mentioned earlier that Dr. Gross initially did not get the surgical internship that he wanted, and eventually I found out more about that from Bill Clatworthy. Dr. Bill Clatworthy was a pediatric surgeon in Columbus. I was privileged to get close to Dr. Clatworthy and work on some national committees with him. He was a captivating, smart man. When he finished his residency, he was Dr. Ladd's last resident, and he went on to be Dr. Gross's first resident, but then he needed two more years of general surgery training. Since he was from the Midwest, he wrote to Dr. Wangensteen at the University of Minnesota and said, "I would like to come and train in your program and finish there, if there is such an opening." Then he went to Dr. Ladd and said, "Would you write a letter to Dr. Wangensteen?" And he went to Dr. Gross and said, "Would you write a letter to Dr. Wangensteen?" They both said they would be happy to do that. About a week later, Clatworthy got a letter accepting him into Wangensteen's program. He finished in Boston and went out to Minnesota. He had his interview with Dr. Wangensteen, who told him where to go and what to get started on. As he was leaving he said, "Dr. Wangensteen, when I went back to thank Dr. Ladd and Dr. Gross for sending letters of recommendation to you, they both admitted that they hadn't sent them yet, and I wondered why you went ahead and accepted me." Dr. Wangensteen said, "Well, I got an application one time from a young fellow from Boston named Gross, and I turned him down. I said to myself, 'I'll never do that again.'" That's what happened to Dr. Gross's application for an internship with Wangensteen.

I went to the Massachusetts General Hospital, and I spent three years on the house staff there. The program there was the exact opposite of the Hopkins program, where they took twelve interns and then selected only two to go through the Halsted residency. Massachusetts General selected eight interns and took them all the way through five years, so that they were then board eligible. This later came to be known as a rectangular program. Many, many Massachusetts General senior residents went out to practice or to work on faculties without being the chief resident, so it was a block program rather than a pyramid. I went there and started as a third-year resident, and I went through my third, fourth, and fifth years there. It was an engaging and a happy place. They had so many good people, both on the faculty and on the house staff, just good people to be around.

I had to negotiate with Dr. Gross to see if he would accept me for the senior residency at Children's once I had finished my general surgical training at Massachusetts General. He agreed to do that. My path was constructed in such a way that when I finished general surgery at Massachusetts General, I would then go back and be a senior resident at Children's Hospital. The senior residency there was a very involved two-year program. Most of the graduates of the senior program would go out to responsible jobs in pediatric surgery around the country. But if Dr. Gross kept you to do the chief residency, you had independent responsibility. It was almost like being a young staff person, as you ran a really busy service for a year under his direction. That prepared me very well for working in Washington later.

I did the chief residency and stayed on the faculty for two and a half years. There were about five of us on the Children's Hospital staff, including Dr. Gross. He was totally involved in cardiac surgery by then, so he allowed those of us who wanted to do other things freedom for other pursuits. In 1961 nobody was paying much attention to the great need for tumor surgery that was evolving along with chemotherapy, so I went to work in the tumor clinic with Dr. Sidney Farber. I ended up doing most of the tumor surgery at Boston Children's, and Dr. Frannie Moore had me work at the Brigham in cancer surgery. I might have very well just stayed and enjoyed that life, but when an opportunity to start my own program came along, I wanted to give it a shot.

Washington, D.C., was almost the last major city in the country that didn't have pediatric surgery, and the Children's Hospital there wanted a director of their fledgling program. The Children's Hospital was a funny little old hospital. A marvelous man named Bob Parrot was made the medical director of this hospital, and he recruited an endocrinologist, a hematologist, and some other medical specialists that the whole community wanted and needed badly. A pediatrician in Chevy Chase would like to send a child to an expert at this growing little facility, but the surgeons in town didn't want a chief of surgery there. They didn't want somebody coming in there to mess up their deal where they worked in the clinic for a month and took all the patients who had insurance. I was not welcomed by the surgical community when I first came to Washington, but the pediatricians were glad that I was there, and gradually things worked out.

The general surgeons in Washington were not doing the really complicated pediatric cases, such as heart surgery or complicated chest surgery. Mostly the surgeons were doing hernias and things like that, and they had a fairly simple OR schedule. I wanted it to evolve into an imitation of the expanded work at Boston Children's, and it took a while to get it going.

When we started an open-heart program, everybody was critical. They thought they could still send patients to the Mayo Clinic and up the road to Johns Hopkins. There was a wonderful old man there named Bill Jameson, a surgeon who had worked with Charlie Bailey. He had made a pump with his own ingenuity in his workshop in Manassas, Virginia. One day he asked me to go look at it. I did so, and I said, "It looks pretty interesting, let's move it down to the lab." We took it to the lab and did some dogs on it. Then I got some money to buy a new pump from a company in Boston. We started clinical cardiac work with several simple cases. Dr. Lou Scott, the cardiologist, who had come to Boston Children's in cardiology while I was there in surgery, very carefully picked out some patients with simple ASDs, some with pulmonic stenosis, and some other things that should go well. The operations did go very well, so we started open-heart surgery at Washington Children's Hospital.

I continued to do the cardiac surgery until it got so busy that I knew that I had to do only that, or else do noncardiac surgery and develop a training program in that field, but not both. We had persuaded a navy surgeon, Dr. Edward McClenathan, to come to Washington Children's to do the children's heart surgery. He was quite good, but he had no experience with babies and children. I kept doing the babies and children for some years until finally we got yet another cardiac surgeon. It was very hard to walk away from cardiac surgery, but I had to make a conscious decision. I decided that my real goal was the education and training of pediatric surgeons so that they would become chiefs of surgery elsewhere. Thus in 1974 I stopped doing the cardiac surgery and concentrated on educating young pediatric surgeons.

In 1991 I retired from the position at Washington Children's Hospital and came back to Nashville. I began working at Meharry Medical School. People at Vanderbilt, Skip Neblett and others, were very warm and welcoming, and I could have done some kind of work at Vanderbilt in the lab or the clinic or in teaching. It was obvious that they had plenty of power at Vanderbilt and that there was a great need at Meharry. I went to Meharry and began to work in the surgical department under Henry Foster, who was the dean at the time. I went to Dr. Frist and Ken Roberts and said, "I need some money to help these young people." They gave me a very generous grant so that I could take a fourth-year student and send that student out to a prospective training program for a month as an elective during his or her senior year. That way the student had a better chance of getting a residency position there. I managed to get a lot of internships and residencies for young people that they might not have gotten otherwise. That was a real labor of love, and I still hear from those young people. Meharry was going through some real changes at that time. David Satcher came, and he was very supportive.

There have been many people who have been important influences in my life. First, I had a wonderful father. He was a newspaperman and didn't know anything about medicine, medical school, or medical training. The intern match program started in 1952. I was in the second year of the match, in 1953. Dr. Scott had come to Vanderbilt, and he had everybody all revved up. He did me the great honor of saying that he would like for me to stay at Vanderbilt and be on his house staff. My best pal in medical school, Bill Edwards, was going to stay, and we were just getting all excited. I went home on Sunday to eat dinner, and my dad said, "Now let me see. You went to Stokes Elementary and Hillsboro High School, and then you went to Vanderbilt for your college education, and Vanderbilt Medical School. That's all within about two miles of each other. Don't they have anything else out there somewhere?" I came right back down to Vanderbilt the next day and I went to Dr. Daniel. I said, "Dr. Daniel, you've got to get me out of town. You've got to get me somewhere else. I don't care where, but I've got to go somewhere." He had a friend named Earl Mahoney who was a cardiac surgeon in Rochester. Dr. Daniel must have said something to Dr. Mahoney about me to get him to accept me, so I got out of the match and went to Rochester. I was very happy there, and I had intended to stay, until I got the chance to go to Massachusetts General.

All of us who went through the Vanderbilt undergraduate-premed program liked Dr. Chadwick. Dr. Chadwick was a biology professor. We called him Chad Daddy, and he was a wonderful, warm, inspiring person. As for the medical school faculty, nobody could come up to my assessment of Dr. Shapiro, but there were a lot of great people on the faculty in those days, just one giant after another. Vanderbilt was better than many other places I think. During our training, a Vanderbilt product was looked on as a good product. We had a small number of students, and they were well trained and knew how to do practical things well. I think we should always be proud of that. I was scared to death when I went to Massachusetts General because it was so high-powered, but I found that my Vanderbilt training stood me in good stead and let me measure up. One time at a big fundraiser in Washington I remarked, "I learned to be a surgeon at Harvard, but I learned to be a doctor at Vanderbilt."

In the Department of Surgery at Massachusetts General, there was Dr. Churchill, who was a great pioneer thoracic surgeon. He brought in people to do different things, and they did those things well. Dr. Linton developed vascular surgery there, and he was matchless in the things he did with all the vascular problems we came to know about in the fifties, sixties, and seventies. Dr. Richard Sweet was a great surgical technician and a pioneer in noncardiac thoracic surgery. He had an interesting aura about him. He stood up very straight when he operated, and he swung his needle holder like a conductor leading a band. He had a marvelous technique. Earl Wilkins was his associate and younger helper for years and years, and Wilk became very skilled. When he first went to work for Dr. Sweet, Dr. Sweet would put the first needle in the subcutaneous tissue or the skin in the middle of the long chest incision and start sewing in one direction. Then Wilk would start in the middle too and sew in the opposite direction. But Wilk got so good and so fast that Dr. Sweet began to start his sewing a little further toward one end. By the time he retired he was only doing a third of the incision, and Wilk was doing the other two-thirds, but never a word was said about this. Dr. Sweet was a great inspiration to a lot of his younger trainees. In those days it was a kind of preceptor training. You asked a man like Dr. Sweet, "Could I come and be your assistant for a year or two?" and that was a way to train.

That way of training was being phased out at Massachusetts General when I went there for my training, but they had Marshall Bartlett, who was a master of the upper abdomen, and Claude Welch, who wrote fundamental treatises on intestinal obstructions. Oliver Cope was the man who started parathyroid surgery and other endocrine surgery, and he figured out the basis of why you do it and what has gone wrong. He was a great pioneer. Bill McDermott was working on shunts because of portal hypertension, and he was also a great teacher and surgeon. Hermes Grillo did some really fundamental things with the trachea, as did Paul Russell with transplantation. The front row of surgical rounds at Massachusetts General was august, and the second row was all young brains.

Dr. Churchill was the chairman, and when he stepped down, Dr. Cope was the interval chairman for a year. Then Paul Russell was selected to succeed Dr. Churchill. He was a young tiger in transplantation. He had worked not only with Rupert Billingham but also with Medawar in England. He was the chairman for five years, and then it was decided that he should concentrate on transplantation, and Jerry Austen became chairman. His education at MIT had been in fluid dynamics, and he trained at the NIH with Glenn Morrow. Then he came back to Boston and started the whole open-heart program at the Massachusetts General Hospital. He became a master not only of cardiac surgery, but also of training young people. He presided over those older surgical icons, and yet he handled it beautifully and so deferentially. It's not surprising that he took that department of surgery further and deeper.

Residency training is changing today, of course. The change to the eighty-hour week is appropriate, but we have to figure out what other changes are needed. We used to work thirty-six on and twelve off, and we had all kinds of demands on us for years. There was a study in the *New England Journal of Medicine* years ago that described the psychological and neurological changes in young people who were working for thirty-six hours straight. They monitored them the first twelve hours, the second twelve hours, and the third twelve hours. By the third twelve hours, the subjects hardly knew what they were doing. It is right that we make some restrictions, but I am not sure eighty hours is enough. The problem is, we say, "OK, it's eighty hours, it's time to quit, you go home," but then continuity is lost and the residents don't follow the patient. We learned a lot by following a patient through, into the night, and on to the next day. I am worried about the ultimate educational outcome of the rigid eighty-hour week. The general public thinks, "Well, that's twice what most people work, so why isn't that enough?" I think a lot of attention should be paid by medical and surgical educators to the problem of how we can meet both the rational and reasonable limitation of hours of work, and also meet our obligation to educate and train young people. We were trained to stay with our patients and guide our patients through their difficult times. The question has to be enlarged, and the medical educators of our day have to figure it out so that we don't lose the precious doctor-patient contact in the educational setting.

It's true that when we worked thirty-six hours at a stretch, we were doing a lot of noneducational work. When I was a surgical intern working at night and a patient was admitted, we had to do all of the basic lab work, the blood work, and urinalysis. One time, I had worked all night and then all the second night. I was up for the third evening in a row, and I had a flask of urine in my hand. The lab was down at the end of a long corridor. I said to myself, "My eyes are burning so bad, and I just have to walk straight down to that lab. I believe I can close my eyes and walk down this hall." I went to sleep walking down that hall. I woke up bumping against the wall, and the urine leaked all over the floor. We can correct that by having other employees doing that work, instead of our house staff.

I had a wonderful wife and partner, and we have five marvelous children. My wife, Comfort, worked and put me through residency, but as I got into the senior years in residency, we decided we would borrow money and have a family. When I was chief resident of surgery at the Boston Children's Hospital, we had four boys. The oldest was four, and three were in diapers. That was a headache for Mrs. Randolph, but she carried it off quite well. I thought the boys were going to kill each other, but they grew up and love each other today. Then we moved to Washington and had a little girl, who is very dear to her daddy's heart.

Bibliography

Moncrief JA, Randolph JG. Congenital Tracheoesophageal Fistula without Atresia of the Esophagus. A Method for Diagnosis and Surgical Correction. *J Thorac Cardiovasc Surg.* 1966; 51:434–442.

Lilly JR, Randolph JG. Hiatal Hernia and Gastroesophageal Reflux in Infants and Children. *J Thorac Cardiovasc Surg.* 1968; 55:42–54.

Randolph JG, Hung W. Reduction Clitoroplasty in Females with Hyperthrophied Clitoris. *J Pediatr Surg.* 1970; 5:224–231.

Anderson KD, Randolph JG. The Gastric Tube for Esophageal Replacement in Children. *J Thorac Cardiovasc Surg.* 1973; 66:333–342.

Randolph JG, Lilly JR, Anderson KD. Surgical Treatment of Gastroesophageal Reflux in Infants. *Ann Surg.* 1974; 180:479–486.

Randolph JG, Altman RP, Anderson KD. Selective Surgical Management Based upon Clinical Status in Infants with Esophageal Atresia. *J Thorac Cardiovasc Surg.* 1977; 74:335–342.

Randolph JG. Total Surgical Reconstruction for Patients with Abdominal Muscular Deficiency ("Prune-Belly") Syndrome. *J Pediatr Surg.* 1977; 12:1033–1043.

Randolph JG, Altman RP, Arensman RM, Matlak ME, Leikin SL. Liver Resection in Children with Hepatic Neoplasms. *Ann Surg.* 1978; 187:599–605.

Guzzetta PC, Randolph JG. Antireflux Cologastric Anastomosis following Colonic Interposition for Esophageal Replacement. *J Pediatr Surg.* 1986; 21:1137–1138.

Randolph JG, Newman KD, Anderson KD. Current Results in Repair of Esophageal Atresia with Tracheoesophageal Fistula Using Physiologic Status as a Guide to Therapy. *Ann Surg.* 1989; 209:530–531.

Anthony R. C. Dobell, MD

(b. 1927)

It took enormous gumption to be a real pioneer of cardiac surgery. Some surgeons just went ahead regardless of the risks; one of those was Charley Bailey.

— On the first cardiac surgery operations

Interviewed May 1, 2000

I was born in Montreal in 1927, in the same hospital where I have worked all my life. My father died suddenly when I was twelve. My mother let me bring myself up; she was an artist and a very stimulating and original woman. There wasn't much in the way of a paternal influence on me. I think I flourished under this self-education. My mother used to tell me to get out more and have more fun. Perhaps I was kind of boring or dull.

I went to McGill University, and I was involved in a lot of extracurricular activities. I played on the McGill hockey team, which was one of the great feats of my life, a terrific experience. In fact, whatever I did seemed to work out well. I did well in mathematics. That was the era of early nuclear physics, and I thought I wanted to be a physicist. During the summers I actually worked in the atomic energy plant of Canada at the research station in the exciting years of 1945 and 1946, but I did not like working for the government.

When I was an undergraduate, I worked one summer as a lifeguard, and I met an older gentleman from Philadelphia. He was actually a judge and in his seventies. He had helped another young student through medical school at Jefferson, and he wanted to help me. I said I already had a scholarship at the time, and I really didn't need financial help. He introduced me to a surgeon, Joe Stayman, who was a member of the American Association for Thoracic Surgery. I later visited Joe in Philadelphia when I was a medical student at McGill. I also had the occasion to meet Dr. Gibbon, and so it was after graduation that I became interested in surgery. I hadn't focused on surgery during my medical school career, but in those days we had rotating internships, and during my surgery rotation I became very impressed by a single surgeon. This was a surgeon who paid great attention to his patients and performed operations with meticulous technique.

Having become interested in surgery, I wrote to Dr. Gibbon, whom I had already met. I was just an intern who hadn't done anything, but I had read those papers about the heart-lung machine. Dr. Gibbon published a paper about the original heart-lung machine in 1949 after he returned from the South Pacific. It was a pretty horrendous device, a Rube Goldberg apparatus. It only became more refined after IBM became involved, in the person of Mr. Thomas Watson.

Mr. Watson got involved through a chance meeting. One of the residents or students at Jefferson brought Dr. Gibbon to the attention of the older Mr. Watson, and Dr. Gibbon had an interview with him. As a result of that meeting, Mr. Watson said that IBM would support the development of a heart-lung machine and that IBM would have no commercial interest in it. They would not produce it, but their commitment to its development was total. They assigned three or four of their brightest young engineers to the project, including an engineer who had been one of the original quiz kids. In the 1930s they had quiz programs on the radio, where unusual young people answered questions, and he was one of them. At any rate, IBM made this commitment, and by 1949 or 1950, they produced a working model of the heart-lung machine. They changed the rotating-cylinder oxygenator to a vertical-screen oxygenator. That machine was used in the laboratory in 1951 and 1952, and then it was used on the first patient, Cecelia Bavolek, in 1953.

I am getting a little ahead of my story. I joined the Jefferson surgical residency in July of 1952. I did the first year of residency rotating through the wards and the private area, and through the TB hospital, where I worked with Jay Ankeney. He was my mentor, who showed me how to do my first thoracotomies. We did a lot of those for TB in those days, the early 1950s.

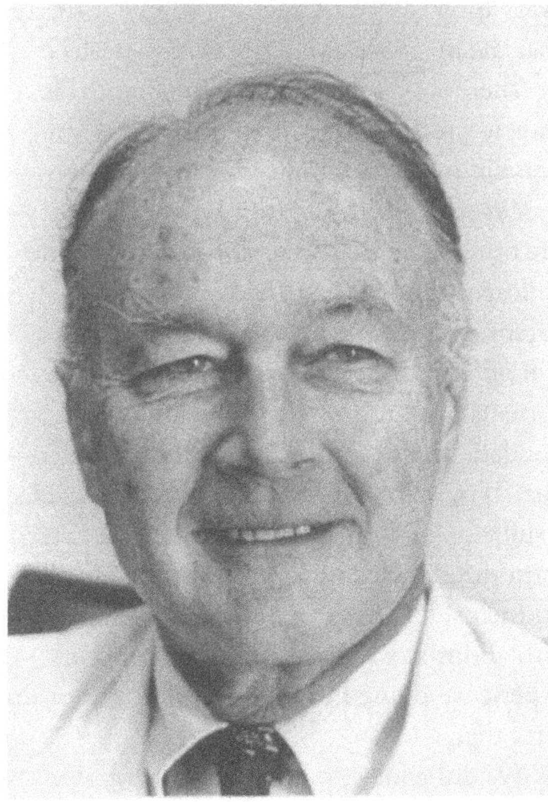

Anthony R. C. Dobell

It was in May 1953 that the first open-heart operation was done. I was actually at the TB hospital down the street, so my role was insignificant, but I was the babysitter during the night. I was allowed to come up from the TB center and sit beside her. She was an eighteen-year-old girl who had had an ASD repair, and she was doing pretty well, so I didn't have much to do. Of course, in those days there were no intensive-care units, or special facilities for intensive care. There were no indwelling lines. You took a patient's blood pressure with the cuff.

Coagulopathy was a problem in Cecelia's case because not quite enough heparin was given. The dosage of heparin had not been perfectly worked out. Toward the close of her time on the bypass, the oxygenator began to clot. It was a near thing. They terminated the bypass with the defect closed and there wasn't a general coagulopathy. Fortunately she got through the operation quite successfully, and is still alive today.

Jefferson was not a cardiac center, nor a pediatric center. It didn't have anesthesiologists until 1954. Instead we had nurse-anesthetists, who were very capable, but we intubated the patients before they were put to sleep. I think that was a huge failing. The diagnostic studies were done by one of the surgical residents using ureteral catheters, and of course these were only right-sided studies. Doing the oxygen tensions by the Van Slyke method took about an hour, so everything was retrospective. Suffice it to say that the diagnoses were not always perfect.

There wasn't much publicity about this case; it wasn't in the newspapers. Dr. Gibbon did not write about it until three or four years later. I think this was because of the other cases that were done on four little children. One of the patients had a large patent ductus. The focus at that time was still on atrial septal defects, but one of the patients had an AV canal. The lungs were just flooded. The operations were quite ponderous. They were done through what was called a suitcase incision, transverse across the sternum through the fourth or fifth interspace on each side. The operations did not work out, and that was the end of Dr. Gibbon's experience doing heart surgery. He gave it up after that.

We did a lot of pulmonary surgery. Dr. Gibbon's principal operation was pneumonectomy. He was an excellent pneumonectomist, and that was the result of the fact that the bronchoscopies were done by Louis Clerf, who succeeded Chevalier Jackson, the great endoscopist. There was an endoscopy service, a bronchoscopy, and esophagoscopy service. There was also a thoracic surgical service, but the thoracic surgeons did not do endoscopy. Nevertheless, it led to a tremendous number of referrals. A pneumonectomy was done virtually every day, and an esophagectomy every week.

Esophagectomy was a grim experience in those days. It was catastrophic, and the survival rate was not good. I had the unpleasant experience of following the esophagectomy patients, and I found that the number of survivors for three years was in the single digits. We had a very high mortality rate from the operation, close to 30 percent, largely due to the lack of intensive care. The residents had to make rounds every two hours at night, after we had worked all day. Those rounds consisted of endotracheal suction to try to prevent atelectasis and pneumonia. We would wake up the poor patient, pull out his tongue, introduce a tube into the airway, flush it, aspirate it, and inject saline to try to suck out the secretions. That was intensive care. One resident would be on one floor, and another resident on another. It was unpleasant.

We had the same kinds of wards at Jefferson that had been laid out by Florence Nightingale, the wards that you see in Civil War photographs where there are big long wards of forty beds, with each bed six feet from the next bed. Our patients would have decreasing magnitude of operations as you went down the ward. It was general and thoracic surgery, so the first patient would have had a mitral commissurotomy. Then there would be three or four lung resections, then you got to the gastrectomies and cholecystectomies, and at the end of the ward, you had the appendectomy or hernia patients. This system provided great experience for the residents, but it was a far cry from the system today.

Residency was fairly intense. We had long hours and worked every second night in the hospital. We would come in at seven in the morning, or at least I did. One of my fellow residents came in about six every morning; he was terribly eager. I lived over in New Jersey, took the bus in, and was on the job by seven. We would make rounds first and then start the cases at eight. We were there all that day, that night, and the next day. Then I would go home. At night we had emergencies and those resuscitative rounds.

My wife and I were beginning to have children then. Sometimes I wouldn't see them for quite a while, even though I slept in the same house with them. My wife told me that my son hugged the milkman and called him daddy once. That was a little traumatic. But when I think back on those days, they were good days. I think my wife looks back on them not unpleasantly. She knew I wasn't around too much, but she was busy. We were in Philadelphia for four years, and we had three children, so she was pretty much occupied with their care.

We were young, and I often think of the Wordsworth poem in which he wrote, "Bliss was it in that dawn to be alive, But to be young was very heaven." The times were so exciting because in my second year I was in the lab. I had a four-year residency and only three clinical years of general and thoracic surgery. Dr. Gibbon did not rate technical prowess as the top requirement for a surgeon. That was clear. He did not have much surgical training himself. He went to Massachusetts General with Churchill and worked in the lab. His role model was Landis, the physiologist, with whom he worked. He accomplished a great deal in the lab with his wife Maly, who had been Churchill's research assistant. Maly later became Dr. Gibbon's assistant and then his wife.

Dr. Gibbon had an incredibly broad knowledge about surgery. When he was professor and chairman of surgery, it was very impressive to hear him give a talk on any subject, any subject at all, hip fractures or whatever. I remember having lunch with him once at a meeting of the American College. He was giving a talk right after lunch on pulmonary edema, a sort of esoteric subject. We had a very full lunch, and the talk didn't seem to be on his mind at all. Afterwards he wandered over and gave a great talk.

He was a student, and he was an editor. Being an editor of the *Annals of Surgery* was the job that he took the most pride in, besides being the Samuel Gross Professor at Jefferson. His father had held that same position, which is quite a tradition. Dr. Gibbon was a great editor. I often came into his office late in the day, and he would be reviewing manuscripts and dictating his reviews. He read every manuscript submitted to the *Annals*. On occasion, he would have three reviewers, all unanimous about whether to accept the article or reject it, and he would sometimes go the other way. That didn't happen often, because he had extremely competent reviewers, but he made up his own mind.

He was a poet and a student of language. I think he wrote poems when he was at Princeton, and he was later an artist. My mother was a very artistic woman, and maybe for that reason we had something in common. He was very good to me. As a young resident I would go to his house. He had a constant stream of visitors—Dr. Blalock, Dr. Crafoord, or Dr. Dick Varco—and for a young resident to be able to meet these people was a great experience. He was very kind to young people.

It occurred to me later that I was the only one who went to Jefferson to learn about heart surgery. I really didn't learn very much heart surgery at Jefferson, but I certainly left Jefferson with a commitment to engage in heart surgery because of my work in the lab. In that lab I began to work on dynamic structures. The first thing I worked on was the femoral artery, to cannulate it. Then I started working on the heart, and on the heart-lung machine project. We made ventricular septal defects with a cork borer on these unfortunate animals, and then we would repair them. We would do a little right ventriculotomy, then apply the cork borer with suction on the end of it and suck out a meatball of septum. A few weeks or a month later, we would repair the defect. We had a few survive that year, but not many.

Jefferson was a regional medical school, a great old medical school, founded in 1820. It is one of the oldest medical schools in the country. It had a great surgical tradition. We think of Gross, but there are a lot of other names associated with it, such as the famous surgeon of the superior sulcus tumor resection, Pancoast. There were a lot of other names you would recognize on the faculty of Jefferson. The students came from around the area. There weren't many that traveled to Jefferson from far away, as I did, to do a residency or to be a student there. In fact, the residents were all former medical students of Jefferson. Most of the fellows who went into surgery were planning to go back to Wilkes-Barre or some other local town to practice surgery. It was an extremely good surgical residency, but it was not a preparation for a career in cardiac surgery.

Of course, in those days there was no cardiac surgery. At Jefferson as chief resident, I did some pulmonary valvotomies, some ductus operations, and some coarctation repairs. I didn't learn heart surgery at Jefferson, but I did have the opportunity to work with an extremely capable surgeon, John Templeton. He had marvelous surgical ability, and he did all the toughest cases and made them look easy, something I could never do. I regard him as a tremendous mentor. He was on the faculty then, and he was also a partner of Dr. Gibbon, in the partnership of Gibbon, Albritten, and Templeton. Dr. Gibbon was the teacher, John Templeton was the surgical technique mentor, and George Willauer taught us how to look after people. He was a humanist.

After Dr. Gibbon's short series of cardiac patients, no intracardiac surgery was done for a couple of years. In 1956, when I was a chief resident, Dr. Templeton began doing cardiac surgery. After I returned to Montreal in 1956, I flew back to Philadelphia a few times because Dr. Templeton invited me. I would help out in the operating room. He felt better with me there, and I felt better for being there, but he was the surgeon. I didn't look after the heart-lung machine, but he may have wanted me there because of my knowledge of it. It was the old Mayo-Gibbon machine. We had very good technical help with the heart-lung machine, and we worked with it in the lab.

In 1956 I went home to Montreal. I had been at Montreal General Hospital before as an intern and felt an affiliation with it, but the chairman of the department had no interest in cardiac surgery. I volunteered to work in the lab to try to develop it, but he said, "Surgeons don't work in labs; they work in the OR. That is ridiculous!" So I went down the street to the other hospital, the Royal Victoria Hospital, and there the chief surgeon said, in response to my proposal, "That sounds like a good idea. You can come and work in the lab here." He gave me a lowly position on the faculty; I was not official faculty, but rather a teaching fellow. I think I was paid $3,000 a year, and I began working in the lab. Of course you need support to work in the lab, and support came very quickly from the Children's Hospital.

David Murphy, the chief surgeon at the Children's Hospital, had been doing closed-heart surgery. He was an expert in pediatric cardiac surgery as it existed at the time. He said, "I'll teach you how to do closed-heart surgery, and you get us into the inside of the heart." We formed a liaison. He had an associate, Gordon Karn, a surgeon who worked with him, and at first I would help them, and then they would help me do patent ductus and coarctations. We worked together to develop heart surgery. We used to do some extraordinary things. The animal facility was separate from the hospital, so we would put the animals to sleep in the animal facility, put them in the trunk of the car, drive them to the hospital, bring them up a freight elevator in the evening, and then do operations on the animals in the patient operating room. We would transport them back to the animal facility in the trunk of the car and look after them there. Of course that couldn't be done today.

We started with a bubble oxygenator, which was a most horrible machine and noisy. We had a finger pump, the Sigmamotor pump. It had been constructed for the milk pasteurizing industry in Minnesota, and that was why it had been available to Dr. Lillehei. It was a terrible pump. We made the DeWall oxygenator out of a coil of tubing and sprayed it with antifoam. It had steel wool in there coated with antifoam. It was a pretty horrible machine. Our results were terrible. The first five cases were especially bad, not just because of the machine, but because of everything. The cardiologists wouldn't let us operate on anybody unless they were pretty darn sick, almost moribund. We did not have the gumption to do a good case, for example a simple VSD. The patient had to have a lot of pulmonary hypertension and right heart failure. My memories of those cases are pretty sad.

Then we got a screen oxygenator made by the Mark Company, the Mark IV screen oxygenator, which resembled a cheap Mayo-Gibbon machine. It had a screen oxygenator and roller pumps. I think this heart-lung machine sold for about $4,000, and it was made near Boston. We felt better with that screen oxygenator and began to do better. That was about 1958. Of course, we still started with very difficult cases, but in time, thank God, things improved.

During that time I coauthored a paper with Arthur Vineberg. He was the first to receive a PhD in experimental surgery at McGill under Dr. Archibald, and he was committed to experimental work. He came up with the extraordinary idea of implanting the internal mammary artery into the myocardium, and it was effective. That operation did bring some blood to the heart of patients with angina.

Arthur had a problem of having an ego that had to be maintained. He didn't take criticism very well. He had a lot of energy and a commitment to his operation, the internal mammary implant, and he was attached emotionally to it. It became obvious that the operation did not bring immediate relief, because the implant had to arborize and nourish the myocardium around it, and this happened rather sluggishly. It took a couple of months before the benefit of the operation was realized. He began adding other things, like an omental flap, which was supposed to bring more blood to the heart. I think he damaged his operation by tinkering with it. Of course, his internal mammary implant was done before coronary angiography was available. People have mentioned that he might tighten a hiatus hernia at the same time and thus relieve some chest pain that may not have been ischemic. He didn't do that all the time; he did his operation. It had to be a big operation for Arthur, so it had to take a long time, and it took him about six hours. He used just one mammary artery. I began putting in two mammary arteries. I had to do something a little different.

Arthur was difficult to work with, and he had his own service. He had one resident that he had hired. He was within the surgical department, with his own little service, and he had an operating room a couple days a week, all because he was so difficult. He was a wonderful host and very hospitable, and he could be charming, but when anything went wrong, it was someone else's fault. He usually blamed things on a nurse or a resident. I really didn't work with him very much. I was a friend and neighbor of his, and we got along very well. I think he needed me, because we started doing intracardiac surgery at the Royal Victoria Hospital a couple of years after we started at the Children's Hospital. We were almost neighbors, and later on we became neighbors. He was always charming, but he believed in a hierarchical system, and he treated people at the bottom pretty poorly. I think he also treated his operation pretty poorly in that he kept modifying it. Yet the implant was successful. There's no doubt that Mason Sones put the implant on the map by doing the angiography on an internal mammary that had been implanted, and this showed that it arborized and nourished the myocardium to some extent. It didn't always work.

I was a great admirer of Arthur in many ways, and I also recognized his limitations. He lived to see coronary artery bypass surgery, but that was after his active career. He was indefatigable, and he was still working in the late 1960s. He was never involved in coronary artery bypass clinically.

During that time I divided my activities between congenital heart disease and adult cardiac disease. I began at the Montreal Children's Hospital doing congenital surgery, which is what open-heart surgery was at that time. Then we began to do some operations at the Royal Victoria Hospital, and later we went to Montreal General Hospital. I think of myself as a McGill surgeon, a university surgeon at three hospitals. I still have appointments at all three, and I tried to bring them all together. We did succeed at bringing them together into a single training program, the first McGill program in any specialty. The other programs at that time were hospital programs. Subsequently they all became McGill programs, but our program was the first, by necessity I suppose. So I have always thought of myself as a McGill man.

Before coronary artery bypass surgery became popular, vascular surgery filled out our schedule. Of course coronary artery bypass became popular in about 1970 and began to inflate our schedule. We became quite busy, or our associates did. I never had quite as much commitment to it as they did, because I was always interested in the children.

One of the operations that we reported on in the early 1960s was aortic valvuloplasty. We tried to save the leaflets because we didn't have a good substitute, and we would spend a lot of time chipping calcium out of the valves. Of course that was a palliative operation, and the patient subsequently required valve replacements. We started off in valve replacements with Henry Bahnson's cusps made of Dacron, in about 1960 or 1961. We would sew in the individual cusps. They looked pretty good for a while, but they stiffened up and fractured. We began valve replacement, as did everybody else, in the early 1960s.

We used the Starr valves, and we grew as the specialty grew. We went through those wonderful years when every year the annual meeting of the American Association was just a blockbuster, and you would learn totally new areas that had been invaded by surgeons and new operations. We contributed to some extent. We were second-ranked characters in the great scheme of things but would come up with a new operation every now and then. In those days a series of ten was a pretty good series of something. We were all learning from each other. Thank God, those nightmare days are over. Nowadays the risk is so much less. In those days we practically had to live with the patients. We would give our own blood to the patient in the intensive care unit, such as it was. We didn't even have intensive care units initially, as they were introduced because of heart surgery. We gradually learned our business.

It took enormous gumption to be a real pioneer of cardiac surgery. Some surgeons just went ahead almost regardless of the risks. One of these certainly was Charles Bailey. Some of these people were very difficult individuals, interested only in getting a few patients through. Of course, I knew of Bailey's initial series of mitral commissurotomies. I used to go and visit Dr. Bailey, because Jefferson is not far from Hahnemann, where Bailey worked. When I was in the lab that second year, I visited him and learned a lot of things. I saw some appalling things too; huge risks were taken. The mortality rate was very high. Charles Bailey could talk of an experimental series before he talked of the clinical series, and these were all on patients. You could do that in those days; that was the norm of that era.

There was no solution for aortic insufficiency, for example. Bailey came up with an operation where he put a monstrous tie around the aorta, under the coronaries. If you think of that route, you realize that the ligature has to go in the left atrium and out again, and under a couple of coronaries. Back in 1953 that was pretty horrendous. I think it was one of those operations that led to what he called an experimental series and then a clinical series. He later switched to another technique, and that operation was forgotten. He led the way, in many ways, for closed-heart surgery. He probably pushed it beyond where it should have been pushed. I think it was appropriate that he went into law later on; he became a lawyer.

Dr. Gibbon died after a heart attack on the tennis court in 1971 or 1972. I played tennis with him often when we went to medical meetings. He was nominated for the Nobel Prize, but he didn't receive it. I think he deserved it, but only about three surgeons have gotten it. One of them, Alexis Carrel, wasn't really a clinical surgeon. Emil Kocher and Joseph Murray were clinical surgeons who received Nobel Prizes. Dr. Gibbon would have been a great Nobel laureate. He was an incredible speaker at meetings; he just had an easy way of expressing himself. He was a great teacher.

I published some papers about Maude

Abbott, who was the first pediatric cardiologist. She did not graduate from McGill University, because they did not accept women in her era; McGill did not accept women until 1920. There was another medical school down the street, where she acquired a medical education after pressuring the people greatly; she was a tough woman. She then went to Europe to acquire expertise in cardiology, but there was very little to be acquired at that time. When she came back, McGill didn't know what to do with Maude. She set up shop in Montreal, but she wanted to be on the faculty and to do something important. Finally, they stuck her in the museum to care for it. The museum was terribly important in those days because the faculty then didn't have the visual aids to teach with that they have now. She began studying hearts. She went down to visit Sir William Osler at Johns Hopkins. He told her that she should study congenital heart defects, and he invited her to write the chapter about that in his book. That's how she became an expert on congenital heart disease. She wrote the first classification of congenital heart disease. Of course, nobody cared about that at the time, because there was nothing you could do for congenital heart defects in those days. She classified congenital heart abnormalities and made the first great steps.

She loved McGill, she loved being part of the academic institution, and she loved medical students. Maude Abbott was looked down upon by her male colleagues as "Maudie who worked in the lab," and they probably didn't have much interest in what she did. She was a great stimulus to another gentleman, Harold Segal, who studied cardiology with her in the early 1920s. He was a good friend of mine, and he died at the age of ninety-something a few years ago. She died about 1940.

This was before cardiac catheterization. She had access to the patients and then to the autopsies, but that was all she had. She was a cardiac pathologist, the first one, probably because she could find no other niche for herself. You could say she was the dean of the museum. The specimens were mounted beautifully in all fields, but her specialty was in the cardiac area. Specimens were sent to her from everywhere, because nobody else was interested.

In Canada the training for cardiac surgeons has changed. For us at McGill, it was always important to remain part of the American board system, but we got thrown out of the American system about eleven or twelve years ago. Our trainees were no longer eligible for American board exams, so that freed us up to devise a new curriculum. Since we didn't have to head for the American board, our trainees did not have to be chief residents in general surgery. The program became two core years of basic clinical work, one year in the lab, and three years of clinical cardiothoracic surgery. In time we lost our credentials in pure thoracic surgery, so we became more of a cardiac training center. In that sense we were following Toronto, where cardiac and thoracic have been separate for many years. That's how it is at McGill now. We have three clinical years in cardiac surgery, after one lab year and two early clinical years doing the basic cardiology rotation, emergency room work, ward work in surgery, and so on.

In the United States, thoracic and cardiac surgery are still taught together, and we want to hold them together. The chief residency in general surgery is still a real keystone of the American system, but I don't think it is needed. Our people are selected straight from medical school. This change appalled me, and I have never really been part of that new system because I retired about ten years ago. It is working out pretty well. There are options for the trainees after the first two years, and there have to be, because how do you know if a person, when they first get out of medical school, has the manual dexterity, the fortitude, and the interest that cardiac surgery requires? I have never really believed in the current system of taking students straight from medical school, but I can see that the system seems to be working, because we are turning out some strong trainees. I suppose our trainees are selected on the basis of their grades, which in my view should not be the ultimate criterion for choosing candidates.

The people who first influenced me in surgery were my friends at Jefferson: Dr. Gibbon, who taught me knowledge, was a great student and source of information. John Templeton taught me operative care and skill, and remains a good friend. George Willauer taught me about people. George was a humanist but he didn't treat everybody the same way; he would treat people according to their own personalities.

My role models were mostly people that I met during my residency, except for Dr. Robertson, who came to head up the surgical department at McGill and subsequently became the president of the university. He ran the whole university during that terrible period when students were beginning to occupy presidents' offices. It must have been heartbreaking for him; he probably wished he could have been back in surgery. I have learned a lot from my friends and associates. We look on our friends as equals, but we learn from them, and I have learned from hundreds of them. I have had a balanced life. I worked very hard, but I have been fortunate with my wife and family. We think we have had a pretty full life at home, although my children are all far away right now.

I am sure that cardiac surgery will be different in the future. That's why I always try to prepare people for the broadest possible careers. It's also one of the reasons why we tried to combine cardiothoracic and vascular surgery, but in the end we were unsuccessful at keeping them together. I think it is very important for young people to have the greatest possible breadth in their training.

What is the future of cardiac surgery? Everybody is aware that incisions are getting smaller and that cardiologists are intervening more, and I think that's good. If I were going to be operated on through a keyhole, I think that would be all right. I am sure that in twenty years cardiac surgery will be quite different from what it is today. If I were a young surgeon starting off, I would like to start in a field that was going to open up, rather than one that was going to constrict. I would like to have the broadest possible training, including a lot of training in cardiology. Fortunately, we surgeons still implant pacemakers; that is a surgical procedure. Cardiologists are doing some surgical procedures these days also. I think it is going to be one field in the future. In Montreal, we work very closely with the cardiologists. They do sometimes take cases away, but our volume of cases has not diminished. We should be aware of what the cardiologists are doing, and they should be aware of what we're doing because our cases come from them. We are busy doing what we do, which is trying to repair hearts.

Bibliography

Gibbon JH Jr, Miller BJ, Dobell ARC, Engell HC, Voigt GB. The Closure of Interventricular Septal Defects in Dogs during Open Cardiotomy with the Maintenance of the Cardiorespiratory Functions by a Pump Oxygenator. *J Thorac Surg.* 1954; 28:235–240.

Dobell ARC, Mitrim M, Galva R, Sarkozy E, Murphy DR. Biologic Evaluation of Blood after Prolonged Recirculation through Film and Membrane Oxygenators. *Ann Surg.* 1965; 161:617–622.

Dobell ARC, Wyant JD, Seamans KB, Gloor P. Penicillin Epilepsy: Studies on the Blood-Brain Barrier during Cardiopulmonary Bypass. *J Thorac Cardiovasc Surg.* 1966; 52:469–475.

Dobell ARC, Charrette EP, Chughtai MS. Correction of Tetralogy of Fallot in the Young Child. *J Thorac Cardiovasc Surg.* 1968; 55:70–79.

Dobell ARC, Murphy DA, Poirier NL, Gibbons JE. The Pulmonary Artery after Debanding. *J Thorac Cardiovasc Surg.* 1973; 65:32–36.

Dobell ARC. Editorial: "Correction" of Congenital Heart Disease. *Ann Thorac Surg.* 1975; 19:103–104.

Dobell, ARC. The Human Touch. *Ann Thorac Surg.* 1982; 34:1–5.

Dobell ARC, Jain AK. Catastrophic Hemorrhagic during Redo Sternotomy. *Ann Thorac Surg.* 1984; 37:273–278.

Dobell ARC, Trusler GA, Smallhorn JF, Williams WG. Atrial Thrombi after the Fontan Operation. *Ann Thorac Surg.* 1986; 42:664–667.

Paul A. Ebert, MD

(b. 1932)

While we were at Cornell, we began working on potassium cardioplegia and myocardial protection. It became very clear in the animal laboratory that you could arrest the heart with potassium for thirty minutes at normothermia and have it recuperate and reperfuse for a period of five minutes, and it would show no ill effect.

— On cardioplegia and myocardial protection

Interviewed October 27, 2000

I was born in 1932 in Columbus, Ohio, an only child, and my mother and father divorced when I was an infant. My mother worked, so I really grew up with my grandparents in a modest family. I was fortunate to be fairly good in baseball and basketball, and would otherwise probably never have gone to college. I went to Ohio State. In those days there were really no scholarships, but I was a hometown boy, and they provided me a job working nine hours a week for $100 a month. It doesn't sound like much today, but it paid for my room and board with a few dollars left over. Ohio State was not nearly as large as it is at the present time. I was probably fortunate that I had good advice while in undergraduate school. I began in engineering but decided that it was too exacting, and I was terrible in mechanical drawing. A spotless paper was required and I couldn't do that. I got some advice recommending that I go into medicine. I didn't know much about it, but I went ahead and finished college, and in 1954 I was admitted to the medical school at Ohio State.

In those days, although the professors knew each other, without the air travel and frequent meetings of today's world, they really weren't as close as one might have thought. Dr. Zollinger, who was a wonderful friend and someone that I admired, suggested that I go to New York for my internship because one of his colleagues at Harvard, Peter Vanbergen, was chief of surgery at New York Hospital Cornell. My wife and I made a journey to Baltimore first and visited Johns Hopkins. We then drove up to New York and visited New York Hospital Cornell and Columbia Presbyterian. The reception that we got at New York and Baltimore was like night and day. I don't know why, but Hopkins seemed like they were much more gracious. It was our kind of place, certainly was not low-intensity, and I decided that I wanted to go to there.

As a Hopkins resident we were told that we would have a certain number of patients who would be on different services, but they would be our patients twenty-four hours a day for the year. If I wanted to leave the hospital, it was just like being in practice, it was necessary to have someone that was willing to cover for me to sign out to. I learned quickly that if you did a good job you could get someone to cover for you, because they really didn't have to work too hard. The worst interns and residents always had the hardest time getting anybody to sign out to.

There were eighteen interns, but only two were kept after the first year. Of the interns that were taken, it was obvious that some were selected because of their interest in orthopedics or neurosurgery, although I don't think there was a quota. I suppose out of the eighteen there were probably ten or maybe twelve that were interested in cardiothoracic or general surgery training, which at that time were combined. There was not a separate cardiac or thoracic service, and there was just one residency training program.

Lazar Greenfield and I were co-interns and ultimately became co-residents. We lived next to each other all the way through the program. Rowland Folks was an intern with us and is now chairman of surgery at the University of Illinois in Springfield. Dave Sumner, who is a well-known vascular surgeon, was also an intern at that time. It's always hard to remember who was in my class specifically, but there were a lot of well-known surgeons scattered through the two or three years around me. Dick Anderson and Harvey Bender were the two residents that followed Lazar and me.

I had some contact with Dr. Blalock, but he was in the latter part of his career. He was very pleasant, and he knew the things that might be of interest, such as a journal article that he would send with a note attached. He would meet with an intern about three to four times a year but very casually. We never knew exactly where we stood, but he rarely ever reprimanded anyone. He ran the heart service in those days, but Frank Spencer and Henry Bahnson were the two people doing most of the open-heart surgery. Dr. Blalock assigned the cases and who would assist. We didn't see him every day, and he would get Dr. Sabiston, Dr. Bahnson, or whoever was available to help us in the OR with cases that were complex.

Dr. Blalock limited himself predominately to subclavian pulmonary artery shunts and coarctations. He did a lot of cervical esophageal diverticula, which for some reason he liked to do. He never did any open-heart surgery or operations that required cardiopulmonary bypass. In those days the surgery often wasn't so bad, but the perfusion systems were not nearly as good as they are today, so there were postoperative problems.

In the fifties and early sixties, we used a regular roller pump which had a piece of rubber tubing inserted through the pump head. We didn't believe plastic could be put through the pump head without the pump breaking it sooner or later. I don't ever remember the pump failing, but oxygenators were a real problem. We were using a Gibbon standing-screen oxygenator that looked like a suitcase and had a dozen sheets of high-quality screen wire hanging down with a film of blood flowing down each screen. It was unbelievably difficult to clean and remove all the foreign protein off of the screens. I think most of the fevers and unknown complications that we saw after open-heart surgery were because of the protein residue. These problems disappeared when the disposable oxygenators came into general use.

The majority of the patients had congenital heart defects, but there were quite a few thoracic aneurysms. We didn't have an aortic or mitral valve prosthesis, so an aortic valve operation involved only reconstruction of the leaflets or removal of calcium. It was the same with mitral disease. Most of the operations were for mitral stenosis, and those were mostly done closed without the pump. We were just in the changeover period where people were starting to do open mitral commissurotomy using the pump, because it was felt that this gave a better outcome. One of the major discussions back in the sixties was which way to do mitral valve surgery, either open or closed.

Helen Taussig was still very active. She made rounds every day, and when I was the resident on the heart service I went along with her. She was a wonderful lady, very knowledgeable, and she certainly knew congenital heart pathology and anatomy. She had a terrible hearing problem in those days and used an amplified stethoscope. It was a little difficult sometimes to know whether she heard what you said or whether she heard what the heart was actually doing. She had some type of inner ear surgery later on and her hearing improved dramatically. She really had a different personality after that. She was not into invasive diagnostics because catheterizations came in after she was already established. She trusted her stethoscope a lot, and most of us liked to hear what she said, but we trusted the angiograms and the pressure measurements more. She also used the fluoroscope a lot in making her diagnosis. I think she went by the size and the configuration of the heart. Those patients with right ventricular outflow tract obstruction or diminished pulmonary arteries have a boot-shaped heart, which is diagnostic on fluoroscopy or an X-ray. She liked the fluoroscope, but I think she liked her stethoscope better.

I also knew Vivien Thomas from day one. He was a wonderful, devoted person and very helpful to the residents, especially if Dr. Blalock had suggested that he help. When I was working in the experimental laboratory, he would take care of everything. He was a fine technical surgeon, and at the beginning of my training there, he was somewhat involved with the heart-lung machine. He took care of the cleaning and running of the pump until we got a full-time technician or two. Obviously he had been involved with it in the laboratory. When they began to use the perfusion system in the operating room, Vivien sometimes accompanied the perfusionists, especially if they were uncertain about some aspect of the procedure. These early pumps were held together at times by a lot of improvisations. It wasn't quite as clear-cut as it is today, so we needed someone around who knew where to adjust things if the pump started shaking a little too much during the case.

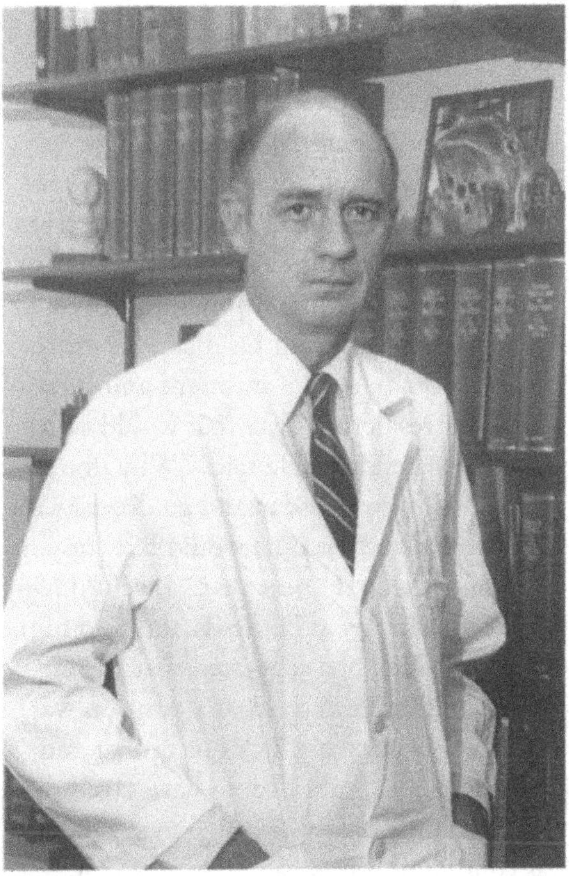

Paul A. Ebert

After I had been at Johns Hopkins for a couple of years I went to the NIH for two years, a common occurrence for residents at that time. I think Glenn Morrow was a resident at Hopkins during the war years in the mid-forties and then became the director of the heart service at the NIH. He was director of both surgery and cardiology. There were four residents per year that went to the NIH. Usually two of them came from Hopkins and two came from other locations. I remember very clearly in my second year at Hopkins being called to Dr. Blalock's office. In those days, you were an intern and then a first-year resident. Today that would be a second-year resident. He said, "Why don't you take off next Tuesday and go down to see Dr. Morrow, and see if he would like for you to come to the NIH next year." I went down to see Dr. Morrow at Bethesda and told him that Dr. Blalock had suggested that I come over and talk to him to see if a position was available. He got a big kick out of that and laughed. He said that I could have saved the trip. When the professor called to say who was coming, it was already taken care of.

In those days the draft for doctors was still in place, and I was fortunate to be able to go to the NIH and fulfill my service obligation. When we filled out the papers and were sworn into the Public Health Service it was a big day for us. They paid for the move to where you would reside, and since you had to be on call for the medical center, the rent was paid and an apartment was furnished for us according to the size of our family. There was only my wife and I at that time, so we only had a small one-bedroom apartment. It was right across the street from the medical center, and I walked to work at all times of the day and night.

Dr. Morrow's predominant work was with congenital heart problems, although he was interested in the disease called idiopathic hypertrophic subaortic stenosis, which today is recognized as a cardiomyopathy. We catheterized and operated on a fair number of people, but I would say that my time at the NIH was just at the beginning of valve replacements. There is a famous story at the NIH about the first total mitral valve replacement. They had tried mitral valve operations in which there were leaflet valves made with chordae that extended into the ventricle, and these chords were attached to the outside of the heart. Getting those two valve leaflets to approximate properly was almost impossible. We did not have echocardiography in those days, which might have made it easier. One day that operation was being tried, and the patient had been on the pump for about two and one-half hours, which was a very long time in those days. We had one Starr-Edwards valve, and it was in the animal laboratory. I was at the lab that day and the phone rang. Dr. Morrow asked me to bring that Starr-Edwards valve over to the OR as quickly as possible. We had been doing some flow studies with it, so we took it out of the pulse duplicator and ran it over to the clinical center. They put it in the autoclave to sterilize it and sewed it in the lady with a minimum number of sutures, and she came right off the pump. It was the most remarkable thing because this solved the problem of mitral stenosis, and she had no insufficiency. Prior to that time, mitral insufficiency was the unsolved problem. That lady survived and came back three years later to have the valve replaced, because the only valve that we had at that time was pretty small, and she had a relatively severe mitral stenosis. She came through the next operation without difficulty and lived twenty to twenty-five more years. I believe she was in her late thirties when she had the first operation. From that I learned that almost anything could be done in cardiac surgery if the patient was left with good hemodynamics at the completion of the operation. That had not been emphasized up to that time. In other words, if the VSD could be closed or the pulmonary stenosis relieved, the operation was a success, but if the aortic or mitral valve were operated on, the valve had better be competent at the end. I think that is why the Starr valve was an instantaneous success. This happened in the spring or fall of 1961.

After two years at the NIH I went back to Johns Hopkins to complete my training, but my decision to go into cardiac surgery wasn't that cut and dried. I guess I took the direction of least resistance. Of my two years at the Heart Institute, I was only on the cardiac surgery service for about six months. Six months had been spent in the laboratory, and one year with Gene Braunwald in the cardiac cath lab. We did quite a bit of hemodynamic research on patients, so I had a lot of experience in cardiovascular physiology that a lot of other people were not lucky enough to have.

When I finished training at Johns Hopkins, the positions offered me were predominantly in the cardiac surgery arena, although when I went to Duke with Dr. Sabiston, it wasn't explicitly stated that I was to do cardiac surgery. We essentially covered the whole spectrum of general surgery along with thoracic and cardiac procedures, depending on who was in town and what was on the OR schedule.

When I went to Duke in 1966, valve replacement had become fairly common. In North Carolina and East Tennessee there were a number of patients who had rheumatic heart disease. They came from the mountains and came down the north side of the hill to Durham, so we had a lot of people with mitral valve disease. Coronary surgery was just beginning around 1969 or 1970 at Duke. It started at different times in different parts of the country. There were also a number of patients with congenital heart disease, many of whom had palliative operations as infants and were coming back for total correction or whatever modifications they might need.

I only stayed at Duke for five years and then went to Cornell as chief of surgery. It was a big job and was an interesting experience. Dr. C. Walton Lillehei had been the chief of surgery at Cornell and for some reason hadn't always gotten along well with the other surgeons or the administration. He was really a nice person, and I always got along well with him. He stayed on after I was appointed chief. When I was interviewed they said that they had to recruit someone who was a cardiac surgeon because they needed someone to hold up their end of the load. I was kind of young, and I wasn't too sure that I was the right choice. It was a really good experience, and I actually learned a lot from Dr. Lillehei. He continued to operate and I don't think he was ever resentful of me. We seemed to hit it off pretty well. There were some very good residents in the program at that time, and I made sure that all of the residents that he had appointed completed their training.

My practice was predominately cardiac surgery and 30 percent vascular surgery. We didn't have a defined vascular surgical service, and we didn't have a full-time vascular surgeon. I inherited a number of people with peripheral vessel disease, abdominal aneurysms, and so forth. There were always a certain number of people in New York that had to be operated on by the chief of surgery, irrespective of what operation was needed. This probably wasn't always the best for the patient, but for that reason I did a moderate amount of general surgery as well.

Practicing in New York was different from the simplicity of a smaller community like Duke, and the referral pattern was more complex. Like all things big, the city was made up of small parts. Each of the major hospitals in New York had a referral base of graduates and physicians that were attached to the hospitals. I learned very quickly that Cornell would always have X number of patients with congenital heart disease. This number probably would never increase very much unless you could draw some patients from around the world. The referral bases were that fixed in New York. I don't mean that this was bad, because on one hand, there were a certain number of patients that went to New York Hospital, a certain number went to Columbia, and a certain number went to NYU. That didn't alter very much from year to year, but it was difficult to build a large practice in any particular specialty or subspecialty. Subspecialization was not nearly as well developed in New York as it was on the West Coast. When I went to San Francisco, it was pretty well decided that you did what the medical society thought you should do and that was it. At that time in New York it was not that way. It may be more specialized now after thirty years.

From Cornell I went to the University of California San Francisco as the chief of surgery. There didn't seem to be a lot of differences from New York, since the chief of surgery position is about the same the world over. In some ways it was probably easier in San Francisco because orthopedics, urology, ophthalmology, and ENT were all separate departments. The only thing that I was in charge of was general surgery, cardiothoracic, pediatric, and plastic surgery, a small service within the medical center. The more difficult part of UCSF was that we had residents in three hospitals: the university hospital, the county hospital, and the veterans' hospital. In New York, Duke, and Baltimore I always worked in only one hospital. There were ups and downs to those arrangements. Figuring out the residents' schedules was much more difficult at UCSF than in New York, where if someone became ill you could shuffle very quickly. You couldn't always do that as easily with three different hospitals.

At San Francisco most of my patients involved cardiac surgical procedures. I can probably count on one hand the number of operations that were thoracic, pulmonary, or esophageal. Interestingly, there were some patients that I had operated on back East that would come across the country to have something modified or to have a secondary procedure. I asked people in the other services to help me if I got into trouble. I had to do these operations because they had come all this way; I couldn't just turn them over to somebody else.

When I was at Duke, Bill Gay was finishing his chief residency and went with me to Cornell. While we were at Cornell we began working on potassium cardioplegia and myocardial protection. Bill and I had been very active in the laboratory at that time, and we could never figure out exactly why the Melrose solution was always such a terrible disaster. Putting the heart at rest should have reduced the metabolism and improved the outcome. We began using different concentrations of potassium. Bill was very interested and did the majority of the work on it. He was interested in different levels of potassium, different osmolarities, and the different ions that were in the solution. It became very clear in the animal laboratory that you could arrest the heart with potassium for thirty minutes at normothermia and have it recuperate and reperfuse for a period of five minutes, and it would show no ill effect. This was considerably different from what most cardiac surgeons had experienced in the early days of open-heart surgery when potassium arrest was first tried. Harold Urschel had done some work at the Bethesda Naval Hospital when I was at the NIH back in 1961 or 1962. He infused cold ringers lactate into hearts in the laboratory, but for some reason that technique never caught on clinically. I think most of the trouble was not with the cardiac arrest techniques, but that we couldn't fix the aortic or mitral valve well enough in those days to get a good hemodynamic result. It was probably overdistention of the heart at the conclusion of the operation that was part of the problem.

We then went to the question of how to administer the cardioplegic solutions. It became rather simple to put it in a plastic bag and to have it mixed in the pharmacy and stored in the refrigerator then to infuse most of it into the aortic root. If the patient had aortic insufficiency, then the aorta was opened and individual cannulas were put into the coronary arteries and the solution was infused that way. I think cardioplegia certainly made the operations safer. I believe it made a lot of cardiac surgeons fairly good very quickly, because they didn't have to bother with putting individual cannulas into the coronary arteries and having someone hold them. There had been several injuries to the coronary ostia because people would retract with these handheld metal cannulas, and the injured coronary arteries were almost impossible to repair.

I don't think anything ever replaces perfusing the coronaries continuously for good myocardial protection, but you always had something cumbersome in the aortic root with that method. The aortic root was sometimes very small when dealing with aortic stenosis. Some surgeons started adding cold solutions around the heart to keep the myocardial temperature reduced. There was no substitute for getting the operation done fairly expeditiously and making sure that the patient had a good hemodynamic result when you finished. Cardioplegia did help a lot of people. There was a lot of controversy at that time and a lot of people did not think that putting a clear crystalloid solution in the heart was good protection. Once they tried it though, it shortened their operating time. You couldn't stand around and be too leisurely; we used to say sixty minutes of myocardial ischemia was about the maximum time. We would reinfuse at around thirty-five minutes if we knew the operation would go for sixty minutes or longer. At that time potassium wasn't the biggest factor, it was keeping the temperature of the heart reduced.

I'm not sure what temperature was used for the cardioplegia solution. It was stored in the refrigerator so it was probably about 40 degrees. I think that is the recommended setting. When I was at the NIH with Gerald Austen, Lazar Greenfield, and Glenn Morrow, we did a lot of studies on hypothermia and isolated perfusion of the heart with hypothermia solutions. We even did some infants using a small heat exchanger and cooling them down to very low core temperatures. It was obvious that hypothermia was essentially the only protection that we had for those patients. The heart used to fibrillate most of the time during the procedure. It was our belief that the addition of potassium put the heart at total rest and thus reduced the metabolic requirements.

When all of these techniques gradually came together, the postoperative ventricular function was almost as good as it was at the beginning of the operation. This was a huge change from cardiac surgery in the late fifties and early sixties. Back then myocardial function was always terrible at the end of the operation. There was a disorder erroneously named "stone heart" where the heart went into tetanic contraction. After surgery it would be impossible to get it relieved. We never had that happen in a heart that had received potassium. At least I never had it or heard anyone report it after potassium cardioplegia. "Stone heart" usually came from anoxia and probably had more to do with how much calcium was available. It was almost impossible to break that sequence once it occurred. There were a number of patients that stayed on cardiopulmonary bypass for an hour or an hour and a half after the time of coronary reperfusion just to try to get the heart resuscitated after a "stone heart" event.

The present status of myocardial protection includes antegrade perfusion, retrograde perfusion, profound topical hypothermia, and modest hypothermia. I was always a believer that we should never rely on a single technique. We should know enough about all of these so we know when and how to use them. I would go somewhere in another part of the country and watch someone close an atrial septal defect. They would use cardioplegia. We would have just fibrillated the heart, kept the perfusion to the heart intact, opened the atrium to repair the ASD, removed all the air from the heart, and restarted it, all at about 32 degrees at the most. I never thought we should learn just one technique, but thought we should understand all of them. I imagine if we were doing a real lengthy operation where we thought we might have two, two and a half, to three hours of aortic occlusion, then retrograde perfusion or hypothermic blood perfusion would be very useful. It probably allows one to go that long. There is a definite limit to aortic occlusion time using potassium and hypothermia. I still believe this, and that is why I emphasize that we have to work within a specific period of time. If you can't get the operation done in that time, then another technique must be used.

In the mid-1980s I received a phone call from the chairman of the Board of Regents of the American College of Surgeons, and was asked if I would recommend three people for the position of director because Dr. Hanlon was going to retire. I gave three names of people that I knew were very active in the College and understood most of its functions. I thought any one of those people would do a superb job. I got another call about three months later and they said it was unanimous. They all decided that I should do it. There were two comments that helped me decide. One was from my friend David Sabiston, who said, "Well, you know nobody ever did anything important after they were forty years old, so you might as well do this." Frank Spencer, who was a regent of the College at the time, made a very key point.

There were a lot of social changes occurring, and he said that the College was the only organization that has the staff and finances to make an impact for surgeons and surgery. He said that all of our other organizations, if they were analyzed, just don't have those resources. I still believe that is very true. We need input from the various specialties, but no one has the voice that the College has and the access to such a large number of surgeons from around the country.

The College got started through the concern of a small number of surgeons about the overall quality of surgery. This group formed a small clinical congress. It wasn't a college at that time. They put on a meeting that was organized by just a few people. They discussed the topic of surgical care and proposed two things that eventually made a big difference in surgical practice. First, they decided that they needed a college similar to the Royal College of Surgeons in England. The College would have a scientific base, and because there were no board examinations at that time except in ENT and ophthalmology, the College would take that responsibility. They felt that the College had an obligation to identify member surgeons that patients could depend upon and feel that they would receive quality service.

Out of this beginning probably fifty or sixty original members of the College observed other surgeons operating. They published a book with a list of names in it. If you were a practicing surgeon, it was very important to have your name in the book because residency training in 1913 to 1916 was pretty sporadic and unregulated. Surgical training was more of an apprenticeship at that time. The second part that the college did was to set up a standard for the operating-room environment. They understood very early that the variety of operating-room techniques, such as the cleaning of the operating rooms, the dangers of explosives, who came in the operating room, and what type of garment they wore, were very important. This really caught on because there were several hospitals that had very high infection rates, and after they took the College's recommendations there were marked improvements within a year. I think identifying surgeons who were doing high-quality work and also setting the standards for the operating-room environment were really major contributions in those formative years.

Today medicine seems to be dominated by managed care, and I don't know the final extent that the College will be involved. I have always believed that the most important thing for the College is to emphasize quality of service and care of patients. There are managed care companies that are providing good service, and there are some that are being very restrictive and not providing good service. I think that the College has a right to keep up with what patients' rights really are and what one can expect, and they have been doing that for the last fifteen years. There have been a lot of positive results. What I think is going to happen in the future is that managed care companies are going to have to liberalize their services more and reduce their profits. I think the public is very much aware of the problems with managed care, and we have done our best to make the public more aware with a lot of statements, advertisements, articles, and testimony in Congress. I think the word is out. We weren't the only ones that did it, but there is no question that someone might tolerate a problem with an office visit, but they won't tolerate low-quality surgery. I think the two worst things that HMOs have done are denying a needed service and, even worse, delaying treatment. They don't recognize, or don't seem to recognize, the danger to the patient when this is done. The College has spoken out very loudly on these issues, and I think this will continue to be very important.

I don't believe we will ever evolve into a single-payer system. We said at one time that a single-payer system was probably the simplest and best way to go, and were severely criticized by about half of the membership. I think if we polled the current fellowship, they would probably agree with us now, although it has taken five or six years for them to understand it. I don't think we will ever have a single-payer system for one reason. If the government could figure out how to arrest the amount of money that private industry and private citizens are putting into health care and recoup that, they could come up with a single-payer system. I don't think there are enough funds in the federal government to fund the whole program at the moment, and I don't think they really want to. I think they are very much afraid of taking on much more than the current Medicare program.

I don't think the malpractice situation will ever disappear even though there is a College course and a very good book about malpractice. I don't think it should wane, because I actually believe that when a patient is poorly served they need to be able to express themselves and have the same access to legal care as anyone else. Surgeons would love to be able to see someone wave a magic wand and have it all go away, but in the year 2000 you could say that malpractice might become the best friend the doctor has ever had. The HMOs are now starting to be assaulted by patients, and the only way they can assault an HMO is legally. They are in business and they learn very quickly if they have to pay a penalty for something that they did incorrectly, then they had better stop doing it since it could be very costly. I think the number of suits against surgeons has decreased, and the amount of many suits has also decreased. I think this is favorable in some way, but I believe many malpractice suits are just being transferred to the HMOs. We have a new enemy now, and it isn't always just the lawyers, it could be the HMOs.

When I was finishing my training, the most interesting aspect of surgery was probably cardiac surgery. There were a lot of new things and new ideas, and it was a dynamic specialty. I believe that young residents should choose what they want to do and not choose a specialty simply because it is thought to have a rosy future. If you really like cardiac surgery and really enjoy it, then I would recommend that you go into it. There are changes in cardiac surgery today, and it might be a little stagnant. I think the biggest change in cardiac surgery is probably that we are moving toward more and more noninvasive techniques. I think technology will continue in that direction; however, there will always be a need for an old-fashioned operation. There is certainly more surgical disease today than there was when I started out. The population has increased in size. People are living longer, and as they get older, we do not turn them down because of age as we did in the past.

Bibliography

Ebert PA, Greenfield LJ, Austen WG, Morrow AG. Experimental Comparison of Methods for Protecting the Heart during Aortic Occlusion. *Ann Surg.* 1962; 155:25–32.

Ebert PA, Allgood RJ, Sabiston DC Jr. The Anti-arrhythmic Effects of Cardiac Denervation. *Ann Surg.* 1968; 168:728–735.

Ebert PA. Relationship of Myocardial Potassium Content and Atrial Fibrillation. *Circulation.* 1970; 41(Suppl II):137–141.

Gay WA, Ebert PA. Functional, Metabolic, and Morphologic Effects of Potassium-Induced Cardioplegia. *Surgery.* 1973; 74:284–290.

Ebert PA, Sabiston DC Jr, Zuidema GD, Weldon CS, Williams GM. Current Trends in Specialization. The Effect of Residency Training. *Johns Hopkins Med J.* 1973; 133:223–235.

Ebert PA. Aspects of Myocardial Protection. *Ann Thorac Surg.* 1978; 26:495–496.

Ellis RJ, Mangano DT, Van Dyke DC, Ebert PA. Protection of Myocardial Function Not Enhanced by High Concentrations of Potassium during Cardioplegic Arrest. *J Thorac Cardiovasc Surg.* 1979; 78:698–707.

Ebert PA, Turley K, Stranger P, Hoffman JI, Heymann MA, Rudolph AM. Surgical Treatment of Truncus Arteriosus in the First 6 Months of Life. *Ann Surg.* 1984; 200:451–456.

Ebert PA. Open Heart Surgery in Infancy. *Ann Thorac Surg.* 1989; 47:321.

Ebert PA. The Importance of Data in Improving Practice: Effective Clinical Use of Outcomes Data. *Ann Thorac Surg.* 1994; 58:1812–1814.

Harvey W. Bender, MD

(b. 1933)

The third person at Baylor was Dr. Stanley Crawford, a very talented surgeon, from a little town in Alabama. He was a low-key person, but was one of the finest surgeons I have ever seen. He was very bright and could operate so fast, and so well, and he could do the most difficult cases with essentially no help. He did a Whipple procedure with the intern and me, a senior student, for help, in an hour and twenty-nine minutes and never stopped talking the whole time. He was really a very good surgeon.

— On the surgical faculty
at Baylor Medical School

Interviewed May 28, 2003

I was born in Corpus Christi, Texas, in 1933 during the Depression. My dad was there trying to get work, and he finally got a job in the oil fields working six-hour shifts. I actually grew up in Humble, Texas, and that was home. Humble had a population of about twelve hundred. The school building was quite old and was the same building that my father attended. Some of the teachers he had were still teaching when I came along. The community was truly like a huge extended family. There was nothing that you did, or thought about doing, that was not known by someone in town, and this pretty much kept us on the straight-and-narrow path. It was a terrific place to grow up, since there was tremendous freedom. Almost every day after school there was an opportunity to go horseback riding in the woods, hunting, fishing, or some other outdoor activity. The agriculture teacher was very important in my growing up, and he encouraged me to attend college. He told me there was more to life than getting out of high school and working in the oil fields, which is what most everyone did there.

I decided to go to college and was one of the few out of my high school who did. My family raised cattle and was in the timber business. I was very interested in the ranching and the cattle business, but I was fascinated by science in high school, so I decided that the thing to do was to be a veterinarian. I went to Texas A & M because at that time it was the veterinary medical school for four contiguous states. There were only twelve vet schools in the country then. Getting into vet school was hard; there were fifty in our class and all were very bright. Most of them grew up in agricultural environments in Texas or the surrounding states, and they were all male. After I got into vet school, it became clear that veterinary medicine was becoming more of a small-animal practice. I was interested in large animals since I grew up around horses and cattle.

At Christmas break during my first year in vet school, I had a friend whose father had died. I attended the funeral in a nearby town on the other side of Houston. As I was driving back (I had my suit on), I noticed that I was driving by the Baylor University College of Medicine. I thought that I would just stop in and see what it would take to become a doctor. It was vacation time and the students were gone. A very nice lady in the administration office talked with me for a while to find out a bit about what I had done in college. She suggested that I fill out an application, and I did. She said that there were a couple of professors there that were on the admissions committee. She asked if I would like to visit with them, and so I took that opportunity. After Christmas break when I got back to A & M there was a letter from Baylor. It said to send $50, that I had been accepted into the new class the following year. More than anything else, this points out the enormous difference in the process of getting into medical school now as opposed to the way it was in 1955. I had to take one course in quantitative analysis that I had not had, and then after dropping out of vet school I took some great fun courses for the next semester before going on to medical school. As good fortune would have it, I wound up in a medical school that was truly on the leading edge of cardiovascular surgery. Baylor was a small medical school and, at that time, not very selective in its admissions process. However, the faculty was incredibly exciting, and it was terrific to be a part of it.

While in medical school I had the opportunity to work in the Department of Surgery, running the heart-lung machine. Dr. DeBakey was a fantastic man. I think he had been in Houston for about six years when I got there. Dr. Cooley had been there about four years. There was a very small surgical faculty and a smaller medical faculty. The full-time medical faculty consisted of two people. The full-time surgical faculty consisted of four people: Dr. DeBakey, Dr. Cooley, Dr. George Jordan, and Dr. Stanley Crawford. At the end of my freshman year in medical school, I got a summer job working as a scrub technician at the Jefferson Davis City Hospital. I came in contact with the

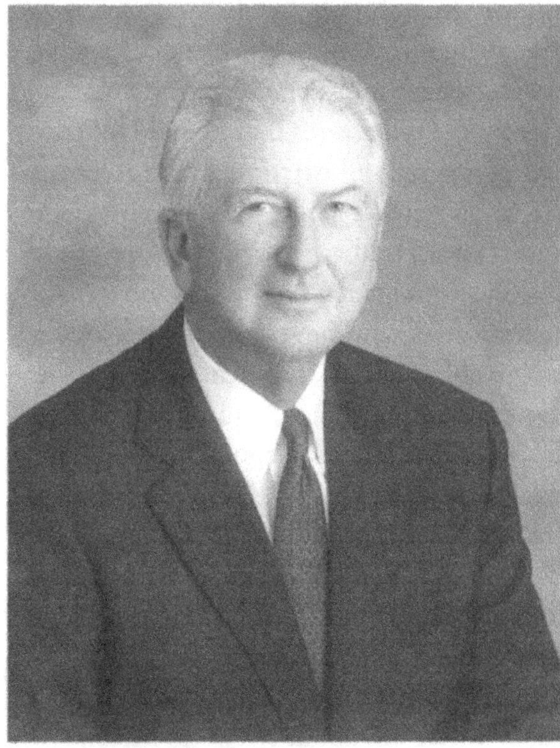

Harvey W. Bender

surgical house officers but not the surgical faculty.

At the end of the preclinical years, Dr. DeBakey had the habit of getting a list from the dean's office of those in the upper part of the class, and he offered those students employment in the Department of Surgery. We were then assigned to one of the full-time people in the department and worked really quite closely with them. My job happened to be running the heart-lung machine for Dr. Cooley, since Dr. DeBakey did no open cardiac surgery at that time. I was running the heart-lung machine when the early cases were done in Houston. I remember a big party, going water skiing, and having a lot of hamburgers and beer when we did the hundredth pump case in Houston. I had the opportunity to work with those people on a daily basis and see the brilliance and enormous energy of both. Cooley and DeBakey were incredibly bright. Dr. DeBakey was very meticulous and very precise in the operating room—the dissections that he did looked like an anatomy illustration. Dr. Cooley had this sort of innate ability always to make the right move. He always knew when he could do something, when he couldn't, how to make it work, and how to do it with the fewest possible motions. His heart-lung machine was simple in its design, and there were very few ways that anything could go wrong. It was not very sophisticated, but with its simplicity, its lack of problems, and Dr. Cooley's speed in the operating room, it all worked, and he had very good results very early in the development of heart surgery.

The pump was originally a stainless-steel bubbler that was about twelve to fifteen inches tall and about five to six inches in diameter. There was a central hollow stainless-steel core, and at the bottom of that was a plate, so that when venous blood and oxygen were passed through that plate it made bubbles. It bubbled up to the top of the central tube and then went around the outside as a helix and debubbled during that transit around the cylinder. It was then pumped back into the patient as arterialized blood. The venous blood and the arterial flow were both pumped at that time.

During this time we were primarily doing congenitals, because we didn't have an artificial valve. The mitral valve operations were mainly for mitral stenosis and were done as closed procedures. There were some attempts to do mitral reparative surgery for mitral insufficiency, but not very many. While I was there the first ventricular aneurysms were resected. Most of the procedures were ASDs, VSDs, endocardial cushion defects, tetralogies, pulmonary stenosis, and things of that nature that were done within about a half-hour. Beyond that thirty-minute time, the risk of being on the pump went up a great deal. We used a low flow rate and there wasn't a really good system of returning blood to the oxygenator, so blood that was lost in the operative field was lost. We hadn't figured that part out yet.

There was one time when I was helping Dr. DeBakey do an aneurysm when there was a moment of uncertainty. This was an instant that I thought was death, not only the patient's, but also mine. Dr. DeBakey occasionally would go to the Jefferson Davis Hospital to do a case. One day the word came that Dr. DeBakey needed a pump the next day at the Jefferson Davis Hospital because he was going to do a thoraco-abdominal aneurysm and wanted to use the pump as a bypass while he did the aneurysmectomy. The pump team consisted of a full-time year-round nurse employee and two students. I was finishing my sophomore year and the other student was finishing his junior year. These two students, my colleague and I, were dispatched to go help Dr. DeBakey. Dr. Cooley kept the nurse, the professional, with him that day. We headed out to the Jefferson Davis Hospital. The plan was to fill a piece of plastic Tygon tubing with saline, pass one end to Dr. DeBakey to put it in the left atrium through a purse-string suture, and the other end into the femoral artery. The blood would have already been oxygenated by the lungs. The blood would be pumped so the aorta could be clamped above and below the aneurysm. We had a Sigmamotor pump, which worked by the progressive massage of the tubing by little metal fingers, propelling the blood forward. I had this Tygon tubing all filled with saline, Dr. DeBakey was operating, and there was great tension in the operating room. I handed him one end of it and said, "This goes in the left atrium." I handed him the other end and said, "This goes in the femoral artery." In a couple of minutes he said that it was okay to turn on the pump. I turned the pump on and the old pump started, but I could see blood coming down the tube connected to the femoral artery going the wrong way toward the pump, which then would subsequently be pumped directly into the left atrium. I had visions of us just pumping the arterial blood back into the left atrium and having the patient go into immediate heart failure. My partner in crime, the student that was one year ahead of me, immediately left the room and was gone. I was sort of hanging onto the table and the lights were going out when the old pump finally caught and the blood started going in the opposite, and correct, direction. Things worked out all right after that one frightful moment.

It is curious that Baylor was using the Sigmamotor finger pump at that time rather than the roller pump which Dr. DeBakey had popularized for use in transfusions early in his career. Since that time DeBakey roller pumps have been standard equipment on all heart-lung machines. A lot of the early perfusion setups used the Sigmamotor pump, probably because it was used in various industrial settings and was readily available. At that time an electric motor-driven roller pump had to be custom made.

The third person at Baylor was Dr. Stanley Crawford, and he was also a very talented surgeon. He was from a little town in Alabama. He was a low-key person, but was one of the finest technical surgeons that I have ever seen. He was very bright and could operate so fast, so well, and he could do the most difficult cases with essentially no help. I remember later when I was a senior student that Stanley had a patient on the schedule that day for a Whipple procedure. He had the intern and me, a senior student, for help. Dr. Crawford did the operation in one hour and twenty-nine minutes and never stopped talking the whole time. Instead of criticizing the way we were helping or whatever we were doing, he was saying things like didn't our mothers teach us better manners and things like that; this went on constantly. Also late one evening when I was a student and we had finished in the operating room, he said, "Harvey, do you have a few minutes?" I said, "Sure, Dr. Crawford. What do you need?" He told me that there was a patient with a big abdominal aneurysm out at the Wright Clinic, which was a little hospital out on the north side of Houston with maybe ten beds. The two of us went there that evening and did the surgery for an abdominal aneurysm. It was just no problem. He was really a very good surgeon.

Baylor had a very large surgical service, and they had great attending surgeons doing a lot of work. At that time it had not been set up as a good training program. They hadn't figured that out, but they were very busy clinical surgeons. Dr. Cooley was young, handsome, athletic, and bright (he was an all Southwest Conference basketball player). He was doing cases that could only be done in a few places in the world. He had trained at Johns Hopkins and was sort of a role model for me. This was the stimulus that I needed to apply to Johns Hopkins for training.

When I got there in 1959, it quickly became very clear that it was a totally different environment. They were doing all kinds of surgery, including heart surgery, and they had a number of good surgeons. The place was set up to train people, and they had a system that worked very well. Many of the pioneers in the field of cardiac surgery came from that program. When I was there, it was the tail end of that golden era which was defined by Dr. Blalock's tenure. I think things had been much more flexible and less organized early on, but when I came along they had developed a structure that I felt was very well thought out and designed to bring people along with increasing responsibility, which resulted in well-trained surgeons. When I went there in 1959, Dr. Blalock was still there, but he died in 1964. I was away a couple of those years, but he was there for part of my training. I was fortunate to get to operate with him a number of times.

Dr. Blalock was a gentleman and incredibly well prepared. I will give you an example. When we arrived in Baltimore, my wife Doris and I had a three-year-old son. Around July fourth, Dr. Blalock had a tea for the new interns and their wives in a small library across from his office. I didn't know whether he had any idea who I was, what I was interested in, or anything about me. When we walked into the tea, my wife was introduced and was talking with Dr. Blalock. He asked her how our three-year-old son was and did he manage the trip all right. This gives you an idea of how he prepared and how thorough he was in everything that he did. This was also the way he approached every patient that he operated on. He got a lot of help from the residents and made it clear that he wanted to get all of the information. The resident would then head to the library and research the problem. Then he and Dr. Blalock would meet and they would go over all of the data. This would refresh Dr. Blalock's memory and the resident learned everything there was to know as well as how Dr. Blalock thought about that particular clinical problem. This process went on every day. Two residents met with Dr. Blalock every day in his office. One was the resident on the cardiac surgical service and the other was the chief resident on the surgical service. It was an incredible learning experience.

Without ever meeting with Dr. Blalock to talk about my plans, I met with Hank Bahnson and David Sabiston and was asked if I was interested in remaining. I received a note toward the end of the year inviting me to become a first-year resident. There were four of us who were selected to stay, so our group went from seventeen to four after the first year. You can't do that now, but in my mind, I think to train really good surgeons or really good people in anything, you don't take just everyone that wants to participate. You take the ones that settle out and appear to have something extra. In the fall, about November of the second year of training (first-year assistant resident) I received a page to call Dr. Blalock's telephone number, which threw me into sheer panic. When I made the call, Dr. Blalock simply said, "Harvey, you have an appointment next Friday at ten o'clock to meet Glenn Morrow at the National Heart Institute; he has a job for you. Call Dick Anderson and tell him he has an appointment, too." So the two of us went to Bethesda, met Glenn, and then the following July we went to the NIH. It was very well structured and all designed the way Dr. Blalock wanted things to be. He had never asked either Dick or me whether we wanted to do cardiac surgery. He just assumed that that was what we wanted to do because that was the thing that was new and the most interesting.

Dr. Blalock had the ability to arrange almost anything, and because his relationships with everyone were so powerful, he could get jobs for people. It is hard to identify the feature that makes one individual powerful and influential even though another individual may have the same intellect. At that time you could see how Dr. Blalock introduced an operation that opened a whole field of surgery that was very exciting. Operating on a human heart caught everyone's attention worldwide. In the next couple of decades he trained a large number of very talented people who were very bright and technically gifted. Those surgeons were scattered around the country doing cardiac surgery and heading important surgical departments, and I think this resulted in his having a great deal of influence.

The program at the NIH was set up so that one year was spent in the research laboratory. It was the easiest place to work that you could imagine. There were no budget concerns and you could study anything that you wanted, there was always funding for it. The lab was well equipped and well staffed. During that year you could crank out papers and do any research that you found interesting. The next six months were spent in the cardiac cath laboratory. At the NIH the cath lab was run by a surgical associate; that's what we were called. During that period of time I did all of the caths, or I would help teach some of the cardiology fellows who were at the NIH to do them. There were four cardiology fellows who became presidents of the American College of Cardiology that I taught to do caths when I had only two years of surgical training and a year in the research lab. Every Sunday all of the new patients were admitted to the NIH, and after they had been worked up, we would meet with Gene Braunwald and review the patient information. We then planned the week's cath schedule, and after the caths were done, the information was discussed on Friday. This process went on for six months; it was absolutely terrific. The last six months at the NIH were spent as the first assistant in the operating room. The surgical results really improved while I was there because the Starr valve became available, first for mitral valve replacement, and for the last three months we had a Starr valve that worked in the aortic position. Suddenly, the patients that had been dying were living; this was an exciting time. Previously, there had been a very high mortality rate. We had been trying to sew in cloth valves, trying to debride valves in patients with aortic stenosis to remove the calcium and make the valve more pliable. This was a time of very high mortality, but it suddenly turned around. With the first cases using the Starr valve in the aortic position the results were very different.

After that I went back to Hopkins and back to a structured program. When I came back from the NIH, I spent six months in surgical pathology. The residents now don't spend any time in surgical pathology. During this six-month period I would cut specimens every other day. There were four pathology house officers that rotated on alternate days. We had a tremendous experience in surgical pathology and an opportunity to read and learn about the things that were going on in the surgical field. The next six months was another unusual rotation that consisted of plastic surgery, and you don't see that in training programs now. Although

Dr. Blalock didn't get along particularly well with the chief of plastic surgery, he thought that the things that you could learn in plastic surgery with respect to handling tissue, rotating flaps, making the flaps so that they would be viable, and learning about spatial relations were very important in surgery. I think he was right. If you wind up doing cardiac surgery, you have got to be able to visualize things in three dimensions, think in three dimensions, and do the procedure in three dimensions. All of the information received before going into the operating room is in two dimensions. I thought it was very helpful to have the six months of plastic surgical experience. In the next six months I was doing pulmonary surgery in a TB hospital, another great experience. The following six months I was assigned to cardiac surgery, which at that time was before Medicare, so there was a big ward service at Hopkins. The patients came into the hospital as patients of one of the attendings, or they just came in on the ward service. During the time that you were a resident on that service, every ward patient that came in was your patient. The heart service had an attending surgeon as an assistant in the operating room, and you didn't do anything on your own, as opposed to general surgery. We always had an attending, but it didn't make any difference as to how easy or how difficult it was, you had responsibility for the patient.

Then there were still two more years of training to go through, and that took place back in general surgery. During the next six-month period you worked three months on the private general surgical service with a lot of private general surgery, big operations, so we were the assistants and ran the private service. The three remaining months were spent in the emergency room doing all of the surgery that came through the ER. During the next six months, three months were spent with each of the outgoing chief residents; they were phasing out. We assumed more responsibility and did bigger and bigger cases. The next year we had a twenty-five-bed ward that was our service, plus we had admitting privileges to the hospital, so any private attending that wanted to could send us a patient and we could admit that patient to the hospital. It was a very good way to train people.

During our first two years in Baltimore, my wife and I lived in a row house right across the street from the psychiatric hospital. My son played in the playground at the psychiatric hospital. We had this row house with a concrete sidewalk with three steps and a little sign that said, "Keep off the grass," but there wasn't any grass anywhere around. It was a three-story building and was a typical shotgun row house. It had a front door and a long hallway that went from the entrance, and there were rooms off to the right. The ground floor was occupied by an ophthalmology resident and his wife. There were stairs that went up to the second and third floor, which is where Doris and I lived with our son. It had a bathroom and kitchen that had been nailed onto the back of the building and was obviously not part of the original building. They were great facilities, but it took a little getting used to the fact that there was someone else, total strangers, living in the house with you. There were no doors that separated your house and their house. After that we lived in the compound. These had the lowest building cost ever and were the flimsiest little apartments. Everyone on the house staff lived there and everyone knew each other. It was tough for the wives, but they were very supportive of each other and became very good friends.

When my resident days were finished, I was asked to join the Johns Hopkins faculty. The pay was miniscule and I was only paid a little more than the chief resident. As the chief resident, I was making about $10,000 to $12,000 a year. At the time I joined the faculty, I was paid $18,000 a year. The salary didn't go up very much over the next several years. I was there for four years beginning in 1967, and I left in 1971. During this time the first heart transplant was done in Cape Town, and I did one in 1968. This was very interesting. It was one of those things that you knew were being done in other centers, and we couldn't wait to do one. We did our first heart transplant before we did our first kidney transplant. We were getting geared up to do a kidney transplant, but we got a heart first. The recipient had had rheumatic fever with mitral stenosis and a mitral valve replacement that had been done elsewhere. He had a lot of trouble and wound up with a heart that was just whipped and had very poor left ventricular function. The donor had a gunshot wound and was pronounced dead in the operating room. This was the procedure at that time. Everyone had problems detecting rejection episodes. We tried to do EKGs and measure the R wave and that sort of thing. The patient lived four or five months and finally died; he was never really well.

My practice there was mixed between general surgery and thoracic surgery. Dr. Blalock didn't really believe that you were going to be one kind of surgeon or another kind of surgeon. He thought he trained surgeons that did different things. He thought that all of their training ought to be pretty much the same no matter what they were going to do. He thought that the cardiac surgical training would make you a better general surgeon or vice versa.

That was not original with Dr. Blalock. For example, during the thirties at Hopkins, the sort of premier rotation for the residents in training was to be on the so-called brain team with Walter Dandy, who was a very prominent neurosurgeon for many years. People spent two years on the brain team. Many times they would finish that and then become the head of the general surgery training program. They thought that was important in their training, and they continued that when we came along. Of the two residents that were a year ahead of me, one did cardiac surgery and one did vascular surgery. My coresident also did cardiac surgery when he finished. The residents the year behind me both did general surgery. The residents the year behind them both did cardiac surgery. It really didn't determine what you were going to do, but the training was pretty much the same for everyone.

Dr. Bahnson and Dr. Frank Spencer had been on the faculty at Hopkins, but they left during the time that I was at the NIH. When I came back, the cardiac surgical service was headed by David Sabiston. Jim Jude, who became well-known for closed-chest cardiac massage and resuscitation, was an attending as well as a fellow named Bob Gaertner, who actually built the first Hopkins heart-lung machine when he was a junior house officer. They were the cardiac surgical service in 1963 when I returned from the NIH.

The next year, in 1964, Dr. Blalock was not well and was nearing his sixty-fifth birthday. He was planning to retire, and they were looking for someone else. When it became clear that this someone was not going to be David Sabiston, he left to head the surgical department at Duke. Jim Jude left to head the cardiac thoracic program at the University of Miami, and Bob Gaertner remained and ran the cardiac service for a short time. Alex Haller, who had come back to Hopkins from Louisville, and Larry Weldon, who had finished the residency a few years ahead of me, were doing the bulk of cardiac surgical work for a number of years. In about 1966 Vince Gott came from Wisconsin as the head of the cardiac program.

After a few years on the faculty at Hopkins, I was invited to Vanderbilt to run the cardiac surgery program. It was being run by Arnold Killen and Hal Collins, along with a fellow named John Sutton. Vanderbilt was having a very difficult time getting their program going. It was kind of a trap in that all the patients being referred were high risk and difficult, so their results were not perfect. They had a group of cardiologists who were very cautious, conservative, and they had no enthusiasm for operative intervention in heart disease. I think they felt that it was some sort of defeat if they had to refer a patient for an operation. When I came, Vanderbilt had decided that they would recruit a new chief of cardiology, a new chief of pediatric cardiology, and a new chief of cardiac surgery all at the same time. Whoever had that idea made a good decision. It brought in three people with enthusiasm. and with no past history that could make things difficult. It was easy for them to work together, and things did improve. Still, there was tough competition in town.

Dr. Scott was the chairman then, and we got along quite well and worked well together. He had gotten over his interest in cardiac surgery by that time and did not interfere at all in whatever I tried to do. I think he had been forced into the situation of bringing in those three new people, as I don't think it was his idea. He wasn't terribly enthusiastic, but at the same time he was totally fair. He kept his hands off and let us do whatever we wanted or needed to do and didn't hinder us in any way. We became good friends through the years, and so I was able to get along with him pretty well. He was a remarkable man in some of the things he did as head of this surgical program. He put together a training program that worked and has turned out a lot of really well-trained surgeons. The bulk became general surgeons, I think, but a lot of good surgeons came out of the Vanderbilt training program during that time. I also worked with John Sawyers, who succeeded Dr. Scott and who is one of my really good friends.

In the early eighties I received a telephone call from Herb Sloan, asking me if I would serve on the American Board of Thoracic Surgery. The board selects the new members of the board, and for some reason my name had surfaced. I certainly accepted. At my first meeting on the board, they said that we had to have someone join the American Board of Surgery. The American Board of Surgery sends someone to the different specialty surgical boards like colon-rectal, pediatric, plastic, and cardiothoracic. This process allowed the board to keep abreast of what was going on in these specialties. They had someone sitting in the board meetings, and it helped them write questions in the specialty areas for the American Board of Surgery exam. For instance, they would have someone from the thoracic board help write the thoracic questions, someone from the plastic board for that area, and so forth. It was a good relationship, and I spent six years on both boards. It was a big time commitment to serve on the American Board of Surgery as it required being out of town about a month each year. There are a lot of exams and a lot of question writing, since those exams are given all over the country during the year.

I also served on the Board of Regents of the College of Surgeons. This resulted from receiving a call from the chairman of the nominating committee for the Board of Governors asking me if I would be willing to serve on the Board of Regents. I had been a governor for a little while and enjoyed that experience. I had a great deal of respect for the College, as I think most of us had an opportunity to present our first work at the forum of the College of Surgeons. It was always exciting to go to the College meetings. I had been involved with them through the years. I said that I would certainly love to serve on the Board of Regents and that turned out to be a nine-year job. The regents are elected for three years and can be reelected twice, so most people would wind up spending nine years in that capacity. I just happened to come along at a time, when I was about two years away from finishing my term, when there was a need for a new chairman for the board, and so I filled the position. From that time it is pretty automatic that the chairman would serve at some point as the president. The president's job is mostly to go around the country to various meetings. It's not a very difficult job and in some ways compensated for having worked on the board in the past.

The Board of Regents takes action on a lot of issues. Education, as well as issues related to the practice of surgery, have been the cornerstone of the College from its inception. They have a heavy involvement in Washington trying to look out for legislation that could make it more difficult to practice and trying to support legislation that might make practice easier and improve patients' access to good surgical care. They are very much committed to the proposition that surgery should be done by surgeons and that you should look for board certification and evidence that the patient has a surgeon who is well trained and well versed in the problem that the patient happens to have. They support a lot of research activity. Up until recently this was done by funding career development grants and fellowships to give opportunities to pursue research in a given area. In recent years the College has also become involved in clinical trials. Initially this was in oncology, headed by Sam Wells. I think this has the potential of giving us a lot of information. It is a very large, broadly based clinical trials program in a variety of specialties and tumor types. I think we can look forward to some real productivity in that area.

The College is big business and has a large budget. There is a lot of money that the board is responsible for shepherding and managing so that the College will be able to continue to do the things that it has done, such as putting on big meetings, traveling symposiums, and various activities that help surgeons. Because of good fortune with the investment of the endowment, the dues are miniscule compared to other surgical organizations. Membership is selective, but not overly selective. It is not automatic, and you just don't sign up and become a member. The selection is based primarily on local input and whether you are viewed as the kind of well-trained surgeon in your community that they like to see.

There are a number of people who have had an influence on my life. I will start with my fourth-grade teacher, Miss Holytski; she really got my attention. In Humble, the fourth grade was housed on the second floor of this little school house. A second floor was a pretty big thing in itself, because that was the only building in town other than the courthouse that had two floors. One night a friend called me to say that there was a new movie at the "picture show," and he said, "Let's go to the picture show tonight." I said that sounded like a great idea, and I talked with my mother and she said, "What about your homework?" I told her that we didn't have any homework and that it was free sailing, so she said OK. My friend and I went to the picture show, and the next day Miss Holytski wanted to know where my homework was. Obviously, my friend and I didn't have it. She grabbed me by the shoulders, walked over to the second-floor window, and held me outside. She said that if I came in one more time without my homework, I was going out the window. She got my attention.

Another man that I mentioned earlier was my agriculture teacher. He had gone to Texas A & M, had been a marine in World War II, and had achieved the rank of major. They were pretty stingy with rank in the Marine Corps. He was a fantastic man, hard as nails, and had tremendous influence on the young boys in our high school. I certainly credit him as someone important.

I also have to say that Denton Cooley was important in that he was a terrific role model. I began to see him work and thought, "Gosh, if you could grow up to have a life like that, then life would be terrific."

Hank Bahnson was someone at Hopkins who I worked with during my internship and during my first year as an assistant resident. I don't think there was a day that went by in my surgical career that I didn't become aware of something during an operation that either Hank told me about or showed me how to do. He was a fantastic technical surgeon. He would finish the cardiac part of the operation and, instead of leaving the operating table for the resident to finish up, he would let the residents take care of the thoracic part, go down to the end of the table and show the intern how to sew the femoral artery back together. All of those details were important. He was an enormous influence on all of us.

Dr. Blalock was a little more removed. Obviously he was very influential, but I didn't feel, and I don't think anyone felt, that close to Dr. Blalock. Of all his residents they say that only Bill Longmire called him Al. None of the other trainees did; it was still a very formal relationship, even after many years.

In the future, cardiac surgery will be very different. I think that one of the things that made cardiac surgery exciting was not just what you did in the operating room. It was taking an incredibly sick, unstable patient to the recovery room, or to the ICU, or whatever, and then using all of your skills as a physician, not a surgeon, to make that patient better and get him or her well. I thought that was a tremendous part of what we did. What we see now, and I see it from afar as I am not there firsthand, is that it seems like surgery is becoming a very technical operating room–based specialty that generates a lot of income. I don't think it produces the kind of physician that we would like to think we were or that we wanted to be when we went into medical school. That is a little disappointing. Whenever I begin to talk like this I feel like I am hearing my grandfather talk about how the world has changed, and that it's all going to hell. I'm sure it is going to work out, but it is going to be different.

Bibliography

Bender HW Jr, Austen WG, Ebert PA, Greenfield LJ, Tsunekawa T, Morrow AG. Experimental Pulmonic Regurgitation. *J Thorac Cardiovasc Surg.* 1963; 45:451–459.

Bender HW Jr, Haller JA, Brawley RK, Humphries JO, Neill CA, Gott VL. Experience in Repair of Tetralogy of Fallot Malformation in Adults. *Ann Thorac Surg.* 1971; 11:508–516.

Bender HW Jr, Fisher RD, Faulkner SL, Friesinger GC. Unstable Coronary Artery Disease: A Comparison of Medical and Surgical Treatment. *Ann Thorac Surg.* 1975; 19:521–528.

Bender HW Jr, Fisher RD, Conkle DM, Martin CE, Graham TP. Selective Operative Treatment for Tetralogy of Fallot: Rationale and Results. *Ann Surg.* 1976; 183:685–690.

Bender HW Jr, Fisher RD, Walker WE, Graham TP. Reparative Cardiac Surgery in Infants and Small Children: Five Years Experience with Profound Hypothermia and Circulatory Arrest. *Ann Surg.* 1979; 190:437–443.

Bender HW Jr, Graham TP, Boucek RJ, Walker WE, Boerth, RJ. Comparative Operative Results of the Senning and Mustard Procedures for Transposition of the Great Arteries. *Circulation.* 1980; 62:I197–I203.

Bender HW Jr, Hammon JW Jr, Hubbard SG, Muirhead J, Graham TP Jr. Repair of Atrioventricular Canal Malformation in the First Year of Life. *J Thorac Cardiovasc Surg.* 1982; 84:515–522.

Bender HW Jr, Stewart JR, Merrill WH, Hammon JW Jr, Graham TP Jr. Ten Years Experience with the Senning Operation for Transposition of the Great Arteries: Physiological Results and Late Follow-up. *Ann Thorac Surg.* 1989; 47:218–223.

Bender HW Jr. Preparation, Trust, and Responsibility. *Ann Thorac Surg.* 1991; 51:351–356.

Bender HW Jr. Omnibus per Artem Fedemque Prodesse: To Serve All with Skill and Fidelity. Presidential Address. *Bull Am Coll Surg.* 2000; 85:8–13.

Denton A. Cooley, MD

(b. 1920)

If young people want to go into a profession that will give them the most reward, spiritual reward I will say, not necessarily financial reward, they should go into medicine.

— On the future of medicine

Interviewed May 4, 1997

I am a native Texan, born in Houston in 1920. My grandparents moved to Houston in 1885 when my father was three years old. My father graduated from the Texas Dental College in Houston when he was nineteen years old and practiced dentistry in Houston for forty-five to fifty years, becoming very prominent. He and my mother had two children: my brother, who is sixteen months older, and me. My brother and I were close friends our whole lives until he passed away. I went to public schools in Houston and then went to college at the University of Texas in Austin. I played basketball in high school and in college, and I continued to play basketball and tennis until I was about forty, when I switched to golf. I still play golf with a wonderful group of other senior cardiac surgeons. There are twelve of us, and all are chairmen of a department of cardiothoracic surgery somewhere in the country. We meet once a year and spend about three or four days with a little scientific program, and then we play golf. It's a wonderful opportunity for us to get together informally.

My father had wanted me to follow in his footsteps and become a dentist in order to eventually take over his practice. I went off to college planning to be a predental student, but dentistry really did not interest me much. I had always most admired the physicians and surgeons in our city. I felt as if my father also wished he had gone on to study medicine rather than getting sidetracked into dentistry. At first I didn't know if I could compete with the better students at a big school like the University of Texas. I soon found out that I could not only compete with them, I could excel. I thought, "Why not go on and do medicine? It is much more intriguing and challenging than dentistry." I switched to medicine.

The first medical school I attended was the University of Texas Medical Branch in Galveston in 1941, and I was there for two years. There were some political problems and the faculty was in a bit of turmoil, so I applied elsewhere for my junior and senior years. I applied to Johns Hopkins, Harvard, Washington University, Duke, and Pennsylvania. I was accepted at all of these schools except Harvard. In the end I was encouraged by friends to go to Johns Hopkins, and I transferred. It was an accelerated, year-round program with no summer vacations.

I knew that a surgical internship would challenge me the most, but I was not sure whether I wanted to do my internship at Johns Hopkins or some other institution. Dr. Blalock encouraged me to do my internship at Hopkins on his service. This turned out to be a very fortunate decision for me, because I had the opportunity to be associated there with a new era in surgery. I was the intern that assisted Dr. Blalock in the first Blue Baby operation in November 1944.

The patient's name was Eileen Saxon. Anesthesia was different in those days, and the nurse-anesthetist, Ms. Olive Berger, used cyclopropane, which is not used any more for a number of reasons. We didn't have an electric cautery. We couldn't use it in the presence of cyclopropane. Also, we didn't know whether the blood would clot in a cyanotic child with polycythemia. There were a lot of other things we didn't know. I remember Dr. Helen Taussig stood at the head of the table behind Ms. Berger, the nurse-anesthetist, and Vivien Thomas, the man who worked in the lab, was also there. Dr. Blalock had brought Vivien Thomas from Vanderbilt to work at Johns Hopkins. Vivien stood behind Dr. Blalock at the table, and Dr. Blalock would ask Vivien questions over his shoulder. He would say, "Vivien, should I do it this way or that way?" Vivien would know the answers as he was used to having those kinds of questions put to him. That was Dr. Blalock's way of getting everybody involved in the whole process. He didn't want to have the whole responsibility for himself or be worrying about who would get all of the blame if something went wrong. Many of us thought this operation was going to be a big disaster, but it turned out to be a success.

Dr. Blalock had arrived at Hopkins a couple of years before I was accepted as a student. Hopkins had wanted to hire somebody more prestigious, like Dr. Evarts Graham from Washington University. Dr. Graham told them that he was not prepared to leave his job, but he recommended a young man from Vanderbilt who was doing some unusual work; that was Dr. Blalock. Dr. Blalock's reputation at that time was based on his research and publications on problems such as hemorrhagic shock and pulmonary hypertension. He was very interested in myasthenia gravis and thymectomy for myasthenia gravis.

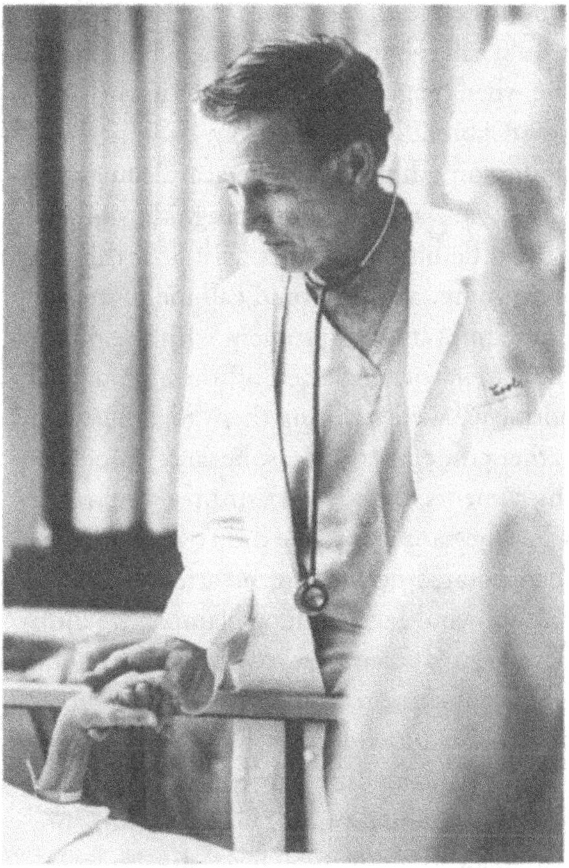

Denton A. Cooley

Dr. Blalock was an unusual person to assist in the operating room. To be honest, he was a whiner. If things weren't going just right, he would say to me, "Denton, why don't you help me?" He could be rather difficult at the operating table. I think he was insecure as a technical surgeon, and he wasn't really adept and sure of himself all the time. He was a determined type of surgeon, but he wasn't gifted technically.

He did begin to trust me, and he also trusted Bill Longmire, who was about four years ahead of me in his training. I think it may have caused a little disgruntlement among my contemporaries that Dr. Blalock would call me to help him. He would call on me when he got into difficulties in surgery when a blood vessel got away, or if he was doing something like a portacaval shunt and there was a lot of bleeding. He would get a little bit out of sorts with how things were going, and he would call me to help. Sometimes it was a problem with the pulmonary artery or the vessels off the arch of the aorta. We were suturing them together with rather crude instruments, because vascular instruments and vascular sutures weren't what they are today. We didn't always have incorporated needles on the arterial sutures, and we would use bulldog clamps. We didn't have vascular clamps; everything was bulldog clamps or some sort of a tie on a vessel to control the blood loss.

Anyway, the Blue Baby operation turned out to be a sensation. It set off an influx of patients with congenital heart disease to Johns Hopkins. Within six weeks we became almost overwhelmed with congenital heart cases of all sorts, not just tetralogy of Fallot operations, but also patent ductus and coarctations. Transposition of the great vessels was our nemesis in those days.

It was very exciting. Our diagnostic techniques were very limited. We really had not started cardiac catheterization, and angiography was just in its infancy. I can remember Dr. Taussig going mostly on physical findings. She just held the X-ray up to the light, looking at what she called the pulmonary window, and if the window looked a little bit open, that meant there was not enough blood going into the pulmonary arteries. That was the only diagnostic test we had other than fluoroscopy.

As a result, when we were doing these operations, we were sometimes surprised to find things we didn't expect. Patients might actually have something like an Eisenmenger with really high pulmonary pressure. A lot of confirmation took place in surgery because Dr. Taussig's fluoroscope didn't quite delineate well enough for us, and we would find something like a big hard pulmonary artery. We would think we were going to put an anastomosis into it, but it wasn't always so.

Dr. Taussig could be difficult, and Dr. Blalock had some friction with her. Yet he always acknowledged her contributions with great generosity, because he was the most humble person in the world. He acknowledged openly that it was Taussig who inspired him to try the Blue Baby operation on a patient, but the friction was there too. In fact, it was due to this friction that I got my step up in the service.

I was just eight months out of medical school. Dr. Blalock called me into his office and said, "Denton, you have the reputation around the hospital of being able to get along with women." This took me aback a bit because at the time I was a bachelor, and I thought, "Uh oh, Dr. Blalock has found out about something I didn't want him to know." But he said, "You know Denton, Dr. Taussig, Mary Allen Engle, Peggy Hanlon, and Ruth Whitemore come around here and worry me so much that—Denton, do you think you could get all of these women out of my hair?" I said, "Well, I'll try, sir." And that's how I got my job with him. I replaced Bill Longmire as his first assistant. Some of the other doctors would get into a confrontation with Dr. Taussig and these other women, and I was sort of the go-along guy. All of those women are now prominent cardiologists.

Another interesting character was Vivien

Thomas. He was a great technician, an ingenious fellow. As I said, we had very limited instrumentation; we didn't have the standard vascular clamps that we use now. In order to control a blood vessel, we would put a snare on it or one of the bulldog clamps, but they would often slip off. Vivien developed new techniques that made these things easier. He operated alone in the animal lab and developed the procedures there himself. Dr. Blalock didn't actually do much surgery in the animal lab. There is no question in my mind that Vivien is the one who invented the atrial septectomy operation, the Blalock-Hanlon procedure. Vivien has written an autobiography, and I contributed to it. His recognition came late, but it was good that he got it. At the end of his life, Dr. Blalock was instrumental in promoting the recognition that Vivien finally got. Vivien only had a high school education, you see, but he was bright enough to have gone to college and medical school if he had had the opportunity. That had been his ambition.

One of my colleagues at that time was another young doctor named Hank Bahnson. Hank went with Dr. Blalock to England where they operated on a blue baby at Guy's Hospital. Dr. Blalock actually invited me first, because I was in the military in Europe at that time. I had just won the tennis championship in Austria, and I wanted to go to Germany to play in the tennis tournament finals there. At the time I thought the tennis tournament was a lot more important than going to England with Dr. Blalock to do a couple of blue babies. He took Hank and Louise Bahnson instead. That is one of the mistakes in my life that I have always regretted, not going with him on that tour. It was very dramatic. Dr. Blalock created a sensation with the European surgeons. Dr. Blalock and Hank presented the details of the Blalock-Taussig operation in the auditorium of the Royal College of Surgeons. The end of the room was all darkened and they shone a spotlight down on a Guy's Hospital nursing sister in her starched blue uniform holding this nice, postop, pink baby in her lap, and everybody just burst into applause. They were so moved by the whole experience; it couldn't have been more dramatic.

Dr. Blalock was a good speaker. He spoke slowly and carefully, with perfect grammar. He wasn't one of those rapid articulate kinds of speakers. I am sure the English were impressed with that Southern talk. In general he was a very popular man, and people just liked him. He was the kind of person who could walk into a room full of people and they would all want to go over and say, "Hello, Al."

In time he became the most powerful surgeon in the United States. He could get people appointed to positions that they wanted, partly because of his honesty and friendship, but also because he was the chief of surgery at Johns Hopkins Hospital, which at that time was one of the most prestigious institutions in this country and abroad. It was the Blue Baby operation that contributed to the reemergence of Hopkins from its previous period of decline. The Blue Baby operation caused a real transfusion of energy; it got Hopkins back into the flow of things, and Hopkins enjoyed a wonderful golden era as a result. The hospital attracted residents who wanted to be part of that, and it attracted visitors from all over the world. It established what I like to call a school of surgery, the Blalock School of Surgery. Since then, there have been successors to that legacy, but all of us who were privileged to train there during that golden era feel a certain comradeship and a lot of pride in having been part of that effort.

I met my wife Louise there. She was a nurse at the Johns Hopkins Hospital, on the service at the Halsted Clinic. I met her when I was in my fourth year of residency, and we got married right before I started my senior residency. We had some happy years there while I was a resident and she was still working as a nurse.

This was after I had been in the military. I went on active duty in January 1945 and immediately was sent to Austria where I had the job as chief of surgery in a 750-bed hospital. I didn't know whether I could handle it. Most of our cases were trauma cases due to misbehavior on the part of soldiers. The war ended in November 1945, so Europe was all torn up from the war damage. The GIs who were still over there were really having a big time misbehaving, and turning over trucks, and having all sorts of accidents and injuries.

I came back to Hopkins in February of 1948 and stayed until 1950. That was when I met Russell Brock. Russell Brock was our visiting professor that year. He had been doing some intracardiac repairs of tetralogy of Fallot, all closed surgery, including valvotomies and valvectomies using some special punches to open the pulmonary valve. He was not yet Sir Russell. He later became Sir Russell and then Lord Brock. Anyway, I was fascinated with him and assisted him in the OR at Hopkins. I asked him if I could visit him for a year in London as a senior registrar, and he said yes. So I went to England and spent a year at the Brompton Hospital with Brock.

We did mostly mitral valvotomoties. He had a sort of knife that he would put on his finger. It was a disaster mostly, but he did a few tetralogies also. He did a lot of tuberculosis surgery, cancer surgery, and pulmonary surgery. I had a chance to meet some very prominent surgeons at the Brompton, like Clement Price Thomas and Norman Barrett, the Barrett esophagus man. Norman Barrett could say some of the funniest things, and I still quote him now and then. One day I walked into the operating theater, as they call it there, and I was looking over his shoulder. He turned to look at me, and I said, "What are you doing, Mr. Barrett?" He says, "Cooley, what I'm doing here should be awfully simple but I'm making it simply awful!" He had a chest full of blood; he had torn the atrium trying to do a commissurotomy with his finger. I have used that quotation several times since.

After my year at the Brompton, I didn't go back to Hopkins. Instead I went to Houston with Michael DeBakey at the Baylor University College of Medicine. He gave me a job there as an instructor, the lowest job there. That was in 1951. We did a variety of cases in general surgery, thoracic surgery, vascular surgery, everything. My special interest was in aneurysms, because I had operated successfully on a couple of big aortic aneurysms while I was at Johns Hopkins. When I came to Houston, sure enough, I had the opportunity to operate on some more. They were mostly syphilitic thoracic aneurysms, which we don't see much any more.

We didn't have any vascular substitutes back then. We repaired the aneurysms. Most of them were sacular aneurysms of the arch or descending aorta. You could put a big clamp on the base and take them out. That was what we called direct surgery, as opposed to indirect surgery, where we would thread a wire in and out of the aneurysm to try to enhance thrombosis, or else we would wrap them with cellophane. We tried all sorts of things.

In 1953 we started using fabric grafts. We had been using freeze-dried, lyophilized homografts, but they didn't last very long. I used to joke and say that they were probably a little worse than the aorta that we were removing. The graft looked bad, but we did use them. At least we showed that the graft could withstand pulsatile circulation, but it wasn't the happiest solution.

John Gibbon's first use of the heart-lung machine also occurred in 1953, but only one of his four patients survived. That didn't seem so outstanding. To my mind the real breakthrough was Lillehei's work with cross-circulation. I visited him and Dr. Kirklin at the same time in Minnesota, at the end of 1955. My pediatric cardiologist, Dan McNamara, went with me, to see what they were doing with congenital heart lesions. We visited Walt Lillehei and watched an operation with cross-circulation, the mother on one side and the baby on the other. It was a complex sort of thing, where they used two pumps in between, one for the venous blood and another for the arterial blood. Sometimes they used the father, but more often the mother had a compatible blood type with the infant.

Tetralogy of Fallot is considered to be reasonably complex, and Lillehei's results were not spectacular. Walt Lillehei took us on rounds, and he showed us some of the results that they had. Some of the children were in bad heart failure, and others had complete heart block. We didn't know that much about the conduction mechanism in those days. Dan McNamara was not thrilled about Dr. Lillehei's results. We went on to Rochester, Minnesota, and visited John Kirklin. John had a big team of people and a big Mayo-Gibbon apparatus about the size of a table. He had cardiologists and physiologists and bioengineers in the operating room, a very complicated setup. John operated very deliberately, closed a VSD, and did it beautifully, of course. On the way back to Houston, Dr. McNamara, who I thought was going to be my source of some cases said, "I'm not going to let you operate on any of my patients until you can duplicate John Kirklin's program at Mayo Clinic." Well, there was no way to duplicate that. We had been struggling with our own efforts at cardiopulmonary bypass. Not too long after that trip, I developed a bubble oxygenator similar to the one used by Lillehei and designed by Richard DeWall. That was the easiest to copy, so within a few months after I got back to Houston, I had my own bubble oxygenator, and we took off.

The first bubble oxygenator we had was just a tube, a vertical column with a big tube of Tygon, with a cork with needle holes to bubble oxygen into the blood. At that time I developed an impression, which has lasted through almost my whole career, that the important thing in cardiopulmonary bypass was to get the patient the hell off the pump as soon as possible. If you wanted to have a living patient, perfusion periods of fifteen to twenty minutes were ideal. Within six months I had done ninety-five open-heart operations. This was more than they had done in Minnesota.

At first the oxygenator was primed with blood. That was the system used in Minnesota and everywhere. Our first case was a postinfarction ventricular septal defect. It happened to be an inferior infarct rather than anterior, and we closed it in a little over twenty-five minutes. The fellow lived for about six weeks, and then he reinfarcted and died. Meanwhile, I had told everybody around town that the open-heart era was here. I got some atrial septal defect cases and ventricular defects to do and some simple things like that, plus a couple of tetralogies, and by the time that first patient died our open-heart program was on the move.

We also soon did the first acute mitral papillary muscle rupture using the same equipment. Then a commercial disposable oxygenator became available, made by the Travenol Company. Vince Gott, who was one of Lillehei's young trainees, designed it. It was like a pillowcase with some avenues in it for oxygenation and defoaming and that sort of thing. We began to use that because it was much easier to assemble, and it worked really well. We made some modifications in the defoaming chamber and put in some steel wool. That was an advance, and from then on the whole industry of creating oxygenators just mushroomed into an enormous project.

Most of our early patients had congenital defects. Our perfusion system was not designed to flow four or five liters a minute; we could flow a liter and a half to two liters. We were worried about getting into high-flow situations with adults. Also, we still had a time limit, about forty-five minutes, in order to have some coagulation left. With a longer pump run than that, the main problem was bleeding and coagulopathy. We had no good means of retrieving blood from the operating field. Hemodilution solved a lot of those problems; it was a real advance in the early 1960s. Nazih Zuhdi had been working with this idea of hemodilution, and Gadboys and Litwak had done laboratory work with it, but I really think that I popularized it, although I didn't invent it. We showed that you could get superior results with hemodilution. One of our earliest papers was on the use of hemodilution, 5 percent dextrose priming, a disposable oxygenator, and keeping the patient normothermic. That was our simplified system. There is now a return of interest in warm-blood surgery. What goes around comes around.

In a short period of time, we were doing several hundred or more operations a year. Once we started using hemodilution, we were not as dependent on the blood bank to supply us, so in 1965 we did one thousand cases in one year, which was unheard of before that time. In 1985 we did five thousand open-heart procedures in my hospital.

The Blue Baby operation had been a sensation when it happened at Hopkins in the forties. In the early sixties, cardiac surgery in Houston was the big event. The next big event was heart transplantation. Many surgeons were poised to do cardiac transplantation, including me, Norman Shumway, and, of course, Christiaan Barnard. At the time we thought the heart was replaceable. We could replace all of its components, such as the valves, and kidney and liver transplants were being done. Also by that time we had Imuran and steroids for treating rejection.

Chris Barnard was the first to recognize that you could harvest an organ after brain death. When I first heard this news, I wondered how in the world he got that beating heart out of a living person. Chris Barnard really showed that there was a window of opportunity after a person's brain had been destroyed. The heart would still be beating, and that was the ideal time to use a donor heart. The mechanics of sewing one in, well, anybody could do that, but to identify the brain-dead donor and not be sent to jail for doing it was his contribution.

That required changing the laws to redefine death. The Vatican law stated that death occurs when the heart stops beating, and that as long as the heart is beating the individual is alive. So legally, and according to Vatican law, death coincided with the stoppage of the heart, but the brain-death laws that came along later accepted the fact that when brain function is hopelessly destroyed, death could be established and organs were then available for transplantation.

The Texas legislature had not yet changed the definition of death when we started doing heart transplants. We got some sort of agreement from our hospital board that we could follow Barnard's precedent. Shumway, too, did one at Palo Alto, and because of that we had tentative, although not complete, approval from our hospital board. We went ahead and did five or six transplants before they could tell us that we couldn't do it again.

One result of this legal confusion was that a very smart lawyer in Houston, Percy Foreman, took advantage of the situation to get his client cleared of murder charges. His client had shot another man in the head, and because the victim had brain death, I had used him as a heart transplant donor. The lawyer claimed that the actual death occurred when the heart was removed, so that his client was not the agent of the victim's death, but rather the surgeon was. I was quite disturbed about this. I thought it was wrong and that the ruling implied that I was the murderer, but the lawyer came up to me afterwards and patted me on the back and said, "Don't worry, doctor, I'll punish him myself." I later found out that he meant that he would punish him by his fees, which included his home, his possessions, his car, and everything.

That was a very stimulating and exciting time. We did twelve heart transplants and had about nine living recipients while everybody else was trying to do one. We thought we were doing great. But then the attrition began because of our inability to combat rejection and infection. Within eighteen months, all of the patients had died. Imuran and steroids weren't really satisfactory. We stopped doing transplants almost altogether. We did do one patient where we used a totally artificial heart as a bridge to transplant. This was a historic thing, but rejection was still our nemesis.

In the early 1980s cyclosporine was discovered. Our local nephrology group under Dr. Barry Kahan had access to cyclosporine, and he came and talked to us and said, "Look, we have a really good new drug. Why don't we reopen the cardiac transplant program?" Therefore we were one of the first programs to get cyclosporine, and we began using it. I had actually turned the transplant program over to Bud Frazier by this time. He has been extremely active in the heart transplant business. In our institution we have now done over six hundred heart transplants. We also did a few heart-lung transplants, but we have not been as active in lung transplantations. I think our pulmonologists have been a little reluctant to go ahead, because we were not satisfied with the long-term results of heart-lung transplants. One of the weaknesses of our transplant program is that we haven't been as active in lung transplantation as some of the other centers.

Before we got into heart transplants, we were successful with the use of several types of artificial valves. The Starr caged-ball valve was the first valve that we used. I had created a few valves of my own design. They were rather crude things with flaps that we would put on top of a calcified aortic valve and that sort of thing. Hank Bahnson and Harry Muller were doing similar things with fabric leaflets. It wasn't until we had the Starr-Edwards valve that I had any real confidence in valve replacement. We tried a lot of different kinds of new valves, and I made some modifications in them. I never wanted to get to the point where I would use just one device. I wanted to try them all and give them a chance, because we had a great clinical resource, a proving ground for these devices. If they showed moderate success in the pulse duplicator, we would try them in a patient. For example, the Surgitool aortic valve was surprisingly successful. I made a few modifications in it, but the mechanism of securing it with claws was really quite ingenious; it was quick. You could do an aortic valve replacement in ten to fifteen minutes on the pump.

In Houston there were several surgeons who developed valves. Arthur Beall had some disc valves, and Dr. DeBakey, working with Surgitool, got his name on several of them. I had two or three different designs with my name on them, but they wouldn't really compare with what we have today. I haven't used a Starr valve in thirty years. The bileaflet valve has certainly changed things, and we are beginning to work on a trileaflet valve that shows a lot of promise. We also use tissue valves in about 20 percent of our implantations.

In addition to valve replacement, we were active quite early in doing coronary artery bypass procedures with saphenous veins. Others, such as David Sabiston, were doing some isolated bypasses, but Favaloro was really the evangelist for coronary artery bypass with saphenous veins in 1968. I was a little bit skeptical about how the heart would respond to some of these manipulations, but looking back on it, I wonder why we didn't think of it sooner.

Still, the Texas Heart Institute has done more open-heart operations than anybody in the world, ninety-three thousand patients using cardiopulmonary bypass. I did perhaps half of those as the principal surgeon, but now I have a team of younger surgeons and they are very busy. Our volume has gone down considerably as competition has increased, but we are still doing twenty-five hundred pump cases a year, maybe more than that. Looking back on that series of cases, I can see that many of them were so much simpler than what we have today, such as a single or double bypass where the patient had never been operated on before. Right now 25 percent of the patients that we are doing have some complicating feature. Often they are reoperations. Those operations take a lot longer.

Cardioplegia is often credited with making a big improvement in our results, enabling us to do complicated cases, and it has made a big difference. I am not inclined to believe it is the sole reason. There is antegrade and retrograde perfusion of the coronary circulation, some people use warm-heart surgery and some hypothermia. It is hard to know what role cardioplegia plays in the improved results with difficult cases. I think it is important to put the heart at rest if you can when you are doing some of these intricate operations. While a lot of other surgeons here are using blood cardioplegia or retrograde cooling, my preferred technique is antegrade crystalloid cardioplegia with potassium chloride as the principal element. I like to get the operation done quickly.

One of my innovations was the idea of a packaged price that a hospital could offer for cardiac surgical procedures. I came up with this idea ten to fifteen years ago, way before everybody else. I got the feeling then that there was too much variation in surgical and hospital fees. I could foresee a day when there was going to be a rebellion against the increasing hospital costs, physician costs, and health care costs. I talked to the health department at one of our local corporations, the Tenneco Corporation. They were complaining that when they send a patient out to smaller hospitals they are getting charged for everything you can imagine, all of these various consultations and treatments that we were not charging for at the Texas Heart Institute. I said, "Why don't you let me work out a package deal for you? I will be responsible for all of those fees, be sure that they are appropriate and at the right level, and that the services that they claim were provided were actually given to the patient. I will be responsible, and we will call it a package deal." The health department at Tenneco felt that that was a fair deal, and we called it Cardiovascular Care. It became popular with many of our corporations there in Houston, and HCFA has adopted it as a demonstration project for cost containment. It gave some uniformity to the chaos that existed when everything was fee for service. Today, I think HCFA is very pleased with it. They keep renewing the contract with us, and it looks as if they are going to extend it to other specialties, like orthopedics, for joint replacements.

We also had some contracts with foreign countries, where we offered to deliver cardiac care at a better rate than they could get at home. One such contract was with the Netherlands. We called it the Dutch airlift. We could bring these patients from Holland over to Houston to the Texas Heart Institute and get them back home within two weeks. They found that it was 20 percent cheaper than having the same procedure done in Holland. We also had no waiting list. It was very convenient for health services there in Holland. We would sometimes get about fifteen patients at a time with their spouses. We would put them in a local hotel near the medical center. Some of them came already worked up, but some of them just had chest pain. Some had valve problems. It was very successful for us. We had translators that could speak all the languages. We did about fifteen hundred patients from Holland on that plan. Finally, the Dutch government and the surgical profession in Holland decided that it wasn't right and that they should take care of their own population.

As for the future of cardiac surgery, I think that minimally invasive procedures are here to stay. Something good will come out of this trend. Maybe some aspects of it will be discarded, but there is no question that we can operate with success on some patients with a lot less invasiveness. We have gotten so comfortable now in wanting to do all of our coronary bypasses in a nice quiet operating field, overlooking the fact that the patient has to go through some trauma so that we can do our operation in a quiet operating field. We need to improve our skills so that we can do some of these operations with the heart beating. There is no question that cardiopulmonary bypass produces some complications that can be avoided by using the off- pump technique.

I hope that someday young residents who are interested in cardiac surgery will read this and consider it as a profession. It has always been the most challenging area of surgical specialty, and I think it always will be. There is nothing quite as exciting or thrilling as operating on an organ like the heart. We can operate on the liver or the lung, but that beating heart is an area of real fascination, and we have not found all the answers yet. There are going to be plenty of areas of new research in the future, and heart surgery is going to be around forever. We have shown that the heart can be manipulated, and most of the elements in the heart can be replaced. They are never going to find anything to prevent advanced heart disease. We may increase the patient's longevity, and patients may have longer and healthier lives, but they are going to have to die of something. Heart disease is always going to be the major cause of death. Young doctors still have an opportunity to extend the average length of life by going into heart surgery. I don't like to hear words of discouragement to young people, words that discourage them from shooting for the highest goal. I think cardiac surgery may interest them the most.

I hear some parents saying that they wouldn't want their child to go into medicine today because of all the intrusions and disrespect that doctors are suffering. This is bad advice. Medicine has always been the noblest profession, and it always will be. This goes back beyond our own century, to many centuries in the past. A physician, no matter how capable or incapable he was, was always a highly respected member of society. I think this is going to be true in the next millennium. If young people want to go into a profession that will give them the most reward, spiritual reward I will say, not necessarily financial reward, they should go into medicine. It may not be as financially rewarding in the future as it has been for the last two or three decades, but they will get their rewards in terms of enjoyment and satisfaction, with nothing to compare to it. I would not in the least discourage anyone in my family or anyone else's family who has the interest and capability from going into medicine.

Bibliography

Cooley DA. Cardiac Resuscitation during Operations for Pulmonic Stenosis. *Ann Surg.* 1950; 132:930–936.

Cooley DA, DeBakey ME. Surgical Considerations of Intrathoracic Aneurysms of the Aorta and Great Vessels. *Ann Surg.* 1952; 135:660–680.

Cooley DA, DeBakey ME. Ruptured Aneurysms of Abdominal Aorta: Excision and Homograft Replacement. *Postgrad Med.* 1954; 16:334–342.

Cooley DA, Al-Naaman YD, Carton CA. Surgical Treatment of Arteriosclerotic Occlusion of Common Carotid Artery. *J Neurosurg.* 1956; 13:500–506.

Cooley DA, DeBakey ME. Resection of Entire Ascending Aorta for Fusiform Aneurysm using Temporary Cardiac Bypass. *JAMA.* 1956; 162:1158–1159.

Cooley DA, Hallman GL. *Surgical Treatment of Congenital Heart Disease.* Philadelphia: Lea and Febiger; 1966

Cooley DA, Bloodwell RL, Hallman GL, Nora JJ. Transplantation of the Human Heart. A Report of Four Cases. *JAMA.* 1968; 205:479–486.

Cooley DA, Liotta D, Hallman GL, Bloodwell RD, Leachman RD, Milam JD. Orthotopic Cardiac Prosthesis for Two-Staged Cardiac Replacement. *Am J Cardiol.* 1969; 24:723–730.

Cooley DA. Ventricular Endoaneurysmorrhaphy: Results of an Improved Method of Repair for Extensive Postinfarction Aneurysm. *Tex Heart Inst J.* 1989; 16:72–75.

Cooley DA, Baldwin RT. Technique of Open Distal Anastomosis for Repair of Descending Thoracic Aortic Aneurysms. *Ann Thorac Surg.* 1992; 54:932–936.

J. Alex Haller Jr., MD

(b. 1927)

> *She felt as so many pediatricians do, that the patients were members of her family. Therefore she was not going to let them be operated on . . . unless she was there.*
> — On the relationship of Helen Taussig and Alfred Blalock

Interviewed October 21, 2000

I was born in Pulaski, Virginia, in 1927 and have a younger brother who became a dentist. I come from a family of dentists. My father, aunt, uncle, and both grandfathers were dentists, or as they call them in the hills of Virginia, "tooth dentists." I guess that makes me a black sheep, since I am the only one who went into medicine.

I always wanted to be a physician. I thought I wanted to be a brain surgeon until I got to medical school and took neuroanatomy. I realized how complicated it was and said, "This is not for me. I've got to find something that I understand." I wanted to be a surgeon, and I ultimately ended up being a children's surgeon.

When I graduated from high school, we were allowed to apply to a number of different colleges. We applied without visiting, as there was not an opportunity to do much traveling because of the gasoline rationing during the war. I applied to the University of Virginia, a couple of small schools in North Carolina, one of which turned out to be a girl's school, and Vanderbilt, because I had heard that it was a good school. I really didn't know too much about it. The reason I came to Vanderbilt was because they offered me a full academic scholarship: a Founder's scholarship. My Dad said, "Son, that's the place to go." I was probably heading for the University of Virginia because in Virginia it is called "The University," but they didn't offer enough scholarship money, so I came to Vanderbilt, sight unseen, along with a high school classmate. I ended up loving the campus, and I met my wife there as an undergraduate.

We came to Nashville by car. My dad had swapped some tires, which were also scarce, and received some extra gasoline coupons. We were able to come in the car with my classmate and his father. This was in the fall of 1944. I had played basketball in high school, so I went out for basketball at Vanderbilt. Because many were in the service, there were few men on campus, so I made the varsity team as a freshman and played for two years. I didn't play my senior year because the organic chemistry and biology laboratories took so much time in the afternoons, and I think I might have flunked if I had taken both laboratories and varsity basketball. We had a fair team. We didn't travel very much because of the wartime restrictions on travel. Vanderbilt, of course, was in the Southeastern Conference, but we only went to regional schools. We went to Southwestern in Memphis, and we played several colleges in the Nashville area. We went to Cookeville, Tennessee, to play the Tennessee Tech team and played in Lexington, Kentucky, and got "murdered" by the University of Kentucky. It was a good experience though. I think we probably ended up losing more than we won, but it was still a great two years.

I was accepted at Vanderbilt medical school along with my wife-to-be, Emily Simms, and several other class members at Vanderbilt. The war was over by that time, and I was no longer in jeopardy of being drafted. My draft board said to do whatever I wanted, so I decided after talking with several of the professors at both medical school and undergraduate school to stay on and get my baccalaureate degree. This would give me a chance to take some of the humanities, which I hadn't had a chance to do before because we were in lockstep as premeds. Therefore, I stayed an extra year and got that BA degree while my wife-to-be went on into Vanderbilt medical school as a senior, in absentia. During that year, several of the faculty in the medical school suggested that maybe I would like to leave and go to Johns Hopkins. I didn't even know there was a Johns Hopkins until they told me about it, but I applied, and went to Birmingham for a "regional" interview. The interviewer was an obstetrician, and he must have recommended that I be accepted, so I went to Johns Hopkins medical school without ever seeing it and without ever even being in Baltimore. The process was much simpler then. People didn't travel as much and you couldn't afford to go, certainly not to fly. I went back and forth to my home in Pulaski on holidays by train. We went from Nashville to Chattanooga, changed in Chattanooga and then went on the Norfolk and Western Railroad right up to Pulaski.

I graduated in 1951, and did my straight surgical internship at Johns Hopkins, where life was pretty restricted. The term "resident" comes from the fact that you were living in the hospital as a resident. "Intern" means that you are gaining supervised practical experience. All of us lived in the hospital or in the immediate environs. The surgical internship was called the "Halsted Internship" because of the first chief of surgery at Hopkins, William Stewart Halsted. The internship was strenuous because we had no time off and were on duty every night. The only way we got out of the hospital was to sign out to a fellow intern. Even at that, we would only sign out for a few hours to go to the movies or just escape the hospital environment. We were really expected to be in-house the whole time.

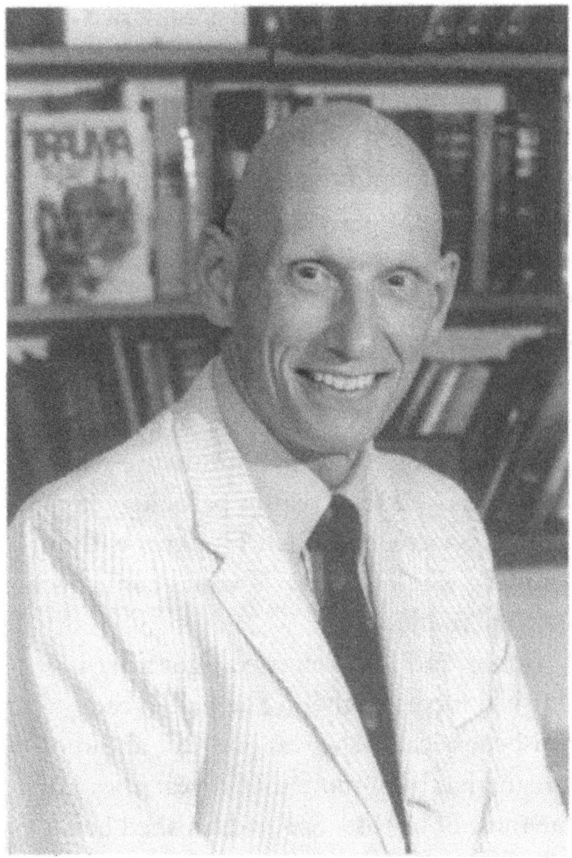
J. Alex Haller

There were ten interns in my group, and,

as was traditional at Hopkins, only two of them would be kept to go through the Halsted residency and finish their final year of training with Dr. Blalock. There was internal competition, but honestly we did not feel it. We were working hard, and we were all good friends. As Dr. Blalock said on a number of occasions, he felt that some of the people he didn't keep in the program did better than the ones he kept. I knew which category I was in. Because I wanted to spend a year in pathology, before the end of my internship I had arranged for a year in pathology in Zurich, Switzerland. I left Hopkins without knowing whether or not I would come back into the residency.

Emily and I had married right after I finished medical school. She had already finished, because she was one year ahead of me and has been more than a year ahead of me most of my life. She had finished her internship at Vanderbilt in obstetrics and gynecology, and she joined the Hopkins ob-gyn house staff. We were on the house staff together. It was very unusual to have married house staff, as it was frowned upon. As Osler said, "Medicine is a very jealous mistress." We lived right there, but they had to make some new living arrangements for us. There were men's areas and women's areas, but they didn't have a place for married couples. They chose one of the single rooms on the top floor of the administration building, which had a big statue of Christ. We were on the fourth floor, so our address was Johns Hopkins, above Christ. That was the first year of our married life, living in that single room on the fourth floor.

This was long before they had the area for married couples called the compound. If a couple lived outside the hospital, they lived in hospital apartments or houses that the hospital owned, primarily row houses with a hospital telephone extension in them. It was like being a part of the hospital, only outside it geographically.

The first Blue Baby operation was done in 1944 at Johns Hopkins and that was, of course, when I was just finishing high school, so by the time I got there in 1947, they had done a number of the Blalock-Taussig shunts. One of the interesting features is that when Dr. Blalock was a resident he had not been kept on in the training program, because he didn't show "promise" in surgery. He had finished medical school at Hopkins and stayed one year as an intern. He left and went to Vanderbilt to finish his training with Dr. Barney Brooks, subsequently stayed at Vanderbilt on the faculty, made numerous important contributions at Vanderbilt working closely with his medical school classmate, Tinsley Harrison. He was very interested in basketball and had been quite an athlete himself, having played baseball in college. When I got to Hopkins, I was lost. Here I was, just a country boy, and didn't even know what this big city was. I was walking down the hall of the hospital just a couple of weeks after my arrival, and Dr. Blalock came down with a number of residents. He stopped and said, "Haller, you are here. How's your basketball going?" I was totally overwhelmed by the fact that he would even know that I had played basketball at Vanderbilt. He had kept up with the Vanderbilt basketball team after he moved back to Hopkins.

There were a number of other people on the house staff whose names became prominent in cardiac surgery. The two chief residents were Denton Cooley and Dick Kieffer. An outstanding general surgeon,

Jack Handelsman, and Hank Bahnson were in lockstep together. Jim Cantrell and David Sabiston were at the next level. There were two residents for each year you went through. Rainey Williams and Bill Reinhoff Jr. were residents immediately in front of me. I came in with Jack Zimmerman, who subsequently became the chief of surgery at Church-Home Hospital in Baltimore. There was really a relatively small house staff considering the size of the surgical service.

About that time the pump-oxygenator was just starting to be used. The first children for open-heart surgery were done in Minnesota by Lillehei and his group. It was done by cross-circulation by hooking up the mother to the child. It could have been the father, but most of the time the mother was connected to the child as the heart-lung support. This was not only courageous, but was also dangerous. Now it would never get by institutional research committees as an acceptable procedure, but that is the way the first procedures were done.

I don't think cross-circulation was ever used anywhere else in the world, at least as far as I know. It may have been tried in other countries, but I just don't know about it. I know it wasn't done anywhere in the United States. I was with Glenn Morrow at the NIH when Walt Lillehei made his first report at the American Heart Association meeting in Baltimore. Lillehei asked for the floor and said that he had some remarkable movies to show. Dr. Blalock was presiding at this particular session, and he said, "Well, you're not on the program, but we will give you five minutes." Lillehei got up and showed the first uncut movie of that open-heart procedure, and there were all kinds of technical problems with the movie. Lillehei went on and on because he was so excited about it, but after about ten minutes, Dr. Blalock said, "Walt, I have to ask you to stop. You only had five minutes as you weren't on the program." Lillehei said, "Dr. Blalock, this is too important. I have to continue," so he went right on. It was about a twenty-minute movie, and it was exciting. At that time we weren't doing any open-heart operations at Hopkins. They were all still closed procedures, and the same was true at the NIH with Dr. Morrow in the Heart Institute. Everyone was beginning to use some of the artificial lungs and pumps that were becoming available, and I got to see some of those in their earliest forms. The one at Hopkins was a screen oxygenator that a fellow resident, Dr. Robert Gaertner, had developed in the Hunterian laboratory. Dr. Bahnson and Dr. Spencer were in charge of the open-heart program. Somebody asked Dr. Blalock, "Why aren't you doing this open-heart surgery, professor?" He said, "I've done my work in cardiac surgery, so I'm going to let the younger men take the anguish and responsibility for the open-heart surgery." He had turned this type of surgery over to the two of them.

The screen oxygenator that was being used was similar to the Gibbon machine, but it was an original design of Dr. Gaertner and used a slightly different pumping mechanism. This would have been in 1955 and 1956. It was very early in the development of open-heart surgery.

The screen oxygenator was used initially for atrial septal defects and some ventricular septal defects. Dr. Blalock was working in the laboratory with Vivien Thomas on a model of a ventricular septal defect, because he had always believed that any clinical surgical procedures should first be developed in the animal laboratory. It was very difficult to create a model of a ventricular septal defect because the conduction system coming from the atrium to the ventricle came right through that septal area where they wanted to create the defect, and any cutting of that tissue would end up with complete heart block. It was Vivien Thomas's technical skill in the animal laboratory that allowed him ultimately to develop a model of ventricular septal defect. He used a cork borer and put it through a purse string in the atrium and then just cork bored a hole right out of the ventricular septum.

From my perspective as an intern, a resident, and then subsequently as a junior faculty member, Dr. Blalock was very personable with all of his friends and his associates. He was not a difficult, overbearing teacher at all. He was relatively kind in his interaction with students and was always extremely well prepared. We had a Friday clinic, and it was called Dr. Blalock's Noon Clinic. The senior students would present one or two cases to him, and he used the cases as examples of whatever he wanted to address in surgery at that time. We would spend all night the night before preparing to be sure we knew all the history and everything that he might ask. The patient was brought in to the conference room and everybody was asked to stop smoking. Interestingly enough, there was not any real knowledge that smoking could cause cancer. It was mainly politeness so that the patients didn't have to have the smoke coming around them. A nurse, in her white uniform and cap, would come in with the patient to chaperone and take care of him or her. Dr. Blalock would say hello to the patient, would ask the student doctor to demonstrate anything that was there to show and give the history, and then use the students as a sounding board for that type of teaching, the so-called Socratic method. It was strenuous on the student, but it was a wonderful teaching environment. He was very demanding regarding accuracy, and he expected you to speak up and stick to your guns if you felt one thing was right over the other. He didn't like people who wouldn't answer him, but he was always the complete gentleman. He always addressed people as Mr., Mrs., or Miss, you responded with "yes, sir" during the teaching conference, and he was the same in his dealings with his interns and residents. He was very meticulous in the operating room, a good technician, but not a brilliant technician. He did a lot of heart cases, but he would also do lung, esophagus, and other surgical procedures as well. He certainly was very competent and knew what he was doing, and liked to have everything just right in the operating room. The lights had to be just right, and the intern's job was to be sure that the lights were in place. The intern and orderlies watched closely to be sure that all of the lines and catheters were out of the way so he wouldn't step on them when he came into the operating room.

It was quite an event when you worked in the operating room with him, and he always asked questions. The resident who was operating with him, the cardiac surgery resident, would be in the fourth or fifth year of the six-year program, and there was an intern who completed the team. When I was the fourth-year resident with him, the American College of Surgeons meeting was in Atlantic City. We had what were called live operating clinics, or "wet" clinics, involving a live operation in Baltimore, shown on primitive television in Atlantic City, where there was a panel of three or four experts in that particular field. They would have the television picture showing the operation and the surgeon would have on a little microphone under his gown and could talk back and forth with them. They asked questions all during the operation. I was helping him do a Blalock-Taussig shunt one of the few times we had one of those live clinics. Of course, I had operated with him many times and knew every move that he was going to make, but I didn't have any way of communicating because he was talking on the little microphone to his friends in Atlantic City. Their conversation was a kind of one-upmanship, because these surgeons would sometimes ask searching questions during the middle of the technical procedure. When Dr. Blalock took off the vascular clamps from the pulmonary artery, there was a lot of bleeding. He leaned toward me and said in a muffled voice, "Suggest something, Alex. I am a very suggestible man." It just came out of the blue as he had not said a word to me the whole time. I said, "Just hold your finger on it." He put his finger down and held it for about a minute, and fortunately it stopped the bleeding. Afterward, several panel members asked what he had said to his resident. He said, "I just said that he was doing a good job." It was a tense moment. Although he had a very warm personal relationship with his residents, he expected us to do the very best at all times.

Dr. Blalock seemed to have a great deal of influence with other doctors all across the United States, and I think that was because of two things. First, he had so many friends in surgery with whom he had grown up who were in important positions around the country. He had been at two outstanding institutions, Hopkins and Vanderbilt, so they would look to him for suggestions about particular personnel and training. Everyone knew that this was a strenuous training program and that some very outstanding young people were coming into surgery, so this was a great source of young faculty members. I think the other reason was because of the people that he chose. He chose not just because they were smart, as I can certainly speak for myself, but because some "B" students make better surgeons than "A" students. He chose them on the basis of how he thought they would relate to other people and participate as part of a team. As a result, in the camaraderie of that close relationship, a lot of things were passed along. I learned so much from the two residents ahead of me, especially from Rainey Williams. You can just imagine what you would learn from that wonderful gentleman, and from Bill Reinhoff, who was another superb human being.

Part of Dr. Blalock's success was related to the Blue Baby operation. It certainly helped open the door for surgery on congenital heart disease, and therefore it attracted some outstanding young medical students and residents who wanted to be a part of the action. It was a very exciting time around Hopkins from the late forties right up through the fifties because of all of this going on. The candidates who applied were top people from their medical schools, and he had the choice of them. When I was the chief resident, one day he said, "You know if we can't turn out good people from the selection we have, we are not doing a good job. We have the best basketball team that you could possibly have, and I would be a bad coach if they didn't all become stars."

In the forties and fifties, Dr. Blalock

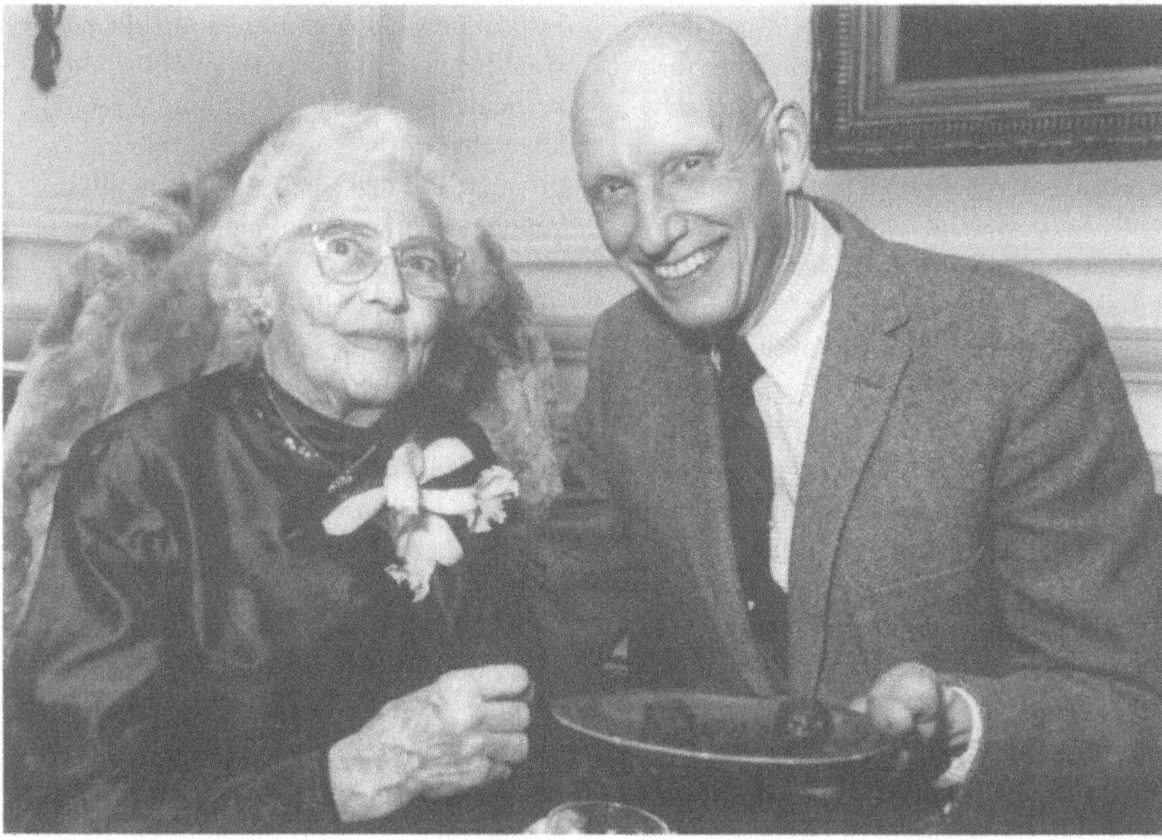

Alex Haller and Helen Taussig shortly before her death in an automobile accident

worked closely with Dr. Helen Taussig, the chief of pediatric cardiology. Relations were not always smooth between them, but that is typically the case with pediatricians and surgeons. Dr. Taussig was a remarkable lady in the sense that she was one of the early female physicians in medicine. It is not often mentioned that Hopkins had the great advantage over other medical schools in that the first class at Hopkins in 1900 had women in it. It was the very first medical school to accept women, and therefore Hopkins had a running start on other medical schools. There were some outstanding contributions from them over the years. Dr. Taussig had applied to Harvard, and they, of course, didn't accept women until nearly a half-century later, in the 1950s. Nevertheless, Taussig applied and was accepted to Hopkins. She was a very soft-spoken woman with a major deafness problem; she wore a hearing aid, and I believe this made her somewhat withdrawn. She was very effective in patient care.

Her chief in pediatrics was Dr. Edwards A. Park, a Canadian whose son now lives in Nashville. Dr. Park had the great insight to divide the Department of Pediatrics into divisions, each with a division chief, something that had never been done before. He selected Helen Taussig to be the first chief of pediatric cardiology because of her interest in the heart and the work she had done in the laboratory, tracing out the conduction bundles. It was that fortuitous choice that gave her the important responsibility of developing the new field of pediatric cardiology, and she went at it with single-mindedness. She had never married, but was married to medicine and particularly to pediatric cardiology. She developed an intense commitment and was so disciplined that the fellows worshipped her because of her intellect, and because of that wonderful volume that she published in the 1940s, which became the bible of pediatric cardiology. Her group of fellows made up most of the leaders in pediatric cardiology for the next several decades.

In her patient evaluation she was very meticulous. She felt, as do many pediatricians, that the patients were members of her family. Therefore, she was not going to let them be operated on, nor have any other thing done, unless she was there telling the surgeon exactly what to do. That didn't always go well with Dr. Blalock. He obviously had to make some of these decisions about the surgical care. She was very much involved in the management of the cyanotic children, the blue babies. There was no good way to treat them, you couldn't give them oxygen outside the hospital, and they frequently died when they reached late childhood. She observed early in her career, in the late thirties, that babies with tetralogy of Fallot seemed to do best, from infancy on for several years, if they had the murmur of a patent ductus arteriosus, permitting blood to enter the pulmonary vessels beyond the pulmonary stenosis. She reasoned that if someone could increase the flow of blood in the pulmonary artery, then the patient might be improved. This was the genesis of her concept of an artificial ductus arteriosus.

While she was mulling that over, Dr. Blalock came back to Hopkins from Vanderbilt in 1941. She talked with him about the possibility of creating a ductus. He didn't know whether that might be technically possible, but as usual he went to the dog laboratory. This was where Vivien, his technician, made such a big contribution. You may also remember that in the early forties the exciting news came that Dr. Robert Gross had divided a ductus arteriosus, the congenital abnormality of a patent ductus, at the Boston Children's Hospital. That was the most exciting cardiac surgery news for a couple of years. Dr. Taussig often told the story (and it was confirmed by Dr. Gross) about going to one of the conferences and meeting Dr. Gross. She told him that she had been thinking about the possibility of increasing blood flow to the lungs, and did he think he might be able to create a ductus arteriosus that would increase blood flow to the pulmonary artery. He stopped for a moment and said, "Madame, I don't create ductus, I close them." That was the end of it. She just folded her tent and silently stole away, so when Dr. Blalock showed up on the scene she talked with him.

The reason Dr. Blalock thought he might be able to do this is an excellent example of chance favoring the prepared mind. Dr. Blalock had been working in the laboratory at Vanderbilt with his outstanding technician on the development of a shunt, a blood-vessel anastomosis to the pulmonary artery, trying to create pulmonary hypertension. Dr. Blalock's good friend and former classmate, Dr. Tinsley Harrison, who became the head of cardiology at Vanderbilt, had a huge interest in pulmonary hypertension, and he asked Dr. Blalock if he might be able to make a model of it so they could study it. Dr. Blalock and Vivien Thomas then developed the technique of bringing the subclavian artery—actually they used the innominate artery—down to the pulmonary artery, making an anastomosis so that all the flow would run into the pulmonary artery. The problem was, of course, that the dogs were mature animals, with a mature pulmonary vascular bed, and the pulmonary blood vessels just dilated and handled this increased flow without a rise in the pressure. The experiment did not create pulmonary hypertension, but it did develop the technique of connecting those two vessels when that type of vascular surgery was in its infancy. As a result, Dr. Blalock was prepared to create a ductus in babies with pulmonary stenosis and inadequate flow to the lungs. It could be anticipated that this would improve the deep cyanosis and not produce pulmonary hypertension. Using the same technique, he and Vivien Thomas went to work in the dog laboratory to create a model. After a couple of years, they were ready to go ahead and try it on a human patient. It is amazing the way those things just fit together. You can imagine the impact on the medical students, the junior residents, and all of us there at that time. This was just astounding. I was only a premed student at Vanderbilt, but I remember hearing about the excitement at Hopkins when they presented the first four cases of the Blalock-Taussig shunt in grand rounds in the Hurd Hall auditorium. There was a sort of awe, then a quiet, and then there was this emotional upheaval and outstanding applause. A lot of people in the audience realized that this was a very significant breakthrough.

This surgical experience spilled out into the community, the country, and all around the world. Dr. Blalock was invited to a number of different countries to do the operation. One of the fascinating aspects is that he had so much confidence in his chief residents (subsequently a number of them were involved in operations on him and other members of his family) that he decided, rather than taking a faculty person with him on his tour, that he would take one of his residents, Dr. Hank Bahnson, as his assistant. They operated all over Europe with accolades up and down the continent. It was a heady time for Hopkins surgery.

Vivien Thomas played a big part in this process. He had started to work with Dr. Blalock when he was nineteen years old. Vivien was a Nashville boy from a poor but hardworking family. It was during the Depression, or the time leading right up to the Depression, around 1930. Vivien desperately needed a job to help support the family, and he heard about a possible opening in the research laboratory at Vanderbilt long before it was called the Light Laboratory. When Vivien came to be interviewed, Dr. Blalock showed him around the dog lab where other technicians were working for Tinsley Harrison and for others, and Dr. Blalock hired him to be his technician. Vivien says in retrospect that he knew nothing about anatomy or anything else, and he had to learn all of that from reading books. He was a very intelligent young man, but he had no medical background and only a high school education. He had been unable to go to college as he had wished because of the expense and the fact there was just no money available in the family. Vivien learned rapidly, had great technical abilities and wonderful hands, and very quickly Dr. Blalock formed a partnership with him, turning over to him the responsibility of keeping the research notes. He recorded everything that went on, and kept meticulous scientific notes of the highest caliber; he also developed various kinds of suturing techniques. He was also responsible for taking care of the animals. He was really the research arm in the laboratory while Dr. Blalock was busy with his clinical responsibilities. They worked together at Vanderbilt from the thirties for ten years until Dr. Blalock was invited back to Hopkins, whence many years before he had been dismissed because he was not felt to have much "promise" in surgery. They invited him back to be the chief of surgery. When he came back he brought two people with him, his secretary, Ms. Grebel, who remained his secretary at Hopkins for many years, and Vivien Thomas, his chief technician. Dr. Blalock thought these two people were essential for his professional career, and I think he was right.

Over twenty years later, Vivien received an honorary degree from Johns Hopkins, but unfortunately it was after Dr. Blalock's death in 1964, so Dr. Blalock was not present to see him receive that degree. Vivien stayed on after Dr. Blalock's death and ran the research laboratory for Dr. Blalock's successor, Dr. George Zuidema, who also had a very active laboratory. It was through Dr. Zuidema's influence and my suggestion that Hopkins gave Vivien an honorary degree. Dr. Zuidema and I contacted the president of the university and asked about an honorary BS degree for Vivien. The president said, "Isn't that the technician who was responsible for the development of the Blue Baby operation with Dr. Taussig and Dr. Blalock?" We said, "Yes, sir." He said, "Well, I think he ought to have an honorary doctorate degree," and that's what he got. I was also instrumental in having a portrait done of Vivien. All of the other important surgeons at Hopkins had portraits. My chief resident at that time, Dr. Jack White, knew of a young artist in New York who had done some wonderful paintings of children, so the artist was contacted and asked if he would be interested in doing this portrait. He said, "Oh, that's a great challenge. I would love to come and do it." The cost of the portrait was underwritten by Dr. Blalock's former surgical residents, referred to as the "Old Hands." He painted a wonderful portrait of Vivien and when it was handed over to the hospital, we thought it would probably hang in the research laboratory. However, when we presented it to the president of the hospital, Dr. Nelson said, "Well, we are very honored to accept this." Then he said, "Vivien, I think you should hang on the wall with all of your colleagues. You are going to be right there in the Blalock Building along with the other great Hopkins surgeons." His portrait hangs today on the wall with all of the other chairmen of the Department of Surgery.

When I finished my training, I went to Louisville and was on the faculty at the University of Louisville and a pediatric surgeon at Louisville Children's Hospital. Dr. Rudolph Noer was the chairman of the department, a wonderful chairman with a strong background in abdominal surgery. The department wanted a cardiothoracic program, but they didn't have anybody trained in cardiac surgery except a couple of people in private practice. It had been difficult to get any kind of an open-heart program underway, although a Michigan-trained surgeon named Dr. Fielding Rubel was starting to do some thoracic surgery at the private hospital.

I brought some of the new technology along with a heart-lung machine and began the first university cardiac surgery program. It was in the Children's Hospital, which was just across the street from the old Louisville General, the adult city hospital. We operated on adults and children there because we didn't want to move the heart-lung machine and all of the equipment back and forth.

We started out with a disc oxygenator and just a roller pump, essentially the same as in a number of other institutions. I had gotten all of the details from Dr. Glenn Morrow at the NIH, and we ordered the same equipment that he was using in Bethesda.

We did only ASDs and simple VSDs. I also did a number of Blalock-Taussig shunts, because we didn't want to try a total correction of the blue babies for the first couple of years. By the time I left, we were doing a few total repairs of the blue babies. I did some aortic valvuloplasties in adults, as there was no good artificial aortic valve available. We did some patients with mitral stenosis, but mainly it was open commissurotomy because there was no good valve before 1963 or 1964. Happily, the chief of pediatric cardiology was Joe Little from Vanderbilt, so I immediately had that tie again with Vanderbilt. He had a number of patients he had been sending to Denton Cooley, but when I showed up, he said, "OK, Alex. These are some cases for you." I said, "Well, let's take some of the simpler cases at first." He said, "All right, but you know ASDs are doing very well now everywhere, we can't afford to have anything happen to the patients." I recognized that we had to be sure we were ready, so we first tried pumping a few dogs to begin preparation. Then I said, "I think we are ready." He lined up ten children with atrial septal defects and said that we would do these ten. Fortunately, all ten of them did well; otherwise, I couldn't have lived with myself, because I knew that these children should do well. We had no technical problems with them and that got us started, but it created a few problems politically. We've all lived through some of those political problems of a new program.

The American Heart Association chapter in Louisville asked if we would do an open-heart procedure as part of their annual fund drive to show how the money was being used to support the congenital heart surgery program. We said that we would. Fielding Rubel and I operated together; he is a wonderful surgeon. We had a child from eastern Kentucky, a really great little patient for the press. He had freckles and red hair, and we operated on him on live TV. This was shown for the television fundraising show in Louisville, and happily everything went well. However, the next day Dr. Rubel and I got a call from the Louisville Medical Society saying that what we did was unethical. We had to appear before them to explain why we did it, and the unethical part wasn't that we were doing the surgery, but that we were advertising. I said to them, "The American Heart Association asked us to do this. We were supporting them, and we are not getting paid anything for it." I told them that there was no other competing team in town and that the closest cardiac program was in Nashville. They said, "Nevertheless." We had to say that we were doing this for the best humanitarian reasons, etc. etc. This was true, but we were put on the carpet for doing this procedure, and it was very uncomfortable being accused of unethical surgery. The little boy is now a pharmacist in Worther, Kentucky.

In 1962 Dr. Blalock asked me to come back to Johns Hopkins to join the faculty. I was having a great time in Louisville, and my wife and our four children loved living there. I realized that one of the areas in pediatric surgery that needed to be addressed was organ transplantation. I asked for a leave of absence to go to Philadelphia to the Wistar Institute to work six months in the research laboratory on transplantation biology with Dr. Rupert Billingham, who subsequently received the Nobel Prize in organ transplantation along with Medawar. I was planning to go back to Louisville and start a liver and kidney transplant program, but then Dr. Blalock got in touch with me and said they were planning to open a new children's hospital. Well, I wasn't sure if that was the right thing for me to do, so I talked with Dr. David Sabiston, who was Dr. Blalock's senior associate and good right arm, and my good friend. David said, "You mean Dr. Blalock has asked you to come back and you can't make up your mind? You're crazy. Why would anybody turn down a Hopkins position?" I said, "Because I am very happy in what I'm doing, David. I am productive, I have a good show, and I have a chance to develop this program in Louisville." Then he said, "Well, you'd be making the mistake of your life if you don't return to Baltimore." I have often thought about how influential David Sabiston was in my deciding to come back, and, of course, I thought I was coming back ultimately to work with Dr. Sabiston. Everyone thought that he was going to be Dr. Blalock's successor, and I had certainly hoped so.

It was a very big disappointment for Dr. Blalock that Dr. Sabiston was not chosen to be his successor. He had been used to recommending people for jobs all around the country. He was a very credible evaluator of surgical people, especially academic surgeons, and he was just sure that the right person to lead that important program at Hopkins was David Sabiston. So, why look any further? Dr. Blalock failed to recognize that you can't pick your successor, and an institution has to decide where it wants to go and chose the right person. Dr. Blalock felt very strongly about this. That was a very good example of his loyalty to his people; he just couldn't accept the fact that David Sabiston was not chosen. He was bitter for the rest of his life over that.

I think it turned out to be a good situation for both places though. First of all, I think Duke needed the kind of leadership that David Sabiston could give them. Look at the result of his stewardship at Duke—he became one of the outstanding surgical leaders in this country, and built that program into a fantastic academic institution. I also think it was good for Dr. Sabiston, because David had grown up completely at Hopkins and Dr. Blalock was his hero, practically his god. He was certainly his professional father, and I think it would have been difficult for him to develop a different program there. He would always be worrying about what Dr. Blalock would have wanted, unable to be himself. David Sabiston is an innovative, dedicated, and very effective person, and he needed to have a place where he could exert his full innovation and be himself. I don't think he could have done that at Hopkins. I was devastated when he decided to go to Duke, but I was resigned to do my best for Dr. Zuidema, who had been a fellow medical student at Johns Hopkins. I thought it was good for both Dr. Sabiston and Duke, and I think time has proved that to be the case.

In my retirement, I still meet and teach medical students and residents. I think the students have changed a lot in their preparation, skills, and the knowledge that they bring to the field of medicine. I believe this has a lot to do with the explosion in medical knowledge in the last fifty years. I don't think they have changed at all in their dedication to what they want to do. They still want to take care of sick patients, and they want to be involved in the care of people who need them. They could be successful PhDs, doctors of science, with perfectly wonderful careers, but they want to be physicians to take care of the sick, and that is a great calling.

Bibliography

Haller JA Jr, Morrow AG. Experimental Mitral Insufficiency: An Operative Method with Chronic Survival. *Ann Surg.* 1955; 142:37–51.

Haller JA Jr, Morrow AG, Roshe J. Combined Aortic and Mitral Insufficiency-Hemodynamic Effects of the Hufnagel Valve. *Ann Surg.* 1956; 144:854–860.

Haller JA Jr, Abrams BL. Use of Thrombectomy in the Treatment of Acute Iliofemoral Venous Thrombosis in Forty-five Patients. *Ann Surg.* 1963; 158:561–569.

Haller JA Jr, Van der Salm T, Rauenhorst J. Effect of Newborn Splenectomy on Homograft Survival in Inbred Mice. *J. Surg Res.* 1967; 7:110–112.

Haller JA Jr, Crisler C, Brawley R, Cameron J, Rowe RD. Operative Correction and Postoperative Management of Transposition of the Great Vessels in Nine Children. *Ann Thorac Surg.* 1969; 7:212–220.

Haller JA Jr. Anna, Vivien, and the King of Cyan(osis). *Johns Hopkins Med J.* 1975; 137:55–56.

Haller JA Jr. Presidential Address: Surgical Heroes, Then and Now, as Preceptors in Medicine. *Am Surg.* 1978; 44:1–6.

Haller JA Jr. Pediatric Trauma. The No. 1 Killer of Children. *JAMA.* 1983; 249:47.

Haller JA Jr, Scherer LR, Turner CS, Colombani PM. Evolving Management of Pectus Excavatum Based on a Single Institutional Experience of 664 Patients. *Ann Surg.* 1989; 209:578–582.

Haller JA Jr. Why Pediatric Surgery? A Personal Journey through the First 50 Years. *Ann Surg.* 2003; 237:597–606.

Valvular Heart Surgery

Albert Starr, MD

(b. 1926)

That same year, 1958, I met Lowell Edwards. He was a rickety old guy, gray hair, a little tremor from parkinsonism, and a retired engineer. He was wearing a little golf jacket and looked pretty casual. He said to me, "The heart is just a pump. We could develop an artificial heart because it is not too complicated, but I can't do it by myself. I need a doctor to help me." I told him an artificial heart was a great idea, and I was certain that some day it would be applied to man, but we didn't even have an artificial valve that would work.

— On his first meeting with Lowell Edwards

Interviewed May 4, 1998

I was born in 1926 and grew up in New York City. I do remember some of the early days of the Depression in New York and the fact that my family had some economic problems, not severe, but I knew that there were limitations of family resources. I was educated through the New York public schools. I had some great opportunities in my early education because we had a rapid advancement system in New York. If you were a bright kid, you moved swiftly through the system, so I saved two years. It was a great opportunity for me to get going early, and I was ready to start college at sixteen.

I enrolled at Columbia University, but I was not sure what I wanted to do. Medicine was in the back of my mind, but I did flirt with the idea of a career in physics. The field of molecular physics was very hot stuff since a part of the atomic bomb was under development at Columbia, a huge program crawling with PhDs. As students, we could sense that there was a lot going on in that particular field. I also flirted with economics, taking some advanced economic courses, and I remember well a discussion I had with the chairman of the department who thought that I should become an economist. However, I was also interested in biology, and it was this interest in the living structure that led me into medical school. A high school biology teacher took us on weekend field trips, and I think that extracurricular activity stirred my interest in biology. Looking back, I feel grateful to him for taking us to the botanical gardens or the zoo or something like that and explaining what was going on there.

In 1945 I graduated from Columbia and entered medical school. I was too young to be called up for World War II, but because of the war, everything was accelerated. We took three semesters a year rather than two, so it was possible to get a bachelor degree after two years. I was only eighteen when I entered medical school, and by the time I was eligible for the draft I was in medical school and was deferred. The war ended shortly after I started medical school. Columbia Medical School was also accelerated, and we went to school during the summer; it was intense, but I learned something from that. I think that the educational system can be accelerated, and we can let people enter their field at a younger age and with more energy. I did well in medical school and was AOA in my junior year. I was a very serious student, but, of course, those were serious

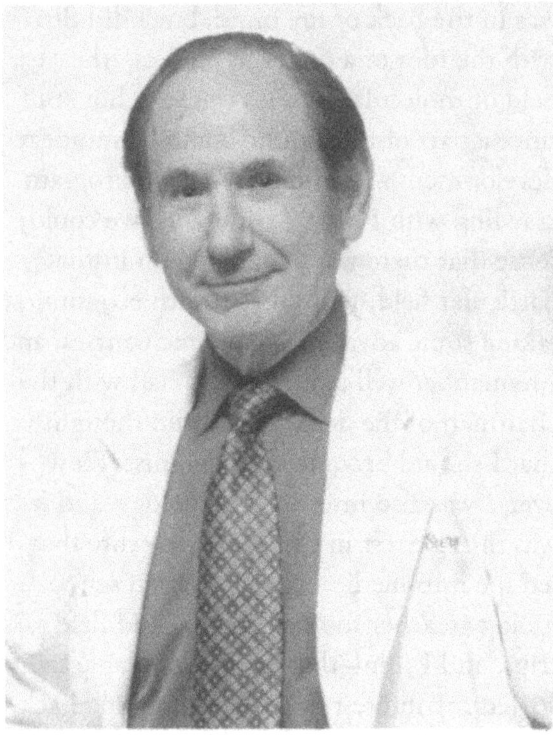

Albert Starr

days. Remember, there was a war, and it was not always clear who was going to win. At any rate, in my senior year I applied for a surgical internship at both the Massachusetts General and Johns Hopkins. I wanted to go to Boston, but when I was waiting to hear from MGH, I was accepted at Hopkins. I received a call from Dr. Blalock, who said in his deep Southern accent, "Starr, we have never had anybody who turned down a surgical internship at Johns Hopkins. What are you waiting for? You have to tell me now if you are coming to Hopkins or not. No one has ever resisted an offer from our program." I had not yet heard from Massachusetts General, but I thought I had better accept his offer, as I might end up with no internship. It was my second choice, but, luckily, it was a great choice and had a tremendous effect on my career.

When I first met Dr. Blalock he was not so sure that I really was a doctor because I looked so young. I matured late in life, and I was at that time shaving only about twice a week. He said he didn't believe that I had gone to medical school and continued to joke about my youthful appearance. He kept the house staff very close to him. He was very much immersed in the surgical service, as it was the most important thing in his life and the people who were on it were very important to him. We all felt like we had a connection to him as part of a common enterprise. That was the element that he created. Another was the enormous sense of excitement about cardiac surgery, because patients were coming to Baltimore from all over the world for the Blalock operation. I had this sense that heart surgery was something really special.

A typical day for an intern at Hopkins would be assisting or maybe even doing a patent ductus operation. This was the most unusual feature of the surgical program. An intern might get to do a ductus, assist on a coarctation repair, and then assist on a Blalock operation all in one day. Dr. Blalock did most of the Blalock-Taussig shunts, but the resident would open the chest and get everything ready. He would place tapes around the subclavian and pulmonary artery so the field would be perfectly dry. Then Dr. Blalock would step in. First he would look at the wound, and he would always find a little bleeding point to put a stitch in. This was to show the resident that he wasn't as perfect as he thought. He routinely put a stitch in an intercostal bleeder, even though it might not be bleeding. Then he would look over the field and complain that there was too much adventitia still on the blood vessels. In those days we had only silk sutures, and silk would not slide through a blood vessel very easily if there was still adventitia left on it. He would meticulously clean off adventitia at the anastomotic site, both the subclavian and pulmonary artery. The silk was oiled with mineral oil, but it was never as slippery as Prolene. The smallest silk that we used was 5–0 for little children, and 5–0 silk was actually too large. By the time I was there in 1949, they had swaged-on needles. When Dr. Blalock did the first Blue Baby operation in 1944, they used straight needles which had to be threaded. Remember that Hopkins was the leader in the development of nonabsorbable suture material. The Halsted tradition was meticulous silk suture technique while others were using absorbable catgut sutures. Halsted set the stage for meticulous surgery by showing the importance of clamping only the blood vessel and ligating it with nonabsorbable silk for hemostasis.

The ordinary postop patient with a coarctation repair or closure of a patent ductus would go back to a room after recovering from anesthesia, but the patients who had had a Blalock shunt would go to the tetralogy room. Here there were four or five beds, sometimes a crib, but most of the patients were toddlers. We didn't see too many infants in the intensive care unit. The tetralogy room was run by a head nurse, who was in charge of the early care of all of the tetralogy patients, and, as interns, we really worked for her. We listened to her carefully because she was experienced, and she would be able to tell a green intern how to take care of these patients. They were all extubated in the operating room at the end of the operation, were placed in oxygen tents, and had their fluid balance monitored very carefully. We had good understanding of electrolyte replacement, so the tetralogy room was very much like a present-day intensive care unit.

The house staff at Hopkins were enslaved for one year. We all had to live in the hospital. There were no outside apartments. The interns' quarters were on the second floor right behind the rotunda. Each of us had a room that was always immaculately kept with clean sheets and a clean uniform each day. Each morning we started rounds at five thirty or six. We were on call every day. The only rotation that included time off was the emergency room, where you worked a day and through that night. The following morning we did outpatient surgery until two or three in the afternoon and then were free until eight o'clock the next morning. After a night without sleep, you had some time off until the routine started all over again. There were thirteen interns for the surgical service. We stayed indoors so much of the time that we got pale to the point that once I got sunburned walking down the street to get a haircut!

As an intern, I was so busy I didn't apply for a residency position, so about the end of May the chief resident, Denton Cooley, came up to me and said, "Where are you planning to go next year?" I told him I had no plans and had not applied as yet, but I would like to stay at Hopkins. He said, "Well, you know there are thirteen interns and we can only keep two of the interns as assistant residents, and those two have already been selected. Dr. Blalock has picked two men who were students here and who have worked with him in the research lab, so you need to start looking for a job. You had better go see Dr. Blalock." He was really quite nice to me, knowing my predicament from having spoken to Dr. Cooley, and he said, "Well, where would you like to go?" I told him I would like to go back to Presbyterian in New York, so he picked up the phone and called the chief of surgery at Presbyterian, and said that he had an intern that he would like to keep but couldn't, and could he have a place as an assistant resident. That was the way it was arranged. With a phone call from Dr. Blalock, I was back in New York at Presbyterian Hospital. Dr. Blalock not only knew all of the academic surgeons in the U.S, but he also had a circle of international friends. For example, while I was there in 1949, Viking Björk was a research fellow developing a disc oxygenator.

Many of the great British surgeons were visitors at Hopkins. For example, the first pulmonary valvotomy done in the United States was done when I was an intern; I scrubbed on that case. Sir Russell Brock came for an extended visit and assisted Dr. Blalock on that first procedure. I remember the episode very well because I was standing on Dr. Blalock's right side and Mr. Brock was on the opposite side of the table. Mr. Brock had brought all of his instruments with him, so Dr. Blalock first put a purse-string suture in the outflow region of the right ventricle. Mr. Brock showed him how to make a little stab wound through which to insert the valvulotome through the pulmonary valve, but when the instrument was withdrawn, it accidentally cut the purse string. The right ventricular pressure was high, and in the few seconds it took for Blalock to put his finger over the hole, I got a face full of blood, because I was hanging over the operative field trying to see what they were doing. Dr. Blalock, who had a sense of humor, turned to me with his finger over the hole, and said, "Starr, your mother should see you now." It was a baptism into cardiac surgery, and I have never forgotten that moment.

Actually, the reason that I wound up in thoracic surgery was not entirely due to Dr. Blalock. When I was back in New York, the cardiac experience at Hopkins faded in my memory; I focused more on general surgery, and also on girls. I could now get out of the hospital and was no longer living like a monk at Johns Hopkins. I was focused on general surgery, the many pretty ladies around, and things in my personal life.

Dr. George Humphreys was the chief of surgery at Presbyterian and he was a different sort of person from Blalock. He was somewhat shy, a nice man, and he ran a very good show, but he was not a charismatic figure like Blalock. The Columbia system had Bellevue, Roosevelt, St. Luke's, and Presbyterian hospitals, and we rotated through all four.

The chief surgeon at Bellevue was Frank Berry, who was a giant figure in surgery. He was very politically oriented and knew everybody in the field. He was highly respected, in the proper New York social niche, a member of all the big clubs, and sometimes he would take us residents for group dinners. He was outgoing and valued his relationships with the house staff. He introduced me to a part of New York that I had never seen before. It was through Frank Berry that I got into thoracic surgery, and he influenced my career enormously.

Shortly after I returned to New York, the Korean War began. Those of us who had missed serving as physicians in World War II were eligible to serve in the next war. Eight months after arriving in New York, I went to Dr. Berry one day and told him I had heard from my draft board and I was going to have to interrupt my training. To me this was a great personal tragedy. Dr. Berry said, "What a great opportunity, Starr. That is great. Where would you like to go? I have a lot of friends in Washington." I told him that we had a number of bases in Europe, and what I should like is to go there and hang out for a while. He looked at me and said, "Starr the opportunity is in war. Why would you want to go to Europe when there is a war in Korea?" I said, "That's why I want to go to Europe, Dr. Berry." He thought Korea was a great opportunity, and I did end up there. I think he had something to do with that, because several of my friends did wind up in Europe, but I ended up going to Korea and that had a tremendous effect on my career.

When I got there the war was quite hot, and our troops were falling back. When they had reached the Yalu River, the Chinese army entered the war in great numbers. The marine divisions suffered a lot of casualties and were in a full-blown retreat. Initially I was placed as a battalion surgeon in the First Calvary Division, Seventh Calvary Regiment. We landed at Pusan and went north by train toward Seoul, which was at the front line. For some time, my battalion was cut off and surrounded by the enemy. I finally reached the battalion, and worked as battalion surgeon for about six months. Working alongside West Point graduates who were running the war very efficiently led me to appreciate the enormous management skills in the armed forces. Then, thanks to Dr. Berry, I was pulled back and assigned to a mobile surgical hospital where I spent the next year. I was put in charge of an abdominal surgical team, which meant I had a corpsman and a nurse-anesthetist. I operated day and night and did about one thousand operations in twelve months. I had calluses on my fingers from the constant use of surgical instruments. It was an unbelievable surgical experience.

We had a very good evacuation system in which patients were brought in by helicopter. Any battalion surgeon had the ability to call a helicopter to evacuate a wounded soldier or marine. Patients would come into the MASH unit fresh off the battlefield with a delay of only three or four hours at most. We would hear the helicopter come in and would go see what was going on. It could be delivering blood or patients or both. We had a triage area where we picked out those that were unstable first, while those that were less ill could wait. We sometimes would get fifteen or twenty perforated abdominal wounds at one time, triage them, and then operate continuously for the next twenty-four hours. We used a lot of O negative blood, which came from Japan. We didn't have time to type and match. When the patient hit the triage tent, the corpsmen would quickly get a 15-gauge needle in each arm and the blood would just pour in. If a patient got into that tent by mistake, he could get a couple of units of blood before someone realized he was not injured. That was how fast volume replacement was done. The overall mortality for penetrating abdominal wounds in Korea was only about 5 percent. If a patient made it to the MASH, the chance of surviving was very good. This was based in part on early triaging and the resuscitation skills of the triage personnel. This was 1950, the early days of vascular surgery, and vascular grafts were not really available. A vascular team would travel around various mobile surgical hospitals, but they were not there on a regular basis, so most patients with vascular problems were shipped to Japan. Only those with problems that required immediate attention were treated definitively in the MASH.

I was in Korea for a year and a half and then spent about six months at Fort Meade in Maryland. After that I was discharged and went back to Presbyterian. I went to see Dr. Humphrey, the chief of surgery, and said, "I have done one thousand operations in Korea and I would like to be promoted to move more quickly through the residency program." He looked at me and said, "Come on, Starr. You are lucky just to have your job back." I put Korea behind me and just continued the residency. Several months later I was at Bellevue doing a lumbar sympathectomy at about three in the afternoon, and I was hurrying along because I had a date that night with a beautiful student nurse. Dr. Frank Berry came in the room without my seeing him and stood there watching me for a while. When I finished and started out the door, he stopped me and said, "Starr, I think you should go into thoracic surgery." I was only a second-year resident, and I told him that. He said, "Well, I know, but we have an opening in our program and I think you should take it." I asked him how I could qualify for my general surgery boards and he said, "Don't worry about that. Next year you will be the chief resident in general surgery (my third year) and then the following year you can start the thoracic residency." It was a great opportunity and that was what I did. I finished general surgery in three years and ended up at the end of five years with qualifications for both boards, with some pretty neat guys helping me, powerful men helping me.

At that time the thoracic surgery program mostly involved tuberculosis surgery. This brought me in touch with Max Chamberlain, who was a tremendous surgeon, fast and methodical, and his principles influenced my own surgical technique more than anyone else. He was also a nice person and had a lot of powerful friends. Clarence Crafoord would come over from Sweden and hang out with him. He had a big convertible with leopard or tiger upholstery, a really garish thing. He was always entertaining foreign dignitaries, and would show up with visitors from South America or Europe. He was a very methodical surgeon and was the one who developed segmental resection. He did lung resections differently from everyone else—he would begin at the back, locate the bronchus, divide it, and, with a clamp on the distal end, lift it up and expose the artery and vein. After each of these was divided, he could just scoop the segment out. It would pop right out the way he did it. He had a reason for everything he did. He would divide the bronchus first because that was the most rigid structure in the hilum, and once it was divided and the lung put on stretch, the vessels are easily visible. He had choreographed every operation in his mind, and it was always reproducible. I found that approach to surgery very useful, and I used it when we began cardiac surgery.

In 1955 and 1956 we were doing mitral commissurotomies and starting to do open-heart surgery in New York. We started with atrial septal defects using the atrial well technique developed by Robert Gross at Children's Hospital in Boston. I assisted Robert Deterling on the first case in New York. The patient had very high right atrial pressures and was in congestive heart failure, not the usual ASD. He sewed the well on the right atrium and then released the clamp and let the well fill with blood. He forgot that the well could overflow because of the high pressure. This was his first case. Blood poured into the well and over the sides and that was it for the patient. Cardiac surgery was high risk during those early days, but we were finally able to do atrial septal defects with a pretty low mortality. We went from the well to a primitive heart-lung machine. Our first pump was a finger pump with a DeWall bubble oxygenator put together on-site. Using the azygos flow principle, the pump-oxygenator could support the circulation with reduced flows for short periods of time, long enough to close an ASD.

One day, during my last year as a thoracic surgery resident, I was assisting with a closure of an ASD. We had a balcony in the operating room, and a visitor in the balcony came down from it while I was putting on the dressing. He said, "Starr, do you know how to do this kind of surgery?" I did not lack for confidence and I said, "Well, yes, I am fully trained." He said, "Well, we don't have open-heart surgery in Oregon, and we are looking for someone to come and start a program." Actually, I was hired by the Department of Pediatrics, not the Department of Surgery, and my job was to start cardiac surgery in the next six months to a year, so I spent the first six months in the animal lab gathering all the equipment and skills necessary.

On my way to Oregon after completing my residency, I first visited Jay Ankeney in Cleveland. Jay had finished the same program that I had a few years earlier, and we were good friends. He showed me the pump that he was using, which was a rotating-disc oxygenator developed in Cleveland by Fred Cross. This was an alternative to the bubble oxygenator we had been using in New York. Next I stopped in Minneapolis. Walt Lillehei was really kind to me; and I watched several cases and hung out with the residents. I met Bill Weirich, for example, who developed the first myocardial pacemaker electrode. This was an important adjunct, since at that time heart block after VSD repair was not uncommon. Then I spent a week at the Mayo Clinic watching John Kirklin. That was my postgraduate course in cardiac surgery. During that trip I had the opportunity to see the rotating-disc, the screen, and the bubble oxygenators. From that experience I decided to go with the rotating-disc as it seemed to involve less paraphernalia than the bubble oxygenator. The screen oxygenators at that time were very complicated and required an engineer. The disc seemed to be simpler and more reliable, and that is what we started with in Oregon. I arrived in Oregon in 1957, and we did the first open-heart operation in 1958. Our first patient had a ventricular septal defect and it went very well.

That same year, toward the end of 1958, I first met Lowell Edwards. He made an appointment with my secretary in the Department of Pediatrics. I looked out the window and saw him get out of his car. He was a rickety old guy, gray hair, with a little tremor from parkinsonism. He was a retired engineer. Coming from New York, I thought men should wear suits and ties. He was wearing a little golf jacket and looked pretty casual. That was because he was a much understated fellow. We got to talking and he told me he had been educated as an electrical engineer, but most of his work was in mechanical engineering. He had worked for Weyerhaeuser and various other lumber companies, and had developed the debarking system that was used in all of the lumber mills in the Pacific Northwest. He had a number of good inventions and some really crazy ones. His most important invention was a fuel injection system for fighter aircraft during World War II. We had developed the P-38 and other high-performance airplanes that could climb rapidly, but as the atmospheric pressure rapidly dropped during the climb, part of the fuel would vaporize and the fuel pumps could not handle mixed liquid and vapor. Lowell Edwards developed a fuel-pumping system that could handle the problem, licensed it to TRW in Cleveland, and traveled back and forth to Cleveland assisting them in its development. The royalties he received from his invention made him a very wealthy man.

He had become interested in medical engineering, and to study the circulation he had built a model that included the concepts of flow and resistance, thinking that if he could build a system, he would understand it as an engineer. He said to me, "The heart is just a pump. We could develop an artificial heart because it is not too complicated, but I can't do it by myself. I need a doctor to help me." He had heard that I had come to Oregon to start the open-heart program, and I was the logical person to whom to turn.

I told him an artificial heart was a great idea, and I was certain that someday it would be applied to man, but we didn't even have an artificial valve that would work. He asked me which valve. Hank Bahnson was working on replacing aortic valve leaflets and Charlie Hufnagel had Silastic aortic leaflets, but no one had anything for the mitral valve, so I said, "Why don't we start on the mitral? That looks like it might be the toughest one." That's what we did.

We did a lot of brainstorming. I met with Edwards at least once a week and spent hours talking about the design. We asked ourselves some very specific questions: What materials are available for use in the human body? How is the valve going to be fixed in place? What valvular mechanism should we use? There are all sorts of valvular mechanisms in carburetors and other devices. We didn't have to invent a valve, we simply had to select the best one for our use. We had a limited choice of materials. Teflon was already available. Orthopedic devices were made of stainless steel and titanium, which is really Stellite 21, a nonferrous alloy used because it had no iron and therefore would not corrode. Silastic was used for shunts in patients with hydrocephalus, and finally there were vascular grafts made of Dacron. Our original plan was to have a cloth sewing ring, nonthrombogenic material for the valve housing, and two Silastic leaflets. We never entertained the possibility of having chordae, which seemed too difficult to design and which would add the problem of finding a material that would not crack or fracture. We thought the valve should be self-contained, and all the surgeon would have to do would be to sew it in without further adjustments.

Our first bileaflet valves failed. We implanted them in dogs, which would come off bypass very well and looked pretty good the night of surgery, but by the next day would get sluggish, and by the second or third day they would die of pulmonary edema. Autopsy would show the valve thrombosed.

Lowell Edwards was retired and he had nothing else to do, so we could go from concept to prototype in a matter of days, something that would take months in a big organization. He had a little laboratory in his home and a small development company in town that was supported by his royalty income, with a machine shop, two machinists, and one engineer named Don Shiley. In early 1959 we began putting caged-ball valves in dogs.

We knew about the early Hufnagel valve, but we were also influenced by the autopsy findings in our dogs. We knew the problem was thrombosis, and it appeared that the thrombus began at the suture line and then spread onto the leaflets. Once the leaflets were immobilized, total thrombosis occurred very rapidly, so we needed a leaflet that would function without being anchored to the base of the valve, and that was when the concept of the ball valve arose. Because it was a free-floating poppet, the results changed dramatically. We did a black Labrador with our first prototype ball valve and that dog survived for years after the operation. After that first survivor, all the dogs would die within two or three weeks of valve thrombosis. The thrombus would begin at the suture line and gradually spread to the orifice, where it would gradually increase in size until it was bulky enough to produce sudden occlusion of the valve. We solved this problem with a circular Silastic shield, which kept the thrombus away from the orifice, and with this modification, we were able to achieve long-term survival in dogs.

This brought us to two questions: Should we use the shielded valve in human beings, and should we use anticoagulation? I wrestled with this and decided that we should start with the unshielded valve since it was simpler. After all, man is so different from dog, and we actually used a valve that had failed in the dog as our first prototype for clinical implantation, counting on the difference in the clotting mechanism to be in our favor.

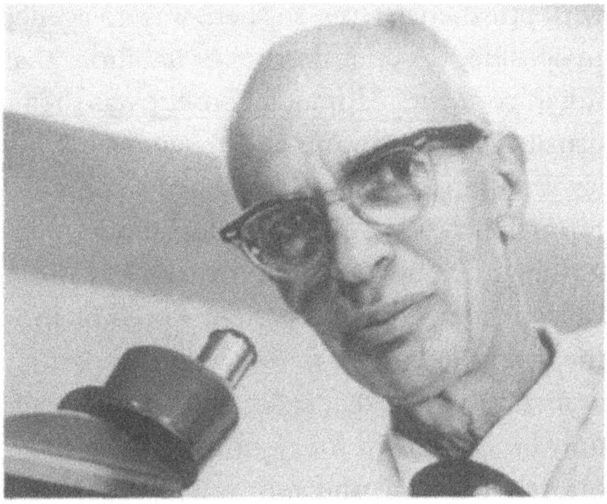

Lowell Edwards

The chief of cardiology at Oregon was Herb Griswold, and he and I worked closely on all of our heart patients. He did not come to the lab very often, but in the summer of 1960 he came by and saw our collection of really healthy dogs with prosthetic valves, and he said, "You know we have patients that are dying of rheumatic heart disease. I think it is time to consider putting this valve in patients." I had not thought we were ready. The chief of general surgery was Dr. Englebert Dunphy, and he was a very progressive guy. I went to see him and said, "Dr. Dunphy, Dr. Griswold thinks it is time to use this valve in man. What do you think we should do?" We went over the results of our valve replacement in dogs, and he said he thought we should go ahead.

Next, I went to Lowell Edwards, who was a very experienced businessperson, and told him about our decision to use the valve in a patient. The FDA was not at all involved with prosthetic valves, so there was no agency to consider the ethical issues or liabilities that might come up. Although consent was then usually verbal, Edwards and I went to his lawyer and together we developed a consent form, which was a one-page disclaimer describing the operation and the status of the valve. It stated that the patient would be in the first group of ten to receive this experimental valve and that successful animals had only been followed for eight months. With informed consent and approval of the chief of cardiology and surgery, we felt that we could go ahead. The first patients were all in advanced stages of heart failure and each decided to go ahead; none refused.

The first patient was a twenty-six-year-old woman who required an oxygen tent twenty-four hours a day. We did the operation through a right thoracotomy and because the left atrium was huge we had perfect exposure. The operation was not difficult and was actually much easier than in dogs. She came off bypass without any difficulty, and for the first time we could hear the opening and closing sounds of an artificial valve in a patient. We sent her to the ICU, and the chief of cardiology and the chief of medicine came in to listen to her heart. Everyone was really pleased and impressed. The patient was doing pretty well and was extubated. I went back to see her that evening and she looked good, and we talked a little. In those days to get a portable chest X-ray we would sit the patient up, the nurse or doctor would stand beside the bed holding the patient while the technician took the film. We lifted this patient up, and while we were holding her, we felt her go limp. We laid her down and tried to resuscitate her, but after a few minutes it was obvious that she was dead. The technician then brought us the X-ray and we could see an air fluid level in the huge left atrium. We had not recognized the need to de-air the heart, and so she died of massive air embolism.

I had known of Dr. Bailey's plan when he first did a mitral commissurotomy. He had five patients scheduled before he started, and it was not until he reached the fifth patient that he had a survivor. We had quite a few other patients waiting in the wings, so we soon did the next one and were able to get a reasonable number of survivors.

The first patient was done in September 1960. Dr. Dunphy became quite interested in this project, and said to me, "Starr, what about presenting some of this work?" I said, "Well, it is still pretty early. I would like to have a larger series and longer follow-up." "Come on, Starr. I think you should present this now, and I think it should be to the American Surgical Association. I will help get the paper accepted, and I will find the discussant for it." He asked Dr. DeBakey, who was a little reluctant, as he hated to talk about something in which he had no actual experience, but he couldn't turn down Dr. Dunphy. He did discuss our paper and made some interesting remarks. He said that if this project were presented to the NIH as a grant application, and he was running the review committee, he would turn it down. This shows how a bureaucratic system can trip itself up and have a negative impact. That presentation created a great deal of interest and soon led to many people requesting a valve.

Lowell Edwards and I began to discuss various options. How are we going to make this available to other surgeons? On what basis? Should it be a commercial project or not? If so, how soon could we assemble the manufacturing equipment and personnel?

Edwards had already obtained patents, which revolved around the sewing ring because the ball-valve principle had been used in many other systems. The evolution of the sewing ring was a very important part of the whole process and, as far as the patents were concerned, was the creative part. We had worked a long time on the sewing ring. I would tell him the physical characteristics that we needed, and he would come up with a way of achieving what we wanted. We went through numerous steps, and the evolution of the sewing ring continued until 1965. Edwards sent the initial sewing ring patent under his own name, but because we had such a close collaboration he then added my name. He then had to decide where to build the valve: Oregon or California. Oregon did not recognize capital gains as a special type of income, but California did. On the basis of the more favorable state tax laws, he decided on California. This is an example of how a state can trip itself up. A huge industrial complex is now located in California, rather than Oregon, because of a more progressive tax law. He started Edwards Laboratories with $25,000 in capital secured from himself and three of his business associates in 1961. By 1962 the valve was available in limited numbers. We needed clinical feedback from experienced surgery centers that were doing a lot of heart surgery, who would use it most effectively. We worked at first with Viking Björk in Sweden, Charlie Hahn in Switzerland, and the Mayo and Cleveland Clinics. They were the early users of the valve, and later longtime supporters because of their favorable experiences.

After the first few clinical implantations, the valve continued to develop, and we had new materials, changing designs and concepts. From 1974 until 1980 we produced a cloth-covered valve, thinking that covering the struts with Dacron would be an improvement. In fact, the cloth cover did not offer a substantial improvement in clinical results, and we discontinued that valve in 1980. We hoped to have a functioning intima growing on the cloth surfaces, but we learned what looked like intima did not function like intima, as the pseudo-intima did not have the same kind of antithrombogenic characteristic as normal intima.

Another early decision we had to make concerned anticoagulation. We were using an unshielded valve that had not been successful in dogs because of thrombosis. Long-term anticoagulation therapy was also relatively rare at that time. Very early we began to see patients with atrial fibrillation or a thrombus in the left atrium that required anticoagulation. Since most of the patients were in atrial fibrillation, we decided to recommend anticoagulation for all artificial-valve patients as a safety measure. Later on we did a series of patients who were not anticoagulated and learned that anticoagulation is essential.

We faced another clinical hurdle. Some of our early patients developed prosthetic valve endocarditis, commonly due to staphylococcus. Prosthetic valve endocarditis was a disease that had never been seen before, and so we had to determine how to treat it and how to prevent it. There were some reports in animals showing that artificial valves could become populated with bacteria. Would it be the same in man? Was endocarditis going to be an inevitable consequence of having an artificial valve? At first it looked like this could be a major problem of valve replacement, but it turned out that by using careful surgical techniques you could implant an artificial valve without it becoming infected. We used antibiotics for the first week after surgery, and it was also important to use prophylactic antibiotics with any kind of dental work or other infections, to prevent valve endocarditis. This turned out not to be as much of a problem as we feared.

By 1965 literally thousands of valves had been implanted all over the world. Remember that from 1960 to early 1970 there were no other prosthetic valves to speak of, and so this valve dominated the field for more than a decade. The peak production was more than fifty thousand valves a year. Eventually we reached the one million mark. The valve is still available and is still used in special circumstances.

At one time we made a nontilting disc valve which was pretty good, another part of the development of valve surgery that was engineered by Don Shiley. He, Warren Hancock, and Jim Bentley all had started with the Edwards Laboratory and were all very entrepreneurial and opportunistic. Shiley designed our aortic prosthesis, the aortic ball valve. We had the concept and Lowell Edwards supervised the development, but the drawings of that valve were done by Don Shiley. He was quite a guy, an experienced valve engineer, and eventually he left Edwards to form his own company. He developed a tilting-disc concept for a prosthetic valve. As he tells it, he was watching football one Sunday afternoon, and he just suddenly thought of it, a valve with an inflow strut and an outflow strut opposite to restrain the disc. He leaped out of the reclining chair and made a simple drawing of it, went to his office, and started tinkering. Within a short time, he came up with the tilting-disc valve that became the Björk-Shiley valve. He first showed it to Denton Cooley, but it did not appeal to him. When he showed it to Viking Björk he became very interested, as he had experienced problems with the caged-ball valve in patients with very small aortas. Björk realized that this would be the answer to the problem of a small aortic root, and thus began their collaboration.

Warren Hancock was always pushing us to use animal tissues for an artificial valve. I felt it was not a good idea because durability is the essential feature of any prosthetic device, and so it never appealed to me. He tried to convince others at Edwards to get into the tissue valve field, but they also declined. He left us to form his own company with the express idea of making tissue valves. He started with formaldehyde-preserved tissue. I think Dr. Litwak in New York and a few others used his early valves. From previous work with arterial graft preservation using formaldehyde, we predicted that heart valves preserved in formaldehyde would not be very durable. However, Hancock learned about using gluteraldehyde from Alain Carpentier. Since he already had a production plant for making valves, all he did was change the solution to gluteraldehyde, and with that came up with the first commercially available tissue valve in the world. It was a great achievement.

Both prosthetic and biological valves now have important roles to play. I think that Carpentier's demonstration of gluteraldehyde preservation was a major milestone in the development of artificial valves, because the valve has enormous utility. The current Carpentier-Edwards pericardial valve is a great choice for aortic valve replacement. In the mitral position, the incidence of deterioration is a little higher than in the aortic position, but it is still a suitable choice for elderly patients. The use of biological valves should be based on the projected life expectancy for the individual patient. For example, I think that for a patient in his mid-sixties who does not want to take anticoagulants and needs an aortic valve replacement, a pericardial valve is a good choice. For mitral valve replacement, I think the patient should have a somewhat limited life expectancy to have a tissue valve. That would be a patient in his mid-seventies with other comorbidities. For a patient in really good shape in his mid-seventies who didn't mind taking anticoagulation, then I would recommend a mechanical valve.

Lowell Edwards originally came to me to discuss an implantable mechanical heart. He asked, "How close are we for that to be feasible?" We had to answer that by separating the technology from the problems of application. The technology was pretty good. The extent to which it could be used is now a complex issue, which has enormous financial and regulatory implications. Certainly, Lowell Edwards's original concept that the heart is only a pump is correct. The heart is itself quite a simple organ that can be replaced. The circulation of the blood and the vasculature is far more complicated.

One thing we learned from valve replacement is this: In the beginning we wondered how a patient would feel about the quality of his life if he knew that his health was dependent on a piece of plastic and metal. We discovered that patients didn't care on what their life depended, as long as they were alive. I have no doubt that a person living with a mechanical heart would have just as good a life, and feel just as good about being alive, as if they had an artificial valve. Considering the alternative, patients will be very accepting of an artificial heart, just as they are with heart transplants.

What we are seeing today in the technology of cardiac, orthopedic, and neurosurgery is development going on in many different sites. We have laboratories in academic centers, we have not-for-profit think tanks, and we have a huge and rapidly expanding for-profit health industry. Edwards Laboratory was the prototype company making life-support implantable devices and was a germinal center from which many other companies sprang, making products such as the pacemakers, disposable oxygenators, and so on. We now have a very creative and rapidly growing interface between surgery and industry, and this interface is where the action is taking place. The industrial component is well financed, sophisticated, and more aggressive than it was in the past. What we are seeing today (1998) is an enormous move of capital into high-risk industries, one of which is the device industry. The venture capitalists have never had it so good in terms of flow of money to finance start-ups. At the same time, the start-up companies are being purchased by larger companies, so there is a lot of ferment and activity, and lot of creative work is being done. The kinds of resources that are now at the disposal of the cardiac surgeon are absolutely enormous and beyond anything that we might have imagined in the distant past. I think that we are on the brink of rapidly changing technology in cardiac surgery.

The two current areas of innovation are left ventricular assist devices and minimally invasive surgery. The ventricular assist devices may be limited by the financial and regulatory process. On the other hand, minimally invasive procedures will probably advance more rapidly. Let's consider the surgical instrument. From the time of the Egyptians until now, a surgical instrument has had two ends, the patient and the surgeon. There has been no deviation in the application of that design for several thousand years, but now we have digital electronics, computers, and robots. When we place a computer between the surgeon's hand and the instrument, the implications are huge. It means that we may be able to get inside body cavities and do things without disturbing surrounding tissue and structures as we have done in the past. I think the potential here is very great.

Simply put, valve replacement has been in the main a very happy story for cardiac surgery, with the heart surgeons leading the way in the development of implantable life-support systems, and setting standards of proper analysis and reporting. Hopefully, it will be emulated by other specialties.

Bibliography

Starr A. Total Mitral Valve Replacement: Fixation and Thrombosis. *Surg Forum.* 1960; 11:258–260.

Starr A, Edwards ML. Mitral Replacement: The Shielded Ball Valve Prosthesis. *J Thorac Cardiovas Surg.* 1961; 42:673–682.

Braunwald NS, Cooper T, Morrow AG. Clinical and Experimental Replacement of the Mitral Valve; Experience with the Use of a Flexible Polyurethane Prosthesis. In Merendino KA. *Prosthetic Valves for Cardiac Surgery*. National Heart Institute; 1961. 307–339.

Starr A, Edwards ML. Mitral Replacement: Clinical Experience with a Ball Valve Prosthesis. *Ann Surg.* 1961; 154:726–740.

Herr R, Starr A, McCord CW, Wood JA. Special Problems Following Valve Replacement. *Ann Thorac Surg.* 1965; 92:403–415.

Anderson RP, Bonchek LI, Grunkemeier GL, Lambert LE, Starr A. The Analysis and Presentation of Surgical Results by Actuarial Methods. *J Surg Res.* 1974; 16:224–230.

Grunkemeier GL, Starr A. Late Ball Variance with Model 1000 Starr-Edwards Aortic Valve Prosthesis. *J Thorac Cardiovas Surg.* 1986; 91:918–923.

Starr A. The Thoracic Surgical Industrial Complex. *Ann Thorac Surg.* 1986; 42:124–133.

Gao G, Wu YX, Grunkemeier GL, Furnary AP, Starr A. Forty-Year Survival with the Starr-Edwards Heart Valve Prosthesis. *J Heart Valve Dis.* 2004; 13:91–96.

Starr A. The Artificial Heart Valve. *Nat Med.* 2007; 13:xii–xvi.

Donald N. Ross, FRCS

(b. 1922)

There was experimental work by Lower and Shumway that showed that when they put a dog's pulmonary valve into the descending aorta, the valve would thicken up but remain intact. Clearly, it did work under aortic pressure and we began thinking of using the pulmonary valve as an aortic valve substitute. The day we did the first pulmonary autograft, we stood back and waited to see if the cusps would tear. Of course, they didn't, and one has never torn, as far as I know.

— On the first use of an autogenous pulmonary valve to replace the aortic valve

Interviewed August 13, 1997

I was born in Kimberly, South Africa, and I think that I still have a South African accent. Some people mistake it for Australian, but it is South African and I am proud of that. My parents came from Scotland. My father was from Glasgow and my mother was from the Highlands. They left Scotland because it was cold and rather miserable, and they were poor. The economy was slow. My father worked in Glasgow on the Clyde, which was the shipbuilding area of Glasgow. I think he was wise to get out. It was a hard, struggling life in Scotland at that time. His brother emigrated to New Zealand and Father went to South Africa to make a new life; my mother followed shortly afterwards. They remained very Scot-oriented for the rest of their lives. For example, my mother's accent was so strong that sometimes she couldn't be understood on the telephone, and the grocer would have to get someone to come to the phone and translate from Scots into English. My father's lowland accent was much easier to understand. They wanted to make a Scot out of me, so when I was six they sent me to Scotland to live with my grandparents for a year. It was too cold for me coming from South Africa, but I suppose they were right that I should be brought up, to some extent, with my grandparents and to understand the environment in which they were brought up.

My father had worked in shipyards on the Clyde and was a handyman. They were called joiners, and when he came out to Kimberly he started a light engineering business. He became well-known for his ability to mend guns and repair machinery, so he developed quite a good business. As you know, those were the days of the Depression. We had everything that we needed and life was reasonably pleasant in South Africa, but basically it was austere and the Depression years really made quite a mark on my conscience and my memories.

My schooling was all in Kimberly, where I went to the Boys High School. It was an excellent school with the emphasis on the classics, mathematics, and Latin. I really wanted to learn about these things and basically enjoyed school.

At that time South Africa was a complex and divided society. The division was not so much between the whites and blacks as it became subsequently, but was within the white community. It was divided between the English-speaking people like me and my family, and the Afrikaans-speaking people, who were the descendants of the Boers. The Boer War was still fresh in people's minds and there was still some rivalry and hatred which has by now subsided, but when I was growing up the white people were strongly divided.

I learned Afrikaans and am fully bilingual and can still speak the language freely. It is similar to Flemish. Now it is not much use to anybody and is seldom spoken. The universities were divided also. Cape Town University was an English-speaking school with English traditions and professors from England and Scotland. Stellenbosch, thirty miles away, was the Afrikaans-speaking equivalent. The same was true in Johannesburg. Witwatersrand University was English speaking and Pretoria University was Afrikaans. There were originally two medical schools, one English and the other Afrikaans. Now there are several medical schools and those language distinctions have been obliterated. The black people were originally not allowed to attend university when I was in school.

I am not sure why I decided to study medicine. I had always enjoyed making models and radio sets. I had an inquiring mind, and I enjoyed using my hands too; I suppose that is why I chose surgery. I studied Latin and did the things we thought you needed to do to become a doctor.

At that time medical school admission was very competitive. Cape Town University accepted about two hundred students in the medical school each year, but only about eighty were allowed to go on to the following year. It was competitive to get in and competitive to stay. I graduated with honours and the university gold medal.

It was part of the requirement of the university that you had to spend a year within its hospital after graduation before you could go into general practice out in the country. I spent my year at the Groote Schuur Hospital, which was the teaching hospital of Cape Town University. As an interesting aside, Christiaan Barnard (of transplant fame) and I qualified together. Altogether we were six years as classmates at the university and spent that next year as doctors together. He was a "good boy" in those days.

After my first year I won an overseas scholarship for two years. It was the L. Oliver Ash Scholarship and it came from Kimberly. I decided to go to England and obtain my fellowship at the Royal College of Surgeons. My plan was to accomplish this in two years and then come back to South Africa and enter practice. When I got to London I worked hard and got the fellowship in two years, and by then I was somewhat established in England. I wanted to stay there for a while because the surgery at that time was very exciting. I did not plan to stay permanently; that just happened. After two years I went to Bath, where I worked under the direction of a Dr. Kindersley, who took great pride in getting his boys through the final fellowship, so I was in luck there. I nearly turned to orthopaedic surgery since I worked for an orthopaedic surgeon in Bath, but the Bath people handed me over to Mr. Belsey in Bristol, because by then I had decided I wanted to try to get into chest surgery, which was also developing into heart surgery.

Working for Belsey really opened the international scene for me. He was well-known for the Belsey oesophageal operation. We had a lot of fun together. He was, and still is, a very intelligent man and very interested in hunting, fishing, and shooting, and he tried unsuccessfully to turn me into a country gentleman. We used to talk over operations and I would say, "Why did you do this and why didn't you do that?" He would say, "Well, if this works well we will call it the Belsey procedure. If it doesn't, we will call it the Ross procedure." We had a good relationship. Mr. Belsey did a lot of oesophageal surgery and also tuberculosis work. He saw a lot of patients with oesophagitis, because he had such a reputation for its surgical treatment. He also did a lot of newborns with oesophageal atresia who would come by ambulance from all over England.

We did a lot of phrenic nerve crushes for tuberculosis. I would drive out in freezing weather in my little open Morris Minor car, hot water bottle over my knees, to the local sanatorium, and do a full morning of procedures, phrenic crushes, and division of pulmonary adhesions. We did thoracoplasties using local anesthesia. Many of the patients were young women with cavitary tuberculosis and positive sputum. The thoracoplasty would close the cavity. We usually took nine ribs altogether. The senior surgeon would take the first three ribs as a first stage, and then I would do the next six at the second stage. The interval would be a month or two between stages. It was a mutilating operation, and it was such a pleasure when we began doing pulmonary resections and stopped doing thoracoplasties. It was streptomycin that made pulmonary resection feasible for tuberculosis. That was in the early 1950s, and was at the end of my period with Belsey.

I was very excited about the prospect of cardiac surgery, so Mr. Belsey handed me over to Russell Brock at Guy's Hospital. Brock was doing pulmonary valvotomy operations and the Blalock-Taussig shunt. Belsey

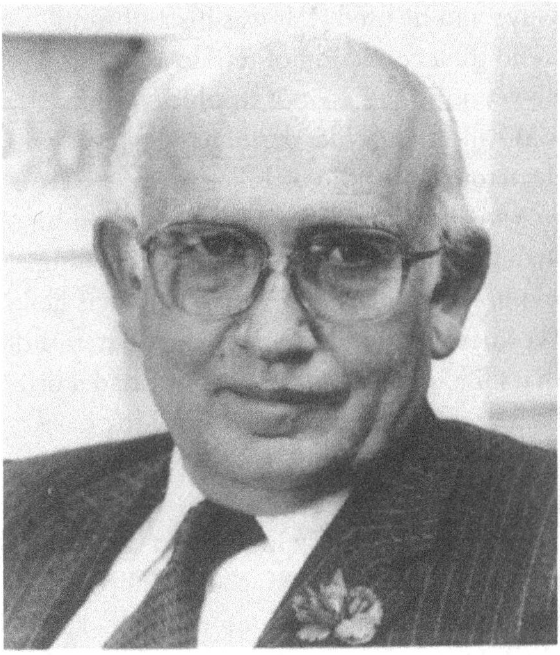

Donald N. Ross

was a great sports car enthusiast and drove an Aston Martin. He took me to Guy's Hospital to watch Brock do a closed aortic valvotomy. He put a valvotome into the left ventricle, and I thought it was fantastically interesting but amazingly bloody. Belsey arranged a job for me as a research fellow with Brock, so I did research for two years; that would be 1952 to 1954. Then I became the senior registrar at Guy's Hospital, where I did a lot of surgery and research. It was a fantastic time. All sorts of things were developing, such as Lillehei doing cross-circulation, and everybody was busy making heart-lung machines.

Lord Brock did a lot of pulmonary valvotomies but he never took to the Blalock-Taussig shunt operation; it was too fiddly. He liked to do infundibular resections, valvotomies, and whatnot. He really was not very dexterous. He liked to do direct surgery but was never really happy with heart-lung bypass surgery. It was developed there at

Guy's and he used it. It was his ambition to do total correction of tetralogy of Fallot; however, he had a lot of trouble closing a VSD and things like that. He was never as dexterous as Kirklin or Lillehei. He used to get so frustrated and cross because of his inability to achieve things in the operating room. At these times he used to give us hell. We knew we could probably do it better, but that's life. He taught me a lot. He had a brilliant and incisive mind, but he didn't have the dexterity that he would have like to have had.

There was a rivalry in London between Hammersmith Hospital where Melrose was developing a heart-lung machine, and Guy's Hospital where Brock was working. We opted for hypothermia first and were pioneers in the use of hypothermia, and from that we started on cross-circulation, but I'm glad to say we never did it clinically. From there, we went on to Lillehei's bubble oxygenator. Melrose was a little bitter and disappointed that we did not use the first British-made machine, but Melrose and Brock didn't see eye to eye. We called the Melrose machine the "Butterchurn," and made our own disc oxygenator in the Guy's Hospital workshop. Brock was also interested in using potassium to stop the heart during surgery, but it sometimes did a lot of harm. We were trying to stop the heart so we could get on with what we were doing, but at the same time we were not supporting the heart properly, so at times it was a bad thing. We used the bubble oxygenator for a time, doing ASDs, VSDs, and AV canal problems, that is, mostly congenital work. Everyone was suspicious of the bubble oxygenator, but it proved useful until we developed our own rotating-disc oxygenator.

I was developing an increasing interest in the aortic side of the heart and began doing aortic valve decalcifications. Brock let me do most of them. At that time Brock was interested in blood vessel replacement for coarctation and abdominal aneurysms. We were going to the autopsy room and collecting aortas and also ascending aortas with the aortic valve attached, trying to work out ways of storing tissue. This was before Dacron grafts were available. At first we stored the tissue in Ringer's solution, but it would soon go bad. Then we used formalin, which turned the grafts into a nasty sort of leather. We struggled with several methods. One was using ethylene oxide to sterilize, followed by freeze-drying. At the same time we stored segments of the ascending aorta including the aortic valve. I had a little pulse duplicator which I used to see how long the aortic valve might last after freeze-drying. At the same time Alfred Gunning and Carlos Duran at Oxford were working on the problem of replacing the aortic valve in animals. They made significant contributions, and, of course, we were all in touch with each other. They felt a bit frustrated in that they did not have the clinical supply that I had. By this time I was getting well-known for decalcifying aortic valves.

There was a famous day when I decalcified an aortic valve and the whole thing finally disintegrated and went down the sucker. There were no prosthetic valves to be had anywhere in England. This was right after Albert Starr had described his first few patients. The patient was going to die, so we reconstituted one of our freeze-dried aortic valves and sewed it in with just a single suture line. We expected to have to send a telegram to Albert Starr to send over one of his valves. We thought this would hold the situation until the new valve arrived. In fact it did hold very well, and he lived another three or four years. In those days the patients were all in advanced stages of heart failure. It was either leave them alone or take a chance and try cardiac surgery. That was how we first started using homograft aortic valves.

We soon changed our valve technique to a double suture line and refined the methods of storing the valves. We put in a lot of homograft aortic valves and had patients coming from all over the country.

Eventually we changed our preservation technique from freeze-dried tissue to fresh tissue, partly through the influence of Brian Barrett-Boyes. I also had a very clever research lady, Dr. Jalabi, from Iraq, working for me then. We used to call her "Jelly Baby." She could do anything with tissue. She could grow it and cultivate it. She did a lot of work on sterilization techniques and viability studies. She did freezing studies many years before cryopreservation became popular. We used a number of different techniques, but basically we used ethylene-oxide and freeze-drying for a long time. Dr. Jalabi also did tissue viability studies and found that tissue taken at autopsy had about 70 percent viability if preserved in tissue-culture medium. This viability persisted for eighteen days. After that, viability started falling off. Sometimes, if there were not enough valves, we would use them up to six weeks rather than discard them, and the patients seemed to do very well.

There was a great argument about what antibiotics should be used. To begin with, we overused the antibiotics. Barrett-Boyes had one formula, we added another formula, Harefield Hospital had another, and so on. Visitors would say, "What is the formula?" We responded, "The formula depends on the dominant organisms in the collecting area." Our aortas were taken from cadavers. The bacteriological flora of London cadavers may be different from that of New Zealand or other countries. It was difficult to convince people that they should formulate their own antibiotic mix.

We put in the first aortic homograft in 1962, and during the next five years there was great excitement and interest. When we started, we thought that the tissue might be rejected so we used corticosteroids and our immunologist was very interested. It turned out that it was more dangerous for the patient to use immunosuppressives and risk infection than to ignore the immunological response, which seemed to peak at about three weeks and then decrease, so we gave up immunosuppressives.

There was a great deal of interest in homograft valves, and it seemed the whole world and his brother came to visit and to learn about homografts. We thought we had the perfect valve, and it was wonderful. But after three to five years, we started hearing new diastolic murmurs, seeing acute failures with torn cusps, and we began to get worried about the long-term outlook for the homograft. We took failed valves out and looked at them under the microscope and found that although the structure was retained, the collagen was totally acellular. Clearly, the writing was on the wall. Within three years, when everyone else was just getting into homografts, it was clear to us that these valves were not going to be a permanent solution. We had hoped that the valves would be repopulated by the patient's own cells, and I am still intrigued that they don't.

Even Dacron vascular grafts get repopulated in a way. There is something in the tissue of the homograft that wouldn't let it repopulate, so we were getting primary tissue failure, decellularization, and lack of collagen replacement—in other words, rejection.

We had been using slightly viable, but not really fresh, truly living tissue. There were only two possible prospects. One method would be to use living tissue from a donor and follow a protocol of permanent immunosuppression, much like a kidney transplant. The other choice would be to use living autologous tissue, so we tried making valves out of the patient's own pericardium, but that didn't work very well.

Next, along with the workers in Leeds we tried making valves out of the patient's fascia lata taken from the thigh, but they really didn't work either. Our conclusion was that the valve had to be not only the patient's living tissue but also had to be of the same or identical structure.

The structure of the aortic valve is unique with its three layers and ability to stretch radially and circumferentially. You can't simulate it with anything else. Everyone has two kidneys and only one aortic valve, but the pulmonary valve is almost identical. If you look at it, it looks like a thin filmy structure that would never work at systemic pressure.

However, there was experimental work by Lower and Shumway that showed that when they put a dog's pulmonary valve into the descending aorta, the valve would thicken up but remain intact. Clearly, it did work under aortic pressure, and we began thinking of using the pulmonary valve as an aortic valve substitute. One could argue that it is logical since during embryological development the aortic and pulmonary valves arise from a common truncus, so their tissues are identical initially. They also develop under the same pressure in the foetus.

It is one thing to say all of that, but to do it was another matter. I suppose I was confident and cocky, and we decided after some thought and deliberation to go ahead and do it without doing animal experiments. One of the things that had held up open-heart surgery was the feeling that a procedure had to be done first in dogs. Dogs have a notorious risk with cardiac procedures, and it is much easier to get survivors in patients than in dogs. I remember someone asking Denton Cooley, "Why haven't you done this in dogs?" He replied, "Because dogs die." Anyway, by that time we had a lot of experience replacing aortic valves. There was, however, a question as to whether the pulmonary valve would stand the sudden change from low pulmonary pressure to high systemic pressure. The day we did the first pulmonary autograft, we stood back and waited to see if the cusps would tear. Of course, they didn't tear and one has never torn, as far as I know. We put the pulmonary valve in the subcoronary position and used an aortic valve homograft to reconstruct the pulmonary outflow tract. That was in 1967. Most of the time we used coronary perfusion for myocardial protection, so we were working with a beating heart. One has to get into the rhythm of the heartbeat. I think Magdi Yacoub still does it now and then just to impress people. I suspect coronary perfusion is still one of the best methods of protecting the myocardium, and we used it. We use cardioplegia now, just antegrade through the coronaries. We did the first operations with beating hearts and placed the valve in the subcoronary position. The first 271 patients were all subcoronary, and the long-term results have been good. I think the first patient is still alive, more than thirty years later.

It was about that time that we did one of the first heart transplants in Europe, and that was also an exciting time. Chris Barnard was my colleague from medical school and was then in Cape Town and doing some really good cardiac surgery. He had some of the best results with total correction of tetralogy of Fallot and was a top-ranking cardiac surgeon. Every year he went to the States to meetings, just as I feel that I should go once or twice a year just to keep abreast, talk to colleagues, and so forth. On these trips he would come through London for a few days. He came for two reasons: He used to like to say hello and visit me in the Heart Hospital, but also because the nurses in the Heart Hospital were very pretty, and he would take them out a lot. He would also come in and nose around in the operating room and ask, "Why do you do this, that, and the other?" We were great friends.

I remember his coming through one time and he said, "You know, I have been watching Shumway's people doing heart transplants in dogs. God! I have got to do that." We chatted about transplants and other things, and I forgot all about the conversation. At that time, we were doing heart transplants in dogs. Everybody knew one could do experimental heart transplants, as it is not a difficult technique, but we didn't have immunosuppressives or anything else. We were all at about the same level of experience. We knew Shumway had the biggest experimental surgical experience and was beginning to put heart transplant techniques on a scientific basis. My friend Barnard went back to Cape Town determined that he was going to do a patient. About that same time a reporter asked me, "When do you think the first human heart transplant will be done?" I replied that I thought it would be within the next few years. Barnard did the first heart transplant a month later, and that was the beginning of really great excitement. All that was needed was for someone to light a match and we would all burst into flames. It was an excitement the likes of which I have never seen in surgery before or since. Not just in surgery, but the media and the public were carried away. Chris Barnard's picture was on the cover of *Time* magazine. It was, however, the end of his surgical career. He turned into a playboy overnight and never looked back. He never did anything useful after that.

I was caught up in the excitement of having done a transplant and the chap was initially doing well, so Chris and I used to go to meetings together. The media was all over Chris; he was the surgical success of the century, but that was the end of his surgical practice. He married a beautiful lady, got a lot of money, and was in the news all the time. He settled down at last and lived in Cape Town until he died two years ago. He had a restaurant and a lot of interests in various things, but not in surgery. The story about his having arthritis in his hands was just a news story. He didn't have any problems eating and drinking with his hands. He had no more aches and pains than I have, I think. His brother Marius, who is also a physician, is now a politician and has nothing to do with surgery. He never really was a surgeon, but Chris made him into one by sending him to Cooley for about a month, and he came back as a "heart surgeon," but his heart really wasn't in it. I think he has given up surgery altogether.

Our first heart transplant was done at the National Heart Hospital in London, and the patient lived for three months before dying of multiple pulmonary emboli. We actually knew so little then, we were telephoning one another, Cooley, DeBakey, or Barnard, all over the world. We really didn't know what to do. We didn't know how to evaluate or treat rejection. We had steroids and Imuran, which we overused, and then we had infections. We lost our patient and then everyone else started losing their patients as well. I had made a decision to try to do three transplants, to be sure whether we were on the right or wrong track. It was a great disappointment when our first patient died. The second patient also died.

By that time there was tremendous public reaction against transplants, and we began receiving vitriolic mail, telegrams, and threats. The controversy concerned brain death and various moral and religious issues. I still have a lot of slides of the headlines and articles in the paper, which would shock you if you saw them. After the death of the second patient, we did the third patient at Guy's Hospital. He did quite well at first because, by then, we knew a lot more. All of us realized that the excitement was over, and it was now time to settle down to real science. At that time most people gave it up. I certainly gave it up deliberately and have never gone back because now it is in the hands of experts. My colleague Magdi Yacoub has done more heart transplants than anyone else in the world, so there was no point in our playing around with it. It was quite an exciting time.

During the 1960s, we had a nice spread of cases—congenital, valve, and some coronary problems. Coronary patients were not flooding the market in those days, so we did a lot of congenital work and a lot of tetralogy of Fallot patients. The Fallot problems became more and more complex as people sent more desperate cases to us. We found that we did not have a good procedure for hypoplastic pulmonary vessels and pulmonary atresia other than a patch of pericardium. What was missing was an outflow tract with a valve in it, and we had plenty of those. We tried one of these in a pulmonary atresia patient and, as sometimes happens with the first case, the outcome was brilliant. That case went very well and we reported it. That was the beginning of right ventricular reconstruction surgery, which spread all over the world. It opened up a whole nest of problems associated with pulmonary atresia and hypoplastic vessels. In fact, it has left me behind and has now gone over to the paediatric cardiac surgeons.

When I first became a consultant, Guy's Hospital sent me on a three-month sabbatical tour of America. Lillehei was still the number one man, and Kirklin was a very impressive surgeon. Kirklin made us all think, and I would say that was his major contribution. I also visited Albert Starr in Oregon and Cooley in Houston. I remember going first to Minneapolis to visit Lillehei and it was like a circus. There was a large gallery in the operating room with about fifty people. People were rushing in and rushing out. They started about seven or eight in the morning and Lillehei came in about eleven. The operating room was chaos with pipes and tubes everywhere. The patient did very well, but, I thought, I don't know if I could do this sort of surgery with so much confusion.

From Lillehei, I went by bus to the Mayo Clinic to visit Kirklin. He and Lillehei were great rivals in those days. Walking into Kirklin's operating room was like walking into a church; there was no sound, no excitement. We sort of sat in pews watching him as he quietly talked. The door opened, the heart-lung machine was wheeled in and connected to the patient, and he then did the operation. I was dumbfounded that you could do this very complex procedure so quietly with no drama. That was a very important lesson for me. Brock had been my teacher up until then, and he was a very noisy and dramatic operator. Kirklin was cool and calm. I learned a lot from him in that respect. I also learned a great deal from Cooley. He makes things look easy because he doesn't mess around. Some surgeons fuss around, pick up things, and put them down. I learned from Cooley just to do it as simply as possible. This was an important lesson. He was very fast, but everyone realized that it wasn't because he was in a hurry at all, he just didn't play around.

We had an Indian trainee who had a motto of K.I.S.S: Keep it simple, keep it safe. His name is Solomon Victor and he works in Madras. He is a very dedicated man and I admire him very much and visit him quite often. He has a hospital there of which he is both surgeon and administrator, which he runs on a divided basis: Half of the treatment is free and the other half of the patients pay. The paying side subsidizes the nonpaying. He is a Christian man, dedicated to cardiac surgery, and he has made many contributions. He has a comparative anatomy museum called the Donald Ross Museum. He is very clever with photography showing embryological development and has hearts of snakes, frogs, fish, elephants, you name it. His wife also trained with us at the Heart Hospital and is now in charge of the AIDS treatment program in that eastern part of India.

For aortic valve replacement there are now several choices: a prosthetic valve, a homograft valve, a xenograft valve, or the autograft valve. I can't visualize many indications for a prosthetic valve. I am not entirely prejudiced, but I can't accept it because the valve is so abnormal, so rigid. I am not downgrading them, as they have saved thousands of lives, but they are not acceptable in my sense of the word. They have to be rigid in order to accommodate the various discs, flaps, or balls. Once you put a rigid ring into a contractile orifice such as the aortic or mitral, you splint a certain amount of adjacent contractile muscle in doing so. There is also a gradient and turbulence, and as everyone knows, you then need anticoagulation. Anticoagulation is like a sword of Damocles. Certainly it can be used in an emergency, and I wouldn't hesitate to use it when there was nothing else available, but I am a biological valve man.

The term "bioprosthesis" is quite a good term, because these valves are not wholly biological but are halfway between the two. You have a rigid mounting ring with a biological valve-closing mechanism inside. You get some of the advantages of the biological valve and the disadvantages of the prosthetic valves. One advantage is that it is easy to sew in place. I like to say that the mechanical valve was designed with the surgeon in mind, not the patient. Take it off the shelf, sew it in, go off and play golf. It is a compromise between the true biological valve, which is either a homograft or an autograft, and the mechanical valve.

One disadvantage of the homograft is that

it does not last forever. You are not going to use a homograft in children since the valve will last only fifteen years, if you are lucky. If you are dealing with someone who is seventy you would say, "Why use an autograft since it is a long and complex operation?" A homograft is going to last your lifetime, especially since the rate of tissue failure slows down as you get older.

When I introduced the autograft we thought there should be clearly defined criteria. The patients should be young adults between twenty and thirty years of age, with at least twenty to thirty years of life ahead of them. That was, of course, before the operation was a success and generally accepted. However, it has been used in much younger patients and also older, as far up as age seventy. The ideal age now is thirty to forty years. I am amazed, astounded, and impressed that it has been done in a one-day-old child. At one meeting they told me about an unborn child, diagnosed with aortic stenosis by transuterine echocardiography. As soon as it was born they operated and put in an autograft. I think that is pushing things too far, but interesting.

I have also been told of patients as old as seventy having an autograft. They are wonderful valves, but for older patients a homograft or xenograft valve may be appropriate. You have to match your patient to what you have and what you think he needs. Some people at forty are old and some at eighty are young.

We started placing homografts and autografts in the subcoronary position, but now most people use the root replacement operation. You have to know how to do the subcoronary procedure properly to avoid problems. Most people don't have the competence or the patience to do the subcoronary operation well. They took up the operation and then said it was not a good operation because the valve leaks. It is not the valve's fault, it is their lack of surgical expertise. The root replacement is easier for the less-experienced surgeon to do, but none of this surgery should be done by amateurs.

It is important to remember that the aortic valve is surrounded by structures which offer support; the left ventricular outflow tract musculature and the fibrous tissue anchors the mitral valve. The proximal suture line of the new root must be placed in this same location so that it will have additional support. If the aorta is divided more distally and the proximal suture line is placed distal to the aortic root, when the new valve is subjected to systemic pressure it does not have the support it once had, and it may dilate and leak. The annulus has been moved to a position where it is unsupported. It is not the fault of the operation; it is a fault of the surgical technique.

There are also some ill-defined diseases that have an inborn tendency to develop dilatation of the aortic root. We all know about Marfan's and we would not do an autograft on a patient with Marfan's, but there are others, like ankylosing spondylitis and lupus, in which the autograft should not be used.

Today aortic valve surgery has a surprisingly low mortality when compared to fifteen or twenty years ago. James Oury reported one hundred autograft operations without a death. Many years ago Dwight McGoon at the Mayo Clinic reported one hundred consecutive aortic valve replacement operations without a death. That was because he was a well-trained surgeon working with a very professional group. Strangely enough, the mortality of the autograft operation is very low in most surgical centers. This is, in part, due to the advances in myocardial protection that have developed from coronary bypass work. The time of aortic cross-clamp is no longer the problem it once was. The other thing, of course, is that when you put in a normal valve, the heart "jumps with joy." The initial response of the heart to the autograft is very satisfying.

One of the recent trends in cardiac surgery has been the introduction of minimally invasive surgery. I am not sure if this is here to stay. Maybe I am just too old, but I think it is a gimmick. I was brought up with the view that one should see clearly what one is doing. You could say that our incisions are too long, and I agree they probably are. If you are just going to do a simple LAD bypass, then there are indications for a small incision and an off-pump procedure, but putting in aortic valves through small portholes doesn't appeal to me.

When I first described the autograft operation, I thought it would be useful for both aortic and mitral valve disease, so when we started we did about eight patients in whom we took the pulmonary valve, put it in a short Dacron sleeve, and then placed it in the mitral position. We then became so involved with aortic valve replacement and its problems that we left the mitral autograft alone and decided to use homografts on stents for mitral valve replacement. At one time we tried replacing the mitral valve with a mitral homograft, but had a lot of trouble with ruptured chordae, so we soon gave that up, but there has been some interest in reevaluating the pulmonary autograft in the mitral position. I have tried to get a follow-up on those first patients with a mitral autograft that we did in 1967. This is very difficult after thirty years with patients scattered all over the world, and some have died. We found one that I had operated on fourteen years before for endocarditis. The valve looked fine except that it had a small healed hole through it. I should have just patched it, but I took it out and replaced it. We found another one that I had done when the patient was eleven years old. She was doing well fourteen years later, but had been referred to another cardiologist and now could no longer be located. A third patient had been treated successfully for endocarditis ten years later, but now is lost to follow-up. Most of the patients were lost to follow-up, but it did seem that the pulmonary autograft in the mitral position might be a useful procedure, especially for children and young people with rheumatic mitral disease.

These days, I often go to operate in Syria, where I have a colleague who is very interested in the mitral problem. Together we have tried the autograft in the mitral position in a number of patients, and so far they are doing fine. The technique is to take the pulmonary autograft, mount it in a short Dacron tube, and put it in the mitral position with a single suture line. Since it could pop back into the atrium, I put a new floor in the left atrium, either pericardium or Dacron. Once the pulmonary autograft has been excised, you hand it to your assistant, who sews it in the Dacron tube with a two-suture-line technique incorporating the pericardium or Dacron. He does this while you repair the pulmonary outflow tract with a homograft conduit. The Dacron tube is then fixed in the mitral position. It is a really neat operation. My colleague Magdi Yacoub gave it the name "Top Hat," and it stabilizes the valve.

I enjoy going to Syria, which is a very interesting part of the world. I also go to Egypt where I operated with my team in the military hospital, and we had a great time. Other areas where I have operated in the past years include Nairobi, in Kenya, where I established a unit, and centres in Europe, India, Japan, South America, et cetera, particularly where rheumatic disease is still common.

Bibliography

Lower RR, Stofer RC, Shumway NE. Autotransplantation of the Pulmonic Valve into the Aorta. *J Thorac Cardiovasc Surg.* 1960; 39:680–687.

Ross DN. Homograft Replacement of the Aortic Valve. *Lancet.* 1962; 2:487.

Ross DN, Somerville J. Correction of Pulmonary Atresia with a Homograft Aortic Valve. *Lancet.* 1966; 2(7479):1446–1447.

Ross DN. Replacement of Aortic and Mitral Valves with Pulmonary Autograft. *Lancet.* 1967; 2(7523):956–958.

Ross DN. Biologic valves. Their Performance and Prospects. *Circulation.* 1972; 45:1259–1272.

Okita Y, Franchosi G, Malsuki O,Robles A, Ross DN. Early and Late Results of Aortic Root Replacement with an Antibiotic Sterilized Aortic Homograft. *J Thorac Cardiovasc Surg.* 1988; 95:696–704.

Ross DN. Reflections on the Pulmonary Autograft. *J Heart Valve Dis.* 1993; 2:363–364.

Ross DN. Aortic Root Replacement with a Pulmonary Autograft—Current Trends. *J Heart Valve Dis.* 1994; 3:358–360.

Chambers JC, Somerville J, Stone S, Ross DN. Pulmonary Autograft Procedure for Aortic Valve Disease: Long-Term Results of the Pioneer Series. *Circulation.* 1997; 96:2206–2214.

Elkins RC. The Ross Operation: A 12-Year Experience. *Ann Thorac Surg.* 1999; 68:S14–S18.

George J. Magovern, MD

(b. 1923)

Dr. Kent said to me, "You know, we really need something that would get the valve seated in a hurry." Myocardial protection did not exist then. The sutureless valve made a huge difference in our survival rate. We had had a 50 to 60 percent mortality rate with the early aortic valve replacement operations, but with the sutureless valve, we did nineteen patients and had eighteen survivors.

— On the development of the sutureless valve

Interviewed September 4, 1997

I grew up in Brooklyn. I have heard that approximately sixty-four languages are spoken now in Brooklyn, and I have heard all of them, I think. Brooklyn has changed, and so has cardiac surgery.

My career was influenced by the local family doctors, Dr. McLaughlin and Dr. Young. Also, my sister developed a rare type of bovine tuberculous infection of the knee after she spent some time out of the country. This stimulated my interest in medicine, and I just always wanted to be a physician. No one forced me into it, but my mother was really very conscious of the fact that people respect physicians; they occupy an elevated position in the community. My older brother and I were both encouraged to go into medicine, and so we both became physicians. One of my early memories is of my uncle, who was an intern at Bellevue. He used to come over and visit us, and one time he came over because he happened to be on the ambulance when the gangster Dutch Schultz was murdered in one of the gangland affairs in New York City. My uncle was kind of a hero to us.

I went to prep school in New York City. When World War II came, I joined the V-12 program. I spent a short time at Manhattan College, and then I went to Union College in Schenectady, New York. Schenectady at that time was the home of General Electric, so Union College was mainly an engineering school. Being there was a great experience, and the navy then got me accepted into medical school while I was a premed student. We got through the entire premed program in two years and then the medical school program in three years. We were able to get through college and medical school in five years.

I had applied to Columbia and was accepted to start in January, but the navy wanted me to go to Marquette because I could start earlier, in August. I wasn't about to tell my commander that that wasn't where I wanted to go, so I went, and it was a very good experience. We had a wonderful faculty; among them were Dr. Beckman, who had written a pharmacology book, and Dr. Quick, the biochemistry teacher, who had invented the Quick prothrombin test.

I came home in 1947 and went to Kings County Hospital, which is now Downstate. At the time the Long Island College of Medicine ran a division at that hospital. I went to the Long Island College division, and while there as an intern I scrubbed on an atrial appendectomy for a woman who had had recurrent thromboemboli. Charlie Bailey at that time was brave enough to put his finger

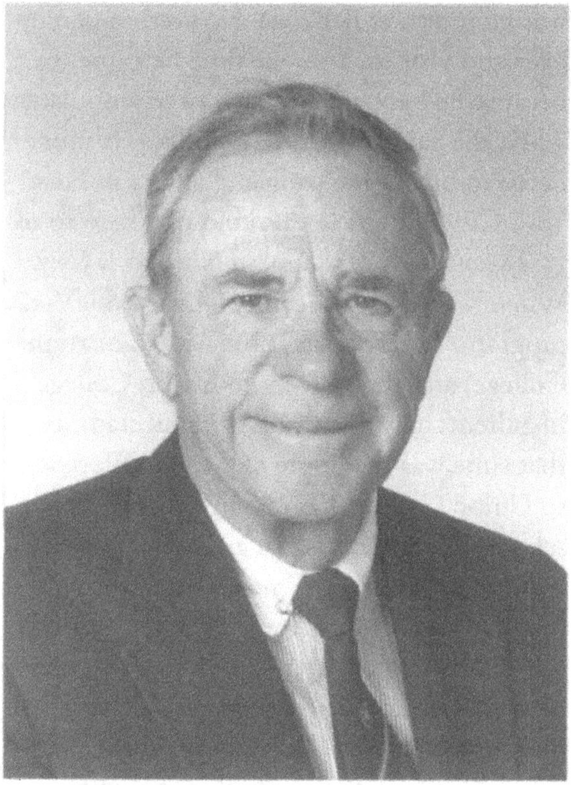

George J. Magovern

into the left atrium. We were only brave enough to put a clamp on it, cut it off, and oversew it. That was done by John Madden, who eventually became a well-known general surgeon and who has written a couple of books about that.

During the last year of my training, Clarence Dennis transferred to Downstate from the University of Minnesota and became the chairman of the department. He brought along with him his heart-lung machine, which was the size of a small refrigerator. Clarence had done the first open-heart surgery using a heart-lung machine, but the patient did not survive. This was two years prior to Dr. Gibbon's first successful case.

Clarence Dennis's heart-lung machine oxygenator had a large round screen, and the blood came into a manifold at the top. It spread out over the screen, and a little motor kept the screen rotating. Oxygen was blown in to arterialize the blood directly. It had a limited surface area with four screens, adequate for young people, for congenital heart disease, atrial septal defects and that sort of thing. To take the heart machine apart, clean it, put in the solutions, siliconize it, and put it all back together took a lot of time, so we could only do one case per week. Dr. Dennis did do three or four cases with it. He put people on it with acute myocardial infarction, on a temporary basis to get them over the period of hypotension. That oxygenator had some serious problems, a lot of hemolysis, and consumption of most of the coagulation products, so the patients had a lot of postoperative problems.

I was a house officer during that time, and I stayed on as an instructor in surgery. I finished my training after the Korean War ended, but I was still on the call list, so I went back in the service. I was sent to the Medical Field Service School in Fort Sam Houston and the Brook Army General Hospital in San Antonio. Based on my experience, they made me an instructor, and I worked at the burn unit of the surgical research division. That had an effect on my career later when I was chairman of the Department of Surgery at Allegheny, where one of the doctors in plastic surgery wanted to start a burn unit. I had seen the tremendous time and resources that it took to take care of burn patients, and I convinced the hospital that it would be better to go into cardiac work instead of burn work. I think that was the right decision.

During my general surgery training, I had met Clarence Dennis and Max Chamberlain, both thoracic surgeons on our faculty. I also met a man in Texas, Larry Schiffs, who had trained at the Barnes Hospital. When I expressed an interest in thoracic surgery, he called a friend of his, Brian Blades, to see if I could get into his thoracic surgery training program. My wife was skeptical about my taking two more years of training, but she eventually agreed, and we went to Washington, D.C., for two years of thoracic surgery at George Washington University.

George Washington was mainly doing closed mitral commissurotomies, but we also got a tremendous amount of thoracic experience. Brian Blades had done a lot of the original work on the anatomy of the lobes and was an early proponent of segmental resections and lobar resections, so we had a lot of patients. The most difficult part of that rotation was the six months that we spent at the Glendale Sanitarium, a tuberculosis resource for the District of Columbia. This was before streptomycin and all the other treatments for TB that later came about. It was difficult surgery, lobectomies for cavitary tuberculosis, invariably the upper lobe and part of the superior segment of the lower lobe, and thoracoplasty.

The George Washington residents went to Children's Hospital of Pittsburgh in their second year of training for their pediatric cardiac surgical experience. Dr. Kent was the chairman, but I also met a man, Don Fisher, who worked at Allegheny General. He was a pediatric cardiologist by training, but he had also become involved with adult patients and was the first in the United States to do percutaneous left heart catheterizations, a unique procedure. Don had the habit of coming to work from 11:00 A.M. until 11:00 P.M. My wife had stayed in Washington because we had a newborn, so I really had nothing to do in the evenings, and I hung around with Don. He advised Dr. Kent and Dr. Harbison to ask me to stay on after my training, which I did.

Left and right catheterization was unique because we did it under fluoroscopy, with glasses so dark you could barely see. There was no image intensifier, just the old fluoroscopy. We stuck long 18-gauge needles in through the back, at about the fifth posterior interspace. Under fluoroscopy we would guide them, and one of the landmarks was to aspirate a little air from the esophagus; then you knew you were on the right track. The needle went right through the esophagus and into the left atrium. Then we got a little bit more vigorous, and we would go into the left atrium and the right atrium, so we would have two needles. We would put two needles into the left side and thread a very fine polyurethane catheter through the needle and into the left atrium. A second catheter went into the left ventricle. We would insert blue dye into the left ventricle and at the same time aspirate blood from the left atrium, and that way we could estimate the degree of mitral insufficiency wonderfully well. It was a dilution technique in which we drew blood and then let it settle out. The plasma of course was blue, and we had fixed controls that we compared it to and graded it one to four plus. It was very helpful in deciding which patients to operate on. Then they would do a finger fracture for mitral stenosis, which caused a murmur you could hear. We found that at three plus mitral insufficiency the finger fracture didn't improve the patient very much. Our best results were in patients in whom the valve was not leaking too badly, and this test allowed for patient selection quite well.

Eventually they began to do the Devilla repair, which involved a long umbilical tape and a long curved needle. We put the patient on bypass, although we didn't open the heart, and externally we would thread this suture with the umbilical tape in the mitral valve, very close to the left coronary and the circumflex. That was the tricky part of it. The operator would put his finger into the left atrium, as you would for a commissurotomy, and then the other surgeon would tie down the suture to the point at which you could no longer feel the leakage coming back. We did that right at the junction of the atrium and the ventricle—a really vascular place. In most cases we probably did not put it in the right place, because most of these acted like a seton in a rectal fistula. We found that after several years the insufficiency usually came back, and the umbilical tape or suture was mostly inside the atrium. We were probably putting it close to the mitral valve but on the atrial aspect of it. It was not an operation that stood the test of time, but it was the one I learned as a young trainee.

We were doing some atrial septal defect repairs as well, but we used the Gross well, which was a funnel, large at the top, coming down to a smaller opening at the bottom. We clamped the right atrial appendage, cut it off, and then sewed the well to the atrium. We then took the clamp off, and the blood would well up in the latex well. With long instruments we could feel the ASD, and then through the blood field we could try to repair it. It worked reasonably well for small secundum defects, but anything more complicated than that was not feasible. We couldn't patch them, and closing them was cumbersome. The needle holder was long, and we worked by feel. I think we perforated our own fingers as much as we perforated the tissue. That was the only way you could feel where you were.

When I first arrived in Pittsburgh, the people at the Allegheny Hospital were doing a huge number of mitral commissurotomies. We had almost as many rheumatic adult patients as we did carcinoma of the lung, which was still very common. Hiatal hernia patients were also common. The Allegheny General Hospital is a private hospital, and when I first arrived, Allegheny and the University of Pittsburgh Presbyterian Hospital had a combined training program. The chairman of the Department of Thoracic Surgery at the university was also the chairman of the department at the hospitals. This was Dr. Ed Kent, a real pioneer. He and Brian Blades had trained together at Barnes under Evarts Graham. He was also president of the AATS and on its board. Ed was the most dexterous person I have ever met. He was truly ambidextrous, a wonderful surgeon, and he treated me like a son and made a big difference in my career. A philosophical difference came about when Hank Bahnson arrived at the university as chairman of the Department of Surgery. The Hopkins tradition had been that general surgery and thoracic surgery were one department, but when Ed Kent was trained at Barnes, thoracic surgery was a separate discipline. We divided the program into two. General surgery remained at the University of Pittsburgh Hospital, and a separate thoracic surgery training program was started at Allegheny General.

Allegheny General is a unique place that has grown phenomenally. When I went there, it had a tremendous endowment for a private hospital, $300 or $400 million, which had been gifts from a lot of steel barons. I had a thoracic surgery lab over at the University of Pittsburgh Hospital, and when they asked me to come over to Allegheny as chairman in 1970, I said, "OK, provided you get me a research lab." That's the only reason I went there. I had worked there with Dr. Fisher and others during my residency, so it was not a radical move. Allegheny is now an eight- or nine-hundred bed hospital, and it has thirteen separate, independent residency training programs. Only four years ago, it became the Allegheny University of Health Sciences when it acquired Hahnemann Medical School and the Medical College of Pennsylvania, and, more recently, the graduate hospital system. It's bigger now in Philadelphia than it is in Pittsburgh. The entire system in the Delaware valley is twenty-three hospitals, and in Pittsburgh alone we have a six-hospital system. It's probably one of the largest private medical universities in the country now.

We were doing aortic and mitral valves, but the mitral valve repair was not satisfactory. Al Starr had just begun to work on his valve around 1960, and everybody was interested in a new heart valve. We put in the first of the sutureless valves in 1962. In 1961 Al Starr had put in his first valve, but we had started working on a valve in 1959. There were many different types of valves in the beginning. We had an ordinary trileaflet Silastic valve, but, unfortunately, unless each leaflet on the valve is exactly the same depth and resistance, we found that one leaflet would open constantly while the other two just sat there; then a clot would form. We worked on a silicone valve and a Silastic mitral valve. The latter was a single leaflet, a flap with a hinge. It was interesting how easy it was to make. We had two Lucite plates, put the Dacron in between them, and then used Lucite glue; we didn't have to sew it on. We had other great ideas, but none of them worked too well. We also had a bileaflet valve with a hinge in the center. Then we got the idea that if you had carbon and a negative charge, it would reduce embolus, so we added carbon to the silicone rubber.

Dr. Kent had said to me, "George, if we could only get these patients off the heart-lung machine faster, we probably would have less pulmonary complications, and we would be able to get a better survival rate." Of course he was still doing aortic commissurotomy by sewing a tube of bovine pericardium onto the ascending aorta and then putting his finger down through it as you would through a purse string, and digitally fracturing it. Charles Bailey and others had a dilator that you put in through the apex of the ventricle. The supra-aortic approach worked reasonably well, but if you got into any problems and the bypass was prolonged, the patients developed a number of pulmonary complications. There were no ventilators. We would leave in the endotracheal tubes, and a resident would sit there the entire night and ventilate for them by squeezing the bag of an anesthesia machine.

Dr. Kent said to me, "You know, we really need something that would get the valve seated in a hurry." He said, "You will be doing surgery all your life, why don't you forget about it for now and go over to the lab and develop a valve?" Can you imagine? He provided the complete stimulus. I said, "OK, if that's what you need, that's what we'll try to do." We did begin to develop some new valves at the University of Pittsburgh at that time. The first thing we did in the lab was to put in a little serrated valve of Silastic.

We just pushed it down into the aortic position. We put the serrated valve in there and sutured around it to hold it in place. It had pins, a bit like the old Hufnagel device, but internal pins. Then we got the idea that maybe the Silastic would do well. This was a mitral valve. We just took the Silastic valve and put Michelle clips on it, and then we would close the Michelle clips on the mitral annulus to hold it in place. This was all done with dogs. There was leakage in between clips, so it didn't work exceptionally well. We were trying to develop a sutureless valve.

Things were a little discouraging at this point. I was working with one man who knew how to make the dies for Silastic, but then we got into the concept of some kind of mechanical valve. I was driving home one evening and I stopped in at a little machine shop, Pennsylvania Alloy Machine. I went in and told them I was interested in getting a mechanical valve made. I showed them some drawings, but the shop owner didn't seem too interested because he had no idea how many of these we would be able to sell. One of his machinists was standing by listening, and after our conversation was over the machinist said, "Doctor, I think I can help you if would like to work on that, but I can't do it in this shop." We purchased some equipment for his garage, a lathe and some other things, and we started coming up with concepts of how to make a sutureless valve. His name was Harry Cromie.

The initial one had teeth coming out in a horizontal plane, and it fit reasonably well into the aortic position. It had a ball valve, and it was streamlined, but the streamlining actually contributed to thromboembolism rather than preventing it. The ball was in the cage, and you could retract the teeth. We would then turn the inner circle in the annulus, and the teeth would go in and out. After we had them properly fixed, there was a little screw that you tightened with an Allen wrench so that you could fix them in place and lock it.

The single plane didn't seem to do the trick, so we thought more fixation points were needed. We went to a double layer of teeth coming out. They were very sharp, and we would fix them in position once they were in place. The concept that really worked was the idea of the teeth coming out in a vertical plane. This was a very difficult valve to make because it was all titanium, and at the time you could not mold titanium; it had to be machined from a solid block of titanium. It was expensive to make, and it took a while. It had a disc rather than a ball. We had both, but the disc seemed to work better because it didn't occupy so much space in the ventricle. It had a central cylinder with a right-handed thread on the upper aspect and a left-handed thread below. If you held the valve at the external part and turned the cylinder, the two plates would approximate, and as they did they would project out teeth which grabbed the tissue.

It worked remarkably well. The mitral was the first sutureless valve, coming first because the design lent itself to the mitral valve and there were alternatives for the aortic valve. We put these in many patients, and sometimes we did not excise the mitral valve leaflet. This practice has come back now.

In 1962 the valve cost about $300, relatively expensive because the Starr valve could be molded at a much lower cost, about $8. They were selling them for the fantastic price of maybe $500. I think that still goes on today.

Clinically, the most successful valve we designed was the sutureless aortic valve. The first group were not totally cloth-covered; they had Teflon on top of the titanium. With the mitral valve, you could put the valve in, and the ball was in the cage. The problem with the aortic valve was how to get that valve in there with the mechanism to fix it, and yet the ball was not in it. If the ball was not in there, it was easier on the aortic side because it was a straight shot down. When we made the opening of the aorta, you could go right down into the aortic ring, and when you turned the valve, the two plates would come together and the teeth would come out and grip at the same time. After the teeth are out and fixed in place, we would push on the bayonet, turn it, and release it. That's how the teeth held it. Then you would take the ball and just insert it into the cage.

That design turned out to have several serendipitous advantages. Because we had to push the ball in, we had an open cage at the top, so we had less thromboembolism from that. We also had to make the ball a bit softer so that you could squeeze it in between the struts of the cage. The result was that we had better clearance than the Starr valve. We cured the ball differently; it was less hard. As a result, the ball didn't absorb cholesterol and serum in the postop period. With the Starr valve, that was a major problem, because it produced ball variance. The ball would get too big for the cage, and the cage cut through the ball after a while. We had no ball variance, and at first people couldn't believe it. We sent the valve over to Carnegie Mellon and had it analyzed, and we found that the degree of absorption of the body fluid into the Silastic was much less than in a Starr valve. We didn't have any major problems with variance; it was not a major concern with us.

At that time, if a patient was on bypass for more than forty-five minutes, things started to fall apart. For example, the lungs would fail. We were able to take out the bad valve, insert the new valve and anchor it, very quickly. I remember doing an aortic insufficiency case, and the total cross-clamp time—from the time we opened it, did the aortotomy, put the valve in, and closed the aortotomy—was twenty minutes. It made a tremendous difference. Myocardial protection did not exist. All we did was put in potassium to stop the heart. The valve made a huge difference in our survival rate. We had had a 50 to 60 percent mortality rate with the early aortic valve replacement operations, but with the sutureless valve, we did nineteen patients and had eighteen survivors.

That set the whole thing off. The valves were used all over the world. Mr. Cromie formed a company called Surgitool, and it was the largest valve company in the world. There weren't very many valves at that time, but his company was the largest. He made new valve designs for Denton Cooley, Christiaan Barnard, Mike DeBakey, and Arthur Beall. All of them had their own valve made at Surgitool. Eventually the company was acquired by Baxter, so we lost another industry in Pittsburgh. We lost steel, but we should have held onto the medical device industry. That would have been quite helpful.

We had a reunion of people who had had this valve put in. The valve had to be in place for twenty-five years. About forty-five people showed up for the reunion out of about sixty patients who are still walking around with them in western Pennsylvania. Some of them are quite elderly now, and some of them have died of other things.

With minimally invasive cardiac surgery nowadays, it's possible that this concept could be revived, but the valve had some real drawbacks. The biggest problem was that the toothed mechanism takes so much of the outside diameter that the opening is small compared to other valves. At a six- or seven-liter cardiac output, there is probably a twenty-millimeter gradient, which is certainly acceptable. We don't really operate until it is about fifty. I think today people want no gradient across the valve. I'm sure that with refinements and different metals, the concept could be revived and utilized again.

I was still using the sutureless valve as recently as four or five years ago. We had a case as recently as three years ago, a complicated case of bacterial endocarditis on a valve that had been replaced two or three times. There was a huge aortic ring, with nothing you could really sew onto. With the valves we use now, you can approximate the tissue to it when you suture it, but with the sutureless valve, you have to have six or seven sizes because the valve has to fit the aortic annulus. We reached back into the cabinet and found a number seven, which was probably built for elephants, I think, and we put it in that huge aortic ring, and the thing caught like mad and saved the day.

At the last count, I personally put in twelve hundred of those sutureless valves, and my associates used a number of them too. I would say that probably twenty to thirty thousand were used worldwide. I had an interesting letter from Dwight McGoon, the premier surgeon at the Mayo Clinic, and he published a report of one hundred consecutive aortic valve replacements. With number forty-nine, they had trouble with the oxygenator and had to get off bypass. They had a sutureless valve, and they put it in and got out; the patient survived. They used ninety-nine Starr valves and one sutureless valve, which kept the series intact. Dr. McGoon was rather grateful to have the continuous one hundred successful cases.

That was a thrilling time. You could try almost any idea, without going through the FDA, and we didn't have much in the way of institutional review boards at that time. Instead we worked heavily in the research lab. I was accused at one point of trying to destroy all the dogs in Pittsburgh, because I was putting valves in so many. It was a very difficult procedure in a dog.

We have been working on myoplasty recently, because of our interest in the ventricular assist devices. We were using muscle wrapped around the left ventricle as an assist device. The problem was fatigue. We couldn't overcome that problem, and I have to give a great deal of credit to the people in Europe, Dr. Carpentier and his group, and the Medtronic Company. Larry Stephenson at the University of Pennsylvania worked on it as well. There were two investigators, Salmons and Streter in England, who showed that the difference between muscle varieties was based more on their electrical stimulation than on the chemotherapeutic agent that was active at the motor end. If you stimulated the muscle at a high frequency, you could convert it from a type-two fiber, which is ordinary skeletal muscle, to a type-one muscle fiber, which is more fatigue resistant. On the basis of that research, Larry Stephenson did a lot of work on the biological ventricular assists, and we got interested in that as well. Then Dr. Carpentier came up with the cardiomyopathy wrap.

We did the first three of our cases without the cardiomyostimulator that Medtronic developed. We just took an AV sequential pacer, and we put the atrial lead on the ventricles to pick up the R wave, and then the ventricular lead was placed around the long thoracic nerve. It worked just as well, except that it was a single stimulus. I think that the experimental work indicated that probably burst stimuli, or multiple stimuli, worked better. In fact, now, ten years later, we're going back to the single bursts because it does the same kind of conversion, except that it does it over a two-month period instead of over six weeks.

I think the future is in using skeletal muscle power. Your eyelid, for example, is rapid muscle, but it fatigues because it is a type-two fiber, whereas your back muscles, which are erect most of the day, are a type-one fiber from being used constantly. The Olympic runner can literally change his fibers so that they become less fatigued. Our research lab is working now on a project where if we stimulate for twelve hours and rest for twelve hours or even six hours or any period, the muscle will not fatigue. If you stimulate constantly, the muscle finally gets to the point at which it enlarges, outgrows its blood supply, and begins to fibrose. With all of the cardiomyoplasties that we have done, the results looked wonderful for the first couple of months, but then not many of them have shown continuous improvement over the long term.

I think that everyone knows that you can train the muscle fiber to do better, but until our protocol is done on two hundred patients, we can't alter it. We are doing a separate protocol on training the fiber and giving it rest periods, and I think those results are going to be much, much better. We are using the latissimus muscle, which you can divide into three segments, and you then have a long, narrow muscle fiber that you can wrap around the aorta three or four times. It works like a ventricular assist device or like an intra-aortic balloon. The muscle contracts during diastole to help propel the blood, so it is diastolic augmentation. One of our former residents, Bob Lazarra, is working on that with Al Starr's group. They use the descending aorta and put the assist just beyond the arch. It is a little tricky because you do have to preserve the intercostals to the blood supply of the spinal cord, but I think this procedure has a place in the future.

Another interesting thing came up with that study. The muscle physiology people have found that in skeletal muscle, you can isolate what they call satellite cells, which lie close to the fibers just under the connective tissue and which produce new myoblasts after muscle injury. We created a cryoinjury on the wall of the left ventricle and injected two billion cultured satellite cells at the injured site. They grow like a weed, so to speak. Over six weeks, and certainly after six months, those satellite cells will develop into myocardial cells. We have the genetic typing to show that a skeletal muscle cell can start out as a satellite, or a very primitive cell, in the cardiac environment, and in that environment it will grow into a myocardial cell. I think there is a big future for the genetic alteration of muscle cells. In Europe, they are using skeletal muscle with a pacemaker around colostomy sites. You can wrap the rectus around the colostomy, and stimulate it to keep it closed. Then when you turn the pacemaker off, it relaxes and the colon can evacuate. They have also treated young people with congenital fecal incontinence, using the gracilis muscle.

I think that the immediate future for cardiac surgery lies in assist devices. We are getting away from the pulsatile devices into a continuous mean flow with a centrifugal pump. They have a big future because there are no valves in them; they just pump the blood, and the peripheral resistance determines the pressure. If it is low, they flow more. We have had experimental animals on a small centrifugal pump with an internal volume of about five cubic centimeters, which takes seven watts of energy, has a single electrical cord that you bring out, and is totally implantable, going from the left atrium to the descending aorta. We are going to get FDA clearance for human application within the next few weeks, and we're excited that we can make it for $500 to $700, in contrast to the $250,000 for the other devices.

I think that implantable devices have to be a major part of cardiac surgery in the future. The government will realize that the amount of money being spent on medical therapy for congestive heart failure is $9 billion a year, just in the United States. Despite all that expense, they've increased the lifespan maybe by a year. The patients feel better for a time, but they don't really live that much longer with medical therapy, so using small implantable devices would be a lot cheaper than all the medical therapy that is going on.

I have two sons who are cardiac surgeons. I grew up in a time when there were so many challenging things we could do; we really did help people. Harvey Bender and I were on the golf course yesterday, in a match with some other fellows, one of whom asked us what we did, and we told him we were cardiac surgeons. He had had mitral insufficiency and a mitral valve ring repair, an annuloplasty. He was out there driving the ball 250 yards, getting eagles and birdies, and everything else. I felt like taking the thing out! I couldn't believe how healthy and strong he was, but he was a good example of how a person's life can be improved. He was in his mid to late fifties, and probably he would not be doing very well otherwise; certainly he would not be out on the golf course.

I think there are a lot of good things going on. I think assist devices will be present in the future. They are learning more and more about vein grafts. One of the big weaknesses of vein bypass now is the ten-year prospects of the vein grafts. There are enzymes available now that can be applied to the vein to prevent the overgrowth of the fibromuscular portion and the neointima formation, so that the grafts will last much longer. They will probably have two- or three-millimeter prosthetic grafts in the future.

Mr. Cromie is still around and perhaps he could work on that. When Baxter took over the company, they kept the development division in Pittsburgh, and Harry worked on the ambulatory dialysis system. Then he worked on a number of devices for administering controlled doses of morphine, self-controlled medications. He has been busy in a number of areas, but he just retired from Baxter. Maybe I can get him to work on something new.

Bibliography

Magovern GJ, Cromie HW. Sutureless Prosthetic Heart Valves. *J Thorac Cardiovasc Surg*. 1963; 46:726–736.

Magovern GJ, Yates A. Human Homotransplantation of Left Lung: Report of a Case. *Ann NY Acad Sciences*. 1964; 120:710–728.

Magovern GJ, Kent EM, Cromie HW, Cushing WB, Scott S. Sutureless Aortic and Mitral Prosthetic Valves. *J Thorac Cardiovasc Surg*. 1964; 48:346–361.

Magovern GJ. Replacement of Aortic and Mitral Valves with Sutureless Prosthesis; Results in 100 Patients. *Dis Chest*. 1966; 50:415–422.

Begg FR, Magovern GJ, Cushing WB, Kent EM, Fisher DL. Selective Cine-coronary Arteriography in Patients with Complete Heart Block. *J Thorac Cardiovasc Surg*. 1969; 57:9–16.

Dixon CM, Magovern GJ. Evaluation of the Biopump for Long-Term Cardiac Support without Heparinization. *J Extracorporeal Tech*. 1982; 14:331–336.

Magovern GJ. How Shall We Then Practice? (Presidential Address). *Ann Thorac Surg*. 1985; 40:103–112.

McGovern GJ, Heckler FR, et al. Paced Latissimus Dorsi Used for Dynamic Cardiomyoplasty of Left Ventricular Aneurysms. *Ann Thorac Surg*. 1987; 44:379–388.

Magovern GJ, Liebler GA, Park SB, Burkholder JA, Sakert T, Simpson K. 25-Year Review of the Magovern-Cromie Sutureless Aortic Valve. *Ann Thorac Surg*. 1989; 48(3 Suppl 3):S33–S34.

Magovern JA, Magovern GJ Jr, Magovern GJ, Palumbi MA, Orie JE. Surgical Therapy for Congestive Heart Failure: Indications for Transplantation Versus Cardiomyoplasty. *J Heart Lung Transplantation*. 1992; 11:538–544.

Savage EB, Clark RE, Griffin WP, Davis SA, Hughson MS, Conway CJ, Magovern GJ Sr. The AB-180 Circulatory Support System: Summary of Development and Plans for Phase I Clinical Trial. *Ann Thorac Surg*. 1999; 68:768–774.

Robert B. Wallace, MD

(b. 1922)

Dr. DeBakey demanded perfection of himself and those who worked with him, and he did not hesitate letting you know when you fell short of his expectations."

— On working for Dr. DeBakey

Interviewed May 5, 2003

I was born in Washington, D.C., and attended public school until high school when I was fortunate to have the opportunity to attend St. Peter's School in New York. I had thought about medicine as a career, although I am not sure what prompted me in this direction. Following graduation from prep school, I was invited to attend tryouts with two major league baseball teams. This was exciting and made me question my career goals, but only for a short time. I had received a scholarship to attend Columbia College, and much to my parents' delight I elected to go to Columbia rather than accepting a minor league offer.

The decision to go to Columbia was one of the better decisions I have made. My brother was a year ahead of me at Columbia, and we had the opportunity to play two seasons of football together under Coach Lou Little, and this experience proved beneficial to me throughout my career. I took a premedical course, but as I approached my senior year, I had real doubts regarding medicine. I finally decided that I would apply to one medical school, the College of Physicians and Surgeons at Columbia, and if accepted I would go to medical school. If not, I would pursue something else. Coach Little took a great deal of interest in those who had played for him, especially those interested in medicine or dentistry, and I am sure that he had a great deal to do with my acceptance at P & S.

I had a difficult time deciding on the field of medicine that most interested me. I had pretty much decided on internal medicine and had completed my applications and interviews for internship in that specialty when I had my first clinical rotation on a surgical service. The chief residents on the service were Drs. Keith Reemtsma and Jim Malm, and they both influenced my decision to pursue a career in surgery. As this was only a week or so before the intern matching deadline, I had to scramble. Dr. David Habiff, my advisor, arranged for me to meet with Dr. Louis Rousselot, who was head of surgery at St. Vincent's Hospital in New York. Fortunately, Dr. Rousselot was a Columbia graduate, and he remembered me from my football days. I did my general surgical training at St. Vincent's. I was unsure as to what surgical subspecialty I wanted to pursue until my third year of residency when Dr. George Morris from Baylor visited St. Vincent's. He spoke about the exciting things that were being done in vascular surgery in Houston and this piqued my interest. With the support of Dr. Dan Mulvehill, a thoracic surgeon at St. Vincent's, I received an appointment to spend one year with Dr. DeBakey and colleagues in Houston. We went to Houston in 1962 with the expectation of returning to St. Vincent's.

The first three months in Houston I

worked with Dr. Stanley Crawford, who I found to be not only an exceptional surgeon but an outstanding individual from whom I learned a great deal. Working initially with Dr. Crawford gave me the opportunity to adjust to the environment at Baylor, which was a bit different from that in New York.

The next three months I worked with Dr. Ed Garrett on Dr. DeBakey's service, and this was a real experience. Dr. DeBakey had a very busy operative service doing eight to ten cases a day. Ed and I spent essentially all of our time in the operating room. The service was also responsible for performing the aortograms and arteriograms. At that time Dr. DeBakey was not doing much cardiac surgery but was doing all types of vascular cases and doing them superbly. He demanded perfection of himself and those who worked with him, and he did not hesitate letting you know when you fell short of his expectations. He could be very intimidating, and it was necessary to develop the attitude that you were going to do your job as best as you could, and let the criticism roll off when it came. There were some who did not get the full benefit of working with Dr. DeBakey because they could not accept his criticism. One had to recognize that his criticism was not personal but more a reflection of his compulsive perfectionist personality.

The residents in Dr. DeBakey's program had tremendous demands placed upon them, especially when they were on his service. The residents on his service generally did not spend time in the operating room but were assigned to work on the floor or the intensive care unit. During the six-week period in the intensive care unit, the resident was expected to be in the hospital at all times; a meal with the family was a meal in the hospital cafeteria. Residents generally accepted this as part of becoming a cardiovascular surgeon, and there was keen competition for positions in the residency.

Dr. DeBakey, out of the hospital and work environment, was a delightful, charming individual, and only those who worked with him could appreciate his dual personality. On the first occasion that we were invited to a reception at the DeBakeys' home, my wife, Betty, was overwhelmed with Dr. DeBakey's charm. As we were leaving, Dr. DeBakey accompanied us to the door, and as we walked away, Betty turned to me and said, "How can you say such things about such a nice man?" She had not spent time with him in the operating room. Over the years I have developed a very good relationship with Dr. DeBakey, as have most of those who trained with him. I have great respect and admiration for his accomplishments and work ethic, and appreciate the opportunity he provided me.

I next spent time working with Dr. Cooley, and that was my first real exposure to cardiac surgery. Dr. Cooley ran a large surgical schedule doing mainly congenital heart cases, but also valve and vascular cases. Valve surgery at that time was mainly mitral valve procedures and aortic valve debridement. With the availability of the Starr valve, replacement became the preferred procedure. Dr. Cooley was one of the best technical surgeons I have ever worked with. He operated with confidence and ease and effortlessly completed operations in a minimum of time, all the while entertaining the many visitors that always seemed to be in the operating room. I enjoyed working with Dr. Cooley and learned a great deal from him; it was he who stimulated my interest in cardiac surgery. Although I had planned to spend only one year in Houston, Dr. Cooley encouraged me to extend my stay and get more experience in cardiac and thoracic surgery so that I might meet the training requirements for the thoracic boards, which I did. It was still my intention to return to New York and develop a program in cardiovascular surgery.

In April 1963 the American Association for Thoracic Surgery met in Houston. Dr. Dan Mulvehill invited me to attend a breakfast which he was having for a group of surgeons. I was seated next to Dr. John Kirklin, which I suspected had been arranged by Dr. Mulvehill. I, of course, knew of the Mayo Clinic and Dr. Kirklin, but didn't know too much about the institution. I had a very pleasant visit with Dr. Kirklin, and he suggested that I might visit the clinic. I was greatly surprised when two days later he telephoned and formally invited me to visit. I had planned a trip to New York to finalize my plans to return there and arranged to spend a couple of days in Rochester on my way to New York. What a surprise it was to find such a huge institution in such a small town. I was greatly impressed and found the environment quite different from that in Houston. Before leaving Rochester, Dr. Kirklin asked me if I would be interested in coming to Rochester and spending a year with him. He indicated that he would design a program that he felt would benefit me and perhaps fill in some of the gaps in my training. I completed my trip to New York, and Dr. Rousselot accepted my spending a year with Dr. Kirklin before returning to New York. Although I knew what I wanted to do, I could not give Dr. Kirklin a definitive answer before talking it over with Betty. It took me a while to broach the subject of another year of training, but, as always, she was supportive. When I finally told Dr. Cooley of my plans, he jokingly asked what I might learn at the Mayo Clinic that I had not already learned from him. Before I left, he did say that he thought that it was an excellent opportunity and that he had the highest respect for Dr. Kirklin.

That year in Rochester was the most educational year I had experienced. I spent most of my time with Dr. Kirklin, and he never stopped teaching. I also worked with Drs. Dwight McGoon, F. H. "Bunky" Ellis, Phil Bernatz, and O. T. "Jim" Clagett, each of whom contributed significantly to my development as a surgeon. I also spent time in the cardiac cath lab with Dr. Jeremy Swan and worked with the pump technicians learning both the complexities of the Mayo-Gibbon pump-oxygenator and the physiology of cardiopulmonary bypass.

When I arrived in Rochester in 1963, the Mayo cardiac surgical service was well established and was well regarded throughout the world, and the individual most responsible was John Kirklin. He grew up in Rochester; his father was a professor of radiology at the Mayo Clinic. He attended the University of Minnesota and Harvard Medical School. His surgical training was at the Mayo Clinic, following which he spent a year in Boston working with Dr. Robert Gross. After a period in the army where he worked primarily as a neurosurgeon, he returned to Rochester. At that time Dr. "Jim" Clagett was the senior thoracic surgeon at the clinic. He had performed one of the first corrections of coarctation of the aorta using the turned-down subclavian artery. He felt that further development of the cardiac surgical program might better be done by a

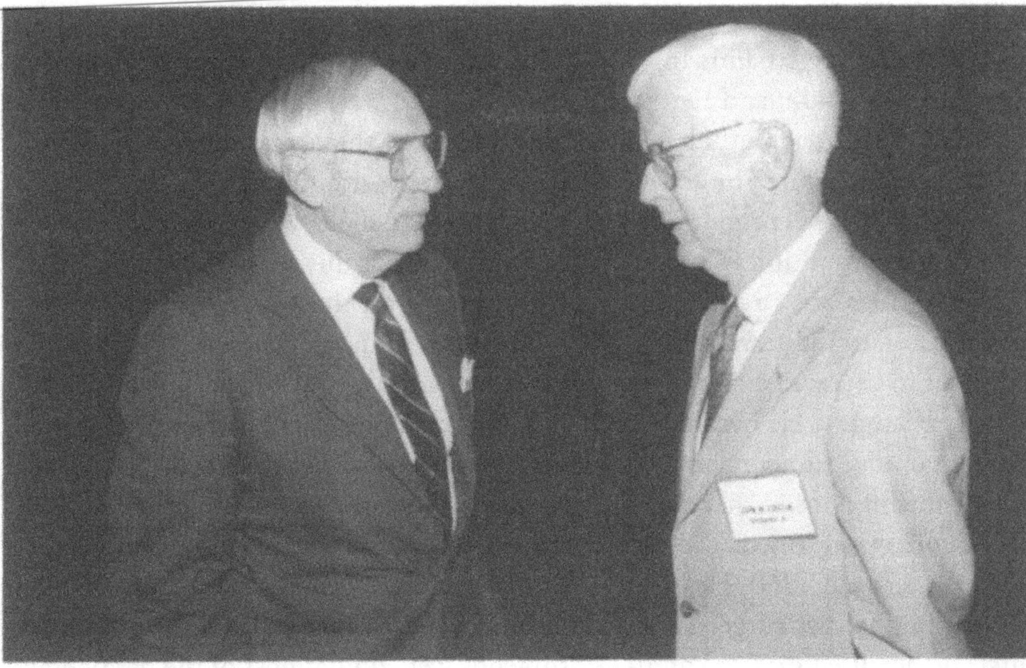

Robert B. Wallace and John W. Kirklin

younger surgeon, and Dr. Kirklin was designated with his full support. Cardiac surgery was limited to closed procedures and repair of atrial septal defects using the "well" technique. Sixty miles away, Drs. Walt Lillehei and Richard Varco were developing a cardiac program at the University of Minnesota, and for many years there was a friendly and beneficial rivalry between the two institutions. The University of Minnesota surgeons were using hypothermic arrest to perform certain intracardiac repairs, and then introduced the dramatic human cross-circulation technology. Although these procedures were quite successful, there was concern about putting the donor as well as the patient at risk. In 1953 Dr. John Gibbon performed the first successful open-heart procedure using a mechanical pump-oxygenator, but abandoned this technique after subsequent failures and discouraged its further use. Dr. Kirklin was convinced that this technique was the way to go. He visited Dr. Gibbon in Philadelphia, and although Dr. Gibbon was not encouraging about the future of his machine, Dr. Kirklin, using the principles of the Gibbon machine, with the help of Richard Jones of the engineering department and engineers from IBM, modified the original Gibbon machine and developed the Mayo-Gibbon pump-oxygenator. This was a large, complex machine that was expensive to build and maintain. Six to eight units of fresh blood were required to prime the system, which made it impractical for emergency cases.

In 1955 the cardiac team, with the approval of the governing board, embarked on a project in which eight patients with ventricular septal defects would be operated on and then the results would be carefully studied before proceeding. There were five survivors in this group; the first patient operated on spoke at the fiftieth anniversary of open-heart surgery at the Mayo Clinic in April 2005. In 1960 Dr. Kirklin and Dr. Jim DuShane, head of pediatric cardiology, reported on 108 patients operated on for tetralogy of Fallot with a 10 percent mortality, which was exceptional at that time.

Dr. F. H. "Bunky" Ellis was an early member of the cardiac surgical team. His primary interest was in thoracic surgery, especially esophageal surgery. He became quite expert in mitral valve surgery and made significant contributions in that area. Dr. Dwight McGoon, who trained at Johns Hopkins, joined the team in 1960. He became an outstanding cardiac surgeon for both congenital and acquired cardiac conditions and made many significant contributions in both areas. In the early days of aortic valve replacement, Dwight did one hundred consecutive aortic valve replacements without mortality, an outstanding feat at that time. Unfortunately, Dwight's surgical career was cut short by the onset of Parkinson's disease. He continued to make major contributions to the specialty, especially as editor of the *Journal of Thoracic and Cardiovascular Surgery*.

Toward the end of my first year at the Mayo Clinic, Dr. Kirklin asked me if I would be interested in joining Dr. McGoon, Dr. Ellis, and him as the fourth cardiac surgeon. I was overwhelmed and there was no doubt in my mind about what I wanted to do. Betty and I had become very fond of Rochester and considered it an excellent place for our family to grow up, and I could think of no better place to develop my career than at the Mayo Clinic. I joined the staff in October 1963, the same day that Dr. Chuck Mayo retired, although I never considered myself a replacement for him. When I informed St. Vincent's of my decision, the people there thought that I was making a major mistake, as they did not think that the Mayo Clinic would do well with the changes that were taking place in medicine at that time. I have often thought of this as I watched the Mayo Clinic grow over the years.

In the early days of cardiac surgery at the Mayo Clinic, the cardiac surgeons also did thoracic surgery, vascular surgery, some general surgery, and even gynecological surgery. As the cardiac cases increased, the surgeons began to limit their operations to cardiac, vascular, and thoracic cases. It was of interest to me that in 1963 the orthopedic surgeons were doing most of the peripheral vascular surgery, no doubt due to the influence of Dr. Joe Janes, an orthopedic surgeon who had had an early interest in peripheral vascular surgery. Because of my experience in Houston, I had an interest in peripheral vascular surgery and suggested to Dr. Kirklin that he invite Stanley Crawford to be a visiting professor. Dr. Crawford was an excellent visiting professor and generated a good deal of enthusiasm for this area of surgery. In a short time, all of the vascular surgery was done by the cardiac surgeons along with Drs. Phil Bernatz and Spencer Payne. Likewise, there was little interest in carotid artery surgery, but an active program developed in the cardiac surgical service following Dr. Crawford's visit. This continued until Dr. Thoralf Sundt, a neurosurgeon with major interest in cerebrovascular disease, was recruited to the clinic. He did an excellent job in further developing the program, including both extra- and intracranial vascular procedures.

In 1963 the cardiac surgical service was doing six to eight cardiac procedures a day.

The Mayo-Gibbon pump-oxygenator required a large amount of fresh blood. Most of the Mayo employees who could give blood were regular donors, as were many of the local residents. Donor blood was collected at 5:00 A.M. the day of the operation, and despite the inclement weather that can be present in Rochester, I don't think a single case was cancelled because of donors failing to report. It did, however, make emergency surgery difficult. I had had experience with the disposable bubble oxygenator while working with Dr. Cooley, and I suggested to Dr. Kirklin that we try using it for emergency cases, to which he agreed. Shortly after obtaining the bubble oxygenators, a patient was presented with what was thought to be an acute dissecting aneurysm. I had seen Dr. DeBakey perform what I think was the first successful repair of an acute aortic dissection; ironically, the patient was a Mayo resident on vacation in Louisiana. Dr. Kirklin suggested that I perform the operation while he worked with the pump technicians. Much to our surprise, and perhaps relief, on opening the pericardium we found an acute hemorrhagic pericarditis. The bubble oxygenator was subsequently used for all of our emergency cases.

When the Cleveland Clinic began its coronary surgery program with the Vineberg procedure, Dr. Kirklin suggested that I spend a week with Drs. Mason Sones and Don Effler to learn about the Vineberg procedure, when and how to use it. We decided to do one hundred cases and then evaluate the results. We could not identify a definite benefit of this procedure. Fortunately, by this time, direct coronary artery bypass had been introduced and was adopted as the procedure of choice for coronary artery disease.

In 1962 Dr. Kirklin was appointed chairman of the Department of Surgery. Prior to that time there had not been a formal structure in the department. One of Dr. Kirklin's accomplishments as chairman was to restructure the training program, which had been criticized because the residents were not given sufficient opportunity for independent operating. Despite this, many fine surgeons came out of the Mayo program, suggesting that there might be more than one way to train a surgeon. Because of my experience in other programs, I agreed with Dr. Kirklin that some changes were indicated to provide the residents more operating experience under staff supervision, and I worked with him to implement these changes. Chief residents had their own services and with full disclosure to the patients operated independently, albeit with close staff supervision.

In 1966 Dr. Kirklin announced that he was leaving the Mayo Clinic to become chairman of the Department of Surgery at the University of Alabama in Birmingham. This came as a great surprise and disappointment to me; I just could not understand why he would leave the Mayo Clinic. Later on, after several discussions with Dr. Kirklin, I think I began to understand. He had accomplished a great deal in many areas; he had served on the Board of Governors, the Board of Trustees of the Mayo Foundation, and if the clinic were to follow their policy of five- to eight-year tenure for chairmen, he would soon have to relinquish that responsibility. Although I am sure the institution would have been better had he not left, the Mayo Clinic is bigger than any one individual. Dr. Kirklin wanted to build a surgical department and an institution that would reflect his concepts. He was able to do this at the University of Alabama, and today that institution exemplifies this. Had he gone to Mass General, it still would have been Churchill's program; at Boston Children's, it would have been the Gross program, but at the University of Alabama, it was the Kirklin program.

Following Dr. Kirklin's departure, Dr. George Hallenbeck, a general surgeon with major research interests, was appointed chairman of the department. I don't think that Dr. Hallenbeck really enjoyed the chairmanship and its responsibilities, and he left a year later to join Dr. Kirklin in Birmingham as the head of general surgery. Subsequently, in 1968, at the age of thirty-seven, I was appointed chairman. I was never quite sure why the board made this decision, as there were so many others in the department who could have done an outstanding job. It might have been that I had had experience elsewhere, and I did bring some different ideas on education and resident training. I will always be grateful for the support I received from Dr. Clagett when my appointment was announced to the department.

I served as chairman from 1968 until 1979. During this period, Dwight McGoon was the head of the Division of Thoracic and Cardiovascular Surgery, and one could not have worked with a better person. Shortly after Dr. Kirklin left, we recruited Gordon Danielson as the fourth cardiac surgeon. He had trained at the University of Pennsylvania and was head of cardiac surgery at the University of Kentucky. He was a great addition to the group and made many contributions over the ensuing years. We also recruited Larry Hollier to head a division of vascular surgery. Although Larry stayed at the clinic only a short time before leaving to become chairman of surgery at the Ochsner Clinic, the vascular division developed into a world-class group.

In 1979 I was invited to become the chairman of surgery at Georgetown University. I had never thought seriously about leaving Rochester, but the opportunity to return to Washington, where my family still lived, was very tempting. Georgetown represented a challenge to restore the program to the high level that it had once been. My tenure as chairman at Mayo was soon to end; I had served on the Board of Governors of the clinic and the Board of Trustees of the Mayo Foundation. After much thought and family discussion, I decided it was time to take on a new challenge, and so in 1980 I began a new career at Georgetown. It was difficult to leave the Mayo Clinic, as I have always considered it the ideal medical institution and an ideal place to practice medicine. I hoped to bring some of those ideals and practices to Georgetown.

Much has happened in medicine and surgery in the years since I retired, and I am sure that the science and technology of medicine will continue to progress. What can be done technologically is truly amazing, and I think that the real challenge of the future is to utilize the new technology appropriately to the benefit of the patient and health care in general.

When asked about those who have had the most impact on my professional life, it is difficult to name a few, as there have been so many who have influenced me or helped me in my career. I think it is quite likely that I would not have pursued a career in medicine had it not been for Coach Lou Little, who was so supportive. Denton Cooley was the reason that I became a cardiac surgeon, and I attribute any success that I have had as a cardiac surgeon to John Kirklin.

Since my retirement in 1996, I would be wrong to say that I have not missed my work. My relationships with patients, colleagues, residents, and students have left a void, but I have been able to pursue other activities not available to me when I was working. These activities are also very gratifying.

Bibliography

Wallace RB, deChantal Sister Jane, Mitty WF Jr. Morbidity and Mortality of Subtotal Gastrectomy: A Review of 500 Cases. *Am J Digestive Dis.* 1964; 9:745–754.

Kirklin JW, Wallace RB, McGoon DC, DuShane JW. Early and Late Results after Intracardiac Repair of Tetralogy of Fallot: Five-Year Review of 337 Patients. *Ann Surg.* 1965; 162:578–589.

Kirklin JW, Wallace RB, Burchell HB. Surgical Treatment of Acquired Valvular Heart Disease. In Hurst JW, Logue RB. *The Heart.* New York: McGraw Hill; 1966. Part 4, 610–621.

Kirklin JW, Wallace RB, DuShane JW. Surgical Treatment of Congenital Heart Disease. In Hurst JW, Logue RB. *The Heart.* New York: McGraw Hill; 1966. Part 4, 453–491.

Wallace RB, Rastelli GC, Ongley PA, Titus JL, McGoon DC. Complete Repair of Truncus Arteriosus Defects. *J Thorac Cardiovasc Surg.* 1969; 57:95–107.

Rastelli GC, Wallace RB, Ongley PA. Complete Repair of Transposition of the Great Arteries with Pulmonary Stenosis: A Review and Report of a Case Corrected by Using a New Surgical Technique. *Circulation.* 1969; 39:83–95.

McGoon DC, Rastelli GC, Wallace RB. Discontinuity between Right Ventricle and Pulmonary Artery: Surgical Treatment. *Ann Surg.* 1970; 172:680–689.

Wallace RB, Giuliani ER, Titus JL. Use of Aortic Homografts for Aortic Valve Replacement. *Circulation.* 1971; 43:365–373.

Wallace RB, Londe SP, Titus JL. Aortic Valve Replacement with Preserved Aortic Valve Homografts. *J Thorac Cardiovasc Surg.* 1974; 67:44–52.

Wallace RB. Truncus Arteriosus. In Sabiston DC Jr, Spencer FC. *Gibbon's Surgery of the Chest.* Philadelphia: WB Saunders; 1976. 1066–1075.

Francis Robicsek, MD, PhD

(b. 1925)

The use of muscle flaps has greatly reduced the mortality of sternal wound infections. The surgeons who first described the use of muscle flaps should get the Nobel Prize, and every cardiac surgeon should mention their names in evening prayer.
— On sternal wound infection

Interviewed April 19, 1999

When I talk about my life, I have to be a little bit schizophrenic. This is because my life has been divided into four segments: one, before the war in Hungary; two, during the war in Hungary; three, after the war in Hungary; and four, finally in the United States. Each segment somehow has very little to do with the others. I have the feeling that I have had four lives, and I hope that I am like a cat and have a few more left.

I was born in a small town in Hungary in 1925. My father was a Shell Oil executive and my mother was an English teacher; she was educated at Oxford. Early in my life we moved to Budapest, and it was there that I went to medical school. In Europe, as you know, students finish high school and then go directly to medical school. I guess this is true in every country except the United States. Anyway, I received my MD degree at age twenty-two and my PhD at age twenty-four. By the time I was twenty-eight, I was an associate professor in charge of cardiac surgery at the University of Budapest. This was not because I was that smart, but because we grew up faster. Cardiac surgery was just beginning, and I was just beginning also. I happened to be at the right place at the right time.

We were doing only closed procedures, but there was an inexhaustible supply of patients with rheumatic heart disease, and so we did two or three mitral commissurotomies a day. We did coarctation repair using French-eye needles, which was very interesting. We did Blalock-Taussig shunts and, of course, repaired patent ductus.

In 1955 I went to Sweden and spent some time at the Karolinska Institute in Stockholm. I watched Ake Senning do his second open-heart operation using a pump-oxygenator, a left ventricular aneurysm repair. Their heart-lung machine looked like a little washing machine and the oxygenator had rotating discs. Clarence Crafoord was the chief and he had with him Viking Björk and Ake Senning; they hated each other. Björk wouldn't let Senning in the research lab and Senning wouldn't let Björk in the operating room. Crafoord was just leaning back and laughing at both of them; it was an interesting time.

I went back to Hungary and built my own heart-lung machine. It was an interesting contraption made mostly of glass. We used a bacterial filter for the oxygen and this turned the blood into foam, which overflowed like the magic porridge in the children's fairy tale. To everyone's horror, it almost filled the room. I began doing heart surgery, if you could call it heart surgery, without much experience. I had books and journals and had had a brief trip to Sweden.

When I went to Sweden in 1955, I saw what was outside of Hungary, and I decided then and there that I would get the hell out of Hungary. In 1956 I received an invitation to move to East Germany. All of the surgeons in East Germany had fled to the West, and they wanted someone who was versatile in cardiac surgery. They asked me to establish a cardiac surgery unit in a university in East Germany, but the Hungarian Revolution broke out and all travel came to a halt. When the Russian troops came back into Hungary, I told my wife, "That's enough. We are leaving." We packed up; my wife was six months pregnant. I had papers to get us as far as East Germany, and we crossed over into Berlin. My East German friends told us to take the subway and as soon as we saw a *Life* magazine in the newsstand to get off, and we would be in West Berlin. From there we went to West Germany and on to the United States. I had some of my publications, but we left almost everything else behind. When we first reached West Berlin, I decided that I was not going to leave my brand-new double-breasted suit to the communists, so I went back and brought it out. That was my baggage. All of the displaced Hungarians were placed in Camp Kilmer in New Jersey, and we were there for a while. My father's brother had lost everything in a poker game in Hungary, had immigrated to the United States, and was a contractor in Charlotte, North Carolina. We went there from New Jersey and have been there ever since.

My uncle in Charlotte had become acquainted with Dr. Paul Sanger, a thoracic surgeon. He was interested in getting a cardiac center established in Charlotte, so he took me on as a fellow. My duties were to do the cardiac catheterizations, run the heart-lung machine, and assist with surgical procedures. I also ran the research laboratory. I was a fellow for six months and then entered the residency training program. On the side, I worked as Dr. Sanger's partner; it was more like a partnership than a surgical residency. I believe I am the only foreign graduate in the United States who was allowed to take the general surgery board examination with no general surgery training in the United States. The board was very generous and gracious. When I took the board exam I was thirty years old, younger than most candidates. I

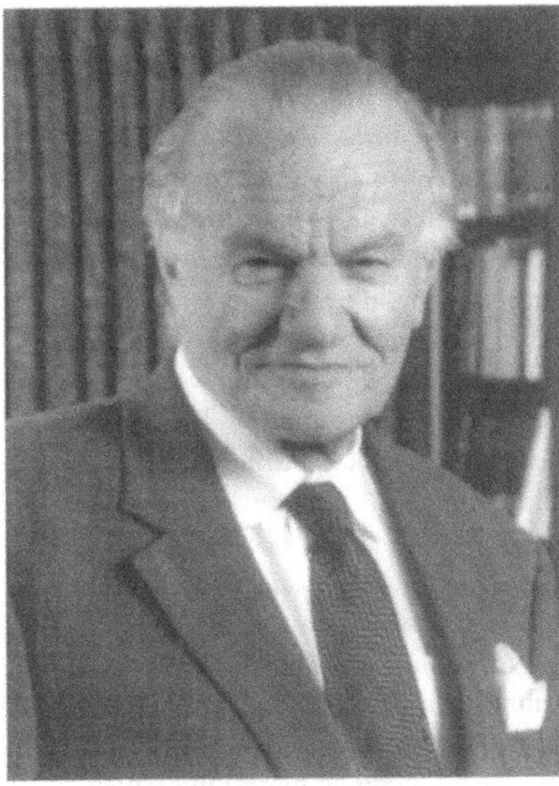

Francis Robicsek

really didn't lose any time. I finished the thoracic training program at Charlotte and took the Thoracic Board Exam.

In the late fifties, we did not have a pump. I went to Cleveland and visited Don Effler, Earl Kay, and Fred Cross. I got some parts from the Pemco Company and built our first pump in my garage. I still have it, and it is still in working order. I had an engineer working with me, and we built a very pretty pump with a rotating-disc oxygenator. We had ultraviolet lights mounted on the pump, so the OR personnel called it the "purple people eater." We used it for four or five years, and then changed to the disposable bubble oxygenator.

We did mostly congenital heart procedures, but we also did some rheumatic hearts. When the Starr valve became available, we began doing more adult patients than children. It took us ten to fifteen years to work off all of the rheumatic disease heart patients from the North Carolina mountains. Dr. Sanger also had a very large thoracic surgery practice. There was a very busy tuberculosis sanatarium next to us, so we were involved with both thoracic and cardiac surgery.

If you could say that my career was mainly with cardiac surgery, it was because I knew a fair amount of cardiology. When my surgical group developed a little later on, we did our own heart catheterizations until 1968, when we hired our first cardiologist. We would go to the cath lab first thing in the morning, do a catheterization, run upstairs to the operating room, do a mitral valve replacement, and then go back down to the cath lab. When we hired a cardiologist, we wondered what we would do all day. As a result, I knew more about surgery than the cardiologists and more cardiology than the surgeons. If I had just tried to be a surgeon I would not have been able to accomplish as much, and the combination of the two specialties has opened a lot of opportunities for me. That is what I have tried to teach my children. Learn something well, and then take up something else, so that you can always be between two specialties. That principle has worked well for me, and this concept is valid in all fields of life. To be prominent, you have to be exceptionally good in your field, and very few people can do that. If you are good in your field and then you develop knowledge in another field, you can advance to a higher position.

In the 1960s, I became interested in archaeology. I have never enjoyed a vacation where you just go and sit around, and I never enjoyed walking around a golf course. I have always needed an excuse or a reason for going from A to B. I saw an advertisement from a hospital in Honduras in the *Annals of Thoracic Surgery* for a surgeon experienced in tuberculosis surgery, and started spending my summer vacations there. The hospital could only manage one thoracotomy a day, so in the afternoons I began to prowl around the ruins. Before long, I began to make some discoveries. One of my discoveries was that archaeologists don't know a damned thing. My second discovery was that they don't know, but they write about it anyway. I began to approach archaeology with the same method that you would use for medical research; it was a lot of fun. I knew more medicine than any archaeologist, and more archaeology than any surgeon. I made my own photographs. My wife, son, and my other children came with me. It gave us an opportunity to travel and use our minds while also visiting beautiful sites, at the risk the occasional scorpion bite. I had a pre-Columbian collection, which is now housed in a wing of a local museum in Honduras, but I still have a few pieces. It gives me a lot of joy, and I was able to publish a book about the Mayan civilization.

During the 1980s, we had an outbreak of nosocomial sternal wound infections caused by atypical mycobacteria. Five patients died and the others all eventually were cured. The source of the infection was never really solved, but we now think it was tap water. We were using topical ice slush for myocardial protection. I think Charles Hufnagel, Norman Shumway, and I were the only three people who started using topical hypothermia very early, and continued to do so until everybody began using hypothermia again. The bacteria may have been in the ice that was used to produce the slush in glass bottles. If this had happened more recently, we would have used muscle flaps after debridement, and the outcomes would have been much better. Their use has greatly reduced the mortality of and recovery time from sternal wound infections. The surgeons who described the use of muscle flaps should get the Nobel Prize, and every cardiac surgeon should mention their names in evening prayer. The sternotomy incision has been a subject of great interest, and I just completed a chapter in Harold Urschel's book on complications of median sternotomy. The management of mediastinitis with muscle flaps has changed the whole scope of that problem.

In 1937 medical advances in Hungary came to a complete stop; everything came to a halt. When the war ended in 1945, we practiced a high level of excellent 1937 Hungarian medicine. By that I mean we treated pneumonia with suction cups, and we used leeches for thrombophlebitis. We had never seen a Levine tube. Gonorrhea was treated with irrigation of dilute carbolic acid. From 1945 to 1957 we jumped two generations in medical progress. I will never forget the first time I saw penicillin used. All I could say was, "God!" As an intern, I worked in the venereal disease clinic, and the syphilis patients were given salvarsan twice a week for six weeks, and then six times a week for six weeks. Someone gave us penicillin and syphilis was cured in a week. In a way, from 1947 until now, there have been three generations of medical progress. I feel like I started out in the Middle Ages and ended in the twenty-first century.

I have been a compulsive writer all of my professional life. When I was a very young surgeon, I did orthotopic heart valve transplantation in an experimental animal with a four-year survival; that was in 1952 or 1953. I was not the first, but was among the first to do a vena caval–pulmonary artery anostomosis. I have published five hundred or six hundred papers; some of them are pretty good. Somehow one of the articles that is best known is a modification of the sternal wound closure called sternal weaving. It states that most problems with sternal closure came from the sutures cutting through the sternum, and so the solution is not some new closure technique but in strengthening the sternum so that the wires do not cut through when the patient coughs. I suggested that weaving a wire in and out of the interspaces at the edges of the sternum would add strength to the sternum and prevent cutting by the wires. Most people seem to know me because of this small modification.

Of the people who have had an influence on my life, I would put my chief of surgery in Budapest, Professor Monor, and the chief of thoracic surgery, Professor Littman, at the top. Paul Sanger also had a great influence on my training, and I became his partner. Our group of six surgeons and fifty-two cardiologists in Charlotte is called the Sanger Clinic. I was lucky to get to know Dr. Churchill and Viking Björk. Denton Cooley has always been a role model. I have met most everybody in American and European cardiac surgery, and when you walk close to them, something sticks to you for all time. I have known Donald Ross for decades. It is hard for me to name one particular person. I was not schooled in heart surgery and did not come up through Johns Hopkins or Harvard. I am from Charlotte, so I had the ability to pick up this and pick up that and just make my own gravy. I guess Paul Sanger influenced me greatly, probably more as a friend than a teacher.

It may be that the golden days of cardiac surgery are over. At one time you could come up with some new earth-shattering innovation, and you could try it. You had free hands, and they were restrained only by your own standards and your own morals. I think that time is over. All of the cardiologists are becoming more like surgeons and the surgeons are more like cardiologists. I still have questions in my mind, and, to some degree, I am glad that I don't have to be among those who will have to solve them. The problem of coronary artery surgery was defined by one of the speakers at a national meeting who said, "The only problem left is to keep the grafts open; everything else is solved." I don't think we should concentrate on how to do coronary surgery through a smaller incision. We need to concentrate on how to make the grafts last longer. The new developments in cardiac surgery will follow new technology rather than new theories or ideas.

Our department did twenty-four heart transplants last year, and we could have done twice that many if we had the donor hearts. Like everyone else, we are limited by the number of donors. This is a social-political problem, not a medical problem. The same will be true for left ventricular assist devices. It will be limited by the cost. A large number of patients could benefit from an LVAD, but who can pay for it all? On one hand, you cannot deny treatment just because it is expensive, and on the other hand we will have relatively less money for basic health care. How society is going to solve this is not yet clear. One of these days, we are going to have to face the basic issues. One of those issues is the length of medical education. At the present time, it is too long and too expensive. My residents are at their peak when they are thirty, when they have the keenest minds and sharpest eyes. Yet, they are in training until they are thirty-four or thirty-six and start practice at age thirty-six or thirty-seven. We need for them to finish at a younger age, and the easiest way is to cut short the time spent in college.

I still go back to Hungary to visit, although my mother died recently. I go back and visit the old institutions with my boys. Things have changed there like everywhere else.

Bibliography

Robicsek F. Cardiac Valve Transplantation. *Acta Med.* 1954; Book 5:Fasc 1–2. PhD Thesis.

Robicsek F. Intravascular Catheterization for the Diagnosis of Aortic Coarctation. *Acta Cardiol.* 1956; 11:474–479.

Robicsek F, Temesvari A, Kadar RL. A New Method for the Treatment of Congenital Heart Disease Associated with Impaired Pulmonary Circulation; An Experimental Study. *Acta Med Scand.* 1956; Fasc II, 154:151–161.

Robicsek F, Sanger PW, Daugherty HK, Lesage MA. Heart Surgery in Normothermic Body Perfusion. Interruption of the Coronary Blood Flow and Topical Cardiac Hypothermia. *Ann Thorac Surg.* 1967; 4:232–241.

Robicsek F. Cigarettes Are Threat to Vascular Grafts. *Modern Medicine.* 1975; 12:122.

Robicsek F. Biochemical Termination of Sustained Fibrillation Occurring after Artificially Induced Ischemic Arrest. *J Thorac Cardiovasc Surg.* 1984; 87:143–145.

Robicsek F, Daugherty HK, Selle JG, Cook JW, Hess PJ. Patency Rate of Bifurcated Aortic Grafts. Comparative Analysis of Woven versus Knitted Prostheses in the Same Patient. *Ann Thorac Surg.* 1985; 40:172–174.

Robicsek F, Thubrikar M. The Freedom from Atherosclerosis of Intramyocardial Coronary Arteries: Reduction of Mural Stress—A Key Factor. *Eur J Cardio-thoracic Surg.* 1994; 8:228–235.

Robicsek F. Complications of Midline Sternotomies. In Urschel H (Editor). *Thoracic Surgery* (2nd Edition). New York: Mosby; 2002. ch 51.

Robicsek F, Cook JW, Reames MK Sr, Skipper ER. Size Reduction Ascending Aortoplasty: Is It Dead or Alive? *J Thorac Cardiovasc Surg.* 2004; 128:562–570.

Robicsek F, Thubrikar MJ, Cook JW, Fowler B. The Congenitally Bicuspid Aortic Valve: How Does It Function? Why Does It Fail? *Ann Thorac Surg.* 2004; 77:177–185.

Alain F. Carpentier, MD, PhD

(b. 1933)

One day when I was going through the entrance to the hospital, the idea of a prosthetic ring came to me in a few seconds. I developed a prosthetic ring. The idea was to rebuild the valve orifice, to remodel it, rather than just narrow it.

— On the technique of mitral valve repair

Interviewed September 16, 2000

I was born in 1933 in Toulouse, France, but I grew up in different cities because my father was an engineer who constructed roads and bridges. We moved every five years, so although I was born in Toulouse, I grew up in Ile-de-France in the center of France. During the Second World War, the Germans wanted my father to construct an airfield, and he didn't want to, so we moved to Algeria. I spent four years there during the war, and then we came back to eastern France, where my father reconstructed the city of Epinal.

These were the conditions in which I grew up. I became interested in medicine during the early German occupation, when we were living in the center of France, because I developed peritonitis, which I remember very well. I was eight years old, and I was operated on by a surgeon just one or two hours before he had to leave to go to another place. If this surgeon had not delayed his departure, I would have been dead, because there was no other surgeon in the city. It was a very painful operation, but as a result of that experience, I decided to become a surgeon.

I started medical school in the east of France, in Nancy, but then my parents moved to Paris, and I finished medical school there. I had all of my surgical training in Paris. I had decided to become a surgeon from the very beginning, so there was never a question of medicine or obstetrics. I went to medical school so that I could do surgery, the only question being the type of surgery. I was fortunate to work with Robert Chudet, an orthopedic surgeon who is very well-known as the inventor of the first artificial hip. We had an excellent relationship, and he wanted me to continue working with him. He was a marvelous surgeon and a very important innovator with a new idea every minute; it was really something to see. I already had a few ideas at that time, so he wanted me to stay in orthopedics. During my residency program, I had to spend six months in cardiac surgery. I selected the service of Charles Dubost, who was, of course, the leading cardiac surgeon in France and Europe at that time. At the end of the six months, he said, "OK, I've decided that you are going to stay with me." I had a difficult time choosing between Dubost and Chudet. Both of them were really remarkable surgeons and excellent human beings. I decided to stay with cardiac surgery, because I could see that in 1965 there were still a lot of new things going on. All of my subsequent training was with Dubost. He was a marvelous person, looking and behaving like a Roman emperor, but we had an excellent partnership, and he gave me strong support

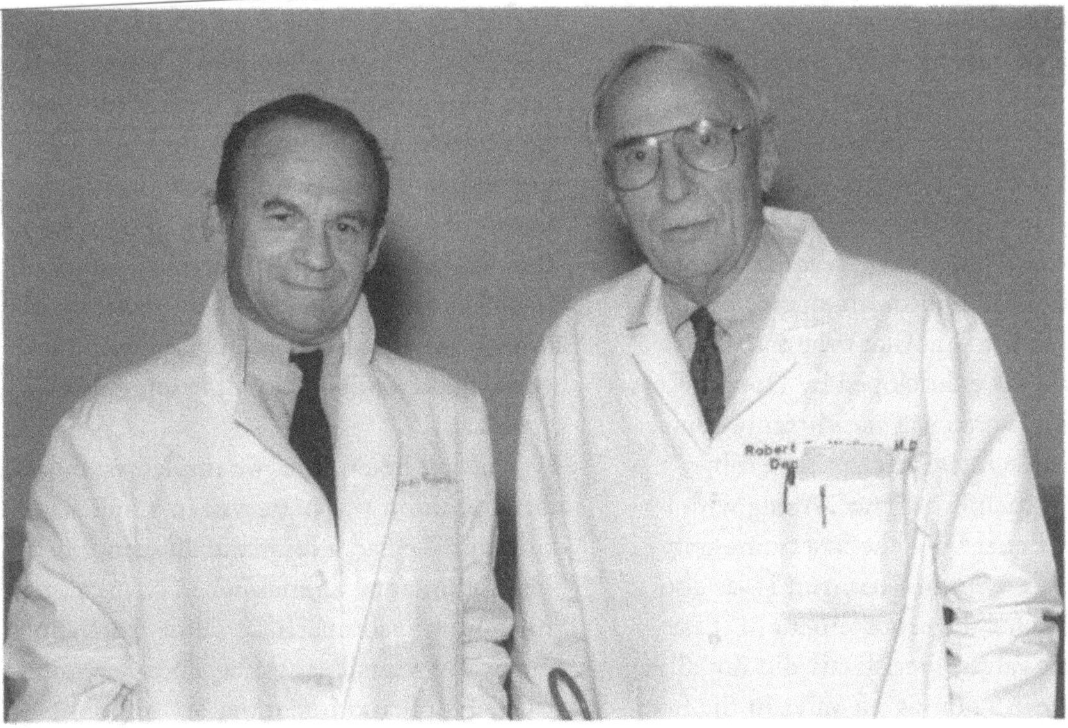

Alain F. Carpentier and Robert B. Wallace

and the necessary freedom to develop what I wanted to do.

When Charles Dubost heard Dr. Blalock give the first lecture on the Blue Baby operation, he decided then and there to give up general surgery and devote himself entirely to vascular and cardiac surgery. Not only did he decide that, but he also invited Dr. Blalock to Paris in 1947 after the war. Blalock came to the Hospital Broussais and did the very first Blue Baby operation in France, and Charles Dubost assisted him. He was influenced by the personality of Dr. Blalock. I still have photographs showing Blalock operating on a child at Broussais. After Dr. Blalock's visit, Dr. Francis d'Allaines was able to raise funds to build the clinic at Broussais Hospital, where I have been working most of my life.

I began full-time cardiac surgery in 1965 and extracorporeal circulation was just beginning, and in the surgical world there were no frontiers between countries. I visited the U.S. frequently, and when something new happened in the U.S., in the following months it was transferred to France. In 1965 we operated on most of the congenital cardiac abnormalities, and for valvular heart disease we used the Starr-Edwards valve; surgery was not yet an option for coronary artery disease.

Although we could obtain marvelous results with the Starr-Edwards valve, I was struck by the fact that in some patients we had severe complications. When you are a young surgeon and you have completed a successful valve replacement operation and then the patient has hemiplegia from an embolic event related to the valve, it is a very emotional and discouraging event. I had two or three patients with hemiplegia after valve replacement. I became interested in trying to develop techniques that would allow the patient to be free of the risk of embolic complications and the risks of anticoagulation. That's why I became interested in what I called nonthrombogenic cardiac surgery. We knew at that time that the homograft valve developed by Donald Ross and Carlos Duran was nonthrombogenic, and I became interested in tissue valves because of their experience. Along with Jean Paul Benet I did the first homograft valve replacement in Paris, and I was also responsible for the procurement of these homograft valves. French law did not allow us to retrieve a homograft valve in the first forty-eight hours after death, allowing time for the family to give or withhold permission. After forty-eight hours, many of the valves were contaminated; even though we used antibiotics, they probably were not safe. The procurement process was very difficult, and we did not have enough, and so I became interested in using pig valves because of both the French law and the limited number of homografts available.

The first homograft valves were freeze-dried, and we obtained them from England. Carlos Duran prepared them for us. I visited Duran who had done the first experiments with heterograft valves. He found that they were associated with an acute rejection process if they had not been pretreated. It was apparent that heterograft valves would be ideal except for this problem, and I began working to find a solution to rejection. I was fortunate to have worked with the orthopedic surgeon, Robert Chudet, in the past. He used homograft skin in operations to reconstruct the knee. Skin is very antigenic, much more so than cardiac tissue, but after these orthopedic operations, there was only a minor inflammatory response to the homografted skin. They soaked the skin in a mercury solution for sterilization, which apparently decreased its antigenicity, and I became interested in reducing the antigenicity of heterografts with chemicals.

The first heterograft we implanted in the aortic position was preserved in a mercury solution. We had a dramatic difference in the experimental animals when we used this solution, compared to saline alone, but one or two years later we began to see some degeneration and inflammatory response in the heterograft valves. I realized that mercury was not the best preservative and continued to investigate different products. I became interested in aldehydes, which are used to preserve leather.

I investigated all the aldehydes, and believe me, there are more than fifty of them. Most did not work at all, and only glutaraldehyde worked really well. I know today why it worked and the others didn't; it was a question of chemistry. I was fortunate enough to discover that glutaraldehyde was able not only to reduce the antigenicity much more than the mercurial solution, but in addition it reinforced the strength of the tissue by intramolecular cross-linkages. Glutaraldehyde is a dialdehyde, and it can bind to additional molecules of collagen. The aldehyde group combines with the immuno group to form what we call in chemistry a shift base. Now I am talking about chemistry, so I should add that in the meantime I had gone back to the faculty of science to improve my knowledge of chemistry. Otherwise I wouldn't have been able to do those studies.

The Edwards Laboratory has a long history of believing in mechanical valves, but they became involved with us in developing a biological valve because of Albert Starr, who is a great man. In 1968 I had just discovered how to use glutaraldehyde to sterilize the valves, and we began to do the first operations with these treated valves, with Charles Dubost. One year later, in 1969, Al Starr visited us and asked Dubost what was new in his laboratory. Dubost said, "Go and see Carpentier." Al Starr came to my laboratory, and I told him everything about the new method of preserving heterograft valves. He was extremely interested in the experimental results and in the fact that we had already started using them. He said, "You have to visit me in the United States." I had already visited the United States, but I went again, and during this visit he introduced me to the people at Edwards Laboratories and told them, "This may be very important to you; you need to work with Carpentier." I got the red carpet treatment at Edwards Laboratories, and I told them everything about how to make these valves. The only condition I asked of them was that they would not sell the valves for three years, because of my prior experience. Although the glutaraldehyde was achieving better results with experimental animals, I didn't want to expose patients to something that might turn out badly like the mercury valves, so Edwards Laboratories promised me not to commercialize the product until 1971.

The vice president of Edwards Laboratories was a man named Warren Hancock, and he attended my presentation. Six months later he left Edwards Laboratories and because he was not bound by the promise to delay production, he developed the first commercially available heterograft valve, the Hancock valve. Actually, Edwards Laboratories had produced the first valve in the United States just for us, for clinical investigation only. The Hancock valves failed after a few years. Hancock was not a scientist, and people finally realized that I was the inventor of the technique. Eventually Edwards Laboratories acquired a very important reputation in the development of the valve, facilitated by their running a very ethical and responsible business. It is interesting that today Edwards Laboratories, which is now called Edwards Lifesciences, produces biological valves almost exclusively. They also still produce a few mechanical Starr-Edwards valves.

Also about that time the Shiley Company produced the first Ionescu valve, which was also a frame-mounted pig aortic valve, preserved in gluteraldehyde. Two years later they began to produce bovine pericardial valves mounted on frames. The first ones had been treated with formaldehyde, and the results were disastrous, but then they adopted our preservation technique and had better results. However, his mounting of the valve was not appropriate, and there were many early failures. This led to a lot of disenchantment with the Ionescu valve and it was removed from the market. The Shiley Company actually went out of business because of both that and the problem of strut fracture of their Björk-Shiley mechanical valve.

I have learned something that I hope will interest younger people: When you have invented something, try to eliminate it yourself rather than letting other people abolish it. I began looking into valvular reconstruction in order to eliminate valve replacement, even with my own valve. I told myself I should try a valve made of bovine pericardium, maybe it would be stronger tissue, and I thought I could do a better job of mounting than the Ionescu valve. I told Edwards Laboratories that we had to develop a pericardial valve as well as the pig valve. This caused a big fight, because the people from Edwards Laboratories said, "The pig valve is very successful. Why should we develop a pericardial valve?" I told them, "If you don't want to develop it, I am going to develop it with another laboratory," so they were obliged to do it. It turned out that the pericardial valve today is better than the porcine valve, as we have been able to improve its durability in older patients to up to almost twenty years.

We are still trying to improve the pericardial valve. I have been working in research all my life, with the help of my wife Sophie, and in the past ten years we have tried to develop a complementary technique to minimize calcification in tissue valves. We have been successful in doing that by introducing a technique of preservation using surfactants, but the bioprosthesis still develops calcification, particularly in young patients. This is very sad, because a nonthrombogenic valve would be particularly useful for children. Today we have new valves, which we call pediatric valves, and we have been investigating them clinically for eight years with promising results. It is a bit too early to say how well they will work. I would like to wait ten years before comparing the so-called pediatric valves with our previous experience using porcine or pericardial valves in children.

In the very early 1960s, before a mechanical valve was available, there were some surgical techniques used to repair mitral valve insufficiency, and there were commissurotomies for mitral valve stenosis. Then when the Starr-Edwards valve became available, most surgeons began replacing abnormal valves, and valve reconstruction became a rare procedure. My ideas began evolving in the techniques of valve repair. Very often a single patient is a trigger for trying to develop something new, and for valve repair that trigger was a young patient, a sixteen-year-old fellow. I was very proud of this patient because I did my first mitral valve repair on him. At that time we were using the Wooler operation, or the Reed operation, squeezing the two commissures to reduce the size of the orifice, even trying to achieve some degree of stenosis to make sure we had a competent valve. The early result was excellent, but when I examined this patient one month later, the whole repair had broken down. When you are a young surgeon, you do not accept this kind of failure, and that is good. I told myself I should do something to avoid this kind of thing happening again. It became obvious to me that these palliative operations were not really reconstructive operations. I kept this patient in mind for months, trying to find a solution. One day when I was going through the entrance to the hospital, the idea of a prosthetic ring came to me in a few seconds. This was after having thought about it and searching for an answer for months. This is the mechanism of invention: When you are thinking about a problem, you have to think about it for days and nights, and then suddenly in an unexpected few seconds you find a solution.

I developed a prosthetic ring. The idea was to first rebuild the valve orifice, to remodel it, rather than just narrow it. This is why when I see a new technique, such as suturing one valve leaflet to the other, it makes me very distressed, because this is what I wanted to avoid. After I developed the prosthetic ring, it became obvious that complementary techniques had to be developed: the chordal shortening, quadrangular resection, and chordal fenestration, and all the techniques that young surgeons now know very well. We organized a course to teach the various techniques of mitral valve repair and called it the Club Mitrale. It was given three times a year for several years and eventually more than a thousand American surgeons came to France and participated in the course. The percentage of American cardiac surgeons who have attended the Club Mitrale is very high. I should give credit to two people who have helped introduce these techniques in the United States. The first is Frank Spencer, who invited me to give the honored guest lecture at the American Association for Thoracic Surgery. The second one is a surgeon, Larry Bonchek. Larry visited us several times. He wrote to me before the first visit saying that he would like to see what I was doing, and I replied that he would be welcome. He watched the surgery, and then six months later he wrote me a letter saying that he wanted me to operate on him, because he had a mitral insufficiency. He had visited ten different surgical groups and had selected our hospital, so I repaired his valve. It was one of the most difficult operations I have ever done, because he had an extreme form of myxomatous degeneration. After I repaired the valve, rather than hiding the fact that he had undergone operation, he promoted the technique of mitral valve repair. Each time he had the opportunity to speak from a podium, he would say, "I've had this operation, and it's a beautiful operation." When he visited the Edwards Laboratories, he took some rings and put them on his ear for people who were taking pictures. So these are the two men who helped promote these techniques, as well as Al Starr, who has also been a very helpful spokesman for this surgery. With the help of Promedica, I developed the Club Mitrale, and we put on a course three times a year for foreign and French surgeons, limiting the audience to twenty people. The participants enjoy it very much, and they ask me to continue doing the courses; I will continue until I can't do them any more.

The pathology of mitral valve insufficiency that lends itself most successfully to repair is degenerative valvular disease, because although the valves are fragile, there is pliable tissue. In rheumatic valve disease the tissue is thicker than normal and repair is more difficult. Degenerative valve disease is the most common form of mitral disease in this country and in Europe, and it is with this disease that we have the best results. In degenerative valve disease the reoperation rate is 0.6 percent per patient-year, which is to say that at the end of ten years, only 6 percent of the patients had to be reoperated, so it is a pretty stable and reliable technique. The incidence of reoperation in rheumatic valve disease is higher at 1.4 percent per patient-year. If you read the literature, you will see some papers saying that valvular reconstruction is no good for rheumatic valvular disease, but that is not our experience with our own techniques of repair. However, when you have destruction of the valvular apparatus, fibrotic tissue, or calcified valves, then valve replacement is indicated, and we still do valve replacement in about 10 percent of our mitral valve patients.

The Alfieri repair is a palliative operation, in the sense that you transform a mitral valve insufficiency into a mitral valve stenosis, or some degree of mitral valve stenosis. It reminds me of the old days, when we did something similar. Every one of us sutured a commissure, and we know now that it works short-term, but not long-term. I am a little bit worried because the Alfieri repair is such an easy operation. It would be extremely sad if young surgeons were tempted to say, "Well, forget these complex operations; in ten minutes I can fix a mitral valve." They are not going to have a good long-term result. By contrast, the reconstructive operation has achieved a degree of perfection in long-term stability over thirty years. I know that, because I started thirty years ago. It is the first time in the history of valve disease that we can talk about definitive cure of the disease. You cannot obtain a definitive cure of the disease by any type of valve replacement or palliative repair; it is only cured if you make the effort to reconstruct the valve, to restore the mobility, to reshape the orifice as it should be, as designed by God Himself. Only in that way can you hope for long-term stability.

I have also worked on dynamic cardiomyoplasty. The first attempt to use muscular tissue to replace a part of the heart was done by René Leriche in 1933. Of course, it was not successful. Then several research fellows, particularly in the United States, have tried to develop the concept, first by using a vascularized muscular flap transposed around the heart. They found that the latissimus dorsi was the most appropriate muscle, but still, all these attempts failed. They did show in experimental animals that you could enhance contraction when stimulating the muscle at the rate of the heart. They failed to transform this experimental experience into clinical practice, because of the fatigue of the muscle. In other words, these operations worked for several hours, but after several hours the muscle became fatigued.

One day I was approached by a man named Juan Carlos Vasquez, who was a plastic surgeon. He thought that using the latissimus dorsi on the heart was an interesting problem, and he came to work in my laboratory. I had the problem in my mind for several months, and then one day in a few seconds I discovered the solution: Rather than stimulating the muscle from the very beginning at the rate of the heart with electrical current, why not do progressive stimulation of the rate over a period of two months? This idea turned out to be the solution. Together with the Medtronics Company we were able to develop the technique of progressive sequential stimulation, stimulating the muscle once every four heartbeats, for example, with small currents.

There was a trio of people who made it possible to do a successful cardiomyoplasty, but it has not really become a viable operation. There are two reasons: In the first place, it is a tedious operation. You have to dissect the latissimus muscle, then you have to close the chest, turn the patient, open the sternum, wrap the heart, et cetera. It is a ten-hour operation. In the second place, there is the disappointment of the cardiologists. They thought that the results should be as good as cardiac transplantation, but I compare this operation to a stick used by someone who has some difficulty in walking. It is not a leg replacement, it is a walking stick, but still I call it successful because these operations really do enhance cardiac contraction and continue to do so for many years. My first patient is still living and well after fifteen years and is on no medication. The cardiologists have been reluctant to recommend these operations, the surgeons are reluctant as well because they are tedious, but there is no question that this operation works. In addition to that, it is a very interesting physiological or muscular concept, because, for the first time, we demonstrated that we could transform ordinary muscle into fatigue-resistant muscle. I remember very well giving a piece of stimulated latissimus muscle to the pathologist who did some specific staining of the tissue and then said, "This is myocardial tissue." The latissimus muscle was completely transformed into fatigue-resistant myocardial tissue.

This is really something very important. What doctors call cellular cardiomyoplasty today was developed from the concept of cardiomyoplasty. Dr. Chu in Canada was one of the first to develop cardiomyoplasty. He came up with the idea saying, "Let's try to develop an operation that is less tedious and then use stem cells," but it is still the same concept, transforming muscular cell into myocardial-type fatigue-resistant cells. I can't say that it is a very practical operation, but maybe someday it will be.

Video-assisted and robotic operations are practical today. It is extremely important for young doctors to look around, particularly into other fields than their own, to see what technology, techniques, or chemical products could be used for the benefit of their patients. I became interested in robotic surgery fifteen years ago. I told myself that robotic technology was everywhere and one day it would be used in cardiac surgery. When Frank Spencer asked me to deliver the honored guest lecture, he asked me to talk at the end of the lecture about what would go on in the future. I went completely crazy describing an operating room in the year 2020, with a robot helping the surgeon to operate. Later, it turned out that I had the chance to co-develop this with the Intuitive Surgical, Inc. company. They knew what I had dreamed of, and they asked me to help adapt their system to cardiac surgery.

I did the very first computer-assisted operation a few years ago, and I think it will become common. I wouldn't have said this two years ago, or even one year ago. I don't know how long it will take, but soon robotics will be used routinely by surgeons for some operations. Today there is a tremendous development of the Intuitive system in surgery. Recently I was in a hospital where we used the Intuitive system for a prostatectomy for the first time, and it was a marvelous operation. The urologist who did the operation said, "I will never use the conventional technique again." It is much more difficult to use this system in cardiac surgery, particularly intracardiac surgery, but I think the Intuitive company was right to set the bar at a very high level, at the level of cardiac surgery, because that stimulated the development of robotic surgery.

People wonder also about the future of

the total replacement of the heart. Will there be mechanical hearts, or genetically altered biological tissue hearts? The history of science in cardiac surgery would suggest that very often when you have several techniques, they are complementary rather than in opposition. I think that genetic manipulation is very promising, and one day it will succeed, but it's like the Concorde jet in that it's very vulnerable to one mistake. If one disease is transferred from a pig heart to a patient, then that will be the end of the operation. One accident like that would be just like the tire that blew up on the Concorde and ended its utility, although it was a marvelous machine. This is why, even if the biological heart is developed, ventricular assist devices should be continued also.

When I succeeded Charles Dubost in 1982 as the chairman of our department, I told my group, "We're going to have one program every four years to help a developing country." I didn't want it to be like the program I had seen in the past, where Charles Dubost and a team went to Egypt, operated for ten days, and then left, leaving nothing at the hospital except a few patients saved. That was a tremendous disappointment for the local physicians. I decided to explore other types of humanitarian aid, although I call it "transfer of knowledge" because I don't like the term "humanitarian." I wanted to have a very serious program, selecting good people in a developing country, assisting the development of facilities, and then helping the people, when back in their own country, to learn to perform cardiac surgery by themselves. The most successful experience was the Saigon Heart Institute, which we developed eight years ago. I followed my original principles: We had Vietnamese cardiologists, nurses, and surgeons come to train in France with me for two years, and we taught them. This is a real transfer of knowledge, because when I go to Vietnam (I go three times a year and spend two or three days there), they do the operations themselves, five children a day. They do reconstructive operations in children and some young adults, and they have the same low mortality rate that we do in our department in France.

I am among the people who like to admire other people, who like to give credit to masters and to people who have influenced me. Admiration is very important because from admiration you can acquire the energy of trying to do something by yourself. My masters were Robert Chudet and Charles Dubost. In addition to them, I have admiration for several surgeons from other countries. Needless to say, Al Starr is at the top. There are several others: Dwight McGoon influenced me quite a bit, particularly for his human aspect. Walt Lillehei and John Kirklin also were very influential. I was fortunate to become friends with them, although I was very young at the time. That was a big honor for me, and they have a part in what I have done.

Bibliography

Carpentier A, Blondeau P, Laurens B, Hay A, Laurent D, Dubost C. Mitral and Tricuspid Valve Replacement with Frame-Mounted Aortic Heterografts. *J Thorac Cardiovasc Surg.* 1968; 56:388–394.

Carpentier A, Lemaigre G, Robert L, Carpentier S, Dubost C. Biological Factors Affecting Long-term Results of Valvular Heterografts. *J Thorac Cardiovasc Surg.* 1969; 58:467–483.

Carpentier A, Deloche A, Dauptain J, Soyer R, Blondeau P, Piwnica A, Dubost C, McGoon DC. A New Reconstructive Operation for Correction of Mitral and Tricuspid Insufficiency. *J Thorac Cardiovasc Surg.* 1971; 61:1–13.

Carpentier A, Guermonprez JL, Deloche A, Frechette C, Dubost C. The Aorta-to-Coronary Radial Artery Bypass Graft. A Technique Avoiding Pathological Changes in Grafts. *Ann Thorac Surg.* 1973; 16:111–121.

Carpentier A. From Valvular Xenograft to Valvular Bioprosthesis (1965–1977). *Med Instrum.* 1977; 11:98–101.

Carpentier A, Chauvaud S, Fabiani JN, Deloche A, Relland J, Lessana A, D'Allaines C, Blondeau P, Pinwnica A, Dubost C. Reconstructive Surgery of Mitral Valve Incompetence: Ten-Year Appraisal. *J Thorac Cardiovasc Surg.* 1980; 79:338–348.

Carpentier A. Cardiac Valve Surgery—The "French Correction." *J Thorac Cardiovasc Surg.* 1983; 86:323–337.

Carpentier A, Chachques JC. Myocardial Substitution with a Stimulated Skeletal Muscle: First Successful Clinical Case. *Lancet.* 1985; 1(8440): 1267.

Carpentier A. "Glue Aortoplasty" as an Alternative to Resection and Grafting for the Treatment of Aortic Dissection. *Semin Thorac Cardiovasc Surg.* 1991; 3:213–1214.

Carpentier A, Loulmet D, Aupecle B, Berrebi A, Relland J. Computer-Assisted Cardiac Surgery. *Lancet.* 1999; no.353 (9150):379–380.

Carpentier A. The Surprising Rise of Nonthrombogenic Valvular Surgery. *Nat Med.* 2007; 13:xvii–xx.

Vincent L. Gott, MD

(b. 1927)

The hinged leaflet design . . . was Dr. Bhagavant Kalke's idea. He had seen passive flood gates along the coast line in India . . . which would open and close with the tide to keep water from rushing into the fields.
— On the development of the bileaflet valve

Interviewed August 26, 1997

I was born in Wichita, Kansas, in 1927. I went to high school in Wichita, graduated in 1945, and, like everyone else at that time, went straight into the military, serving in the navy. After I was discharged from the navy I returned home and enrolled at Wichita State University to do my premedical training. I went to Yale Medical School after that and graduated in 1953.

My interest in cardiac surgery first developed when I was a medical student at Yale, and a young faculty member named Bill Glenn gave some lectures on the only heart operations that were being done at that time, in the late forties and early fifties: the Blalock-Taussig shunt, the closure of the patent ductus, and mitral commissurotomies. Dr. Glenn was a wonderful lecturer, and I vividly remember as a junior medical student watching Dr. Glenn do a coarctation repair. It was then that I thought I might like to go into surgery. We had had a close family friend back in Wichita, Dr. Abe Hiebert, who was a plastic surgeon, and as a high school student I used to go over and watch him operate and sometimes scrub. I always thought I would like to go back to Wichita in private practice, maybe general surgery or plastic surgery. When the time came for me to do my internship and residency, I applied to Barnes and interviewed with Dr. Carl Moyer. They had a very severe pyramid system at Barnes, where they took twelve interns and only finished one or two residents. I knew I didn't want that kind of competition, so I also interviewed with Dr. Wangensteen at the University of Minnesota. He had a program where almost all the interns finished their residencies. I was very fortunate to be accepted there. I started my internship in 1953 and met my wife-to-be, Iveagh, there. She was a dietetic intern at Minnesota, and we were married in September 1954.

I think the most fortunate aspect of my career was having been an intern on Dr. Lillehei's service in March 1954. On March 26 he was the first surgeon to close a VSD. As an intern, I wasn't at the table, but I was standing on a footstool behind him with Norm Shumway standing next to me. Norm was a third-year resident. It was a very exciting day, probably one of the most important days in the history of open-heart surgery. The first child did not survive, but the third child, done just a few weeks later, did survive. Then over the course of the next year, from March 1954 to April 1955, Dr. Lillehei repaired very complicated congenital defects in about forty-five children, with remarkable results. Two-thirds of those children survived. No other surgeons in the world were doing open-heart surgery at that time. All of those first operations were done using cross-circulation, using the child's parent as an oxygenator.

That year was an exciting time because we had chest surgeons coming from all over the world to watch Dr. Lillehei do these cases. Dick DeWall, working in Dr. Lillehei's laboratory in 1954, developed the early DeWall bubble oxygenator. I had the good fortune to be invited by Dr. Lillehei to go into his lab in September 1955. That again was an exciting time, because now he was using the DeWall oxygenator. Again, every day there might be ten or fifteen visiting surgeons up in the dome watching him do his cases. Then in the afternoon these visitors would come down to the dog lab, and we would try to do a mitral valvuloplasty using the DeWall oxygenator. So it was a very exciting time. I wouldn't be where I am today if I hadn't been in Dr. Lillehei's operating room in March 1954.

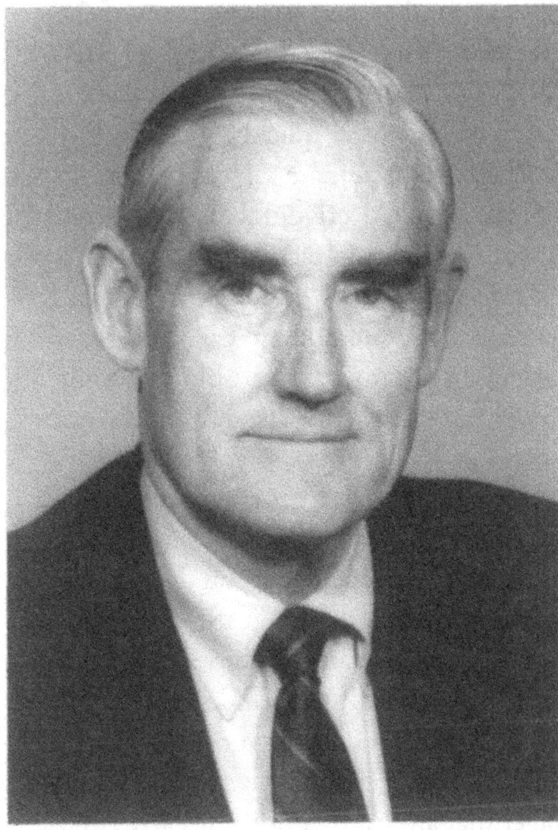

Vincent L. Gott

Cross-circulation lasted just a little over a year. I don't think that any other centers took up cross-circulation, because it took a lot of courage to connect a parent, either the mother or the father, to the child. Walt Lillehei tells the story that Conrad Lam looked in and said, "You know, Walt, this is the only operation that carries the risk of a 200 percent mortality rate." Yet there was only one parent during that time that sustained a cerebral-vascular incident. It happened before they had even connected the parent to the child. In those days they had a glass bottle for blood, rather than plastic containers. The anesthesiologist was pumping air into the glass bottle to push the blood in, and he accidentally pushed some air into the mother. Unfortunately, she sustained a pretty significant stroke. Dr. Lillehei stopped the operation and didn't proceed; he did subsequently repair that child, who had a tetralogy of Fallot, using the DeWall oxygenator. But there were no deaths from the donor participant using the cross-circulation operations.

Dr. Lillehei was the first surgeon to do a variety of open-heart operations: the closure of a VSD, the total repair of tetralogy of Fallot, and the total correction of an atrioventricular canal. In doing these operations, he had to work out a number of things, such as patching the pulmonary outflow tract. Those first VSDs were closed without a patch, but with direct suture. In fact, I have a copy of one of the earliest videos of the operation—the closure of the VSD without a patch and then closure of the ventriculotomy using just a straight needle with a loaded suture. It took about fifteen to seventeen minutes for the open-heart portion of the operation. They really didn't have a good cardiotomy sucker system and so everything had to be done very quickly.

The first patch material was Ivalon sponge; it wasn't very durable, but it seemed to work all right. In fact, I think that of those early defects closed without a patch, very few developed any subsequent leak. The principal cause of death was heart block. About 15 percent of the patients developed heart block.

Air embolism was initially not that great of a problem because Dr. Lillehei started off repairing ventricular septal defects; Dr. John Lewis was still doing ASDs with hypothermia. However, by the time I was in the lab, Dr. Lewis had stopped doing his atrial defects with immersion hypothermia, and Dr Lillehei was closing the ASDs. I would wager that almost half of those early ASD patients suffered some kind of air embolism problem; this was well before cardioplegia. We did develop a little device that looked like a flexible screw that Dr Lillehei used to put through the ASD and through the mitral valve. It kept the mitral valve incompetent; he would close the ASD and then screw this device out. There is a publication on that. Very quickly cardioplegia came along, but air embolism was a problem in the early cases.

Another interesting development was the introduction of the pacemaker. As I indicated earlier, about 15 percent of Dr. Lillehei's early VSD patients developed heart block; it was a universally fatal complication. It started in 1956, before Earl Bakken made his contributions. I remember we had our mortality-morbidity conference every Saturday morning, and in the fall of 1956, a child was presented with fatal postoperative heart block. I attended this mortality-morbidity conference, and behind me was a young professor of physiology, Dr. Jack Johnson. Dr. Johnson suggested, "You know, we have been pacing frog hearts in the physiology lab for twenty years. Why don't you borrow my Grass stimulator and pace these hearts?" That was on a Saturday; I went over the following Monday and borrowed Jack Johnson's Grass stimulator. It was pretty easy to create a heart block in a dog. We could stain the canine septum with iodine and this would delineate the bundle of HIS. We were able to create heart block by placing a ligature around the bundle. We placed one wire in the myocardium and connected it to the negative pole of the Grass stimulator and a skin wire was connected to the positive pole, and sure enough, it worked. A few weeks after we started working on this pacing system, Dr. William Wierich from the University of California joined us to work on this pacing project in dogs. Then in January 1957 Dr. Lillehei called down to the lab and said, "I have a patient here in the OR in heart block. Would you bring up the Grass stimulator?" We took it up, and Dr. Lillehei put one wire in the myocardium and a second wire in the skin, and sure enough, the patient did fine. The heart block was usually temporary and would clear up after ten days or so, and then we could take the wire out. It did require a very long extension cord, about fifty yards long, to go from Dr. Lillehei's operating room to the intensive care unit to insure continuous pacing while the patient was being moved.

The Grass stimulator worked fine, but the extension cord was a problem. There was a young electronic technician, Earl Bakken, who would come by the operating rooms and labs in order to repair and adjust the Sanborn monitors that we had. Dr. Lillehei, being the innovative man that he was, asked Earl Bakken, "Could you make us a battery-operated pacemaker?" Earl had this little company called Medtronic, and at that time their main product was a impedance meter. Earl, being a very creative engineer, came back within a month with a battery-operated pacemaker. That was the start of Medtronic. He had a little shop in a garage on Central Avenue NE in Minneapolis, and that's where it all started. Last year their sales were $2.5 billion, and they have thirteen thousand employees. It all started in Earl Bakken's garage. (Update: In 2005, Medtronic's sales exceeded $14 billion, and they had thirty-two thousand employees.)

At that time, miniaturization technology for implantation was not yet available. Those first pacemakers were about three by four inches in size. The patients had wires coming out of their chest, and they would frequently get infected. We had some patients that were on the pacemaker for months, and they always got infected. It was a tremendous step forward when the Buffalo engineer, Wilson Greatbatch, working with surgeon William Chardack, developed the implantable pacemaker in the early 1960s. It was a few years later that Medtronic purchased the patent rights from Greatbatch and Chardack. Who would have thought, back in the mid-fifties when we had all this heart block in children after having a VSD repaired, that the eventual primary use of pacemakers would be in adults with nonsurgical heart block?

Bubble oxygenators had a similar interesting history of development. The first ones were made in the laboratory, and everybody copied that model. Eventually Dick DeWall developed a commercially available oxygenator. He was working in Dr. Lillehei's lab in 1954. During that year, while Dr. Lillehei was utilizing cross-circulation, Dick was working on various types of bubble oxygenators. Dick was using a helical coil, attempting to bubble oxygen into blood, but he couldn't get the bubbles out of the blood. One day he decided to use his helical coil as a debubbler, and he found that if the helical coil was half full of blood, then the blood with oxygen bubbles coming down an inclined plane would not progress; the bubbles would be trapped. The Germans had constructed a bubble oxygenator as early as the 1920s, but nobody could figure out a way to get rid of the bubbles. Dick, using his helical coil with the inclined plane, was able to do that.

For the first DeWall oxygenators, people would buy Mayon tubing from a plastic store in Minneapolis. The name Mayon came from "mayonnaise," because the tubing was used to pump foods. The first pump that Dr. Lillehei and Dr. DeWall obtained was the Sigmamotor pump; it was a simple industrial finger pump that was used for pumping milk and other liquids. It worked beautifully in combination with Dick's bubble oxygenator.

The surgeons (five hundred or more) who came in 1955 to observe Dr. Lillehei's surgery would then go downtown to buy the plastic tubing and take it back to their heart centers around the world. That was how it all got started. Dr. John Kirklin did his first VSD repair in March 1955, exactly a year after Walt did his first case. Kirklin used a

Mayo-Gibbon oxygenator, but it was very expensive. The DeWall bubbler was very reasonable to construct and easier to use, particularly in some of the foreign countries.

When I got to Dr. Lillehei's lab in September 1955, Dick DeWall had started working on what we called the unitized sheet oxygenator, a two-dimensional oxygenator. I worked with him on that, but he deserves all the credit for that oxygenator. The sheet oxygenator was about two and a half by three and a half feet and stamped out so that the vertical bubble column was on one side, and the inclined-plane debubbling channel came down at an angle. This sheet oxygenator was used at various centers around the country. The next step was to get the unitized oxygenator commercially fabricated. It was DeWall's idea to come up with a disposable, hard-shell, fabricated, unitized bubble oxygenator; he was able to get Jim Bentley to commercially fabricate this new oxygenator.

In 1960 I finished my training at the University of Minnesota, and I joined the faculty at the University of Wisconsin in Madison as an assistant professor. I was there from 1960 to 1965. Dr. William Young was the chief of cardiac surgery, and there were two of us who were assistant professors. We only did three cases per week, so I had a lot of time to work in the lab. At that time, in the early sixties, the only prosthetic heart valve we had was the Starr-Edwards valve with a silicone ball. It is a great concept, and it is still manufactured and used in some centers. We found, though, that in some patients who had mitral stenosis and a normal-sized left ventricle, the valve cage could impinge on the ventricular septum and cause ventricular irritability and death in rare cases. By 1961 we realized that this could be a problem, and so I worked with a plastic engineer at the University of Wisconsin, Professor Ronald Daggett, who had a great talent with extruded plastics. We were looking for a low-profile valve and came up with some leaflet ideas. Our first valve for canine use had three hinging leaflets, and it really wasn't very successful. We then came up with a bileaflet valve. It had fabric leaflets coated with silicone rubber, and it really worked very well. But we found that when we put this valve in the canine mitral area, it clotted in a few hours. The valve housing was made out of a polycarbonate plastic. So we thought, let's investigate various plastics for thrombo-resistance. We started using little streamlined rings, like little napkin rings that we would implant in the inferior vena cava of the dog; we found that all of the polymer rings that were implanted in the IVC would clot in two hours.

We knew that Philip Sawyer had determined that the lining of a blood vessel had a negative charge, and it had been determined earlier that the lining of red cells and platelets had a negative charge, so we thought that if we could put a negative charge on our valve, we might be able to minimize clotting. Ron Daggett said, "I have a conducting paint in my basement—graphite paint." So we coated these little rings with the graphite paint and then, using an insulated wire, connected the ring to the negative pole of a nine-volt battery; a wire from the positive pole went to the skin. We rinsed the rings in the common hospital sterilizing solution, benzalkonium chloride, because we couldn't autoclave them, and then we rinsed them in heparin. It turned out that the rings coated with graphite and a negative charge did not clot for two weeks. One day the wire to our ring broke, and the results were just as good. It took us a year to determine what was happening: Our graphite paint was bonding benzalkonium chloride with its strong positive charge, and the heparin we rinsed them in had a strong negative charge, so just accidentally, the graphite was bonding heparin. By 1963 we had a bileaflet valve that could be used clinically in the aortic or the mitral area, and it was coated with graphite and heparin. We had serendipitously stumbled onto a way to bond heparin to polymers. This valve was used in about five hundred patients around the world from 1963 to 1966. We took it off the market in 1966 because some of the patients developed thrombosis on the central cross-strut. We were not aware of any patients having an embolus from this valve. Incidentally, I have had some Gott-Daggett valves sent to me after twenty years, and they looked great. I am not aware of any leaflet failures.

In 1965 Jack Bokros, working at Gulf Atomic, developed a new material called pyrolytic carbon, which was used to encapsulate nuclear fuel rods. Jack sent some of his pyrolytic carbon to us in the form of IVC rings to see if we could coat them with heparin. We found that his carbon would not coat with heparin, but it also turned out that pyrolytic carbon was the best rigid material we had ever tested. So very quickly Jack Bokros started making leaflets from his pyrolytic carbon, such as the leaflet for the Björk-Shiley valve. The next step, of course, was the bileaflet valve of Kalke's, and then the St. Jude valve using pyrolytic carbon. And so our bileaflet carbon-coated valve was a precursor of the St. Jude valve.

The really big step was going to the hinged-leaflet design. This was Dr. Bhagavant Kalke's idea. Dr. Kalke worked in Dr. Lillehei's lab in the late 1960s. He had grown up on the west coast of India, and he had seen passive flood gates along his coastline in India. These passive gates would open and close with the tide to keep the water from rushing into the fields. They were peripherally hinged metal floodgates. He knew we were taking our valve off the market because of the thrombus, so he made a valve like those floodgates. The peripheral hinging didn't work very well, so he then very quickly made a valve out of titanium with central "butterfly-wing hinging." Dr. Lillehei implanted that titanium valve in a patient at New York Hospital of Cornell in 1969. Then it was Manuel Villafaña at St. Jude who, being aware of pyrolytic carbon, took the Kalke design and made his bileaflet valve. Through this interesting series of developments, we got to the place where we are today with very reliable St. Jude bileaflet valves constructed of Bokros's pyrolytic carbon.

When we realized we had a way to bind heparin to plastic, we began to look for other applications of this technology. At that time, it was thought the best way to bypass a thoracic aneurysm was with left atrial-femoral bypass using a pump. But this required systemic heparin. Our fabric vascular grafts weren't very good, our sutures weren't very good, and postoperative bleeding was a significant problem, especially since the patients had been heparinized. So we thought, "Let's just coat polyvinyl tubing with this graphite and heparin and eliminate systemic heparin."

So we created homemade polymer tubes coated with the graphite and heparin. We did our first descending thoracic aneurysm repair here at Hopkins in 1966, using a left atrial-femoral artery shunt with this graphite-heparin coating. The only problem was that the tubing was opaque, and so we couldn't see if there were bubbles. About this time, two surface chemists, Dr. Richard Falb and Dr. Robert Leininger at the Battelle Laboratories in Columbus, had come up with a way to bond heparin to plastic without graphite. You'll recall that we had used graphite and then benzalkonium chloride and then heparin. They were able to bond the benzalkonium substance right to plastic without the interposed graphite. That meant that they were able to fabricate clear plastic tubing bonded with heparin. When we heard about that, we went to the Argyle Company in St. Louis and asked them to help us design a heparinized left atrial-femoral shunt. And so Argyle came up with our tapered, clear vinyl shunt coated with heparin. That was a big step forward, getting away from the graphite and being able to bond heparin onto almost any plastic. That led to the heparinized oxygenators that are pretty widely used at the present time. This is all because polymer engineers were able to bond heparin directly to the oxygenator polymer tubing. The coating is a proprietary coating, but I believe it is similar to benzalkonium chloride that in turn bonds heparin.

After I came to Johns Hopkins, I became interested in the Marfan syndrome, particularly patients with a thoracic aneurysm. At Hopkins, we have a very strong genetics group headed by Dr. Victor McKusick, one of America's foremost medical geneticists. Dr. McKusick established a Marfan clinic here at Johns Hopkins Hospital almost fifty years ago. Unfortunately, we did not have a good operation for ascending aortic aneurysms until the Bentall operation came along in the late 1960s. It seemed like a very difficult operation, and we didn't do our first Bentall procedure until 1976.

In the early 1970s, Dr. McKusick and Dr. Reed Pyeritz, who headed our Marfan clinic, were following about five hundred Marfan patients. There are only about ninety thousand Marfan patients in the country, and because of our Marfan clinic we see a lot of patients. Over the last twenty years, we have done 220 aortic root replacements in Marfan patients using mainly the Bentall technique. I am not active in surgery right now, but Dr. Duke Cameron has picked up our Marfan work and is very active in this area of surgery. If a young woman with a Marfan aneurysm wants to carry a pregnancy through and can't be on coumadin, Dr. Cameron would use a homograft to replace the aortic root. A few of our patients have had the new valve-sparing procedure, but the great majority have had a Bentall or a modification of the Bentall procedure. I have done 150 or so of those aortic root replacements, but the other 75 have been done by at least fifteen other surgeons, including Dr. Reitz, Dr. Baumgartner, and Dr. Cameron. We have been lucky in that we have only had two hospital deaths in that series of 220 patients.

(Update: As of September 2006, twenty-three surgeons have performed aortic root replacement in 371 Marfan patients. Of those, 271 had the Bentall composite graft, 84 had a David valve-sparing operation, and 16 children had a homograft or xenograft aortic root. There have only been two hospital deaths in this series; both patients who died arrived in the OR with an acute rupture of the aortic root.)

Dr. Pyeritz has moved on to Allegheny Hospital in Pittsburgh, but Dr. Hal Dietz. one of our pediatric cardiologists here, is a world-class geneticist. He has actually been able to produce mice with Marfan aneurysms. There have been tremendous strides in Marfan genetics. Dr. Dietz was the first to determine the location of the mutation in the Marfan gene. It is the gene that allows for the proper development of the fibrillin protein, which is the main structural protein in connective tissue. He has been able to alter that fibrillin gene in a mouse and has developed mice with aneurysms that rupture at about eighteen months of age.

I have been very fortunate to have lived through the golden years of heart surgery. First, I had the good fortune of being trained by Dr. Lillehei and was there when open-heart surgery got started. I have seen the introduction of coronary artery bypass surgery in the late 1960s. It seems as if there have been tremendous developments in just the last few years. From my point of view, one of the great developments is in the area of congenital heart surgery, in that surgeons are able to get remarkable results in newborn children. But in the future there will still be lots of problems to solve. For example, we have great artificial heart valves now, but the patients who receive them have to be on an anticoagulant for the rest of their lives. This is certainly a problem for a young woman who might want to carry a pregnancy to term. So there is still a lot of room for improvement in prosthetic valves.

The whole area of heart and lung transplantation has come a long way. Obviously, there are not enough human hearts out there for heart transplantation, so the possible use of a primate heart, a xenograft, seems like a big area for future development. There is great enthusiasm, too, for the development of the artificial heart; a number of surgeons are working on this. There are certainly some excellent temporary devices being used for left heart support, as bridges to transplantation, but that is another area of research. Someday we will have a completely reliable, implantable four-chamber artificial heart, but I think it is still years away.

I would encourage any young surgeons who are thinking about cardiothoracic surgery to jump in and proceed with their training. We may well have a slight overabundance of cardiac surgeons right now, but I think our field has a great future, as does the whole field of medicine in general.

Bibliography

Gott VL, Lester RG, Lillehei CW, Varco RL. Total Anomalous Pulmonary Return: An Analysis of Thirty Cases. *Circulation*. 1956; 13:543–552.

Gott VL, DeWall RA, Paneth M, Zuhdi MN, Weirich W, Varco RL, Lillehei CW. A Self-contained Disposable Oxygenator of Plastic Sheet for Intracardiac Surgery; Experimental Development and Clinical Application. *Thorax*. 1957; 12:1–9.

Gott VL, Sellers R, Lillehei CW. The Development of an Epicardial-Endocardial Electrode for Permanent Placement in Stokes-Adams Disease. *Surg Forum*. 1960; 11:250–252.

Gott VL, Whiffen JD, Dutton RC. Heparin Bonding on Colloidal Graphite Surfaces. Science. 1963; 142:1297–1298.

Gott VL, Daggett RL, Whiffen JD, Koepke DE, Rowe GG, Young WP. A Hinged-Leaflet Valve for Total Replacement of the Human Aortic Valve. *J Thorac Cardiovasc Surg*. 1964; 48:713–725.

Gott VL. Heparinized Shunts for Thoracic Vascular Operations. *Ann Thorac Surg*. 1972; 14:219–220.

Gott VL, Daggett RL, Young WP. Development of a Carbon-Coated, Central-Hinging, Bileaflet Valve. *Ann Thorac Surg*. 1989; 48(Suppl 3):S28–S30.

Gott VL. C. Walton Lillehei and His Trainees: One Man's Legacy to Cardiothoracic Surgery. *J Thorac Cardiovasc Surg*. 1989; 98(5, Pt 2):846–851.

Gott VL, Greene PS, Alejo DE, Cameron DE, Naftel DC, Miller DC, Gillinov AM, Laschinger JC, Pyeritz RE. Replacement of the Aortic Root in Patients with Marfan's Syndrome. *N Engl J Med*. 1999; 340:1307–1313.

Gott VL. Lillehei, Lewis, and Wangensteen: The Right Mix for Giant Achievements in Cardiac Surgery. *Ann Thorac Surg*. 2005; 79:S2210–S2213.

Alden H. Harken, MD

(b. 1941)

During that era you could invent a valve, develop it with a company, and go ahead and use it; there was no device regulatory agency.

— On the development of the first artificial valves

Alden H. Harken interviewed May 7, 2001, with recollections of his father, Dwight E. Harken

I was born in 1941, and I grew up in Boston. Shortly after I was born, my dad went away to England and served in the army for four years. I don't have much recollection of that time or of my dad in that period. He came back in 1945 and joined the faculty at Harvard. He had a very active practice at multiple hospitals, including the Boston City Hospital. I remember learning how to ride a bike in the parking lot of the Boston City Hospital. Everything I did as a child was focused around hospitals.

My dad got up early to go to the hospital and came home after dark. I didn't see much of him, but he was so enthusiastic and suffused with the importance of what he was doing that I got a sense that the time I had with him was special. On weekends we would go to the hospital with him. I remember going to the Boston City Hospital and the Peter Bent Brigham Hospitals; I spent a lot of time in parking lots. We would put my bicycle in the back of the car, and I would ride around the parking lot while I waited.

I remember going to the hospitals and seeing both preoperative and postoperative patients. My dad would introduce me to the patients and their families. The relationship that he had with the patients and their families was really very special. Clearly the patients had life-threatening conditions, and surgery was risky. There was a 50 percent mortality rate for mitral valvuloplasty at that time. They would go into surgery essentially moribund, but if they made it through an operation like mitral valvuloplasty, their lives were significantly improved. My dad had this phenomenally charismatic and exhibitionist way of demonstrating the improvement. Prior to surgery the patients would become very dyspneic just walking twenty yards across the floor, but four or five days after the operation, he would walk them up a flight of stairs. I remember seeing these women, most of them between thirty and forty years old, just overwhelmed by emotion at the obvious improvement in their exercise tolerance and breathing. The importance of being able to do that, to help somebody in that fashion, was not lost on me, nor was the importance of the bond my father had with the patient and family. I thought that was what everybody did. It was gratifying, rewarding, and fun for me to watch this as a little boy, to see that kind of relationship, and to understand why my dad was so excited by what he did.

I did not make a conscious decision to study medicine; I floated into it, which I think young people should do. There was absolutely no pressure from my family to go into medicine, although my grandfather and father were physicians and surgeons. In reality I went through all the same career choices that most other people did in that era. I thought engineering was exciting, because the space program was developing, and I thought it would be fun. I don't think I decided on medicine at any moment; I just evolved into it.

I went to Harvard for my undergraduate education. I seemed to be able to relate better to the biological sciences than to the humanities. I majored in biochemistry, and I think that was probably an inappropriate major. In retrospect I can see that I didn't take full advantage of all the opportunities of being at Harvard. Now when I go back to Boston, I love to indicate to people from Harvard that I think it's a curable disease. There was a phase in my life when I thought that the intellectual world certainly began and ended at Route 128, the circle route that goes around Boston. It is a very interesting place to collaborate with other people, but I really didn't take advantage of that as an undergraduate.

I went to Case Western Reserve Medical School in 1967, which was a time when there was a lot happening across town at the Cleveland Clinic. I was not aware of René Favaloro and the early coronary artery bypass operations. When I first went to medical school, Western Reserve had started a program in clinical medicine for the first couple of years of medical school. I met my patient on the first day, and she was pregnant. As a student I was her "physician" and was the interface between her, the obstetricians, and pediatricians. My patient, Diane Spites, was a delightful person. I was twenty-one at the time and she was seventeen. We were supposed to be linked up with an obstetrical patient during her first pregnancy, so that both the patient and the medical student could learn together about the whole process of childbirth, but at seventeen, Diane already had three children. She was one of eleven children, and two of her brothers were cellmates at the Ohio State Penitentiary. She had packed a lot of life into her seventeen years, much more than I had in my twenty-one years, but we learned a lot together about medicine, childbearing, and delivery. I remember staying in Cleveland over the Christmas holidays, hoping that she would deliver, and, in fact, she did.

I had access to some extraordinary pediatricians. Dr. Spock was the pediatrician at Western Reserve, and as students we had contact with him. Spock was a very charismatic guy. I could call him when Diane had trouble with her children. He was able to communicate not only with the lay public but with medical students as well. Because a child's heart beats so fast, I am still not sure I have ever heard a diastolic murmur, and I had certainly never heard one in a child under two. He could tell you what you were supposed to be listening for and make the sound, and then it was lot easier to identify. Those kinds of communication skills were extraordinary. He used to say that the only thing that a child was willing to share with everyone was a communicable disease and his mother's age. He had a lot of delightful observations like that.

With all that pediatric influence, I suppose it is surprising that I decided to go into surgery. The way in which students decide on their choice of specialty has been studied a lot. People have wondered if the deciding factor is the biology of that specialty or the lifestyle, the material reward, or the philosophy. Almost every time it has been studied, the overwhelming, most robust influence on a student's choice of specialty is his working with a person or a group of people that he wants to emulate. I saw surgeons doing diagnostic things that I thought were intellectually exciting, and then I saw that surgeons were able to *do* something about their patients' conditions. I could participate in the therapy as well as make the diagnosis, and I found that very appealing. There was a wonderful, charismatic guy named Reed at Western Reserve at that time, who had developed a problem-oriented medical record. He made outpatient medicine so exciting that I almost took a medical internship. I decided not to at the last minute and went to the Brigham as a surgical intern.

I have always thought that there were advantages and disadvantages to having the same last name as somebody who was well recognized. It really does change the relationships that you have with other people, and it was clearly an advantage in getting my internship and residency. I don't think there was any way I would have landed at Brigham had my dad not been there. Nepotism is alive and well at Harvard as well as in Boston. On the other hand, in a surgical internship, you really have to get in there, roll up your sleeves, and participate. The other surgical residents really don't care who you are. If you participate and pull your weight, they are very comfortable with you. If you don't, it doesn't make any difference what your last name is. I learned a huge amount from the other residents. I remain convinced that I learned more from my senior residents than I did from the faculty, in a fashion very similar to the way students still learn today. Surgical residency is really an apprenticeship, not a didactic teaching system. I looked to my mentor, Bob Bartlett, who was the first senior resident I had on the private service. I thought he knew everything, and there was good reason to believe that he did. He was very generous in bringing me along, offering me responsibility and authority, and backing me up when I made errors. I was very fortunate.

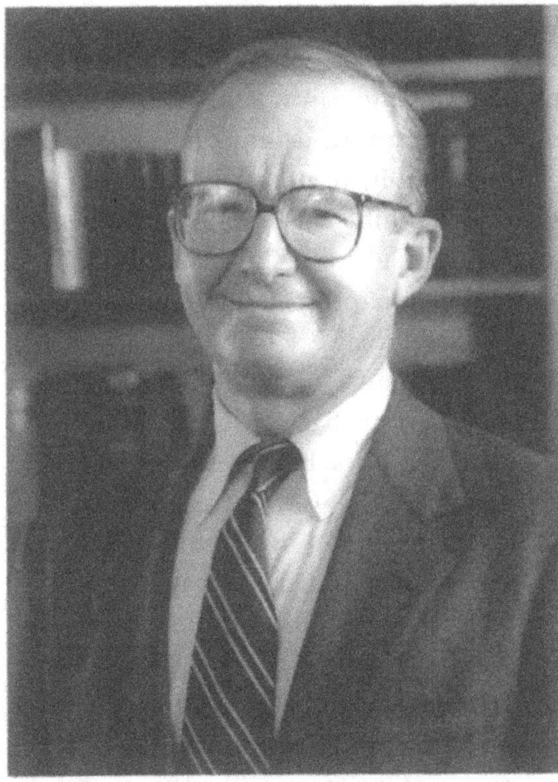

Alden H. Harken

The thoracic surgical program at the Brigham at that time was run by my dad, and he treated me exactly as he did everyone else. I did rotate through his service. He had a special relationship with the other residents, the fellows, and the other faculty. It was a kind of critical relationship, and he was eager to point out flaws. I was used to that from my childhood, and so I could deal with it a little better than most, maybe. There was a kind of morbidity and mortality conference going on over the dinner table all the time at our house, and I thought that was kind of fun. I didn't realize that other families did anything any differently. As a surgical resident, I liked and trusted the other surgical residents, and my relationship with my dad was really not different from my relationship with the other members of the faculty.

After my internship and two years of residency at Peter Bent Brigham, I went to the Boston Children's Hospital. I had an opportunity at the time that I thought was based on my own abilities, but in retrospect I think it was a fluke. In May of my second year of residency, I was called to Dr. Robert Gross's office. Dr. Gross, in that era, was a very extraordinary person and controlled surgery at the Boston Children's Hospital. I think he can be credited, along with Dr. Ladd, with developing the whole specialty of pediatric surgery. He called me in and asked me if I would like to be the chief resident on the children's service starting that July. I thought this would be absolutely fantastic, and so I went to talk to Dr. Moore at the Brigham, assuming that he would think that it was wonderful that one of his boys had made good. He said, "If you take that job, you're fired." I talked with my wife, and then Monday morning I went back to his office and said, "I've thought about it, and I think I am going to go ahead and take that job." What I didn't realize at the time was that somebody else who had accepted the job with Dr. Gross had decided at the last minute not to take it. I thought I had been offered it based on my abilities and didn't realize that I would be leaving a vacancy in the surgical residency program at the Brigham.

I started working at Boston Children's Hospital in July, and it was an extraordinary experience. At that time, Dr. Gross funneled everything through the chief resident. To my knowledge, he never talked to a referring physician, never talked to a family, and didn't even talk to the nurses. Unlike interns today, I spent 365 straight days on call at the hospital. I was able to go home, but it wasn't for very long. I got to do everything. His favorite operation was an undescended testicle. He would do one of those in the morning, and then the next case would be a tetralogy of Fallot. I would get to do that operation. He was a very generous person, but a very shy person. I think the reason he coordinated his service in the way he did was so he could relate to a chief resident that he knew well and trusted, and then he didn't have to deal with the outside world.

Dr. Gross did three or four pump cases a week. He also did closure of patent ductus and coarctation repair, mixed with a reasonably active general pediatric surgery schedule. It was just all thrown together. He was very sensitive to operating room and personal decorum. One's relationship with Dr. Gross was very stiff and formal inside the hospital, because he rarely spoke to or communicated with people other than his chief resident, who thus had a very privileged position in the hospital. Dr. Gross always wore a very stiff, starched white coat, but he would walk directly into the operating room with street clothes on under that white coat. He was the only person allowed to do that, but it was clear that nobody would challenge him.

I remember a case that I did fresh out of my junior residency. I was placing a Blalock shunt in a "blue baby" who already had a Glenn shunt. I had taken down the subclavian artery, and I was going to put it into the left pulmonary artery. When a child had a Glenn shunt, it meant that his right pulmonary artery was disconnected from the main pulmonary artery, and the more distal pulmonary artery on the right side was put into the superior vena cava. What I didn't realize was that when they divided the right pulmonary artery, the stump retracted back into the left chest. When I went back in to try to dig out the left pulmonary artery, I got into the right pulmonary artery and met a moderate amount of bleeding. I called Dr. Gross and said, "Dr. Gross, I think you probably need to come on in here; I am in trouble." The call came back that no, he wasn't coming; he thought I could probably handle it. I called back and said that I wasn't sure I could handle it. It turned out that he was out in Framingham, and he had already taken the carburetor out of his car. There was no way he was going to be able to come to the hospital, but the patient did fine. Those were the kinds of maturing experiences that Dr. Gross gave me. He had an extraordinary way of knowing what the limits of his residents' abilities were. I really think he was very conscious of patient safety, but that residency was an extraordinary learning experience in which I had a lot of responsibility.

I had been fired from the Brigham when I went to Boston Children's Hospital. I didn't think that was going to be much of a problem until about November, when I realized that when July came around, I wouldn't have a job. In January I didn't have a job. Then February came, and I still didn't have a job. At that point, some of the senior residents at the Brigham helped me, Bob Bartlett, Gordy Vineyard, and Roger Christian. I said to Gordy, "This is March, and in July I am going to be unemployed. I don't have a residency position." Gordy told me what we needed to do. He said, "You and I will go in the surgeon's lounge at the Brigham, and we will wait until John Brooks, the residency program director, comes in. At that time what you need to do is ask me how to deal with your interview tomorrow at the Massachusetts General." I didn't have an interview at the Massachusetts General, but we played out that charade. We had the discussion, and Gordy gave me some sage advice about how to deal with my interview. Within fifteen minutes after our conversation, I received a call to come to Dr. Moore's office. He said, "What are you doing in July?" I told him that I didn't have any idea. He asked me how I would like a job at the Brigham, and I told him that I would like a job there very, very much. I got back into the residency program that way, but I would not have been able to do it without Gordy's advice. In retrospect, I could see that I had done something that really destabilized the residency program there, but at the time I didn't realize that.

When I finished my residency, I wanted to be a pediatric surgeon, because Dr. Gross had had an extraordinary influence on me. I applied for a job at Great Ormond Street Hospital in London. I would be the senior registrar, and they would give me not only an apartment, but also a car and six weeks vacation. Three weeks later I received an acceptance letter from London. Then a similar letter arrived from the U.S. Army, offering me the opportunity to go either to Korea for two years or to Walter Reed for three years. I elected to go to Walter Reed to their institute of research. Again, I had an extraordinary opportunity to meet many of the people with whom I have subsequently spent a lot of time. It was a fortuitous opportunity to spend time doing surgical research in an environment where you didn't have to write a proposal; they just let you do whatever you wanted. I didn't get a lot of direction, but I had all the support systems anyone could ever dream of. It turned out to be a phenomenally rich experience for me.

After my time at Walter Reed, I thought it would be interesting to be a cardiothoracic surgeon. That was in 1975 or 1976. I finished my general surgical boards, and in December 1975 I took my thoracic surgical board examination. I looked at a number of job opportunities and wrote lots of letters. The only job offer I got was at the University of Pennsylvania, and I took it. Hank Edmunds couldn't have been nicer in recruiting me. I don't know how desperate he was, but I know how desperate I was. I started on the faculty at the University of Pennsylvania without ever having taken a thoracic surgical fellowship. I had put in one aortic valve, no mitral valve, and I had never even seen a circumflex coronary artery anastomosis. It was a relatively busy cardiac service.

I did ninety-one pump cases my first year there, and developed a good relationship with some of the referring physicians from outside, so things improved. Hank Edmunds was wonderfully supportive in helping me with my on-the-job training. I was alone in the operating room, but he thought that was appropriate, and it was certainly the way Dr. Gross would have run things. It worked out pretty well.

I was at Pennsylvania for seven years, from 1976 to 1983. During that time, I was also carrying on a research program, trying to develop a project out of what I had done in the army. I was interested in augmenting oxygen delivery. The idea was that we might be able to shift the oxyhemoglobin dissociation curve and therefore deliver more oxygen. It was a hot topic, and one of the ways we could do that was with the pump-oxygenator. We could have a fixed flow rate and hemoglobin level, so we could control many of the variables. I tried to alter the position of the oxyhemoglobin dissociation curve in order to deliver more oxygen to the tissues. It turned out that as soon as I did that, I changed so many other factors that it was hard to make the case that it was the oxyhemoglobin affinity that was altering oxygen consumption, but in doing that research I learned a lot about basic science and was very fortunate to get funding from the NIH. This was similar in some ways to the research that my dad had done; he used the heart-lung machine to assist patients who were in heart failure.

My mom and dad knew each other in high school in Osceola, Iowa. One of my grandfathers was a country doctor and had delivered both of my parents. He and his family lived in the basement of the Harken Hospital, a seventeen-bed hospital in Osceola. You walked into the front lobby of it, and the pharmacy was on the right side. It had that kind of old wood pharmacy look that is right out of a *New Yorker* cartoon, and it had a very characteristic antiseptic smell. The second floor was the medical ward, and the third floor was the surgical and burn wards.

Both of my parents were very eager to move out of Osceola. My dad was sent east to Harvard College, which would accept you if you were in the top 10 percent of your high school class. It was a big change from Osceola High School to Harvard. My mother went to the University of Chicago, but after they were married she transferred to Radcliffe, where she began a personnel administration course that rapidly evolved into the Radcliffe Business School, but at the time it was the only business administration school for women. Dad went to medical school at Harvard and then did his internship at Bellevue, which, despite being rotating, was very prestigious, although it was a rotating internship. He did surgery, medicine, OB, and everything. He had some very colorful stories about the month that he spent on an ambulance as the Bellevue doctor. He would take his brown bag and race all over the city, answering calls to come resuscitate people, deliver babies, and all sorts of things, most of it outside the hospital. The era in which the patient had to come to the hospital for most emergencies had not yet occurred, so doctors provided therapy in the kitchen or on the street. He has stories about marching up six or eight flights of stairs because there was no elevator, carrying a heavy bag, only to find that the people at the top had called him to punish their children, to prevent child abuse, or to deliver a baby. There was no good communication system, so when he went somewhere, he did not have a clear idea what he was going to be confronted with.

After Bellevue, he went to NYU and Roosevelt Hospital for two years, and then he spent some time with Tudor Edwards in London. It was a big step, because nobody in this country was really identified as a thoracic surgeon, but Tudor Edwards called himself one. Thoracic surgery was really the surgery of tuberculous disease, bronchiectasis, and empyemas. Lots of thorocoplasties being done and, to a lesser extent, resection of destroyed or infected lungs.

After my father finished his thoracic fellowship in England, he was offered separate opportunities to return to Boston and New York, and he decided to settle in Boston as a full-time faculty member on the Harvard service of the Boston City Hospital. In the late 1930s before the advent of antibiotics, subacute bacterial endocarditis and acute bacterial endocarditis were uniformly fatal, and he thought that if he could surgically remove the vegetation from the valve it might be possible to cure the infection. The availability of the sulfonamides and some of the penicillins in the early 1940s made his investigation irrelevant, but his research had given him some experience in intracardiac procedures.

Then he went into the military and was sent back to England until the war ended. During that time, he established a thoracic surgical unit with some help from Tudor Edwards. I have seen some pictures of it—several large tents, MASH-style, with beds and operating rooms inside the tents. He used the Brompton Hospital as his tertiary care base. When he was in England during World War II, he operated on 131 consecutive soldiers with bits of shrapnel either around or inside their hearts. The assumption was that a bullet in your heart was probably bad, so he would take it out. In those 131 young, healthy Americans, he was able to pull shrapnel from various locations in the mediastinum, from inside the pericardium, and also from inside their hearts without a single death. That was extraordinary, because if the patient developed ventricular fibrillation, it was all over. In World War II military hospitals, they were unable to measure blood gases or serum potassium, and they didn't have any antiarrhythmia drugs. I remember seeing pictures of his spraying lidocaine on the epicardial surface of the heart to try to quiet cardiac ectopy. That was basically the only treatment they had.

Some of the missiles were actually inside the ventricular cavity. He would make an incision in the heart and introduce an instrument; it was pretty rudimentary. Dr. Beck in Cleveland had developed the "Beck maneuver": If you have a small hole in the heart with blood shooting out, you put your finger over the hole, not a complex concept. By X-ray, my dad would identify where the missile was. If he thought it was in the right ventricle, then he would make a partial thickness incision down through the myocardium, and then put several stay sutures around the incision in an elliptical fashion. When he got down through the endocardium, blood would shoot out. He would grasp the missile with an instrument introduced through the incision, pull it out, pull the stay sutures across, and then close the incision in the myocardium.

Blood grouping had been described by Landsteiner in 1900 and the Rh factor in 1940. Blood banking and blood transfusions were common in regular hospitals during World War II, but not in the frontline mobile hospitals. Blood was collected in glass bottles, and after placing a large needle in the patient's arm, they would pump air into the inverted glass bottle to build up pressure. With the tubing clamped, they had a rapid infusion device at the ready. As soon as all of the bleeding was over, they would take the clamp off and blood would rapidly be pumped into the patient. They had some extraordinary hurdles to overcome: using mask anesthesia, very few cardiotonic and hemodynamic-altering drugs, and no ventilators. My father published articles about the procedure in both the *Annals of Surgery* and in *Surgery, Gynecology & Obstetrics* in 1946, when he was out of the army. He joined the Harvard service at the Boston City Hospitals, but he began to do more and more work at the Brigham and the Mount Auburn Hospitals.

In 1946 and 1947 he recognized that there were a number of patients in the Boston area with mitral stenosis secondary to rheumatic heart disease. This was causing the death of many young people, primarily women. Typically, they would have their first symptoms during their first pregnancy, and with the hemodynamic stress of pregnancy, they would go into congestive failure. They would deliver the child, and if they survived that, they would then get progressive symptoms. It seemed like a straightforward plumbing problem. If you could isolate the left atrial appendage, place your finger through that left atrial appendage, and then break open the mitral valve commissures, you ought to be able to greatly improve their outlook.

Dr. Charles Bailey in Philadelphia had a very similar concept, developed completely independently. He was a very innovative surgeon. He did the first left ventricular aneurysmectomy through the left chest. The patient had a great big left ventricular aneurysm. Before cardiopulmonary bypass was available, Dr. Bailey took a big clamp and just went squish, right across the base of the aneurysm. I can't imagine how much thrombus that must have dislodged when he did that, but that's what he did. He amputated the aneurysm and oversewed the cut edges. He had several patients who survived and were improved.

Dr. Bailey scheduled two mitral commissurotomy patients in early June 1947 on the same day. He was quite concerned that one, or both of them, might die. He thought if they did die, he could be cut off by the hospital from doing this kind of surgery again, so he scheduled one in the morning in one hospital, and a second in another hospital, with the plan that if the first patient died, he could get the second operation started before word of the first death traveled across town. The first patient did fibrillate prior to the operation, just as Dr. Bailey was starting the thoracotomy. At that time, a patient that fibrillated usually died. He tried to resuscitate the patient, but it didn't work and the patient died. He immediately went over to the other hospital and did the second operation, which worked out fine.

That was six days before my dad did the same operation at the Brigham. Both he and Bailey had the concept of putting a knife on their finger in the initial phases. They had tried early on to just put a purse string around the left atrial appendage, slide a finger into the left atrium (you can actually feel the mitral valve very easily), and then fracture the commissures. My dad and Dr. Bailey loved to argue in public about what was really going on here. Dr. Bailey felt that he was fracturing the commissures back to the annulus on both sides, whereas my dad felt that he was fracturing those but also freeing up the chordae in the subvalvular apparatus. So he called it a finger fracture valvuloplasty, whereas Bailey said he was just doing a commissurotomy. My dad thought there was a difference, but I'm not sure there really was.

Five or six of my father's first ten patients did not survive, but, of course, they were end-stage patients. This was the type of patients who were presented for surgery and were definitely at the very end of life. There is a story, perhaps apocryphal, about my father going up in front of the Massachusetts legislature when the antivivisection laws were being debated. He made the point that of the first ten patients on which he performed some sort of intracardiac procedure, 100 percent had died, but of the subsequent ten patients, 100 percent had lived. The first ten patients were dogs. He wanted to make the case that it was very important to do animal experimentation, and during his lifetime that was still a very serious issue. I think he did it responsibly and well. The patients and the medical community in that era were still very frightened by this kind of invasive intracardiac work, and patients showed up in the late stages of heart disease, with significant fatigue, shortness of breath, weight loss, and dyspnea on exertion. They were very orthopneic. Many had to be anesthetized sitting up, and they had some very frightening abnormal cardiac rhythms, primarily because they were so hypoxic and had been nutritionally depleted for so long. It was a very difficult group of patients. I remember how devastated my father would be when a patient succumbed. He spent a lot of time with the patients and the families, both before and after the operation. I remember what a wrenching experience it was for him, especially in the cases that didn't do well. I remember the letters that he would get from families, both when patients did well and when patients succumbed. The relationship he formed with the families was so strong that they were very grateful for his attempted intervention. I think there is a real message there, which I have certainly learned and tried to communicate to the residents in my department. We are being forced to spend less time with our patients now, but the opportunity to do so is gratifying, rewarding, and fun, and it's something we need to continue to do.

Mitral commissurotomy began to be done by Charles Bailey in Philadelphia and by my father in Boston, but Henry Souttar had actually done the same thing once before in London in 1925. My father wrote to Dr. Souttar inquiring why he didn't keep doing this, since the patient did very well. Dr. Souttar's very cogent response was that another patient was never referred to him. The medical doctors didn't think that this was a good operation, even though it had worked once. They were frightened about sending him another patient, so he only did one mitral operation.

Mr. Russell Brock from England had come and watched these operations in Boston and at Johns Hopkins. He went back to England where he devised a similar operation for pulmonary stenosis, the Brock procedure, using a valvulotome. People came to Boston from all over the world to learn about mitral commissurotomy, and they frequently stayed at our house. At the time I didn't think this was unusual; I was only about ten years old. I remember that Sir Clement Price Thomas came over, had dinner, and stayed in our guest room. He had just done a pneumonectomy on King George V. Mr. Norman Barrett, who first described Barrett's esophagus, came over frequently. He loved to play a word anagram game, so he and my mother would spend long hours playing a kind of Scrabble game. I didn't think of him as being different from anybody else. I got to know many of these people from around the world: Australian, Japanese, and English surgeons. It was a small community, and a very hospitable community. When these various surgeons visited Boston, they invariably not only had dinner with us but also stayed at our house.

In 1952 my dad reported using a heart-lung machine as an assist for patients with heart failure. He knew John and Maly Gibbon very well because the cardiac surgery community was small at that time. Dr. Gibbon was unlike most of the others, much more of an academic physiologist, and he spent eighteen or twenty years developing his pump. He really did only one single successful case with it. The deaths of three other patients were a devastating emotional experience for Dr. Gibbon, and he never did another operation using his pump, but his thought was to share his ideas with other people, and my dad was one of them. At that point, the heart-lung machine used either a roller pump or a finger pump. My dad began experimenting with different ways of excluding the heart and lung from the circulation in the early fifties using femoro-femoral bypass. At that time there were many variables and very few things that you could actually monitor accurately. They were still sometimes using mask anesthesia, and they were rarely able to obtain blood gases, so they had very little information about what was happening, and at the same time they were taking on very sick patients.

My father was also instrumental in founding Mended Hearts, before he started doing open-heart cases. The surviving patients suggested that they come back and help other people through the experience of heart surgery. Dad recognized the value of having a support group made up of people who had survived one of these psychologically and physiologically trying experiences. It became apparent that the therapeutic value of this kind of support for both patients and families was huge. A chapter of the Mended Hearts was started in Boston, and I think Mended Hearts now has twenty-five thousand members across the nation. It is still a major supportive organization in which former patients make a real contribution to other patients. Of course, patients now accept cardiac surgery pretty much as routine, but it's still frightening, and any cardiac surgical procedure is a major event, so the value of a support group for both patients and families can be very real.

In the latter part of 1950 my father developed the caged-ball valve, which had a stainless-steel cage and a Lucite ball. The first patient to receive this valve died, but the second valve was placed in a patient named Mary Richardson in 1960 and was a long-term success. In 1950 Charles Hufnagel, who was my dad's first trainee, had placed a somewhat similar caged-ball valve in the descending aorta. I believe Mary Richardson was the first patient that had a caged-ball valve in the subcoronary anatomic position. She survived for the next twenty-five years with that valve in place, and then had it replaced with another mechanical valve and lived another ten years. Shortly after this first operation, the Starr-Edwards caged-ball mitral valve became available and was widely used. It was a similar design but used a Silastic ball which would expand slightly after it had been exposed to blood for a while. In some patients the poppet would crack and have to be replaced at a second operation. The initial idea was that the poppet might catch in some of the periaortic tissue, so one of the early experimental valves was a double-caged-ball valve to keep periaortic tissue away from the mobile poppet. It turned out that this double cage was unnecessary, so they used a single-caged ball in Mary Richardson. The problems of long-term anticoagulation, bleeding episodes, and thrombosis became the Achilles' heel of the system. Starr-Edwards developed cloth covers for the struts of the valves, hoping that these would endothelialize, and they did, but with continued use the cloth would fragment and pieces of cloth would embolize. Eventually the cloth-covered cage was withdrawn from the market.

During that era you could invent a valve, develop it with a company, and then go ahead and use it; there was no device regulatory agency. That was exactly what happened with the caged-ball valve: Dad worked out a mechanical valve device and put it in a patient. Back then people were very liberal in sharing their intellectual property; nobody expected any kind of material reward for their inventions. As soon as he could, he told everybody what he was doing. Nowadays, in order to make any change in a valve, you have to put it in two hundred experimental animals for a year, which inhibits innovation to a certain degree. Back then, they could change the design almost weekly.

My father used the caged-ball valve for replacing valves in both the mitral and aortic positions, but he realized that the mitral cage extended into the left ventricular outflow tract. If you have a patient with a great big dilated heart, having that high-profile valve in the left ventricular outflow tract was not a big problem. Most of his early patients were like that, but as the valve technology got better and the patients referred were in better condition, the left ventricular outflow tracts were smaller, then a high-profile valve tract became more obstructive. Ten years later, they switched to low-profile mitral valves, built first by a person at the Bingham, and eventually the Surgitool Company in Pittsburgh. Back then, nobody thought of owning any patents.

My father got interested in medical malpractice issues toward the end of his career. He thought that medical malpractice lawsuits had a constraining influence on medicine. He was even more interested in the regulatory components of surgical and biotechnological innovation, and he thought these were very constraining also. He was active within legislative bodies as a provivisection advocate and also, to a more limited extent, on the issue of medical malpractice. I don't remember his ever being personally involved in a malpractice case.

He was the first editor of a journal called *Medical Instrumentation*, which evolved from an organization of engineers and physicians called the American Association of Medical Instrumentation, or AAMI. Their goal was to develop a collegial relationship between regulatory bodies and the engineers and physicians that they regulate.

On the subject of residency training, I disagree with most people who are involved in this issue right now. I believe that surgical training should not be didactic; it should be on-the-job training. You need to learn some principles, but once you know those principles, you need to be able to apply them to surgery. Surgery is not just a skin incision; it is a way of thinking, a way of dealing with problems with the clock ticking. That's the difference between us, the surgeons, and the internists. They have enough time to be able to diagnose a problem with great precision and then apply a therapy that is perfectly tailored, so they are less likely to make an error. A surgeon always has the clock ticking; you have to be able to do something without all the information you need, which means you are going to make some mistakes. You have to have the ego strength and self-confidence to deal with those errors and to admit them when you make them.

Really good surgeons make everything look easy, and that's because of their knowledge base, not just technical skill, so I think the general surgical training as it currently exists is the best possible way of training people in surgery. To force people into specialty niches before they're capable of deciding on a specialty is inappropriate. Moreover, to cut back on the basics of general surgical training and push people off quickly into a surgical specialty is doing the surgeon a huge disservice, because twenty years later they're going to be limited in what they are able to do. The two biggest jumps in medical surgical education are the jumps from fourth-year medical school to internship, and from resident to chief resident. The chief resident year in general surgery is absolutely invaluable. To cut that out of a training program and have people move into cardiothoracic surgery prematurely is a mistake; it does the surgeon and ultimately the patient a great disservice. I would love to see general surgery training stay at five years, with an obligatory chief year responsibility, because that's where half of surgical education occurs. After that, residents can go into some kind of surgical subspecialty.

I am optimistic about the future of medicine. Katherine Graham said, "The luckiest people in the world are people who are doing something that they think is important and that the rest of the world thinks is important." That's us. That's surgeons, specifically cardiothoracic surgeons. We are willing to address, identify, and take on a problem before we've got all the data; that's what surgery is. Surgeons will be necessary for the next fifty to one hundred thousand years. Their training has to be an apprenticeship in which you watch people address evolving problems. I can't imagine a luckier or more fortunate situation than being a cardiothoracic surgeon. I don't know what would be second best, but being a surgeon is so much better than whatever is second best. I feel as if I have lived a very privileged life, working with patients.

Bibliography

Harken DE. Foreign Bodies in and in Relation to the Thoracic Blood Vessels and Heart. *Surg Gynec Obstet.* 1946; 83:117–125.

Harken DE. The Surgical Treatment of Mitral Stenosis. *N Engl J Med.* 1948; 239:801–809.

Harken DE, Black H, Taylor WJ, Thrower WB, Soroff HS. The Surgical Correction of Calcific Aortic Stenosis in Adults; Results in the First 100 Consecutive Transaortic Valvuloplasties. *J Thorac Surg.* 1958; 36:759–773.

Ellis LB, Harken DE, Black H. A Clinical Study of 1,000 Consecutive Cases of Mitral Stenosis Two to Nine Years after Mitral Valvuloplasty. *Circulation.* 1959; 19:803–820.

Harken DE, Taylor WJ, Lefemine AA, Lunzer S, Low HB, Cohen ML, Jacobey JA. Aortic Valve Replacement with a Caged Ball Valve. *Am J Cardiol.* 1962; 9:292–299.

Lown B, Perlroth MG, Kaidbey S, Abe T, Harken DE. "Cardioversion" of Atrial Fibrillation. A Report on the Treatment of 65 Episodes in 50 Patients. *N Engl J Med.* 1963; 269:325–331.

Harken DE. One Surgeon Looks at Human Heart Transplantation. *Dis Chest.* 1968; 54:349–352.

Harken DE. Surgery of the Mitral Valve. *Cardiovasc Clin.* 1971; 3:215–241.

Harken DE. Bifocal Demand Pacing. *Chest.* 1971; 59:355–356.

Harken DE. The Emergence of Cardiac Surgery. I. Personal Recollections of the 1940s and 1950s. *J Thorac Cardiovasc Surg.* 1989; 98:805–813.

Harken DE. Pacemakers, Past-makers, and the Paced: An Informal History from A to Z (Aldini to Zoll). *Biomed Instrum Technol.* 1991; 25:299–321.

Coronary Artery Surgery

René G. Favaloro, MD

(b. 1923)

We should always think that the responsibility to be honest is enough in our life.
— On how physicians should practice medicine

Interviewed March 3, 1997

I was born on July 14, 1923. My father was a carpenter and cabinetmaker. My mother was a dressmaker. If I had to judge the status of my family, it would be low middle class. My father was a real expert in making fine furniture, and I would assist him by doing small jobs, and sometimes very delicate work. My mother helped to support our family with her sewing. We lived in the city of La Plata, a university city fifty miles south of Buenos Aires, and the whole city was connected to the University of La Plata in one way or another. We lived in a small suburb in the southwest part of the city, where I went to a public elementary school. In Argentina, we had elementary school, secondary school, and university, similar to the education system in Europe. This meant that we had six years of elementary school, six years of secondary school, and then medical school. We called secondary school college, and it was while I was there that I really grew up and began to mature. I was lucky because the best professors did all of the teaching. These were not secondary-level faculty nor graduate students; they were from the top level, department chairmen. We had first-class teachers in the humanities, mathematics, and engineering, and we thought they were a collection of the best teachers of the whole system. Some of them had very strong humanistic and altruistic ideas, and we were all greatly influenced by them. They were all interested in freedom, justice, and responsibility. They encouraged us to maintain a commitment not only to our profession, but also to look at what is going on in society, and to try to help those in our country who were suffering. When you are growing up and between the ages of twelve and eighteen, it is a special time in your life. The professors at that school made a lasting impression on me. We were involved with the school seven days a week, really. The campus was very large, and we spent Saturdays and Sundays there, walking, sitting under the trees, and talking about the problems of the world. This would surprise today's students, since we didn't have any interest in such things as rock music and the other things of society today. We were interested in philosophers and teachers. For example, I read the life of Louis Pasteur, which really impressed me and was one of the main reasons that I was inclined to the field of science and decided to go to medical school.

My experience in medical school was similar. Our class had only 120 students, and the curriculum was for six years. The first three years we spent in the classroom; the third year we began working in the hospital; and for our last two years, we were expected to be in the hospital twenty-four hours a day. It was the same as secondary school in that our professors worked closely with us, and our medical education was excellent. It is not like that today and, in my opinion, is not anywhere near as good. Now anyone can go to the university, and they have thousands of students, no selection process, and few regulations. I think that we need to go back to the time when an entrance examination was required, and I think we are losing the quality that we once had.

I try to spend some time talking to students. We have an auditorium here in the Favaloro Foundation, and once a month we invite small groups of secondary students to visit our facility. I meet with them for an hour or so, usually talking for ten to fifteen minutes, and then take questions. I try to impress upon them the importance of their responsibility to society. Nowadays everything is "lite." We live in a "lite" society; even Coca-Cola is "lite" now. I try to tell them that little can be accomplished without hard work, responsibility, and effort.

I was influenced in my decision to study medicine by my father's brother, a doctor who practiced in a suburb of Buenos Aires. He was a bachelor and lived alone, and in the early 1930s I would stay with him for two or three weeks during school holidays. He had a small car, and every afternoon we would go visit his patients in their homes. There was not a lot a doctor could do compared to today, but the family doctor was very important to his patients. I would be with him all day, watching him see patients in his office and in their homes. Many of his patients were quite poor, and I was really impressed with his commitment to his profession. I thought he had a wonderful job.

When I finished medical school in 1948, I was convinced that I would stay at the university and teach, to which I was really drawn, but for several reasons that did not work out. My younger brother was also in medical school, but he was involved in an accident and lost his left leg, bringing unexpected expenses. My parents were not very well-off, so I began thinking of going into practice to help with the family finances. There were plenty of doctors in La Plata, so I was considering going to a smaller town where it would be easier to start a practice. One other thing happened that caused me to give up the idea of a university career. There was a real lack of freedom in Argentina in 1948 and 1949 under the leadership of Juan Perón. With each new job or appointment, you had to sign some papers saying you were in favor of the National System, the Peronist party. I remember the director of the hospital sent for me and said, "Look, you were number one in your class. There is an opening in the surgical training program, and you are the one we want." Then he gave me a paper and said that I had to sign it. I asked him what was going on. He said the paper affirmed "that you are in favor of the National System," and you agreed this was the best thing for our country. On the other side, a member of the Peronist party also had to sign. I asked him to give me twenty-four hours to think this over, and I went back to him and said, "If you think that I have been working hard, I have been studying hard, and was number one in my class, then why do I need to sign this kind of a paper?" He explained that if I did not sign, the job would not be open for me. The atmosphere was really unpleasant. I decided not to sign, and very soon left to exile myself in the country away from La Plata and Buenos Aires. That is how I wound up in a rural practice.

I went to an area southwest of Buenos Aires in the Pampas, a town called Jacinto Arauz. It was similar to West Texas or Arizona, where the desert begins. My brother was still in medical school, and when he graduated, he joined me. This was a very poor area and there was no hospital. We set up an emergency room and would take care of fifteen or twenty emergency patients a day, all kinds of accidents and injuries. We had no real equipment at first, and one memory still stays with me—a young boy was injured playing soccer, and it was fairly clear that he had a ruptured spleen. He was dying in front of me, and I could do nothing, as we had no instruments for major surgery. However, soon after, my brother and I bought one of those typical long, large, old homes that you find in rural Argentina, and we started our own clinic. We had an operating room and twenty-three beds. I bought the best X-ray equipment available, so we also built a laboratory, and then we were really able to take care of the majority of the problems. I worked there from 1950 until 1962, and after I left, my brother stayed on for another year. We had a chart and clinical history for each patient, and when I left, we had over eleven thousand operative notes.

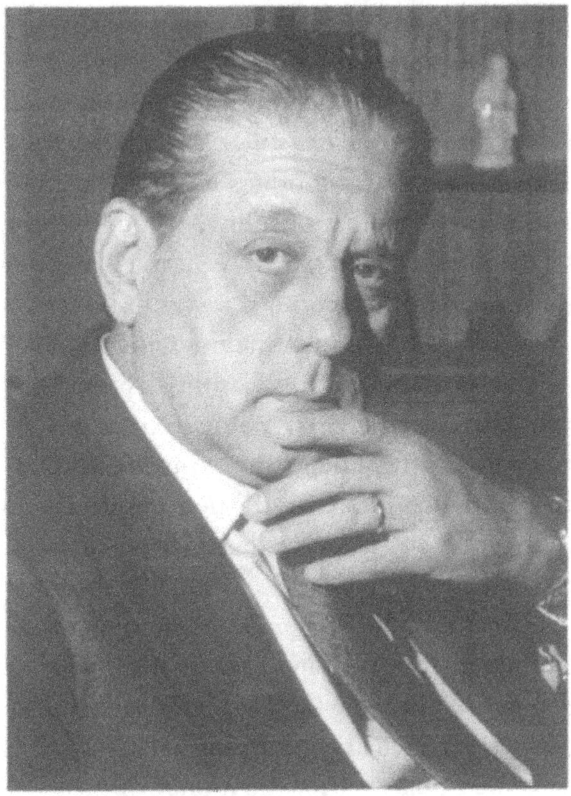

René G. Favaloro

Our practice was primarily surgical because we had the only surgical facility for a region of about 150 miles from our clinic. We did operations day and night, all types of surgery, a lot of abdominal operations, and a lot of trauma. At the same time, our practice was like other country doctors. We delivered babies and did a lot of general practice. We had an educational program to teach patients how to take care of their problems. In the summertime, there was a lot of pediatric diarrhea, typical of rural areas where the water supply might become contaminated. There was, at that time, a high mortality among children in Latin America due to diarrhea, as high as 150 to 200 deaths per thousand children in the worst areas.

The mothers did not know how to take care of their sick children. We invited small groups of mothers from different areas to come to our clinic and showed them how to prepare the bottles of milk. The water should be boiled at least twice a day, and all meats should be boiled. For a sick child, we suggested boiling a mixture of half milk and half water, increasing the amount of milk as the child improved. I started a plan for our pharmacy to supply every family a small bottle of atropine drops. It would sometimes take six or eight hours to bring a child to the clinic, and by that time severe dehydration could occur. We taught them to start the atropine drops, one drop every three hours, along with frequent spoonfuls of boiled water; the babies would arrive not completely dehydrated. Within one or two years, the death rate for infant and childhood diarrhea decreased dramatically.

The majority of the deliveries were done by midwives, but if something went wrong at the last minute, they would call us. Sometimes this was too late, so we asked them to bring the expectant mothers to the clinic for one or two examinations three or four weeks before the delivery date, to see if the baby was in the right position. If it was the second or third child, then the midwife should deliver the baby, but if it was the first pregnancy, we asked them to come to the clinic, and this greatly reduced the complications and mortality. We changed the community so that they began to see that they could improve their care.

To be a family doctor is very complicated and never simple. In my visits to the United States, I see that the family doctor is now the gatekeeper. Actually, what this means is that he is the gatekeeper for the money of the health management company. What he really should be is the gatekeeper of the health of his patients.

During this time, I still maintained an interest in the field that I had first planned to enter, thoracic surgery. When I finished medical school in 1948, only two places in Argentina were doing thoracic surgery. The most famous was the service of Dr. Enrique Finochietto in Buenos Aires. They had a postgraduate session every Wednesday that one could attend, making rounds and observing in the operating room. It started at eight in the morning and often went on until ten at night. They were doing lung resections and esophageal surgery, and I became interested in this new field. Clarence Crafoord from Sweden came as a visiting professor to La Plata, and he and my professor, Dr. Mainetti, did several lung resections and a coarctation of the aorta. I was one of the assistants, and many years later at a meeting of the AATS, I reminded Crafoord of his visit to Argentina and told him what an important event that was for me. During the years that I was a rural doctor, I continued to read of the advances in thoracic surgery and in the new field of cardiovascular surgery. My brother and I did all kinds of surgery: gastrectomies, cholecystectomies, and even some operations for carcinoma of the esophagus.

I have a nephew who is a surgeon, and he used to go to the United States once or twice a year. He had connections in Boston and at the Cleveland Clinic. I told him that I was planning to give up being a country doctor and that I wanted to go to America and finish my training in thoracic surgery. I asked him to look at training programs while he was there, and help me decide where I should go. When he returned, his advice surprised me. He recommended the Cleveland Clinic, but I have to confess that nobody in Latin America knew anything about it. Everybody knew the Mayo Clinic, the Lahey Clinic in Boston, Johns Hopkins, and Harvard, but nobody knew about the Cleveland Clinic, so I asked him, "Why?" He had really analyzed it well, and said, "I saw Mason Sones in the cardiac cath lab, he is doing very advanced work, and they have an excellent service. I also saw Willem Kolff in their research lab, and he is working on a heart-lung machine. The chief of thoracic surgery, Donald Effler, is a very good surgeon, and I think this is the right place for you because of these three brilliant men." My nephew's recommendation of the Cleveland Clinic changed my life.

This was the winter of 1962, it was my first trip to America, and actually the first time my wife and I had ever traveled in an airplane. Coming from Argentina, we thought Cleveland was very cold. We checked into a hotel, and Monday morning I went to the clinic. I had an appointment to see Dr. George Crile, whose father had been one of the founders and chief of surgery at the Cleveland Clinic. The success of the Cleveland Clinic before World War II was based on its reputation for thyroid operations, and its continued success today is associated with its excellent cardiac surgical reputation. George Crile Jr. was also a good surgeon and became an advocate against unnecessary surgical procedures, being one of the first to question the wisdom of radical mastectomy. He had many interests outside of medicine, and eventually we became really close friends. When I first saw him, he was very nice to me; we talked for a while, and I apologized for my poor English. He was interested in my plan to resume surgical training, but he asked me if I had taken the ECFMG examination, and I had not, since I had never heard of it. He made one or two telephone calls, and then told me that since I had not taken the ECFMG exam, they could only let me be an observer, but in the meantime I could study, and take the exam later in the year. He then sent me down to meet Donald Effler, the chief of thoracic surgery, who was very nice. After we talked for a while, he suggested that I register as an observer with the education department, and there I had a big problem. The man in charge clearly did not like foreigners. He told me that a year or two before, an Argentine doctor had applied for a position in the experimental surgery department and signed a contract for a year, but after three months he left the clinic and took another job without saying anything to anybody. He was still quite upset about this, and he began saying a number of unpleasant things about foreigners, especially those from Argentina. He was very insulting about Argentina, and I stood up and said, "I cannot listen to this anymore. One example is not enough to insult the entire country. You are offending me. I am leaving." I walked out of his office intending to go back to the hotel and tell my wife we were going back to Argentina, but I returned to Dr. Effler's office and told him what had happened. He laughed and said, "Forget it. You don't need to register. I will expect you in the operating room at seven thirty tomorrow morning." I never had any problems from there on. The man in the education department who did not like foreigners was dismissed soon after that.

I started out observing, but very soon I tried to make myself useful by helping the orderlies bring patients to and from the operating rooms. After about a month, Dr. Effler asked me if I would like to scrub, and I was really very anxious to do so. It was a pneumonectomy. I can see it today. He started to dissect one of the pulmonary veins and his first question was for me to identify the vein. That was easy. There were several young surgical residents, but you must remember that I was thirty-nine years old and had a lot of experience from my practice in Argentina. Within three months Effler and I became friends, and remained good friends for many years. His wife Joanna and my wife also became friends. In July, the Efflers went to Canada for a month's vacation and Joanna called my wife and asked if their daughter Gretchen could stay with us while they were away. We seemed to have many things in common, and from that I sensed a freedom to pursue my work. He gave me an open field, and I was able to develop many things. I always talked to him about ideas, and his advice was always helpful. We never had a single problem between us.

We did cardiac operations three days a week, mostly valve replacements and some congenital heart procedures. Don Effler was really a master at doing pulmonary surgery, having trained with Brian Blades at George Washington University. He never used blunt dissection, always sharp dissection with scissors. He was very good with lung resections, esophageal surgery, and mediastinal tumors. He had started the cardiac surgical service with the help of Willem Kolff, who had worked on developing a heart-lung machine. We used a Kay-Cross rotating-disc oxygenator, modified and improved by Kolff. Mason Sones was our main cardiologist. Many times I had the privilege to be in the OR where Mason Sones was checking on the hemodynamic status of the patient, and Kolff was running the heart-lung machine. He had not yet started working on the artificial heart. Part of my duty was to clean the heart-lung machine and put it away after each operation. It was very difficult to do more than one open-heart operation a day, because it took at least two hours in the morning to get the machine ready. It was big and complicated; we called it the monster. It took a long time to clean and resterilize, and only the plastic tubing was disposable. Because of Kolff, extracorporeal circulation was very dependable. Today young surgeons don't know how much we suffered to develop good extracorporeal circulation. Coagulopathy and postoperative bleeding were big problems, and we watched the clock all the time. If the operation lasted more than one hour, we knew that even if the operation was done well we would have postop problems, especially bleeding.

My surgical training at the clinic lasted two years. I was an observer and studied at night. Five or six months later, I passed the ECFMG exam and was made a junior fellow. I started in 1962, and in the fall of 1964 I was the chief resident.

The first selective coronary arteriogram was done by Mason Sones in 1958, by accident. Prior to that time, everyone carefully avoided injecting dye directly into a coronary artery as it was thought that it would produce ventricular fibrillation or myocardial infarction. Coronary arteriograms were done by aortic root injection, and the quality of the visualization of the coronary arteries was poor. Mason Sones was doing an aortogram on a patient. The fluoroscope was at the lower end of the X-ray table and the film changer was three or four feet toward the head; they had no cine films. With the patient under the fluoroscope, the catheter was positioned in the aortic root, and then the patient was moved up the table to be over the film changer. During that move, the catheter accidentally changed position and entered the proximal right coronary artery. Without knowing of the position change of the catheter, dye was injected rapidly and a huge amount went directly into the right coronary artery. As soon as they realized what had happened, they opened an instrument tray thinking the heart would fibrillate and they would have to do a thoracotomy for resuscitation, but nothing happened. There were no arrhythmias and no EKG changes. Mason Sones recognized the importance of what had happened. Selective coronary arteriograms could be done safely, and the quality of the selective arteriograms was an enormous improvement. I don't know how soon he did another selective arteriogram, but it was within the next few weeks. His first publication on the topic was in 1959 or 1960.

He then began working to design a proper catheter and to develop the cine X-ray equipment. He was working with the Phillips Company, so one of their people was in the cath lab all the time. He was almost living in the cardiac laboratory, working day and night, and later he developed bilateral cataracts from radiation exposure, requiring operation. He was not very interested in writing papers, but he worked very hard. When you first met him he could appear to be unfriendly, but he was a very sensitive person and a dedicated teacher. He always had crowds of visitors, and always took time to explain the whole process to everyone.

My wife and I were living in a small apartment on the other side of the clinic, in a place named Palace Royale, which was a crappy old building, and at first we had only one room, but it was very convenient. When I finished my duties at the clinic around five or six o'clock, I would take some of the cineangiograms home and look at them in the evening trying to interpret what I was seeing. My relationship with Mason started at that time. I could not always interpret the films, and the next morning I would ask him to help me. He always said, "Sure," and we started looking at the cinearteriograms together. He began to teach me how to interpret the films, and from there on our friendship began to grow. You can imagine the excitement each day as new information was developed. I have always emphasized that everything done at the Cleveland Clinic was a team effort. We had the leadership of Don Effler in the thoracic surgery department who gave us freedom. At the same time, he was always pushing ahead. Mason Sones and his team in the cardiac laboratory worked with William Proudfit, the chief of cardiology. Mason Sones was the father of the new cardiology, where they developed the relationship between the clinical picture and the abnormalities shown on the cineangiogram. One of the big hurdles was that we were talking two different languages. When I tried to discuss coronary artery surgery with some of the cardiologists, my impression was that they did not have any concept about cineangiography; they only knew the clinical findings and symptoms. They were sometimes reluctant to move ahead and see what was going on with coronary arteriograms and how they correlated with the clinical course. It was the work of William Proudfit that brought these two groups together, so we worked together as a team. Sometimes we had disagreements, but the final result was a better understanding of coronary disease. This was not just the development of coronary artery surgery, it was the development of a whole new concept of cardiology.

The Vineberg operation, in which the mammary artery was tunneled into the myocardium, played an important role. I was lucky because I started at the Cleveland Clinic in 1962, and just at that time Mason Sones did coronary arteriograms on two patients from Canada who had had a Vineberg operation, one done by Arthur Vineberg and the other by Wilfred Bigelow. With selective injection into the mammary artery, dye immediately filled branches of the anterior descending coronary artery in each patient. This confirmed Vineberg's theory that after implanting the mammary artery into the myocardium, collaterals would develop with the nearby coronary artery, and proved that we could increase myocardial flow. Just as I started working at the Cleveland Clinic, Effler was starting to do many more Vineberg operations.

We did the Vineberg procedure through a left thoracotomy. Every time we did a midline incision for valve replacement, I would identify the mammary arteries and dissect a short length of artery to see if it could be done. As a consequence, we soon changed to a midline incision for the Vineberg operation, which had two advantages. The first was that now we could implant both mammary arteries, one anteriorly and the second in the distribution of the right coronary artery on the diaphragmatic surface of the heart. The second advantage was that we could combine a Vineberg procedure with valve replacement or with left ventricular aneurysm repair. George Green should be recognized as the first to advocate direct anastomosis of the mammary artery to the coronary artery. In 1966 and 1967, we were combining the Vineberg procedure with valve replacement and other cardiac operations.

The next development in coronary artery surgery was the use of a patch graft, first suggested by Ake Senning, who was with Crafoord in Stockholm and later went to Switzerland. It was very simple, involving a longitudinal incision in the artery across the area of obstruction and a patch graft of either pericardium or saphenous vein sewn in with a running suture. The idea was excellent. In arteries with very sharply localized obstruction and good distal runoff, it worked well. It actually worked well in the right coronary artery, but on the left the mortality was too high. Everybody recognized that left main coronary stenosis was the number one problem, the highest risk. We tried to do the patch graft operation for left main stenosis and it was a disaster. I was the one who did most of them, and, as I remember, there were only two survivors from the first ten patients. Because of the success rate for the right coronary artery, we then began to do patch grafts for more complicated and longer areas of stenosis, two to four centimeters. We did not try to remove the atheroma, and there were areas of crevices and other irregularities. This produced turbulence and eventual thrombosis, and it seemed that the longer the patch, the higher the thrombosis rate. If the obstruction was localized, the success rate was very good with a low mortality, but as the patch grafts increased in length, the thrombosis rate was higher.

Saphenous veins were being used to bypass areas of obstruction in the peripheral arteries, and the urology department was using saphenous vein grafts to repair or bypass stenotic renal arteries with renal artery disease. We started to do interposition grafts for right coronary obstruction, removing the diseased segment, but we realized very soon that this had limitations and could only be used for very limited localized disease. The proximal anastomosis was a problem because of atheromatous disease, and we switched to the bypass technique so that the proximal anastomosis was done on the aorta. My first paper reported fifteen patients with a saphenous vein bypass to the right coronary artery. The evolution took place in just a few months from patch graft to interposition graft to bypass graft.

In the beginning these were simple cases, a single graft to the right coronary artery or a single graft to the anterior descending coronary artery. Many of these first patients were done with the heart beating, and we also did some patients without cardiopulmonary bypass if it was a single graft to the right coronary or to the proximal anterior descending, but I think the off-pump technique should not be used if you are going to use arterial grafts. Later, we would fibrillate the heart to do the anastomosis using normothermia without cross-clamping the aorta.

As in other things, you start slowly. Looking back over thirty years, I think that one of the most important developments in cardiac surgery was the evolution of cardioplegia, combined with techniques of myocardial preservation. I believe that retrograde perfusion and cardioplegia that we use now are the number one advances in cardiac surgery that occurred during my career. Protection of the myocardium has extended the safe aortic cross-clamp time to two or even three hours, and it took me by surprise. I remember when Donald Ross came to Argentina in 1966 or 1967; he tried to convince me to try his operation, but we thought the cross-clamp time would be too long. Today we are doing the Ross operation frequently on young adults with aortic valve disease, and the mortality rate is very low. Unbelievable!

My time at the Cleveland Clinic was a happy time. During those nine years I made many friends, and it was certainly an exciting time to be involved with cardiac surgery. I had freedom and great respect for my colleagues. Looking back, it was the peak of my career.

In 1970 the World Congress of Cardiology was held in London, and it was an important landmark. I was scheduled to discuss coronary bypass with some of the cardiologists. The room was jammed with people when we began the debate, and the doors were closed, but the doctors out in the foyer began pushing to get in, and after four or five minutes, they broke the handles off the doors and crowded into the room. It was an important meeting because there were cardiac doctors from all over the world, and I think that at the end everybody was convinced that coronary bypass could prevent heart attacks and prolong life.

At the end of the meeting, the moderator was entertaining everybody with a few jokes and remarks to make things less serious. He said, "Surgeons are all the same. If there is a hole in the heart they sew up the hole. If the heart doesn't have a hole they make a hole." He then said that it was difficult for him to accept such low mortality figures for coronary surgery. My Latin blood flared up, so I said, "I cannot accept that somebody doubts our numbers. They are true numbers and the doors of the Cleveland Clinic are open if you want to review our records." Later, some visitors did want to see our records of ventricular aneurysm repair, and we were able to show them the charts and the data.

It was at this meeting that I began thinking that I had done my job in America. I had trained many people. Floyd Loop, who was the best resident we ever had, is now the chairman. I began thinking that they needed more help in Latin America than in the United States. It was a big decision for me. I composed a letter of resignation, but every time I read it, I would wonder if it was the right course. In that letter, I made it clear that I wanted to return to Argentina to reproduce the things that I had learned at the Cleveland Clinic. I wanted to continue to do surgery, but also I wanted to organize

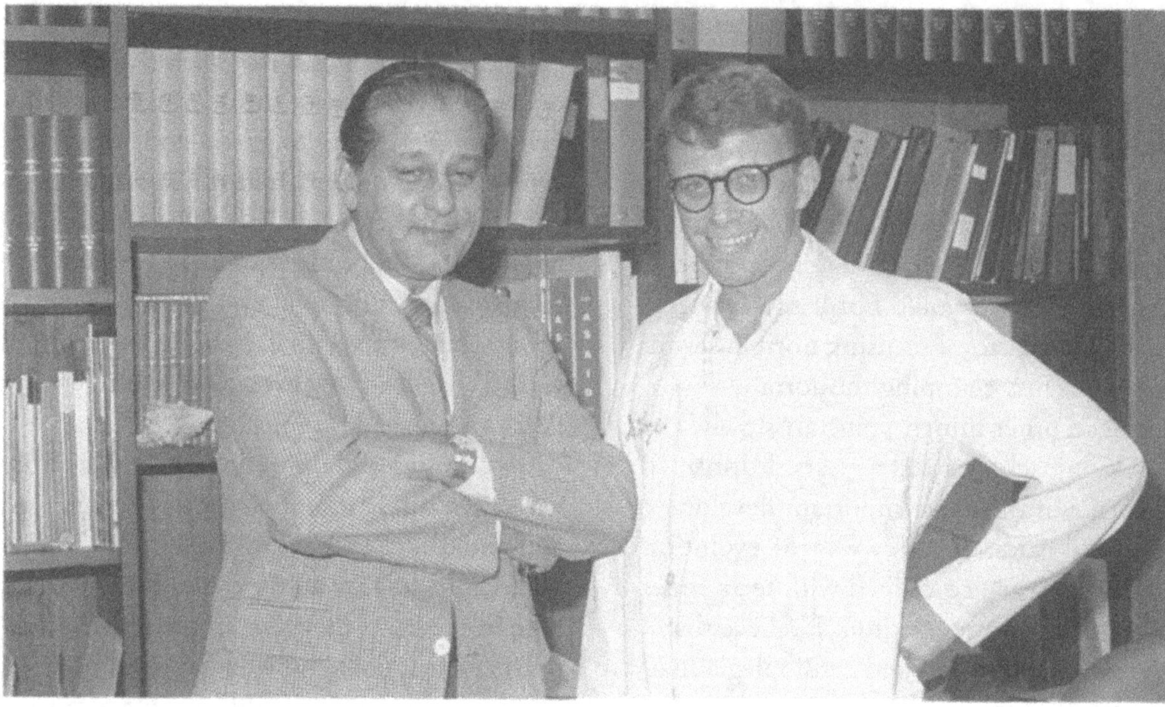

René G. Favaloro and Floyd Loop

a teaching and research program. It was very difficult to convince my colleagues, especially Mason Sones. He was very upset, and we discussed it several times. After I sent my resignation, things became difficult for me. Everywhere I went, someone would try to convince me that it was the wrong decision. Finally I told Mason Sones, "There is only one thing to do, you come with me," and he really considered doing that. I don't have any regrets. I am still a member of the Cleveland Clinic, and I go there often, but not in the last two or three years. I still think of America as my home. My country is Argentina but my second country is America. When the plane lands, I feel like I have landed in my home country.

I was very lucky after coming back to Argentina. We have trained over 350 fellows at the Favaloro Foundation, and the head of the surgical department in the Mexico Heart Institute is one of our fellows. In a country such as Ecuador, there was no cardiac surgery and only the rich could go somewhere else for care or training, but now we have three teams there that we trained. We trained not only doctors but also nurses and technicians. In every single country in Latin America there are fellows from our foundation. All my life I have said I hope I will be remembered as a teacher more than a surgeon, because my life has been dedicated mainly to teaching. I still do some surgery and still enjoy it, but most of the time I start on the other side of the table so that I can teach one of our young fellows. I feel peace in my soul when I see young people with potential whom I was able to help. It is a very rewarding thing.

When I first returned to Argentina in 1971, I worked in a private clinic, but we started a teaching program for residents in cardiology and cardiovascular surgery, funded by our fees. Finally, the new clinic was built by the Favaloro Foundation, which gave me all of the needed facilities, and our residency training program continues there. We then established a big international meeting called Cardiology for the Consultant, which we sponsor every two years. It lasts for one week, we usually focus on about fifteen subjects, and we invite faculty who are known all over the world. For example, a speaker talks for thirty minutes on acute myocardial infarction, and then we have questions and open discussion for the next hour or two. I no longer favor lectures without discussion. When I am invited to be a speaker, I always ask the host if I can talk for forty-five minutes and then have the next hour for questions and discussion. With this format, Cardiology for the Consultant became one of the most important meetings in Latin America.

We started with clinical research, but by 1977 and 1978 we began to build our basic research department and now they are doing an excellent job. This led to the development of our transplant service, which does heart, kidney, and liver transplants. I think transplants are more difficult in Latin America because of the reluctance of families to agree to donate, in part due to the influence of religion.

In 1967 we occasionally did a single bypass with the heart beating. Today, one of our surgeons is doing a similar procedure, the MIDCAB operation, using a small incision to dissect a short length of the mammary artery and then completing an anastomosis to the anterior descending without using cardiopulmonary bypass. Since the anterior descending is the most important coronary artery, I think this procedure will continue to be useful. Some surgeons will not like it since you have to get used to the motion of the beating heart. On the other hand, I am not so sure about multiple grafts with the heart beating, the off-pump bypass procedure. It has become apparent that the best long-term results are with the use of arterial grafts, bilateral mammary artery grafts plus radial artery, and maybe the epigastric artery grafts. These small vessels require precise suture lines, many of them on the lateral or inferior ventricular surface. This can only be done well with a quiet heart on the pump.

After twenty years, 35 percent of the vein grafts are still functioning well and 65 percent have developed problems. We tend to blame the vein, but progression of disease in the vein graft may well be related to the usual risk factors. Studies have shown that only about one-fourth of our patients continue to be careful about cholesterol and other risk factors after a coronary bypass operation. There is no question in my mind that some people continue to eat anything, continue to smoke, and do not exercise. From the beginning, we have always said that this is a palliative operation. There is no surgical cure for coronary disease.

I have recently been collecting all of the data on angioplasty and coronary surgery, and, of course, there is still a lot of controversy. Angioplasty alone has not really been that successful. The use of stents has made a significant improvement, but in small arteries the restenosis rate may still be significant. I think that when there is diffuse disease, coronary bypass is the better choice. Another problem is the variation in management of patients after acute myocardial infarction and the variation in treatment based on availability of services. The delivery of care can be confusing. On top of all that, our society has moved toward money. Power, pleasure, and money seem to be the most important issues, and medicine has been infected. The majority of physicians are doing an excellent job, but many are influenced by our materialistic society. Sometimes, when I attend a meeting and we are having a heated discussion, I don't know if the one who is talking is defending a real issue in medicine, or trying to defend his pocket or the pocket of the company he is working for. I am sorry to say this, but it is true.

I never patented anything. You may know that I designed a retractor for exposure and dissection of the mammary artery, but I did not patent this retractor. Recently they told me that they have sold about five hundred thousand of them, for $2,000 each. I wish I had all of that money for our foundation. Money has never been a god for me; other things are more important, and I operate on a lot of people who are unable to pay. I don't feel particularly noble if I operate on such a person, because the only thing I have done is spend some time in the operating room, and it has not taken anything from my pocket. I work in our outpatient department on Tuesdays and Thursdays, and our patients come from a variety of backgrounds; some can pay and some cannot. Our policy here has been to take care of everybody who comes regardless of their ability to pay. In medicine, we should compete by trying to help our fellow man, and competing for profit should not be the real sentiment. We should always think that the responsibility to be honest is enough in our life.

Bibliography

Effler DB, Sones FM Jr, Favaloro R, Groves LK. Coronary Endarterectomy with Patch-Graft Reconstruction: Clinical Experience with 34 Cases. *Ann Surg.* 1965; 162:590–601.

Favaloro, RG. Saphenous Vein Autograft Replacement of Severe Segmental Coronary Artery Occlusion: Operative Technique. *Ann Thorac Surg.* 1968; 5:334–339.

Favaloro RG, Effler DB, Groves LK, Fergusson DJ, Lozada JS. Double Internal Mammary Artery-Myocardial Implantation. Clinical Evaluation of Results in 150 Patients. *Circulation.* 1968; 37:549–555.

Favaloro RG, Effler DB, Groves LK, Westcott RN, Suarez E, Lozada J. Ventricular Aneurysm—Clinical Experience. *Ann Thorac Surg.* 1968; 6:227–245.

Sheldon WC, Sones FM Jr, Shirey EK, Fergusson DJ, Favaloro RG, Effler DB. Reconstructive Coronary Artery Surgery: Postoperative Assessment. *Circulation.* 1969; 39(5 Suppl 1):I61–I66.

Favaloro RG, Effler DB, Cheanvechai C, Quint RA, Sones FM Jr. Acute Coronary Insufficiency (Impending Myocardial Infarction and Myocardial Infarction): Surgical Treatment by the Saphenous Vein Graft Technique. *Am J Cardiol.* 1971; 28:598–607.

Favaloro RG. The Developmental Phase of Modern Coronary Artery Surgery. *Am J Cardiol.* 1990; 66:1496–1503.

Favaloro RG. Heart and Lung Transplantation in Argentina. *Transplant Proc.* 1996; 28:3398–3399.

Favaloro RG. Landmarks in the Development of Coronary Artery Bypass Surgery. *Circulation.* 1998; 98:466–478.

George E. Green, MD

(b. 1932)

In 1989 there was a session at a meeting where Bruce Lytle said in public that he thought it was malpractice to do a bypass operation and not include a mammary anastomosis.

— On the use of the internal mammary artery

Interviewed May 5, 1998

I grew up in Brooklyn, New York, in a great neighborhood that was only about a block away from Ebbets Field where the Dodgers played. I had a great passion for the Dodgers and for baseball, but it disappeared; the Dodgers moved to California. I went to school in Brooklyn and then attended college at Yale. I didn't like college very much. I wanted to get out and go to medical school. I was lucky. I was able to start medical school before I finished college, and I hardly had to leave town. I went to Yale Medical School and loved it. It was the best place I had ever been and so different from anything I had ever known. That was in 1952.

Yale Medical School was unusual for its time in that it had no examinations within the curriculum, and there were no attendance requirements. You had to be at the discussion sessions, but nobody said you had to read any particular thing. However, you had to be able to talk about a subject. I remember the first comments of the professor of anatomy, Bill Gardner, who was a great guy. He said that they would work very hard to teach us all they could about gross anatomy and about microscopic anatomy, and that it would be hard work for us to learn it, but it was very important. Then he said, "But you must realize that there is probably a more important anatomy than we can teach you and it may exist somewhere between gross anatomy and microscopic anatomy." That kind of teaching was in the nature of that school. It was a wonderful place.

When I finished, I wasn't sure at first what I wanted to do, but surgery became my choice because it seemed that I could have a clearer sense in surgery of what I was doing. If I thought somebody had appendicitis and they didn't, then I would know it right away and wouldn't have to worry about it too long. That appealed to me. I went into general surgery and back to New York to Bellevue Hospital for my internship at New York University. I then went to St. Vincent's Hospital because a close friend from medical school was the chief resident. I was there for two years and then went across town to the Veteran's Hospital. William McPhee was chief there and was a wonderful man. He was then seventy years old, but he was still a wonderful surgeon and teacher. He had many interests, one was head and neck surgery. I learned a lot about head and neck surgery from him.

I planned to go into the navy at the end of my residency. In the sixties, everybody had to do military service. At first the navy said, "Oh, forget about it, we don't need you," so I started putting together a career in New York teaching anatomy at New York University and trying to piece together a surgical practice. Then the navy said I did need to join. I couldn't ignore that, and after a while, in

1962, I ended up in Oceanside, California, at the Naval Hospital at Camp Pendleton. My interest was general surgery and head and neck surgery. I had taken the written part of the surgical board examination, but not the oral part. A friend who was also a reserve naval officer went with me to San Francisco to take the oral exam. We weren't in the same examination sessions, but we met afterwards, and he was quite upset. He said he was asked questions that were outlandish. "Like what?" I asked. He said, "Well, you know, they asked me, 'What is the role of surgery in the treatment of ischemic heart disease?'" I laughed so hard I thought I would fall on the ground. That was ridiculous. I had never heard of such a thing.

About a year later I was out of the navy, back in New York, and I had no idea how to make a living. We had one child and were expecting another. I had to do something, so I took a job as an assistant to a surgeon in New York City, Max Som, who had a very busy practice in head and neck surgery. This was the summer of 1963, as I had been discharged from the navy early. Dr. Som had a number of patients with serious problems, cancers of the oropharynx and hypopharynx. The only thing you could do when the cancers were big was to remove the larynx and esophagus. The reconstruction was the "Wookey" procedure with skin flaps, and it would take four, five, or even six months before someone could swallow. As I recall, there were three such patients in the hospital at the time and Dr. Som said to me, "This is just awful; we have to do something better. You go up to Mt. Sinai where Julius Jacobson is and learn how to sew small blood vessels. We're going to take out sections of small intestine for vascularized interpositions and stop this craziness of six months of skin flaps."

Jacobson was great. He had a microvascular lab. I spent just one day there and went back to Beth Israel where Max Som was working. This was in 1963 or 1964. Beth Israel had a laboratory, so I could practice the sewing technique on small vessels, at first on rats, and then I started doing interpositions in dogs. It took a long time, about eighteen months, before we had a bunch of dogs that had interposed segments of the esophagus. Dr. Som said, "Oh, this is wonderful. Now you must give a paper at the hospital about that." So I did, but I was young and didn't see what was so wonderful about it, because we had operated on all of the patients that Dr. Som had, and now there were no more. Anyway, I gave the paper at Beth Israel Hospital, and my wife's cousin, who was a physician there, took me aside and said, "You really can sew one-millimeter blood vessels together?" I said, "Yes, sure, just use a lot of magnification, but there is no use for it because Dr. Som doesn't have any more patients that need it." He said, "Well, if you can sew blood vessels that size, you ought to think about the coronary arteries." This was two years after I had been laughing at the idea. I said, "Is that a problem?" He said, "Oh, my God, is that a problem!"

I had some free time so I went up the street to the New York City morgue. It was a great place, run by a fellow who became a good friend, John Devlin. They would do two dozen autopsies every morning, and I could look at as many hearts as I wanted to. I started learning about coronary artery disease. As I looked into it, I discovered that it was a very diffuse disease, but if you looked carefully, when you went down to the one and a half millimeter level, things cleared away. The arteries were open from there, so I started reading about it. Emerick Szilagyi, a distinguished vascular surgeon from Detroit, had written about the pathology of coronary artery diseasc and possible surgical treatment. In 1959 he had published a paper in the *Annals of Surgery*, saying that surgical intervention for coronary artery disease was unlikely because you would have to go to blood vessels at the two-millimeter range or smaller, and the technical facility isn't there. Of course, I got sort of fired up because I thought, using Jacobson's technique, it *is* there, and I should pursue it. Meanwhile, I was also asked by Beth Israel to submit a paper to the American Heart Association on small blood vessel anastomosis using the microscope. I went to some of the meetings, and Don Effler gave more than a paper—it was almost a lecture—on the long-term results of the Vineberg procedure at the Cleveland Clinic. I think they had started doing that in 1962 at Mason Sones's urging, and he was the first person who demonstrated that the Vineberg procedure really worked. As I read more about it, I found that there wasn't that much contention about what happened to the internal mammary artery implanted in the myocardium. My friend Julio Sosa worked with Sones then, and he said that Sones developed coronary arteriography about 1959. Thereafter, in 1962, Vineberg came to him and said, "If you can really photograph the coronary artery, study my patients who have had an internal mammary artery implanted in the myocardium." Sones listened. He was very broad-minded, and he said, "I can study them, but I don't think you'll want to see the results."

Julio said that Sones studied the internal

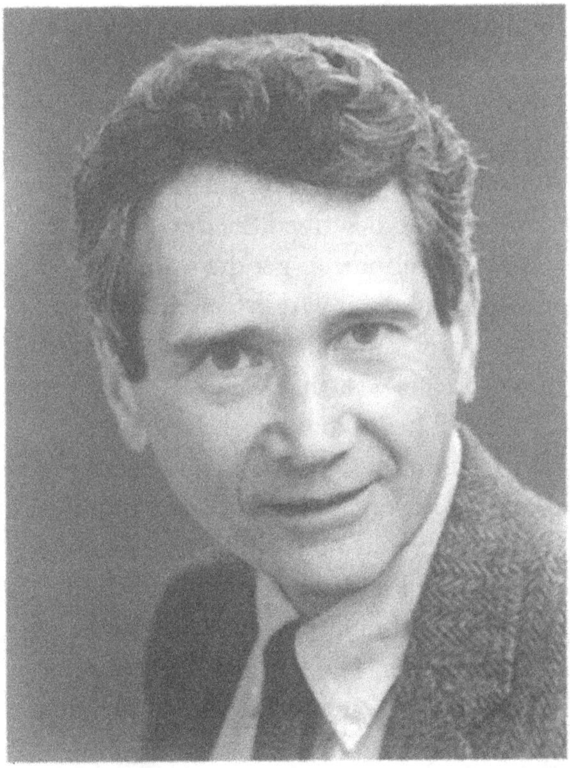

George E. Green

mammary arteries and coronaries of the first Vineberg patients, who had had good results from the implant. On the first one, the internal mammary artery was closed and the coronaries were normal. On the second one, the internal mammary was closed and the coronaries did have some disease. They did another one and the internal mammary was open. It was feeding the coronary artery by collateral vessels, and there was proximal coronary artery occlusion. Sones let out a great whoop and got very excited, and sent Effler up to Montreal to see what Vineberg was doing. He wanted to start doing patients in Cleveland, study them before and after, and to keep track of the results. In 1965 Effler gave a paper, and it was really impressive. They had documented that you could get a good result if the patient not only had significant proximal coronary occlusion, but also had preexisting collateral vessels. If you put the implant in the area of that collateral circulation, you would augment it, and the clinical results showed considerable improvement. He also described the drawbacks: It takes three months to get the improvement, and you can't do it with left main disease. You can't rock the boat that hard and have those patients wait that long.

When I heard that paper, I thought, "With coronary collaterals, you are talking about blood vessels of a tenth of a millimeter at most. I can do a one-millimeter anastomosis, and I know that these people have one and a half millimeter vessels that are open. I thought I could do a direct coronary anastomosis. I went back to New York fired up, wanting to do this. I actually did one operation at Beth Israel on one of the sick dogs. Its heart was beating so slowly that you could put a tangential clamp under the coronary and sew it. I tried a dog that wasn't sick and it was ridiculous, too much motion. Beth Israel had no heart-lung machine, and I wouldn't have known how to use it anyway. I was so excited about this that I went to John Mulholland, the chairman of the Department of Surgery at New York University and the editor of the *Annals of Surgery.* He was a wonderful man; he listened to my idea, and he said, "Well, that's pretty interesting. You go to the laboratory, and George Reed and Roy Clauss will show you how to use the heart-lung machine. If you can show me some meaningful data, then you can go to the operating room with it."

I was just in a frenzy of excitement and started working in the laboratory. They were great about teaching me to use the heart-lung machine, as I knew nothing about it. I said to the technician, "If I can figure out how to put the cannulas here and there on the dogs, all I have to do then is turn on the machine, but when I did, it looked like an explosion. The dog just blew up with air." Eventually, I learned a little bit about heart-lung bypass. It took a long time, though, because we were using blood primes, and if you use that in a dog, they don't do very well. All of those dogs had black and blue lungs by the end of the operation. This was not even cross-matched blood. If we used a clear prime though, things went all right. It took about eighteen months before we had some dogs that were alive and ready to have the first angiograms. By then, from 1965 to 1966, Mulholland had retired, and Dr. Frank Spencer had come to New York University. He was looking around and asked me what I was doing. I told him, and he said, "Well, what do you expect to do with that?" I said, "I will get these data, and then I will want to move to the operating room." He said, "But you don't have thoracic boards." I said, "Well, no, because Mulholland never had a program in thoracic surgery."

Dr. Spencer organized a thoracic training program. He said, "If you are really serious about this, you can be a resident in the program and get qualified to do cardiac surgery." I was in practice at that time and teaching anatomy, and I was also doing mammary grafts to the anterior descending on dogs in the lab. I wanted to do this because Effler had said that arteriolar communication helped patients with coronary artery disease, and he had proved that it did, but Szilagyi had said, "You can't sew vessels this small. They won't stay open." I thought, wait a minute, Vineberg hasn't sewn anything. He was just sticking the mammary artery in the heart muscle, and it hasn't closed off. I thought if you are going to use anything as a graft, then use the mammary artery, because there must be some reason it hasn't closed off. I had no idea what the reason was, but it seemed to me that there was evidence that the mammary artery had some resistance to thrombosis. As my lab work was going on in the late sixties, there was some interest in multiple myocardial implants, not just the internal mammary artery. Ted Diethrich, I think, wrote about using veins and implanting them in the myocardium. Bill Bloomer had talked about using the splenic artery and its many tributaries to make multiple tunnels in the heart muscle.

Dr. Spencer wanted me to evaluate the Vineberg operation (implanting the mammary artery in a tunnel in the heart muscle) in the laboratory. I took vein grafts and splenic arteries and implanted them in the myocardium of dogs, and they all thrombosed, but not the internal mammary; clearly, there was something unique about it. People were saying that you couldn't use the internal mammary because it would clot off, but I thought that if you were going to do a graft, it was worthwhile to use the mammary artery, and that's what led me to try the mammary grafts. By January of 1966 I had started a thoracic surgery residency under Dr. Spencer, but I kept doing the lab work at night, and by 1967 we had all the data in hand. The eighteen-month angiograms showed patent grafts. I was very excited about this, but Dr. Spencer wasn't enthusiastic about internal mammary grafts. I worked with him every day and every other night for eighteen months. He was interested in doing Vineberg implants, which was the standard of those days. Every time we discussed a coronary case, he would ask what I thought should be done. I would say, "I think a direct anastomosis should be done." He would say, "I have told you that you can't do it." One day I replied, "Well, I know I can do it. I have done it." He said, "Yes, but you could never sell it to the cardiologists."

Anyway, he was uninterested in internal mammary grafts. When I put my experimental data together, I showed him the manuscript, which had his name on it too. He said it was a very good manuscript, but he crossed his name off and said, "That's not my work, and I won't have my name on it." I thought, well, this is sort of hopeless. I submitted an abstract of the paper for the meeting of the Society of Thoracic Surgeons, which was to meet in February of 1968. Much to my amazement, it was accepted, and I gave the paper in February.

I finished my residency with Dr. Spencer, and he asked me about my intentions. I told him my plans were to do coronary artery anastomoses on humans. He didn't think it was feasible to do it. I was young and energetic, so I thought I would find someplace else to do it. I thought, of course, of Dr. Effler, so I wrote to him and then went to Cleveland with the angiograms. His office sent me down to speak to Mason Sones. I had met Sones before when I had gone there to look at Sones's late angiograms of internal mammary implants. He looked at my films and got very excited. He called Effler and said, "You need to talk to this fellow and look at these films. This is very important." Effler hadn't seen the films, but I went up and talked to him in the operating room. I told him what Sones had seen and that he said that we needed to talk about this. He said, "I have a busy day. You stay with me, and we will go home tonight and then talk tomorrow." I told him I had to be back at work in the morning. He said, "No, no, you don't have to be anyplace. Stay with me." I spent the night at his place, and he was very charming and hospitable. He looked at the films early the next morning with Sones and said that we had to keep talking. Then he made me an offer that I just couldn't accept, to come to Cleveland to be his resident. I said, "I just finished two years of residency, three years after I finished my general surgical residency. I can't start all over again."

I didn't know what I would do. Back in New York, my friend David Tice, a near contemporary at NYU, knew about the work I was doing in the lab and about my trip to Cleveland. He was the chief of surgery at the VA hospital down the street from NYU, and said, "You don't need to go out of town; just come here. Frank doesn't pay any attention to what we do, and you can start doing it here." He added, "If it works, we're in great shape. If it doesn't, you just get out of town."

I gave my paper in February in New Orleans at the Society of Thoracic Surgeons, and at the end of that month I operated on the first patient at the VA. Through the grace of God it went okay, and so did the second one. By the time I got the proofs for publication of the paper, I was able to add the two patients that had been operated on as a footnote. Dr. Sterling Edwards read the paper, and he came up in May to see the surgery. He became a great friend and sponsor. Dr. Spencer admired him enormously. Edwards was staying at Dr. Spencer's house, and he told me later that he said to Dr. Spencer, "Frank, you don't understand what's happening in your own program." The next month I was told I could work in the University Hospital, and things went along well from then on.

The first patient was a single mammary, and I can't tell you how nervous I was about it. I used the microscope because that is how I learned to sew one-millimeter vessels. I was also nervous because in New York in 1968, I had never seen a good angiogram done on a human being. I had seen good angiograms on dogs, but the human angiograms were foggy. You could tell where an occlusion was, but you couldn't tell where a patent segment was. All I knew was that in a patient with severe coronary disease, if I exposed a one and a half millimeter segment, I should find someplace suitable for an anastomosis. I just hoped to do a little better than a Vineberg, which was supposed to be of some benefit to the patient. The vein bypass graft was still not generally accepted at that time. I had first heard about a vein bypass on one of my visits to Cleveland in September 1967. René Favaloro had done a couple of interpositions, cutting out a segment of the right coronary and putting in a section of vein. I remember saying, "Why do that? Why not sew it to the aorta?" I am sure he thought of that himself, and that is what he started doing thereafter. He was only operating on the right coronary artery. The reason was that Sones was a really smart man, and he wanted coronary surgery to work. He knew Szilagyi's work, and Szilagyi had said that the technique was not possible for working on vessels smaller than two millimeters. Sones thought that with the right coronary, he could pick patients with proximal stenosis. His angiograms were superb. He could judge the distal circulation, and he sent Favaloro patients who had three-millimeter distal arteries. That's why he started with the right coronary.

In addition, by then Effler had had success

with the IMA implant into the myocardium of the left ventricle. He knew all about the risk of left coronary endarterectomy—high mortality and at least 50 percent late failures—and he thought that direct surgery on the left coronary system should not be done. He believed that you could do an implant on the left side and that on the right side you could do a vein graft, so they had not even considered left-sided bypass. I knew that Favaloro was doing veins to the right coronary, but I also knew that this usually wasn't the most important area. I was eager to get to the left anterior descending coronary artery. My operations went well in one way, but the one-year mortality was too high. These were patients with triple vessel disease, and I was doing just one bypass. I think I did fifteen or eighteen patients that first year. There were no operative deaths, but at the end of the year, a third of them were dead. The mammary artery grafts would be open, but the patients would be dead of myocardial ischemia. I started doing vein grafts to the right and mammary grafts to the left. Just adding one graft made a huge difference. The one-year mortality dropped below 5 percent, but there were patients with recurring angina, and when they were studied, invariably it would be the vein that was closed. By then, people were saying that it was silly to do mammary grafts, because vein grafts were bigger and carry a lot of blood. It kept bothering me, because the studies that I saw showed that the mammary graft stayed open and the vein grafts sometimes failed.

As I said, Dr. Spencer invited me to leave the VA and move to New York University Hospital. By then, he had started doing vein grafts, but he actually referred a patient to me, a bilateral amputee. In 1968 I had published my first paper, and in 1969 there were a couple more papers published with more information, but he still wouldn't have his name on them. In 1970 he finally said, "Well, OK, we can work together on this."

I started doing mammary grafts on both the right and left coronary arteries in 1972. I did a few dozen of them that year because of Sterling Edwards. Edwards said that arterial grafts were better. He said, "You know, Edwin Wylie has shown that an arterial graft is far better than a vein graft." Wylie was using arterial grafts in renal revascularizations, and Edwards had even used the splenic artery as a direct anastomosis. He used the gastroepiploic artery as a graft back in the early 1970s. It was because of my mentor, Sterling Edwards, that I started doing bilateral mammary artery grafts. I even did one of his procedures using both mammaries and the splenic artery in 1972. There was a lot of criticism about it. At one time, only 10 percent of cardiac surgeons were using the internal mammary artery. It took eight or ten more years for that to change.

I think there were a couple of reasons that mammary grafts were slow to catch on. The first cogent objection to mammary grafts came from Bob Flemma in Milwaukee. He said that the mammary was a small vessel and that it didn't carry enough blood, and therefore it wasn't as good as a vein. Well, I had my own opinions about that. I started out using a microscope since the mammary artery is a small vessel. Its size depends on how much spasm there is. It if spasms, it can be as small as one millimeter, but if you give enough papaverine, it can be as large as two millimeters or two and a half millimeters at the most. Also, the technique of suturing a mammary artery is very different from the vein-suturing technique. With a vein, a good technique is to take deep bites in the vein, bring it through just a narrow segment of coronary arterial wall, and then include a lot of epicardium to seal the anastomosis. That is a perfectly good technique, and you don't need much magnification in a quiet heart. You cannot do that with the mammary for two reasons. The artery is not as big as a vein, so you can't incorporate great bites of mammary without narrowing the heel and getting a stenotic anastomosis. The mammary artery is more friable, and if you put a lot of tension on it, you are going to disrupt it and get an internal hematoma, causing another stenosis or occlusion. I thought that the low flows seen in mammary grafts were due to technical problems, not due to artery size. I said that because I had done flow studies on mammaries in dogs and in humans. I kept doing flow studies through the sixties, and I didn't get very different flows in veins from the flows that I got in mammary arteries. Every case would vary, depending on the proximal occlusion and other factors, but the flows weren't dramatically different. I didn't think it was a valid criticism to say that the mammary artery was too small to give enough flow.

The other reason that people preferred to use veins was perfectly understandable—it was tedious to take the mammary artery off the chest wall. If you use a vein, one group can take out the vein, and the surgeon loses less time. Also, back in the early seventies, anesthesia was still very difficult. The scariest time in the operating room was during the induction, and I never knew when there was going to be cardiac arrest. There was no appreciation of the importance of keeping the blood pressure down. They would intubate the patient, the patient would get a little blue, the blood pressure would hit two hundred, the heart would get ischemic, and then you would have an arrest. There were good reasons to do an operation that could be done more quickly, like a vein graft.

Eventually, the cardiologists recognized that the mammary graft was superior, and they began insisting on it. In 1989 there was a session at a meeting where Bruce Lytle said in public that he thought it was malpractice to do a bypass operation and not include a mammary anastomosis. My jaw dropped. I don't know if he would say that again, but he said it then.

There are some particular techniques in taking down the mammary artery, and some are better than others. Cautery is fine, but you have to use a low grade of cautery. I used to be horrified to visit some operating rooms because you would open the door and smoke would be coming out from the intensity of the cautery. That's not good. I think that mechanical dilation of the mammary using probes is very bad. Occasionally a mammary artery will have a spasm of unknown origin. Most often, I believe, when a mammary artery is narrowed and spastic, it has been injured. The injury may be subtle, such as avulsing a branch and getting a small hematoma within the wall, or it may be a lot more serious, but it is unusual to see a spastic artery. I dislike mechanical dilation, because I know of cases where the mammary artery has been disrupted because of it. I think it is OK to put papaverine directly into the mammary artery, but not forcefully. Hydrostatic dilation is a mistake, and it's not necessary to achieve a huge flow. The biggest mammary arteries I have seen in the range of three or four millimeter are disrupted ones, dissected ones. They are three or four millimeters because you have ruptured the intima, and it makes me leery when I see one that large.

In the Soviet Union, it was recognized early on that the mammary artery could be used for bypass. In 1967 a Russian named Kolessov published a paper in the *Journal of Thoracic and Cardiovascular Surgery* with a comment by Effler. Kolessov described six bypass operations using the internal mammary artery to the LAD using a direct suture, but there was no postoperative angiography, and Effler was critical of that. He published it because it was important, but he had no idea what had happened. In fact, there was no preoperative angiography either.

In the mid-1970s, I received phone calls from the Soviet Union. Of course, the Cold War was on, and our relations with Russia were very bad. I seemed to get these calls in summer when I was on vacation. I would get a call from Evgeni Kolessov, the son of Vladimir Kolessov, who had done the initial work. He wanted to know about my work. We would talk, and I would say, "Let's meet." He would say, "No, I'll call you." I had a political scientist friend who had been in Russia a lot, and knew the scene there. He said, "Don't make the man uncomfortable. He is going to be in deep trouble if he starts getting calls from an American. Just let him call you."

In the mid- to late seventies, when things were briefly easing up in the Cold War, Kolessov said, "Let's make a joint presentation at the International Cardiovascular meeting in Moscow," which was scheduled to happen in the late 1970s. I was eager to do it, but I couldn't get in touch with him again. I wrote to him, but he never answered. A few years went by, and it was almost 1980. He called again and was very cheery. I was sort of miffed and said, "Listen, I was looking forward to getting material together for a meeting with you in Moscow, and you never followed through on it. What happened?" He said we couldn't do that, and I asked why. He said it would have been embarrassing. I asked why again. Finally he said, "Because we don't yet have coronary arteriography in Russia, and we couldn't present the subject at an international meeting." He added, "But someday we are going to squeeze a machine out of East Germany." So they had no coronary arteriograms.

These mammary artery grafts can last a long time. Some of my patients have had patent mammary grafts for twenty-five years or more. When I registered for a conference recently, Bradley Allen was standing with Gerald Buckberg, and Gerald introduced us. Allen said, "Well, I know Dr. Green because he operated on my father twenty-six years ago, and my father was just restudied, and his mammary artery graft looks fine." I don't know the exact number of patients I have whose mammary artery grafts have lasted that long. What has impressed me enormously is that I have never seen arteriosclerotic changes in mammary artery grafts. I know that they occur in internal mammary arteries, but not in the grafts. I have taken down mammary arteries on rare occasions that I haven't used because you could see the arteriosclerosis, but I have never seen it develop in one that was grafted. I have never seen an angiogram that showed it. I have seen angiograms that show 360-degree twists, some with narrowing from either organized intramural hematoma or cautery injury. I have seen the so-called string sign, which I think is tension. I have not seen arteriosclerotic change with ulceration, or other hallmarks of arteriosclerotic change.

I am not in favor of the use of radial arteries, however, which were first used in 1972 and 1973 by Alain Carpentier. It is a very muscular artery, it spasms, and there is a high incidence of intimal hyperplasia. In 1985, before I started doing a whole lot of bilateral mammaries, I went to the Cleveland Clinic to speak with Floyd Loop about the late results of free grafts. He had just published a paper, with some recent long-term angiograms, and he said he had never seen atherosclerotic change or stricture in a free graft. That impressed and surprised me, because I thought that the pedicle graft worked by carrying its nutrient vasa vasorum with it. I thought, therefore, that the free graft would not work.

I went back to New York and tried to figure it out. I went back to the morgue and injected mammary arteries and radial arteries with a barium gelatin mixture. The mammary artery has a lot of intercostal branches, but from those intercostal branches, there are tributaries that form the vasa vasorum. If you do a free graft with a bit of tissue around it, and if you don't strip all the adventitia, you will immediately reconstitute the vasa vasorum, and you will not have an ischemic arterial graft. On the other hand, the radial artery is thick, a lot thicker than the mammary artery. You can't count on oxygen diffusion from a real thin intima through a thin arterial wall as with the mammary artery. You have to have vasa, but if you inject a radial artery, it's disconcerting to discover that, at least between the wrist and the elbow, the branches of the radial do not contribute to the vasa, and you could have an ischemic graft. I think that is possibly why the radial artery doesn't work. I have not done that kind of preparation with the gastroepiploic artery or the inferior epigastric artery.

My ideal setup for a patient that needs multiple grafts would be, then, two mammaries and whatever vein is necessary. The two mammaries are used for the most dominant part of the circulation. I have had good experience also with sequential grafts in patients that had really inadequate veins. I think they are OK. There is also the concept of bringing a vein graft off the mammary, to avoid having to put a clamp on the aorta. I guess that is OK, but I don't think the vein graft is going to do any better than it would have done on the aorta. The real danger is not using enough magnification.

I have used magnification continuously, for vein grafts and for artery grafts, but when I started using vein grafts, I did not use a microscope. I used loupes with two and a half times magnification, but then I thought it was just ridiculous, it's easier to use a microscope. I have used loupes on peripheral vascular surgery and on carotid surgery, but I just think it is easier to use a microscope for coronary surgery.

I think it is really important to use magnification. When you are making an arteriotomy in the internal mammary artery, you must remember that it is a very friable wall. You have to have a very sharp blade and be very careful not to damage it. The only danger that I see in taking a graft off of it is that you might not be careful enough about the arteriotomy. I usually use the equivalent of ten times magnification. I use magnification also for the aortic anastomosis when I drop down to eight times or even six times magnifications. On rare occasions I will go up a lot higher. I think that even on an endarterectomy, magnification is helpful. I don't like endarterectomies, but I have done them.

For people coming from smaller communities, it may seem difficult to start a practice in a place as large as New York City. It really wasn't that hard because I was doing something that nobody else was doing at the time, and there was a tremendous need for it. I don't know if you could duplicate that now, but it was a procedure that was needed and not available. I had no problem establishing my practice. The only problem was dealing with the fact that I had more patients than I could see.

Nowadays, we have things like MIDCAB and minimal incisions. I think that the whole basis of good bypass operating is sewing a good vascular conduit to a normal vessel. If you sew to an arteriosclerotic vessel, you are likely to get a stenosis. You already have a disease process there. I think that the most important part of the operation is finding a normal vessel in which to make an arteriotomy, and I think that if you use minimal access, you are giving yourself a huge handicap. It is not unusual for the best place to be under a myocardial bridge, and I don't see how you could do that with minimal access. I have never used minimal access, however, so I don't know, but when you are dealing with the back of the heart with open chest and cardioplegia, you can turn the heart any way you want. I don't think you can do that with minimal access, so I think you are working with a tremendous handicap.

I am also amazed at the stent business. The stent can't be better than an endarterectomy. An endarterectomy is a bad operation in a small artery because it is just the beginning of a biologic process that ends up with scarring. The stent in the small vessel isn't going to be the answer, and I am quite certain of that. Angioplasty, too, is a poor procedure. Gruentzig, who introduced angioplasty and had long-term follow-up on his patients, said that it would be appropriate in 15 percent of the patients. I think he was right.

Bibliography

Green GE, Stertzer SH, Reppert EH. Coronary Arterial Bypass Grafts. *Ann Thorac Surg.* 1968; 5:443–450.

Green GE. Microvascular Technique in Coronary Artery Surgery. *Am Heart J.* 1970; 79:276–279.

Habal SM, Fitzpatrick HF, Green GE. Training in Microvascular Surgery. *Surgery.* 1977; 81:596–598.

Green GE, Kemp Alam SE, Pierson RN Jr, et al. Coronary Bypass Surgery. *J Thorac Cardiovasc Surg.* 1979; 77: 48–56.

Green GE. Coronary Bypass Surgery Highlights Blood Vessel Biology. *Ann Thorac Surg.* 1986; 41:235–236.

Green GE, Sosa JA, Cameron A. Prospective Study of Feasibility of Routine Use of Multiple Internal Mammary Artery Anastomoses. *J Cardiovasc Surg* (Torino). 1989; 30:643–647.

Green GE, Swistel DG, Castro J, et al. Sternal Blood Flow during Mobilization of the Internal Thoracic Arteries. *Ann Thorac Surg.* 1993; 55:967–970.

Green GE, Cameron A, Goyal A, et al. Five-Year Follow-up of Microsurgical Multiple Internal Thoracic Artery Grafts. *Ann Thorac Surg.* 1994; 58:74–79.

Cameron A, Green GE, Brogno DA, Thornton J. Internal Thoracic Artery Grafts: 20-Year Clinical Follow-up. *J Am Coll Cardiol.* 1995; 25:188–192.

W. Dudley Johnson, MD

(b. 1930)

We started working on end-stage endarterectomy, revitalizing arteries that had almost no flow and no lumen.

— On his interest in extensive coronary artery endarterectomy

Interviewed May 6, 2003

I was born in 1930 in Madison, Wisconsin. My father had grown up in the middle of Wisconsin on a little farm that had a cheese factory, which was one of many in those days. He worked his way through school and became an electrical engineer. He was a professor at the University of Wisconsin in Madison, and he met my mother there. She was teaching in the home economics department. I have two brothers, one older and one younger, and we grew up in Madison. When I was thirteen, my father left his position at the University of Wisconsin and went into industry, and we moved to Rockford, Illinois. Somewhere around eighth grade, I decided I wanted to be a physician. I went through high school in Illinois and then on to premedical school. One of our close family friends was a family doctor, and I liked and respected him enormously. How much that influenced my wanting to be a physician, I cannot say, but he certainly was a positive influence.

I received my undergraduate degree from the University of Illinois in 1951 and graduated from the University of Illinois Medical School in 1955. My internship was at Cook County Hospital, which at that time was a big city hospital with thirty-five hundred patients. One ward would commonly have forty to fifty patients in a big open room. There was always a significant shortage of nurses, so the interns often took care of many of the nursing functions. I do not think that you could get away with that kind of system nowadays because of the number of mistakes that we made. The lack of supervision of young inexperienced interns was remarkable, and much of the time we were totally on our own. We had to make decisions, and we had to do things. We did not have a lot of backup.

The hospital was so large that the general surgery service had three fracture services, two for men and one for women. When I rotated a month on urology, I did all kinds of cystoscopic examinations and retrograde pyelograms. Every night someone would come in with an obstruction, and we would have to dilate the strictures. It was the same on the fracture service. I had one solid month of fractures, and then one month of dermatology. There was a whole ward for dermatology, end-stage skin problems, plus huge dermatology clinics. By the second year, I could pick the service that I wanted to go on, and I took a lot of different services. I thought this experience was far better than any other general practice residency that I was aware of, because of the exposure to so many different disease processes.

I worked every other night, and an eighty-hour week was a good week. At that time, I intended to be a general practitioner. I did not really like surgeons when I was in medical school, but when I rotated on the surgical service for three months as an intern at Cook County, my senior resident was wonderful, a very good surgeon and a very nice person. He changed my attitude about surgeons, and he is still living and practicing in upstate Wisconsin. I saw him last year, but I had not visited him in many years. That experience got me interested in surgery.

I did two years of a rotating internship at Cook County Hospital. Part of the reason that I spent two years there was that I was awaiting my draft notice, and to be allocated to a service. I was drafted, and assigned to go to the navy. That would have been a disaster for me, because I have never known anybody to have more motion sickness than I do. If they had put me on a boat, I would have been useless to anybody for two years, so I signed up for the Public Health Service, which was one of the uniformed services in those days. I was assigned to work in their chronic disease division, and they sent me to Columbus, Ohio, where I spent two years with the state health department. I met a fellow there whose wife worked as a secretary for Dr. Edwin Ellison, the assistant chief of surgery at Ohio State Medical School in Columbus. In 1958 he left and went to Milwaukee to be chairman of the surgery department at Marquette University. She had such good things to say about him as a surgeon and as a teacher that I followed him there and interviewed for a position as a surgical resident, and I ended up going to Marquette for my residency.

As a general surgical resident, I became interested in vascular problems, although I have no idea why. I did sixty or seventy carotid endarterectomies at a time when no one else had done very many, and I also did aortic aneurysms and the like. We had to do all of our own angiograms in those days, so

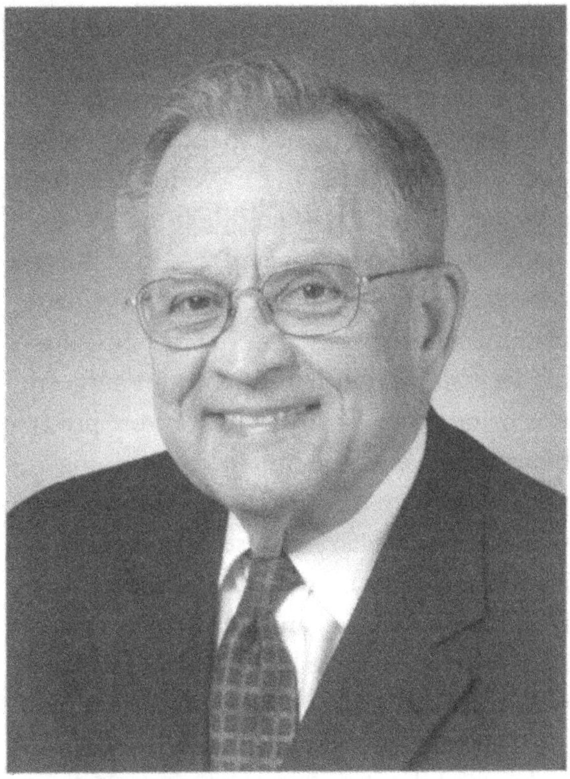

W. Dudley Johnson

we put needles and catheters in, and did our own carotid films and aortograms.

One of the best teachers I had was a surgeon who was in charge of my rotation in thoracic surgery, Dr. Ben Narodick. He was a phenomenally good teacher, and he had incredibly sound judgment. He was a huge stimulus for me to go into thoracic surgery. Of course at that time there was not much heart surgery of any sort. I was not that happy with my experience as a general surgeon, so I thought that if I went through the thoracic surgery program, I would have additional experience to help get a better job in a clinic somewhere when I finished my training. As I was finishing my residency, I had nothing lined up, and Dr. Derward Lepley, who was in charge of the cardiac program, asked me to join him. Until that point, I had

had no illusions at any time about being a heart surgeon.

Dr. Lepley came to Milwaukee from Minnesota, where he had spent a year or two with Dr. Lillehei in Dr. Wangensteen's program. When I was a resident, he was doing a few open-heart operations on children. I took an extra year as a fellow, to have better training before I started in practice just doing hearts, but not that much heart surgery was being done. We thought we were pretty busy when we reached the point of doing a valve case every Wednesday. Obviously, there was a lot of coronary disease, and the mortality rate for coronary disease was higher than it is now. I expressed an interest in it, and Dr. Lepley gave me a free hand to do anything I wanted in the field of coronary artery disease.

In 1966 I started doing the Vineberg procedure and developed a variation on it. Some of those patients are still living, thirty years later. People make fun of the Vineberg operation, but unlike most forms of treatment for coronary disease today, when the Vineberg works, it gets better year by year. In subsequent years, I have had the occasion to reoperate on a fair number of those patients, and I would commonly measure flow through the mammary artery implant, and it would be anywhere from 100 cubic centimeters to as high as 275 cubic centimeters per minute.

It became obvious that if you simply tunneled the mammary artery into the heart muscle, the operation really did not do much. The mammary artery develops collaterals with the distal portions of the coronary system, so I had to do my implants directly adjacent to the diseased coronary artery. A large percentage of patients would develop collaterals connecting to the distal coronary branches. I developed a way of dissecting intercostals and mediastinal branches of the mammary artery all the way down into the epigastric area, and I would wrap this mammary artery around the heart and do five, six, seven, or even eight implants of the branches of the mammary artery, under the different target vessels. On subsequent studies, it was very common to find many different coronary branches being filled from the one big mammary implant. I used a single left mammary, since the right would not reach far enough to revascularize a diagonal or marginal.

Every year, I would go to the thoracic surgery meetings, and every year the Cleveland Clinic surgeons got up and talked, and every year they had a different approach. At first, it was a single mammary implant, then a double mammary; every year it was different. In the mid-sixties, they were doing patch grafts on the right coronary. I think they were using pericardium, or maybe a vein patch. I went down to Cleveland and watched them do two of those patch grafts in the proximal right coronary artery, where they put the patch across diseased areas of the coronary artery. They were very concerned about keeping the patch proximal to the acute marginal branch, and they were putting catheters distally to perfuse the distal coronary artery in order to maintain circulation. When I returned home, I was referred two patients for a patch graft to the right coronary artery. As I was doing the second patch, I said to myself, "This is ridiculous. The disease obviously extends above and below the critical obstruction. If you can cut across the diseased area and sew a patch into it, why not just go down two or three centimeters to where the artery becomes normal, open the artery there, cut the distal vein graft like a patch and sew it to the coronary, then anastomose the proximal end of the vein to the aorta?" This was my concept of the coronary artery vein bypass operation.

Also important at that time was the method of myocardial protection, and everybody was afraid of dealing with these coronary patients. The Cleveland Clinic surgeons had talked about putting a catheter in the distal coronary artery and constantly perfusing the right coronary beyond where you were working. They were also doing intermittent aortic cross-clamping for valve replacement.

I put a number of dogs on bypass, cross-clamped the aorta, and perfused the root of the aorta at three different temperatures and pressures. I think we used forty, eighty, and one hundred millimeters of mercury pressures, and thirty, thirty-four, and thirty-seven degree temperatures, in different combinations. Even under the worst circumstances, the lowest pressure and the highest temperature, the coronary sinus oxygen saturations were still 70 or 80 percent, and most of the other coronary sinus saturations were up in the nineties. It became obvious to me from these simple experiments that once you put a dog on bypass, the heart consumes very little energy, and therefore the coronary patient should tolerate ischemic arrest just as well as the valve patients. If there is enough blood supply in the coronary patient for him to live the way he is, then once we go on bypass and remove the workload from the heart, there should not be any coronary ischemia in a great majority of patients. That was my simplistic reasoning, and it seemed to me that we should be able to cross-clamp the aorta, stop the heart completely, and sew the grafts in wherever we want. That has turned out to be true. I started with ten minutes cross-clamp time, and then went to fifteen and twenty minutes. I did not want to do a study to define the limits of that, but obviously fifteen- and twenty-minute cross-clamp periods work very well. I would totally stop the coronary circulation and have intermittent ischemic arrest. This was critical to doing precise surgery, being able to stop the heart and coronary flow completely.

At first, we only did grafts to the right coronary artery. I did a few of those operations, then several months later I started doing left coronary artery lesions. I remember that I had a patient with a large ventricular aneurysm, which I repaired. The right coronary artery was diseased all the way down to the posterior descending. His heart would not take off after I did his aneurysm, and in desperation I sewed a vein graft into the posterior descending and anastomosed it up to the aorta. The heart took off and did fine. I said to myself, "Well, if I can put a graft into the posterior descending, certainly I can put one anywhere on the left side." The next week, I did a graft to the main circumflex, beyond a 95 percent obstruction, and then I started putting in multiple grafts. Actually, that first patient that I did a vein graft to the left coronary artery is now eighty-five years old and has had no symptoms since the operation. He was catheterized three or four years ago, and the graft is still open after thirty-five years.

I had two or three patients in those early years (1967–1968) who had beautiful grafts to the right coronary artery who died two or three weeks later with an acute anterior infarct. It was obvious that one graft does not save the patient and that we have to bypass all the arteries that are involved. Very quickly the idea of total revascularization evolved. I gave a talk about it then, and I am still talking about the importance of multiple grafts and the better long-term survival of patients with total revascularization.

During the initial phase of the development of the operation, the Cleveland Clinic thought that it was safe to do the right coronary artery but that the mortality was very high with grafts to the left coronary artery. They tried putting vein patches in fourteen patients with stenotic lesions of the left coronary, and eleven of those patients died, so they stopped operating on the left coronary artery. I went down there in 1970, and they had kept a running list of how many patients they had done, and they had just done their one thousandth coronary bypass operation. Of those, forty patients received two grafts, and everybody else had a single bypass. I think that the term "dominant right coronary" is misleading, because it really means that it is dominant to the inferior wall of the ventricle, and it is quite rare that you find a right coronary that is dominant to the whole ventricle. I watched Don Effler put a graft to the right coronary artery, and then he would do a Vineberg under the left coronary.

I did a lot of patients combining the Vineberg operation with vein grafts. I did an occasional Vineberg procedure up until a few years ago, because it works very well when there is ischemia. The most difficult situation, for example, would be a large circumflex with half a dozen marginal branches distally, and the circumflex so diseased that there is no place for a graft. I would do a Vineberg under that whole area as a means of improving circulation.

After we developed the concept of total revascularization, we learned very quickly that the survival rate was exactly the same whether we had done one, two, three, or four grafts as long as we did not leave stenotic vessels ungrafted. More grafts do not increase postoperative mortality. That may not have been true at every center, but it was true for us. There were some centers at that time that used a single cross-clamp rather than intermittent cross-clamp, which for three grafts meant a long cross-clamp time and a longer ischemic time.

In the early seventies, there was a good bit of controversy as to the benefits and long-term results of coronary artery surgery, although there was never any question about immediate relief of angina. In those days, we would see a lot of patients with severe angina and pain at rest. After the operation, the surgical pain was not severe, and they would be smiling from ear to ear because of the relief. I initially insisted that the cardiologists recatheterize all the patients before they went home, which in those days was eight to ten days after the surgery. The cardiologists said that they would rather do it a year later. I said, "If they are all closed now, then I can forget this operation and go fishing. I want to know now. If they are open now, then we will study them again in a year." There were all sorts of predictions that they would all close in months like bypasses sometimes do in the lower legs, so we studied them early and consistently. We found that there was 90 percent patency in early studies, and we studied them again a year later, and sometimes after that.

I started using single and double mammaries in 1971, and did almost seven hundred double mammaries in the seventies. We compared the five- and ten-year survival rate of those seven hundred patients with a double mammary graft to three thousand single mammary graft patients. In ten years, there was no difference in the survival at all. It was clearly better than vein grafts, but after ten years, in no category of patient could we show any contribution of the second mammary artery. After fifteen to twenty years, there is some additional benefit of the second mammary artery for survival, but not very much, and that occurred mostly in younger people. Certainly in sixty- to seventy-year-old patients, there is no big advantage to a second mammary graft. You hear more and more talk at meetings about how multiple arterial grafts are going to improve survival. From our studies, there is very little evidence to substantiate this assertion.

If we are really removing heart attacks as a major cause of death for our patients, then life expectancy for the sixty-year-old who has had bypass surgery should be dramatically higher than in the general population, where half are dying from coronary disease. If we were removing that risk, there should be a strikingly lower mortality rate for people who have had bypass surgery, but that is not the case, and the mortality rate for bypass patients seems to be about the same as that of the general population. Forty-year-old patients with double, triple, and sequential mammaries have a higher mortality rate than the general population. We are not doing nearly enough to change the basic cause and progression of the disease. I'm certain that this is a problem in all of our patients, and it is more obvious in the younger ones.

We started working on end-stage patients, those with arteries with diffuse disease and no lumen, and patients with very poor LV function, and we started in a private hospital, not at the medical school. The cardiologists were a big help in getting it started. A cardiologist brought a patient in and said, "I cannot give him any more digitalis and diuretics; why don't you give it a try?" The patient had a badly dilated heart, and he did fine after surgery. In 1968 we also started aggressively pushing endarterectomy. In those early years, my overall mortality was significantly higher than that of the Cleveland Clinic, but the Cleveland Clinic surgeons were not operating on patients with bad hearts. Of course, in those days nobody understood the difference.

In February of 1969 our local academy of medicine invited Mason Sones to give a talk. This was before I had given my papers. I sat next to him, but I had never met him before. At dinner, I was telling him about what we were doing—double, triple, and quadruple grafts. He said he could not believe it. He tended to pontificate, and it always made for a brisk conversation. He gave his talk about what he was doing, and then, to his credit, he went over to the hospital with me and stayed there until one o'clock in the morning looking at postoperative angiograms, and seeing open grafts all over the place. He sent a letter back to the cardiologists after that, saying that he had witnessed the biggest breakthrough he had ever seen in the treatment of coronary disease. I got along with Mason Sones just fine.

At any rate, we began operating on patients with poor left ventricular function. One of our cardiologists reviewed these after a few years, and in 1977 he presented a paper on coronary bypass surgery with poor heart function. We had an average follow-up of six years on about 400 patients with ejection fractions ranging from 35 percent down to 10 percent. About 250 of the patients went through surgery and 150 patients refused surgery, and he compared long-term survival of the two groups. The relief of angina was far better in the surgical group than in the medical group. They were divided into four groups based on the ejection fraction, with the top group having an average ejection fraction of about 30 percent and the bottom group having an average ejection fraction of 12 percent. He compared the surgery group to the medical group in each, and in every category the surgical patients did much better. Even in the worst category, where the ejection fraction was in the 10 to 14 percent range, we had a 38 percent five-year survival rate in the surgical group, compared to less than 5 percent in the medical group. In conclusion, he could not find a group of patients with poor ventricular function that did better with medical treatment than with surgical treatment. This study was published around 1977, so this is how we began doing bad hearts. In that series, we had an 18 percent operative mortality, but now it would be much lower.

There are many subtle little things that have decreased the operative mortality in patients with poor ventricular function. We have much better perfusion and heart-lung machines than we had in the past. We learned very early to keep the pO_2 normal at one hundred millimeters. I started measuring flows in all of my grafts from the beginning. I measured pressure differentials when we came off bypass. I would occlude the vein graft, insert a needle connected to a transducer into the distal vein, and record the back pressure from the coronary artery. Then I opened the vein and recorded the aortic pressure. It was difficult to make a hemodynamic estimate by just looking at an angiogram. I found that 30 to 40 percent occlusion could produce a severe gradient, and that some 90 percent coronary blockages had no gradient. It was informative to me. I also found out that if there was no gradient, the vein stayed open just as well as those with gradients. We decided to bypass every stenotic coronary; this concept of total revascularization developed in 1968 and 1969.

In our first paper, I pointed out that sometimes when opening the pericardium, I would see yellow plaque further down a coronary artery than was on the angiogram, meaning that disease was forming there, beyond the main obstruction. In such a case, I would purposely cut across the secondary plaque two centimeters or more, and would sew the vein across that, largely bridging the plaque, to try to eliminate that secondary lesion from causing trouble in the future, and I have done this almost from the beginning of our program. I do not see how you can anastomose grafts to the aorta first and know every place you are going to select for the distal anastomosis. I find disease in so many distal places that I vary where I put my grafts. With the right coronary, you can have a severe proximal stenosis, and on the arteriogram the whole distal vessel looks fine. Almost always, if you expose the bifurcation at the posterior descending, there will be thick yellow atheroma forming at that location. I usually cut across it and bridge that plaque, hoping to prevent further disease. Sometimes while doing this, the plaque becomes loose, and then there is no choice but to remove it, especially on the right, so I began doing endarterectomies in the coronary artery system very early in 1968. I could open up both distal branches of the right coronary, and the techniques to do this gradually evolved. By 1974 we began doing the same on the left side, and by 1976 and 1977 we were doing endarterectomies all the time.

The technique of intermittent ischemia worked well for endarterectomy. I would clean the plaque out of the artery and sew a vein onto the coronary, stopping every twenty minutes and reperfusing the heart for five minutes. I would do all the distal anastomosis first. It has not been unusual for us to remove twenty, thirty, or forty centimeters of plaque. The most I ever removed was sixty-five centimeters, and that patient had a beautiful postop angiogram with everything wide open.

We restudied our endarterectomy patients, both early and late. Early restudies showed a slightly lower patency rate, about 3 percent lower compared to conventional grafts; 90 percent overall patency for endartectomy patients. After three or four years, the patency after endarterectomy is exactly the same as with conventional grafts.

In 1989 I developed a relationship with the school of education at the University of Wisconsin in Milwaukee. I had contributed some financial support for scholarships for students, and got to know the dean. He invited me to go to Cuba with him, and I met Dr. Gonzalez, the chief of heart surgery there, who asked me if I wanted to do an operation, and I said no. Heart surgery is a team effort, and I had learned from my first experience as an itinerant surgeon back in the 1970s that to do cardiac surgery alone is a disaster. The real definition of stress for me is being a visiting heart surgeon and having to operate in a strange environment. Since that first time in 1977, in India, I would always take appropriate people with me. I told Dr. Gonzalez that if he wanted me to come back, I would bring a team. Some time later we all went to Havana. I took along my anesthesiologist, my perfusionist, a couple of ICU nurses and OR techs, and we worked for two weeks. It was interesting. We spent one night with Fidel Castro, and that was interesting also. I have been back a couple of times since then.

I first went to Cuba in 1989, and I visited various clinics. Their primary care is phenomenally well-established. Every couple or three blocks, there is a house or building with a primary care physician, where people can go to be taken care of. Even out in the country there are clinics, and it is probably much better than what we have for rural areas. Castro had very detailed knowledge about all kinds of things like the incidence of congenital heart disease per thousand births, and they had a beautiful pediatric hospital, which was built to handle the appropriate number of patients. They were doing adult heart surgery and had done forty or fifty heart transplants prior to our visit.

When we went back four to five years ago, it was much worse, and they had cut down on the volume of heart surgery. They did not have much money and could not get equipment and supplies. Cuba has huge economic problems, but I must say that when I was walking down the streets and meeting people, I did not notice any anti-American hostility. They were very interested in us. They could not understand how we could open the door to relations with China but could not deal with Cuba. I remember what Lillehei told me once, that he had gone to

Havana on his honeymoon back in the early 1950s, and there was so much crime and terror then that he had to hire at least one or two guards to go with him every time he would go out at night. When I was down there in 1989, I could not imagine a safer city in the world. You could go any place at any time; there was zero crime. There were no gift shops; you could not buy fancy things to take home as you do in every other tourist place, but it was unbelievably safe, certainly the safest city in the hemisphere. I do not agree with everything that Castro has done, but there is no perfect culture.

There is a lot of pressure now to have a fast turnover in everything, but I cannot bring in the disaster patients, clean out their arteries, spend six hours on bypass, and send the patient home in three days. I have no reservations about six hours on bypass, even seven or eight. These are long reconstructive procedures. The patients do not go home right away, and have more problems and longer hospital stays. You may get by in doing a lot of these without an endarterectomy, but on a totally blocked right coronary artery, 98 percent of the patients can be bypassed if you clean them out distally with an endarterectomy. A lot of surgeons do not do that; they put all their grafts on the left side and forget about the right coronary. This is a different philosophy, that of total revascularization and cleaning out vessels. I have not seen anybody with disease too diffuse to be surgically treated, and there is no medical treatment for this problem.

Endarterectomy is almost always suitable. The only time it is not is if there have been two or three operations and the arteries are fibrosed and collapsed; then there is not much you can do. We restudied our patients before they went home, so we knew that the great majority were functioning. When new people joined me as partner or when I had fellows, I insisted that we do a cath on their patients before the patient goes home. I have never had problems with insurance coverage for a postop cath. When we see problems with the surgery, such as kinked grafts or narrowings or poorly placed grafts, we learn from that. I learned so much in the beginning about my own grafts from postop caths, but I do not know of a training program in the country where a resident ever sees his own grafts on postop film. I find this astounding. Even when doctors set a simple Colles fracture, they take a postop film.

In regard to stents, I doubt if anybody in the world has referred more people for angioplasty than I have. I think I gave the first paper on antioplasty for postop patients in the mid-1980s. If they can open the artery, it is a lot better than doing a big operation. I have had patients who were really short of vein when doing a third redo procedure, and I opened up the grafts or cleaned out vessels that I knew could not be treated by angioplasty. I would leave one or two vessels where an angioplasty would be appropriate and send them down for it a week or so later. I think that is reasonable; sometimes the two procedures can work together. If they can solve the problem better with stents, that is fine if they can get the artery open and it stays open.

Very early, I became interested in the septal artery. I had patients die from a septal infarct even though there was a functioning distal LAD graft. I did my first direct end-to-end graft to a septal artery in 1972, and from then on, until about 1978, I did close to one hundred direct end-to-end septal grafts. The right mammary artery worked beautifully. It was the most difficult anastomosis of all, but the result was good, and I have a picture of one wide-open septal graft still functioning after twenty-three years. In 1968 it was obvious that atherosclerosis does not involve intramyocardial vessels. The circumflex marginal goes under one millimeter of muscle, and it is free of disease. The septal arteries are the same, so rather than digging down, I would do an endarterectomy of the LAD. I extended my incision in the LAD higher and carefully extracted this big plug out of the septal branch. I have data on close to two thousand patients where we did an upper anterior descending septal endarterectomy, and we have some fifteen-year survivors. Surgical treatment of coronary disease is going to be an important factor for a long time to come. There are times when it is much better than any other treatment.

The single biggest thing I ever did to lower mortality was to introduce the use of allopurinol preoperatively. I went to a meeting in Brighton, England, and Mark Braimbridge was talking about his animal studies of heart muscle. When he used allopurinol, the animals did not fibrillate. Back in 1971 DeWall published some papers on studies with dogs, where he was ligating the upper LAD, and all the dogs fibrillated in three to five minutes. He loaded them up with allopurinol, and they could go eight, ten, twenty, and even forty hours without fibrillating. After we started using allopurinol, patients would essentially never fibrillate. My electrophysiologist did various studies on patients and showed profound changes in threshold potential for fibrillation with allopurinol. Initially, we gave them three hundred milligrams twice, and then we went to six hundred milligrams in the evening, at four in the morning, and three hours postop. This created profound protective effects. It did not help the lungs at all, but it markedly protected the kidneys. Some studies suggest that it does protect ischemic kidneys.

This protective effect of allopurinol is not generally known. We sent a paper to the *New England Journal of Medicine* about it. They sat on it for six months and finally said they would not publish it. The same thing happened with *JAMA*. Finally we got it published. In India, the use of allopurinol is widespread, because I have been invited to speak there many times, and I have trained a lot of the surgeons working there now.

Bibliography

Johnson WD, Flemma RJ, Lepley D Jr, Ellison EH. Extended Treatment of Severe Coronary Artery Disease: A Total Surgical Approach. *Ann Surg.* 1969; 170:460–470.

Johnson WD, Flemma RJ, Harding HW, Cooper GN Jr, Lepley D Jr. Surgical Principles in the Direct Reconstruction of Left Coronary Flow. *Ann Thorac Surg.* 1970; 10:141–152.

Johnson WD, Flemma RJ, Manley JC, Lepley D Jr. The Physiologic Parameters of Ventricular Function as Affected by Direct Coronary Surgery. *J Thorac Cardiovasc Surg.* 1970; 60:483–490.

Johnson WD. Surgical Techniques of Myocardial Revascularization: An Overview. *Bull NY Acad Med.* 1972; 48:1146–1156.

Manley JC, King JF, Zeft HJ, Johnson WD. The "Bad" Left Ventricle. Results of Coronary Surgery and Effect on Late Survival. *J Thorac Cardiovasc Surg.* 1976; 72:841–848.

Hellman C, Schmidt DH, Kamath ML, Anholm J, Blau F, Johnson WD. Bypass Graft Surgery in Severe Left Ventricular Dysfunction. *Circulation.* 1980; 62:I103–I110.

Brenowitz JB, Kayser KL, Johnson WD. Results of Coronary Artery Endarterectomy and Reconstruction. *J Thorac Cardiovasc Surg.* 1988; 95:1–10.

Johnson WD, Brenowitz JB, Kayser KL. Factors Influencing Long-term (10-Year to 15-Year) Survival after a Successful Coronary Artery Bypass Operation. *Ann Thorac Surg.* 1989; 48:19–24.

Johnson WD, Kayser KL, Brenowitz JB, Saedi SF. A Randomized Controlled Trial of Allopurinol in Coronary Bypass Surgery. *Am Heart J.* 1991; 121:20–24.

Johnson WD, Kayser KL, Hartz AJ, Saedi SF. Aspirin Use and Survival after Coronary Bypass Surgery. *Am Heart J.* 1992; 123:603–608.

John L. Ochsner, MD

(b. 1927)

I spent three months in the hospital without leaving. The only time I saw my wife and children was when they would come over for Sunday lunch.

— On being the resident
on Dr. DeBakey's service

Interviewed May 1, 2000

I was born in Madison, Wisconsin, in 1927. Shortly after my birth, my father, who was a prominent surgeon, was invited to join the faculty at Tulane Medical School in New Orleans. He was probably the youngest professor of surgery in history, twenty-nine years of age when he took Dr. Matas's place, so I grew up in New Orleans. In fact, my father was king of carnival in 1948, and I was king of carnival in 1990. In the old days there were quite a few instances of sons succeeding fathers as king of carnival, but it has not been common recently. I think my dad and I were the only two people who were not born in the state of Louisiana who have been king of carnival. When I was in the first grade, the teacher asked the kids where they were born, and I got up, gave my name, and told them that I was born in Madison, Wisconsin, but of course, in New Orleans that wasn't anything to be proud of, so I hastened to add that my father and mother were there on their honeymoon. When I was king of carnival, I told that story and said that the moral of the story is that I would rather be a bastard than a Yankee. As a child, it wasn't a proud thing to be a Yankee; mythically we were still fighting the Civil War.

I went to public high school for a while in New Orleans, and then I went away to prep school, at Darlington in Rome, Georgia. I came back to New Orleans to go to Tulane, but I got caught up in the war and joined the Naval Reserve at age seventeen. I had to get permission from my dad to join. I went through eighteen months of that war never seeing any action, thank God, and then came back to Tulane to finish my undergraduate education. I graduated in 1948 and went into medical school there at Tulane. I graduated in 1952 and was doing my internship at the University of Michigan when I got drafted into the Korean War. Not many people served in both wars, but they had a separate draft act for doctors in the Korean War. If you served in the Second World War, you were normally exempt from the draft, but because I was a doctor, I was subject to a different draft act.

I was in the service then for two more years, and when I left Michigan to go in, I realized I didn't really want to stay there to finish my residency. I knew I wasn't smart enough to get the kind of education that the residents received there. Dr. Collier never turned down anybody coming back from the war, so he would take the normal four to six residents per year, plus all of the people coming back. There were probably sixteen senior residents the year I left, and that meant that each resident was operating no more than one or two months out of the year. I couldn't learn that way; I wanted to go where you were thrown into the trenches. In Houston, at the Baylor-affiliated hospitals, the chief resident spent his time at Jefferson Davis

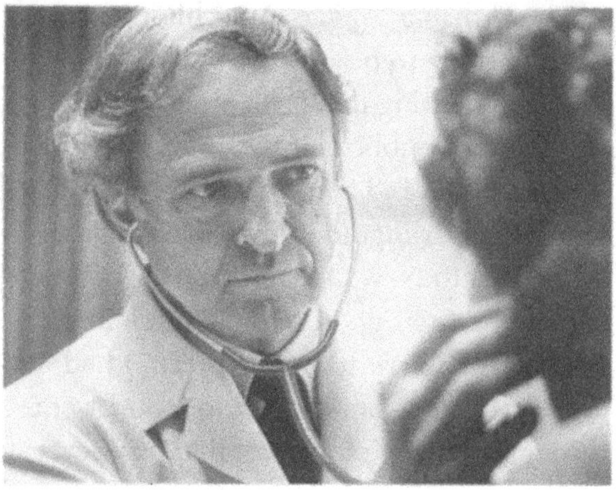

John L. Ochsner

Hospital, the city and county hospital. You could operate to your heart's content, so I went into Dr. DeBakey's program in 1956, and it was the smartest thing I ever did.

Dr. DeBakey's mentor had been my father. Dr. DeBakey spent eighteen years working closely with my father, and he described my father as the principal guiding light of his life, so I had a close relationship with him. He was first a student, then a resident, and then on the faculty at Tulane as my father's young associate, and he held my dad in great esteem. He always referred to my dad as Dr. Ochsner, just as I would always refer to Dr. DeBakey as Dr. DeBakey. When I was a child, he was frequently our babysitter. In fact, he and his wife, Diana, spent their honeymoon in our house while my mother and father were on a trip in Europe. Dr. DeBakey and Diana had just married, and they didn't have any money. None of the residents had any money, so it was nice for them to stay in a house that had the amenities that we had. He and Diana spent their honeymoon babysitting for us, but I don't know how much fun that was for them. I always referred to him at that time as Mike, just Mike.

When I first went to Houston, a few days before I started my training, John Overstreet and Oscar Creech said they wanted to take me to lunch. (John Overstreet was chief of surgery at Methodist Hospital and also trained under my father, and Oscar Creech later took my father's place as chairman at Tulane.) I thought, "Gee, this is very nice of them." They gave me two pieces of advice that helped me a great deal during my training. The first thing they said was, "Forget about calling him Mike, he's nothing but Dr. DeBakey. Don't ever refer to him as anything other than Dr. DeBakey." The second thing was, "Don't ever talk back and don't make excuses." The whole time I was there I never referred to him as anything other than Dr. DeBakey, and I can assure you that I never talked back to him. In fact, all I said was, "yes, sir," and "no, sir." One time he was chewing me out about something and I kept saying, "Yes, sir, yes, sir, no, sir, and no, sir." He grabbed me by the collar and said, "Can't you ever say anything but yes, sir, and no, sir?" I said, "No, sir."

He was tough to work for. He wanted to find fault, but it was for the sake of your training. I recognize now that there was no malignancy behind his actions, but during my training, I would go home and tell my wife how mean he was to me. Back then, if one of Dad's friends was in town as a visiting professor or something, Dr. DeBakey would call me up, and he would want Mary Lou and me to pick up Dr. "So and So" and take him to the Houston Country Club for dinner. My eyes would go up in my head and I would say, "Yes, sir," and we would go. There would be some music playing, and he would ask Mary Lou to dance. He was always so charming when you are out with him. Mary Lou would say, "How can you say that he's mean? He's the most gracious man in the world." Actually if you see Dr. DeBakey now, now that we are not in training with him and he is not trying to make sure that you tow the ropes, he really is gracious and nice to be with. I really enjoy going out to dinner with him, and he is really a lot of fun.

We had long hard hours back then, on call every other night, and when you were at Jefferson Davis, you were up all night when you were on call, so every other night you were up all night. Then when you were on Dr. DeBakey's service at Methodist, which all of us went through, we didn't leave Methodist Hospital at all. Somebody before us had started that tradition, and I spent three months in that hospital without leaving. The only time I ever saw my wife and children was when they would come over on a Sunday afternoon for lunch at the hospital. Finally, my wife quit doing that because she said that I was just too anxious to get away from them to get back to work. We had to keep up with the Joneses, so to speak, because it was a pyramid system. If we didn't do it, the guy behind us or next to us was going to work that hard, so we didn't have a chance. My experience wasn't unique; it was everybody's experience. I lost thirty-seven pounds in those three months. You had to give up something, and it was a necessity for me to get at least six hours of sleep at night, so I just gave up eating. The only time I ate was when I was making rounds. The nurses there would have orange juice and milk and things like that. I would usually get a sandwich at night in the cafeteria, about two o'clock in the morning, just before I would quit.

Dr. DeBakey had a huge service. Believe it or not, he used to run about ninety patients, and he had only one resident. That was forty years ago. Now there are ten residents where there used to be one of us. At least, there were ten residents a few years ago, when he was actively operating and had that big service. Of course, the cases have gotten bigger. We had some pretty big cases, and it was during the early days of vascular surgery, so we had a lot of complications. It was very common for us to have grafts and suture lines rupture and people getting ischemia. When we were first doing peripheral vascular work and abdominal aneurysms, we didn't anticoagulate them during the operation, and I can remember more than one patient who was gangrenous from the belly button down. We had a lot of infected grafts. The grafts were sterilized; we put them in an autoclave, but they didn't go through the tests that they get when they are done commercially. We had a lot of infected grafts that were terrible to deal with. These cases were tougher. The state of the art was immature, and unfortunately we had to face all of those terrible, terrible things.

I was in Houston from 1956 to 1961, which was the beginning of heart surgery. Denton Cooley started doing heart surgery at Texas Children's Hospital because the only hearts anybody operated on at that time were children's hearts. Adult hearts weren't being done. We did a few closed mitral valve commissurotomies, and a few open the last year that I was there, but not many, because we had no artificial valves. We would try some of the damnedest things in the world. We would take a piece of Dacron and make a sail out of it and bring it out of the apex of the heart, thinking that the thing was going to work as a valve. I can remember doing six consecutive mitral valve patients, and all of the patients succumbed. We did six mitral valve operations before we had one survive. With the aortic valves, we didn't have a good operation. Most of the patients that we saw had aortic insufficiency, because we were still operating on a relatively young crowd. We weren't doing the calcified valves then or the complications of a bicuspid aortic valve. I think we only did about one or two aortic valves the whole time I was there. This was all brand new, and it wasn't much fun to see the results.

We used two kinds of oxygenators in Houston. We used a Kay-Cross, and I used that for a long time when I came back to New Orleans. It had 144 rotating discs in it, and every one had to be cleaned, and then you had to fill it with about nine units of blood. Denton Cooley was smart enough to try to get something simpler. Denton really got ahead of the game, because he knew that the important results were the early results, whether the patient survived the operation, not whether they were cured, so he used the bubble oxygenator that DeWall developed up in Minnesota. He simplified it, and we couldn't keep a person on that for more than thirty minutes or it would destroy most of the red blood cells in the body. If we kept them on it for a short period, we could do it without too much destruction of the blood elements and still have a surviving patient. A lot of the VSDs still had holes in them, and there were a lot of tetralogies that still had stenosis at the pulmonary outflow, but they survived. You could report at the time that the patient survived the operation, and that it was a success. Those successes would not meet the criteria for success today, but, at that time, they did.

Dr. DeBakey's first use of the heart-lung machine was directed toward thoracic aneurysms. He got into it right away. I asked him if I could go to Children's Hospital in my last year, since Denton Cooley was operating on the hearts there, and he said, "Yes." He said he would only let me go if I came back and spent another year with him, which I did. I got my general surgery boards and my thoracic surgery boards the same year, general surgery in February and thoracic surgery in October. I finished at Jefferson Davis and then went to Children's. That was a new residency really. It wasn't a true residency, it was really just thoracic training.

At Children's I started doing some hearts, and then I went back and worked with Dr. DeBakey for another year, and we started doing hearts there also. Dr. DeBakey began with thoracic aneurysms, using the extracorporeal circulation.

Once they got a good bubble oxygenator, everybody jumped into it pretty quickly. I think Travenol was the first to patent that oxygenator. It was an adaptation of the DeWall oxygenator, but instead of being metal, it was plastic. It was a big plastic bag, like a window shade, big at the top, and the blood went through a helix to debubble.

I am now good friends with both Dr. DeBakey and Dr. Cooley, and I know very well what the reason for their split was, but I would rather not discuss it. I am privy to both of their personal lives, and I can truthfully say that I love both of these men, and am very happy to be friends of both, and I want to keep it that way. Unfortunately, I believe their friendship has come to a point where I don't think it can ever be patched, which is too bad, but I think that for both men, being in the same place at the same time stimulated both of them to be better surgeons than either would have been without the other. There may be some who disagree with that, but I will have to stick with that assessment. They are gifted in slightly different ways: Denton in having technical ability, particularly in big operations, whereas Dr. DeBakey has great expertise in medical and surgical policy and development.

When you look at Dr. DeBakey's life history and what he has accomplished as a worker, it is just astronomical. You can't conceive of anybody doing that again, yet when Dr. DeBakey was young, at the Ochsner Clinic with my father, operating was not his forte. My dad says that Dr. DeBakey wasn't really interested unless he was working in the experimental lab. He was such a scientist, and there wasn't a lot of science going on in the operating room back then. He preferred being in the experimental laboratory, working on something like a bleeding peptic ulcer, so different from the way his actual career turned out.

Later on, he realized the importance of surgery. He told me that one time my father told him, "If you do more of something than anybody else, then you are the authority." Dr. DeBakey took that to another level. When he started doing aneurysms, he did many more than anyone else. When I was in Houston as a resident, he was invited to go to the Mayo Clinic as a visiting professor to show them how to do an abdominal aneurysm. He was really thrilled because he was going up to Mecca to show them how to do it. That's when he told me that my dad had said that if you do the most, then you're the authority. He was going up there as the authority on aneurysms.

Dr. DeBakey worked really hard, and my dad was a hard worker too. Dad would make rounds every morning at five or five-thirty. My father was the first surgeon to come right out and say that smoking causes cancer. All of his staff smoked, and they all hid it from him. Dr. Gage told me that he burned a lot of holes in his pockets trying to put his cigarettes out when Dad came around. It's unfortunate that Dad didn't live long enough to see his views vindicated, because he was ridiculed throughout most of his young academic years. Evarts Graham was the one who finally proved in his lab that the tar of the cigarette produces cancer, when his associate Wynder took tar from cigarette smoke and painted it on the backs of dogs and produced cancer. Evarts Graham had written Dad a letter at one time, saying, "Al, you have got to get off this antismoking kick. All of your colleagues are beginning to think that you are a kook." Dad wrote him back and said he didn't care what they thought. "I'm telling you, Dr. Graham," he wrote, "that smoking is the cause of cancer of the lung." Dr. Graham had been his professor when he went to school in St. Louis. Some years later Dr. Graham developed cancer of the lung, and he wrote my dad another letter saying that he wished he had listened instead of condemning him.

My father was involved in another controversy when he ran afoul of the governor of Louisiana, Huey Long. When Dad went to New Orleans, the biggest-paying job in the state of Louisiana was that of the director of Charity Hospital; he actually made more than the governor, although the governor appointed him. The chairmen of the different departments at Tulane and LSU were appointed also, and they in turn appointed the subspecialty heads, but Huey Long didn't want Dad to appoint them. Long wanted to appoint the people on my dad's service at Tulane himself. All of them were political appointees. Huey Long appointed a guy to be head of ENT, but he wasn't even sure this appointee was a doctor. The appointments were all ridiculous, just payoff for some kind of political patronage, and Dad told the truth about Governor Long. Also, Dad wrote a letter to the University of Chicago, because they were looking for a new chief and he had trained in Chicago. In the letter, he said that things weren't going as well as he would have liked in Louisiana because of the political patronage problem, and he would like to reconsider the Chicago job. He had the letter in the pocket of his white coat, and he went to operate in the old amphitheater at Charity. The letter was apparently stolen out of his pocket, and he forgot about it, until Huey Long called him into his office and showed him the letter! He said, "I hear you don't like it here," and he kicked Dad out, saying he wasn't sufficiently appreciative of the state's efforts, so he could no longer be appointed to Charity Hospital. Of course, that was devastating to my father, but he made the best of it. He spent two years working in the laboratory and could operate in the other hospitals, but not in Charity Hospital. On surgical grand rounds, they would have to roll the patients across the street on a stretcher to Tulane to have them presented.

I stayed on in Houston for a while after I finished my residency, and things were really popping. We were getting out a lot of papers, and things were going quite well. Dr. DeBakey invited Mary Lou and me to come over for lunch with him and Diana, and he said that if I stayed with him for five more years he could pretty well promise me a professorship any place. It was very tempting; Mary Lou, my wife, really liked Houston because financially we were doing better there than I could have done anyplace else, but my last name was on a clinic in New Orleans. Patients were coming from the Ochsner Clinic in New Orleans to Houston for their heart surgery or vascular surgery, because it wasn't going very well in New Orleans. It was almost an embarrassing thing to me, and I wanted to go back to New Orleans. I have always loved New Orleans—the life of it, and the friends there that I grew up with. Most of them aren't doctors, and they all stayed in New Orleans. Not a lot of people leave New Orleans; in fact, most New Orleans girls return with their husbands sooner or later.

So I went home. I remember walking into the doctors' lounge at the Ochsner Clinic and overhearing an anesthesiologist say, "If he thinks they're going to start heart surgery here again, he's nuts." They had tried heart surgery once and then put a moratorium on it, because there was a very high mortality rate, but I wanted to get it going again, and I did. I had a hard time at first. I could only find two people that were willing to do the anesthesia out of all the anesthesiologists there, and only one cardiologist, so we started from scratch. I picked my cases carefully, and I picked fifty. I wanted to do fifty cases that I knew I could get through without any problem, VSDs, ASDs, tetralogies, a few simple things like that, nothing too hard. All of those patients survived, and once I got that going, everybody accepted it, and it was no problem.

We went through various pump-oxygenators. I started off with a Kay-Cross, and of course, it was a mess. Anything could go wrong. It would take a day and a half to get the thing prepared, to wash it and sterilize it. It had two driving discs, one going perpendicular to the other one. That function went awry one day, and when it did my dad happened to be walking by the operating room. He came in, and throughout that operation, he manually turned the malfunctioning disc. I told him afterwards that this had been beyond the call of duty of a father, but that I surely appreciated it, and that the patient appreciated it even more.

Next, we went to the bubble oxygenator because it was a lot safer, but then one time there was an oxygenator distributed across the country in which they had made the holes too big. A lot of people died from that oxygenator. The case would go well and then suddenly the patient wouldn't wake up, mentally destroyed by air embolism. They recalled those right away, so thank God we only had one patient die because of that oxygenator, but a lot of people across the country died because of it.

The Ochsner Clinic was not the only cardiac surgery center in New Orleans. Oscar Creech was doing heart surgery at Tulane, but we were the only two. Page Acree did a couple of operations at Baton Rouge, but he decided he didn't want to do them and started sending me patients. Oscar really didn't quite get it off the ground either. It was tough for us in New Orleans because geographically we were between two major heart surgery centers. John Kirklin was doing well in Birmingham, Alabama, and of course, there was the Houston group to the west. If a patient went away from New Orleans for surgery, that patient didn't come back to us. Often no one told the patient that it could be done in his own hometown, so we were limited in what we could do.

We did have the crippled children's program. We didn't get paid for those operations, but both the Tulane group and our group would accept patients from that program so that we could keep open-heart surgery going. That was before coronary bypass and the like, which didn't come until later, so we struggled, trying to get valve patients and congenitals. That was all we had. The good thing about it for me, though, was that almost everything I did then was something I had never seen done before. It was always exciting to do something for the first time. I was fortunate enough to have done the first valve, the first pacemaker, the first coronary, the first anything, in my community. I also did the first lung, heart, and liver transplants.

In 1966 we wrote a paper about revascularization, and this preceded the Favaloro operation. Really we were doing two things—Vinebergs, and also an endarterectomy on the right coronary artery—we felt that the LAD system was taboo. When Ed Garrett did the first bypass, it was because he got in trouble doing an endarterectomy of the left coronary artery. He wasn't trying to do a bypass; they converted it to a bypass to save the patient's life. He just took it a step forward. We did all the endarterectomies off bypass. I once made a movie in which I did an entire endarterectomy all the way up into the aorta. I started in the middle of the right coronary artery and went all the way up. I opened up the aorta so you could see the proximal endarterectomy, because I didn't want to dissect the aorta. I didn't know what was going to happen. I was going to show the movie at the Society of Thoracic Surgeons, which always had a movie day, but I decided it was a little too radical and I never did show the damned thing. I had a good angiogram showing the artery open postop, but I am sure it didn't stay open, because all of those endarterectomy sites eventually closed. We did six localized endarterectomies on the right coronary back in the mid-1960s, and in a two-year period all of them occluded.

I don't know how many Vinebergs I did, but I reported on a hundred of them with a ten-year follow-up. It's amazing how well those patients did. If the disease was just localized to that area and you got a good tunnel, it would supply the whole coronary system. I made a slide that Vineberg actually put in his book, showing a heart where, with just one injection of dye into the implanted mammary artery, we lit up the whole heart, all the coronaries.

We started using internal mammary arteries at a very early date. We were used to taking them down, originally skeletonized. We had two to take down, both the right and left. We would put one across the mediastinum parallel to the LAD, and the other parallel to the diagonal coronary artery. Later, we started taking them down as a pedicle and just skeletonizing the distal part, which we brought into a tunnel in the myocardium. We started using the mammary artery as a bypass conduit a few months after we heard that George Green was using them as grafts.

We also used fresh allografts, saphenous veins from cadavers. We were the first to use them, originally to bypass the femoral artery in the leg, but eventually in the heart too. We found out first that there had to be a major ABO blood match or they didn't work very well. Then we found out that if we cryopreserved them ourselves, they did a little better, but still they were very unpredictable. You couldn't tell which ones were going to work and which ones were not. None of them really stood the test of time, and the long-term results were not good. We used them mostly in peripheral vascular operations, and we used a large number of them. In fact, it wasn't uncommon for me to be working in one room and Noel Mills in the other, and one of us would not have enough vein graft. We'd yell over, "You got any graft left?" and send over any extra to the other surgeon. Today if you did that, you'd probably be put in jail. I bet we did that thirty times, but we were just trying to do some good for the patients.

After my father died, the *Annals of Surgery* had an issue dedicated to him, and they asked people to write articles about him. Dr. DeBakey was one, and they asked me to write about him as a son. I just wrote what he was like as a father, and how we went through various stages in our relationship. Dad wasn't really a close father. He worked a lot, very much like Dr. DeBakey, who also wasn't a close father to his boys. Dr. DeBakey is very close to his daughter now, later in life, but both men were so busy that they didn't have time for their children when they were younger. My dad just didn't have time for us, so my mother raised us, but that didn't mean he didn't love us. It was obvious to me that he loved us, but he was a strong disciplinarian. There wasn't one weekend in my life that I didn't get a whipping. When he was home on the weekends, we were always making a lot of noise, and that upset him. I remember being very proud one time when he broke a belt on me, and I took it to school to show to my friends. It was par for the course to get a whipping, just weekly. We were used to those. If you spilled your milk, you got a whipping.

Then I really became a student of his when I was in medical school. When I came back to the Ochsner Clinic years later, I became a colleague, and it was really fun operating with him. He'd say, "Do you mind doing this case with me?" There were some new things that he didn't do or didn't want to do, and he wanted me to do them. He would come in and watch when we started doing heart surgery. He enjoyed seeing things. He went to every medical meeting and sat in the front row. He never missed a medical meeting until he died when he was eighty-five. He kept up with everything and read everything. Later on I became his mentor in a way, because he didn't trust his own judgment as he got older, not just in medical matters but in other things, and he would come to me for advice.

The first time he asked me for advice was kind of funny. My mother died, and he did not remarry for a while, and we had him over for dinner frequently. Once he came over for dinner and said that he was going to run for city council because the Republicans in town had talked him into it. Dad was a guy who liked to be honored, and he thought that this was an honor, and also he was a little bored, because he wasn't operating then. I thought it was a bad idea, and I told him, "Dad, that's below your dignity in the first place, and in the second place, you don't know anything about it, and third, you're going to run against a very good man. I think they're just using you because of your name. The party is using name recognition to try to get a Republican elected in a Democratic city, and that's not fair to you or to the constituents." Oh, he was mad as hell at us, and he stormed out after dinner. The next day I was going down the hall at the clinic, and he saw me. I thought, "Uh oh, what is he going to say?" He pulled me into his office and said, "You know I've been thinking. I don't think I want to run for that office after all." It had to be his idea, though. I thought, "Gosh, this is the first time he's taken my advice." After that, he did everything I advised him to do; it was really kind of interesting. He would call me and tell me he wanted to talk to me about his marriage, when he wanted to get married. We became very close in later life.

We got into heart transplantation relatively early. It was so exciting in the early days, and everybody wanted to get into it. I did the first one in 1970; I think I did about number thirty in the world. We had a patient who was actually a very good candidate, in failure, having angina all the time, and we had a donor who had a pulmonary embolus. He had been resuscitated and was on a respirator but was brain-dead. The cardiologist, Charles Moore, thought that our patient was a good candidate, so we talked to the family, and they were excited about it. We did it one night, and it was a big thing with the news media. I remember leaving the hospital at about five o'clock in the morning, sneaking out to go change clothes. The cameramen and newsmen were flying by me in the hall, and I asked them, "Where are you going?" They said, "There's a doctor up there that has just done a heart transplant, and we're going to get the story." I said, "Oh, good," and just kept going out the door.

Two things were interesting about that operation. The first thing was that when I tried to get the patient off bypass, I couldn't, because his heart was distended. The right ventricle was big. I thought this was due to damage from pulmonary hypertension, but in retrospect what probably happened is that when we came off bypass, we didn't have the heart protected well enough and it dilated. Anyway, I put him back on bypass, opened the right atrium, and did a tricuspid valvuloplasty. I obliterated the posterior leaflet, and he came right off bypass after that. I am sure that this was the first, and maybe the only, transplanted heart that had to be operated on to get the patient off bypass.

The next thing I did was smart. George Burch was a very well-known cardiologist in the country, probably one of the most famous cardiologists, and very conservative. He did not believe in cardiac catheterizations, angiograms, or heart surgery, and he certainly did not believe in heart transplants. Before I did anything else that morning, I called George Burch. I said, "Dr. Burch, this is Johnny Ochsner, and I just wanted to tell you that I have just done a transplant, and I want you to know the circumstances about the patient before you get the news secondhand." I knew the media would go right to him, and he would probably have a fit and say how terrible it was that I had done a transplant, so I called him before the media could. He said, "Well, I'm sure if you thought it was the right thing to do, John, it was." That really helped because then there was nobody that could condemn it locally in our community.

Unfortunately, back then we didn't have the means to diagnose rejection, and we didn't have cyclosporine. All we had was Imuran and steroids. We never knew when the transplant patient was rejecting, and of course that was the big fear. If he had a fever, we'd say, "He's rejecting! Give him some more steroids!" Eventually he was so immunosuppressed that he developed a brain abscess due to a fungus. He lived for about six months, which at that time was pretty good, considering that transplant patients never lived more than a year. The average was probably about two months because so many of them died in surgery, especially from air embolism. People didn't realize then that when you get a heart full of air, it just goes right to the brain. When he was autopsied he didn't have any evidence of rejection of the heart, and the place where we fixed the valve was all healed over. You couldn't even see where it was fixed. I went back years later to look at his chart to see what we had been giving him. He was getting 250 milligrams of prednisone four times a day! He was taking this every day for months. We thought that was the thing to do, and nobody knew the right dosage. Every time we looked at him, we thought he was rejecting. If his heart rate went up, we thought that meant he was rejecting.

We did liver transplants also. We had had a patient with acute yellow atrophy that died. Then we got another patient with liver failure that was also going to die, so Bill McKinnon, who was the general surgeon at the Ochsner Clinic, suggested that we try a liver transplant. He said to me, "You do the vascular stuff, and I will do the liver anastomoses." I don't think we lost two pints of blood, and at the time people normally used a hundred bottles of blood for a liver transplant. We just put the liver in and got out. The patient died about a day and a half later, because all of his organs were in failure by the time we got him. He had a nice liver in him when he died, but he didn't have a brain, a kidney, or anything else.

We took up heart transplantation again

in 1983. By that time cyclosporine was available, and also they had developed the heart biopsy technique at Stanford. That made all the difference. When we started again, the cardiologists didn't want to have anything to do with it, so the surgeons did everything. We went out and picked up the donor heart and put it in. The clinic had a doctor doing kidney transplants, so we got in touch with him and he helped us with the immunosuppression drugs. We did the biopsies also, because the cardiologists wouldn't do them. We would take the patients back to the operating room one or two weeks after surgery, then three weeks and four weeks. We spread it out and we did a lot of biopsies. We were doing it all. Then after we did about fifty heart transplants with no deaths, the cardiologists wanted to get involved. They did, but it was another year before they did any of the biopsies.

The first heart transplant patient we did in 1983 is still alive. He was a boy who had transposition of the great vessels that we had previously repaired, but the right side of the heart, the pumping chamber, had just failed, and he was dying. So we took him back. He wasn't a very good candidate because his liver was practically down in his pelvis, and he had terrible coagulation problems, but he did well postop and is still well, sixteen years later. Of the first ten that we did, six of them survived ten years, so our results were better in that first group than they are now. We haven't improved on those results, but of course there are probably some reasons for that. The average age of the transplants was much younger then, and we had short ischemic times. We used to go get the donor hearts in helicopters; we weren't using any fixed-wing aircraft. Some of our patients now have been on assisted circulation, and they are a lot sicker, so their mortality is high.

I've always been interested in the history of medicine. One time when I was president of the Southern Association for Vascular Surgery, I gave a talk on the South's most famous doctor. Of course, I started my research by looking at people like Marion Sims, Dr. Blalock, Halsted, my dad, Dr. Cooley, and Dr. DeBakey. I went through all the well-known Southern surgeons, but finally I decided that the one who was the best known was a man named Dr. Tichenor who developed a patent medicine, and he sold over a billion bottles. This medicine goes back to the time of the Civil War, and it is still being used as a patent medicine. Now they even have toothpaste using his name.

Dr. Tichenor was quite a famous person aside from his patent medicine. He did a lot in the Civil War as a soldier, and he was a musician, but he is most famous because of his patent medicine. It was mainly alcohol, 70 percent alcohol. It really sterilized things. He didn't know it, but he had just the right percentage of alcohol to make it a sterilizing agent. Most people used it to drink in the early days of Prohibition. Black people drank it because in the South they had a hard time getting alcohol or liquor. People wouldn't sell it to them at times, but they could always get Dr. Tichenor's. A lot of Cajun folks would put it on mosquito bites and things. It was made to be applied, and it was for everything; mosquito bites, itches, gout, everything. People even rubbed it on horses. It is just very cooling. I mix it with bay rum, and I use the mixture as my aftershave lotion. I don't drink it, though.

I also gave the Gibbon Lecture on the history of the scalpel, the surgical knife. It is a fascinating history. The first surgical knife was used by the Cro-Magnon people around 8000 B.C. It was a stone knife, used for trephination, making holes in people's heads. Trephination was done in the pre-Inca era in South America also. The procedure was supposed to cure epilepsy, headaches, and melancholia; it got rid of the demon. It was probably also used for people who were schizophrenic or had other mental problems.

Surgical knives went through different phases. Ambroise Paré made them pretty to look at, with gorgeous ivory handles engraved with human figures. He was the one who invented the bistoury, which looked like a razor blade and clasped open, but the guy who really changed the surgical knife was Gillette, of the Gillette razor. He was an unusual person; he wrote a book describing a sort of utopian society, where instead of the competition that is the cornerstone of American enterprise, there would be cooperation and one company that everybody worked for. Everybody worked in one place where there would be thousands and thousands of apartments. Each person would only work a short time, twenty years or so, and then they would retire to philosophize and do the nice things in life. The setting was to be near Niagara Falls, where they had enough power to manufacture everything. He was actually selling stock in this company to make it a reality when he cut himself badly while shaving, so badly that he wanted to do something about it, so he invented the safety razor, one that you could put in a holder with guards on it. It had to have a very short blade, and, in order to manufacture it, he discovered a way to temper the steel and hone it to make a sharp edge. Then they developed a very thin razor that could be reproduced cheaply, so that it could be disposable.

At that time all surgical knives were just one piece on a handle. Gillette tried to develop a way to put a separate blade on a knife handle. At first there was a third part that you put the blade onto, but then Mr. Parker figured out a way to put a blade onto a handle so that it clicks on and there are just two pieces. That is still the standard knife today, and it was invented in the 1920s. It hasn't changed since that day. There are modifications of it, such as the Beaver blade, but Parker took that big step forward.

The story is ironic because Gillette, who was a socialist and didn't believe in free enterprise, became one of the biggest capitalists in the world. Parker didn't have a job when he invented his blade. His uncle, though, was a surgeon, and he asked Parker to figure out a way that surgeons could avoid sharpening their scalpels all the time. There used to be a course in medical school on how to sharpen blades. John Murphy from Chicago used to put razor blades onto a handle with that third part, but they were regular straight blades. Parker was the one who put a company together to manufacture surgical knives. He needed a medical group to market it, so he looked in the yellow pages, or whatever was the equivalent of the yellow pages at that time, and the first doctor he came to was named Bard, so the company was called Bard-Parker.

We have had a surgical residency training program at the Ochsner Clinic for a long time. It is long on general surgery and a bit short on thoracic training. There is no doubt that one needs more than two years to train a thoracic surgeon. We should increase thoracic surgery training to three years. I don't think five years of general surgery training are needed, but you have to teach a man senior responsibility, and he doesn't get that unless he gets five years of general training. If they get only two or three years of training instead of five, they'll never get to the point where they have much responsibility. You also worry that if a trainee gets into a program that is five years of general surgery and just three years for thoracic surgery, then the thoracic trainees will always be in a subservient position. They're not going to get to do the stuff that the golden boys of the past got to do. That's human nature.

The other problem is that residents who are now going through five years of general surgery training, then three years of thoracic surgery, very rarely take the recertification exam in general surgery. They are recertified in thoracic and cardiac surgery, but not general surgery. There should be a way to teach cardiac and thoracic without requiring so many years of general surgery. I predict that our present system will eventually change.

I also believe that thoracic surgery and cardiac surgery should not divide into entirely separate specialties. The heart surgeons are giving up too much these days. They've given up vascular surgery, which is a very lucrative business; they've given up putting in pacemakers because they don't have time for that; and they've given up general thoracic surgery. There's no reason they can't do those things in addition to heart surgery. There's no doubt that people are going to subspecialize, but surgeons should be well versed in their entire field, because your subspecialty could be gone tomorrow. In the future, coronary disease could be treated by cardiologists, or better drugs and preventive measures. Coronary artery surgery could be eliminated. The same is true for general thoracic surgeons. The day could come when chemotherapy or prevention of cancer could knock them out of a job. People are smoking less, and we will see a lot less lung cancer. The future of cardiac surgery is hard to predict, so it's best to be trained in all of thoracic and cardiovascular surgery.

I have had some great mentors and guiding lights in my life. One of them, of course, was my father. I also had two brothers who were doctors. Both of them died. My younger brother died relatively young when he inhaled a piece of meat. He was at the Southern Urological meeting, at a cocktail party. The urologists are heavy drinkers and cigar-smoking guys, and he was choking at that party, but they didn't recognize it. They gave him mouth-to-mouth resuscitation when he needed the Heimlich maneuver.

My older brother died just this year. He had Parkinson's disease, and it was a sad, terrible death. We were glad when he finally did go, though, because he had had his head on a pillow for six months without moving. Both my brothers were important in my life, particularly my younger brother; he was my best friend.

Both Dr. DeBakey and Dr. Cooley have been my mentors. I can always say that they helped shape my life, and they continue to do so in one way or another.

Bibliography

Ochsner JL, Cooley DA, Harris LC, McNamara DG. Treatment of Complete Transposition of the Great Vessels with the Blalock-Hanlon Operation. *Circulation.* 1961; 24:51–54.

Ochsner JL, Cooley DA, McNamara DG, Kline

A. Surgical Treatment of Cardiovascular Anomalies in 300 Infants Younger than One Year of Age. *J Thorac Cardiovasc Surg.* 1962; 43:182–198.

Ochsner JL, Ochsner A. Funnel Chest (Chonechondrosternon). *Surg Clin North Am.* 1966; 46:1493–1500.

Ochsner A, Ochsner JL, Sanders HS. Prevention of Pulmonary Embolism by Caval Ligation. *Ann Surg.* 1970; 171:923–938.

Mills NL, Ochsner JL. Technique of Internal Mammary-to-Coronary Artery Bypass. *Ann Thorac Surg.* 1974; 17:237–246.

Ochsner JL, Moseley PW, Mills NL, Bower PJ. Long-term Follow-up of Internal Mammary Artery Myocardial Implantation. *Ann Thorac Surg.* 1977; 23:118–121.

Ochsner JL. Superiority of the Internal Mammary Artery as a Coronary Bypass Graft. *Cleve Clin Q.* 1978; 45:81–82.

Ochsner JL. Institutional Variations Influencing Results: Arterial versus Venous Grafts. *Circulation.* 1982; 65:81–85.

Ochsner JL, Lawson JD, Eskind SJ, Mills NL, DeCamp PT. Homologous Veins as an Arterial Substitute; Long-term Results. *J Vasc Surg.* 1984; 1:306–313.

Ochsner JL. Giants. *J Thorac Cardiovasc Surg.* 1993; 106:769–778.

Floyd D. Loop, MD

(b. 1936)

René Favaloro and Dudley Johnson were the two surgeons that really popularized coronary artery surgery, but they were not in communication. . . . It just happened in both places at the same time.

— On the first coronary artery bypass operations

Interviewed March 5, 2003

I was born in Lafayette, Indiana, in 1936. My father was an old-fashioned country doctor, and I used to go around with him to farms and carry his black bag. I had sort of a Huckleberry Finn childhood. It was a very innocent time, and I had a wonderful boyhood. I went to Purdue University after high school because I had a full scholarship, so it was inexpensive. For medical school, my choices were either to stay in the Midwest and attend Indiana University, or to move from the Midwest. I was always seeking something new, so I decided to look at George Washington University, in Washington, D.C., where my father had gone to medical school. I had an uncle who lived in Washington, and I went to see him. He said, "The best way to learn about George Washington University is to go and see the dean." I pointed out that we had no appointment. My uncle said, "That won't matter." So we walked in to see the dean, John Parks, an old football player from the University of Wisconsin, but he was getting ready to go to a commencement. My uncle said, "This young man wants to go to your medical school and would like to meet you." So the dean invited me into his office and sat down and talked to me for a while. One thing led to another, and I did attend George Washington University. I had a wonderful medical education and had a great clinical exposure there. DC General Hospital was the site of a lot of our clinical activities. After I graduated in 1962, I decided to intern there, because I liked the diversity of practice.

After one year of general surgical residency, I was drafted into the air force. I thought that if I went to see a colonel or a general, perhaps he could advise me on where to spend the next two years. They were very affable and talked to me a long time about career opportunities and where I might go to do a little surgery while I was in the air force, but when I got my orders, they said that I was going to Laredo, Texas. I have nothing against Texas, but they had a twenty-five-bed dispensary down there, and I didn't feel too good about that. Nevertheless, I packed my bags and was ready to go. The professor of surgery at George Washington University, Brian Blades, called me in and said, "Where are you going?" I told him that I was going to Laredo, Texas. He said, "No, you're not." He picked up the phone, and within a month I was at Andrews Air Force Base. I was very fortunate when I got to Andrews, because they didn't have any general surgeons. There was another fellow like me who had only one year of surgical training, and we became the general surgeons, under supervision, of course. We did a lot of surgery over the

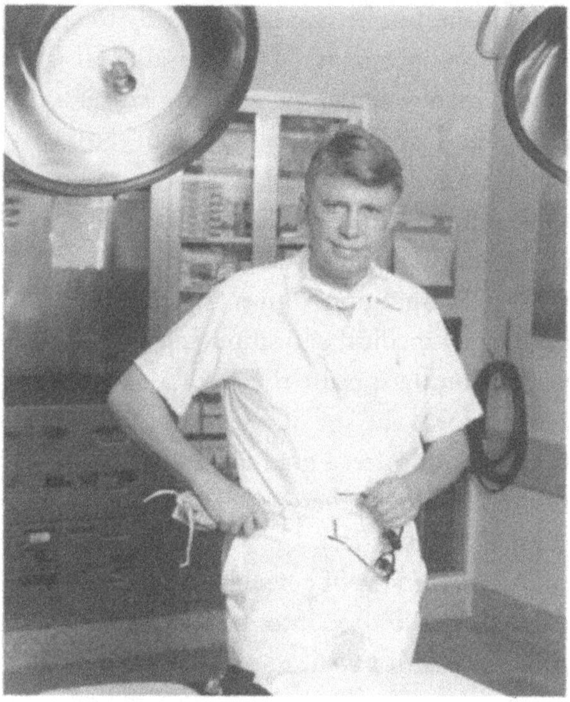

Floyd D. Loop

next two years. I did so much surgery in the air force that I was given a year's credit of residency training.

I went back to George Washington University after I was discharged, and started my third year of residency. One of the chief residents decided to go back into the navy, so I became the chief resident in my third year and consequently gained more experience, again under supervision. I decided at that point that I wanted to go into cardiothoracic surgery. At first I had thought I might like to be a plastic surgeon, but cardiothoracic surgery seemed more challenging. It seemed as if there were more opportunities for research and new procedures. So I talked to Dr. Blades and told him that my plan was to go do research somewhere for a year and to study thoracic surgery in England. He listened very patiently and then said, "You're not going to do any of that. There's a new field that is going to start, called coronary artery surgery." How he knew this, I have no idea. He was a friend of Don Effler at the Cleveland Clinic, but this was 1966 and coronary surgery had not started yet, but he said, "You're going to go to the Cleveland Clinic for a year, and then come back to us for a year. After that, I want you to stay here on the faculty and do heart surgery at George Washington University." All this amazed me because I had no idea about the Cleveland Clinic. I knew some of the advancements that had occurred in general surgery at the Cleveland Clinic, but I didn't know anything about their cardiothoracic program. When you're a young fellow, however, you often do as your mentors advise, so I drove up to Cleveland and met Don Effler, Larry Groves, and René Favaloro. They constituted the Department of Cardiovascular Surgery.

After a year there, I realized that I couldn't learn all of these new advancements in heart surgery in a year, so I asked to stay for a second year. After the second year, I was ready to go back to George Washington University, but the situation there was not right. The cardiologists were not doing coronary arteriography yet. Don Effler asked me to join the staff at the Cleveland Clinic in 1970, and I decided to stay there.

Dr. Effler looked as if he had come from central casting. He was a very impressive man and a good surgeon, having started at the Cleveland Clinic in 1948. He had actually been Brian Blades's first resident, and I was Blades's last resident, so there was some continuity there. Effler gave everybody in the department the ability to create new procedures and to operate virtually every day. At a very young age, I was able to do well over a hundred cardiothoracic procedures a month. Of course, he allowed René Favaloro to develop coronary artery surgery and supported him while those new procedures were evolving.

Effler had been interested in the Vineberg operation for some time. His interest began when Mason Sones selectively catheterized two or three Vineberg implant patients that had been operated on by Bigelow or Vineberg, and found that some of them actually worked. Since there was no direct coronary surgery in the mid-1960s, Favaloro actually started out doing the Vineberg operation before he did his first coronary artery operations.

Mason Sones was a pediatric cardiologist. One day in 1958 he was doing an aortogram on a patient, and the catheter inadvertently slipped into the right coronary artery. They were loading the syringe for a ventriculogram, and they thought that the catheter was in the ventricle. The patient received twenty to thirty milliliters of dye into the right coronary artery. Mason understood right away what he had done, and he recognized that it was possible to selectively catheterize coronary arteries without producing myocardial injury. He then worked with amplification of the imaging system, integrating a motion-picture camera with the process, and thus he was responsible for the evolution of cine-coronary arteriography. It wasn't until four years later that he published his first one thousand cases. Originally nobody believed him, because the results were exemplary, with hardly any complications. The American College of Cardiology sent a group of people, headed by Henry Swan, to the Cleveland Clinic, because they thought this might be false data, but Swan came back and said, "It's all correct, and Sones knows exactly what he's doing. He gets in there and does it, and it's a very slick and quick procedure."

Mason Sones was a very hard worker, a very bright man, and a hard-drinking fellow. He was a great friend of mine and referred literally hundreds of cases to me in my early years. I used to spend most early evenings in Sones's lab, looking at films of potential candidates for surgery. Mason was just a wonderful guy. He used to sit in the cath lab in an old man's undershirt, not a T-shirt, and he always had a cigarette. He would smoke during the catheterization procedure. He was a very heavy smoker, and that was his downfall as he eventually developed lung cancer. It was a different era back then. The connection between tobacco and atherosclerosis was not very firm at that point, so many doctors smoked.

René Favaloro was from Argentina, and he came to the Cleveland Clinic as a fellow. In the beginning he could hardly speak English. He spent a lot of nights and weekends in Mason Sones's laboratory looking at arteriograms, and he performed various indirect operations, such as talc poudrages and Vineberg implants. One day in 1967 Favaloro did an interposition vein graft in the mid-third of the right coronary artery. Sones studied that patient and found that the vein graft was open, and within a very short time Favaloro performed an aortocoronary bypass to the right coronary artery. Simultaneously, Dudley Johnson in Milwaukee also performed aortocoronary bypass grafts to both the right and left coronary arteries. They were the two surgeons that really popularized the operation, but they were not in communication with each other when they did the operations; it just happened in both places at the same time.

The Cleveland Clinic was established in 1921. There were four founders, but Crile and Lower were the principal founders. Crile had a huge practice of thyroid surgery, but there was also a lot of general surgery done there. The pioneering work in colorectal surgery started there also with Tom Jones and then others. It was the early surgical prowess of the Cleveland Clinic that was responsible for its early fame and success.

When Favaloro came to the Cleveland Clinic in 1962, the cardiac surgery program was very modest. It was comparable to other larger academic centers at that time. They mostly did valve and congenital heart procedures. By the late 1960s, though, the experience in coronary arteriography at the Cleveland Clinic was huge. Thousands and thousands of cases had been performed, so there was a massive library of all sorts of conditions from coronary anomalies to various atherosclerotic problems. Favaloro immersed himself, and he soon understood that there was a largely centrifugal distribution of the lesions at the right coronary artery bifurcation. The disease in the anterior descending and the circumflex was usually in the proximal part of these arteries. These findings were anatomically suitable for a bypass operation. The question was whether a vein from the leg, put into an aortocoronary position, would actually stay open for a long period of time. Sones showed that it would. Also, the retrospective study of a patient operated on by Dr. Garrett in 1965 showed a vein graft that was still open seven and a half years later.

Favaloro used an interrupted suture technique. He believed that this was a more precise anastomosis. Some of the vessels that he had to graft into were only a millimeter and a half in diameter, and he didn't want the purse-string effect of a continuous suture. That's why he used interrupted sutures.

Dr. Favaloro was great to work with. He probably taught me more about cardiac surgery than anyone else. He was a very kind man, a good teacher, and an excellent technician; he really cared about his patients. He spent a lot of time with his patients, and he had a huge experience. I attached myself to him, and he taught me every day. He was probably responsible for my career as a cardiac surgeon more than any other person.

In the early 1970s he went back to Argentina, because he had always wanted to return. It wasn't that anything happened at the Cleveland Clinic that caused him to leave. He was very happy there, but he always wanted to go back to Argentina. He started the Favaloro Foundation in Buenos Aires based on the Cleveland Clinic model, and it was very successful for many years. I don't know why he died the way he did. He certainly did not seem depressed to me. I think there were economic problems in Argentina and the Favaloro Foundation was having financial problems, so that may have contributed to the situation. He had lost his wife a few years before that, but I don't know any of the circumstances. He died of a self-inflicted gunshot wound to the heart. The entire country was shocked by his death and mourned the loss.

The first aortocoronary operations at the Cleveland Clinic were done with vein grafts. We started using the internal mammary artery in 1970, and our series really took off in 1971. We did not know of George Green's work, but the internal mammary artery was in such a perfect location that it was a simple matter to detach it from the chest wall. We already knew how to do that from the Vineberg days, so we just sewed it into various coronary arteries. Of course, most of the early cases were the left mammary to the anterior descending. We used interrupted 7–0 silk sutures to do the anastomosis, and then we restudied most of the first few dozen cases. They all looked splendid. We had no idea that twenty to thirty years later, they were going to look the same as the day they were put in.

In 1986 we published an article establishing that the use of the mammary artery had a huge effect on survival. That article was originally turned down because it wasn't a randomized prospective study, but Eugene Braunwald and John Kirklin helped get the paper accepted by the *New England Journal of Medicine.* It was the lead article in January of 1986. The article lent a lot of credibility to the procedure and its long-term results, and it may have opened the path to the goal of all artery revascularization.

Nowadays, almost half of the patients at the Cleveland Clinic are valve patients rather than patients with coronary disease, but ten years ago this was not the case. That increase in valve surgery can be attributed to Toby Cosgrove, who succeeded me as chief of surgery. I consider my tenure as chief very successful because I passed it on to someone who could do it better than I did. Cosgrove built up the valve practice and made it even better through the various minimally invasive techniques that he pioneered.

Small incisions are here to stay; there is no question about that. The question is about how fast robotics and the port approach to coronary surgery and valve surgery will occur. I think it will take off pretty fast now. People are getting better and better at it every day. I wish there were a way in which you could arrest and protect the heart as well as you can with the older extensive exposure, because then the ports would really come in handy. A lot of people believe that the off-pump methods will suffice. However, I think you get into technical acrobatics when you have to do multiple grafts through very small incisions off-pump. It is a big controversy, but surgeons are getting better at it all the time, and the minimally invasive era is here to stay.

The Cleveland Clinic has a large program in assisted circulation. We have a bridge-to-transplantation program with assist devices, and we have the wonderful Kaufman Center for Heart Failure with excellent cardiologists. The first cardiologists were Mason Sones, Proudfit, and Sheldon, and now we have Eric Topol. Each succeeding department chair made a better department, and so we have remarkable cardiologists who help the surgeons and the patients.

The artificial heart is not quite here yet, but I believe it is coming soon, will work well and be miniaturized.

Now everybody is concerned about stents and drug-eluting stents. I think cardiologists will use more stents per patient and will expand the indications for stents. They will use them in smaller vessels, probably eventually in diabetics and older patients too. I know the European results, and clearly the new stents will reduce restenosis to zero. Cardiac surgery is not over yet; it will be a few generations before that happens. The solution lies in pharmacology and genomics.

I decided to study medicine in part because my father was a doctor. My mother was also a very strong influence on me. She lived to be ninety-nine, and saw almost the whole twentieth century. She was a very organized woman who spoke many languages, and taught at both the University of Illinois and Purdue. I emulated her approach to life, her organization, and her drive. I had a very good education and good teachers in high school, college, and medical school. I think Brian Blades influencing me to go to the Cleveland Clinic probably changed my life more than anything else. How he knew what I should do, and why he took an interest in me, I don't know. He and Paul Adkins were good friends, and Adkins was the professor at George Washington University under Brian Blades. I would have joined Adkins in 1970 if conditions had been right there. The cardiologists at George Washington were talking about phonocardiograms rather than angiography, and I could see the writing on the wall, so I did not join them.

Favaloro was also a huge influence on me, as was Don Effler by offering me a job. I had many arguments with Effler over the years, and he certainly didn't want to retire when the time came. There was a mandatory administrative retirement at age sixty at the Cleveland Clinic back in those days, and Effler did not go kindly. We had a few arguments at that time. Nevertheless, he was quite a force in American cardiac surgery and ran a very good department.

In the future, we are all going to have to run a lot faster in order to stay in the same place. Productivity in medicine has to increase, and costs have to go down. It's very hard to do that in this day and age, with the scientific and technical changes that occur every year. I think as there are more and more uninsured Americans, if there is an economic downturn, and if the Democrats get control in Congress and the White House, we could well have a modified form of universal health care in the next ten to twenty years. I don't think it is a good sign for medicine, but I think Americans are smart enough not to duplicate the Canadian health care system, where there is no private practice at all and patients cannot buy insurance. I think it will probably be more like England, with the more disadvantaged people being subsidized.

I chaired the cardiac and thoracic department at the Cleveland Clinic for fourteen years, and I happened to be on the Board of Governors when they decided on a change in the leadership at the Cleveland Clinic. I had no interest in any sort of administrative job other than running a large department, but the selection process wasn't going well. As a member of the search committee, I kept complaining about the candidates for the job, so they finally said, "Well, if you don't like it, give us a plan." So I gave them a strategic plan, and they said they wanted me to be CEO. The first year, 1989 to 1990, was probably the worst year of my life. I had no administration. We made fifty key executive changes within the first five years. We had to change a lot of the department heads in clinical medicine, and we had to change a lot of the key administrative people, but the financial picture changed dramatically in the first year. Now I am heading into my fourteenth year as the CEO, and I am finally, as they say, resting easy in my harness, but it took a long time, and I wouldn't recommend it to anybody.

I didn't stop operating until 1999, so I operated for quite a while after I took the CEO job but Cosgrove had such a good department that I was really going to the OR just to escape my administrative duties. I didn't do a large volume of cases, about 150 to 180 cases a year while I was CEO, but finally things got too busy, and I had to stop. We had some acquisitions of other hospitals, our health system got huge, and I realized that I was just taking up space in the OR. I just walked away from it, which I think is the way to do it.

Bibliography

Loop FD, Spampinato N, Cheanvechai C, Effler DB. The Free Internal Mammary Artery Bypass Graft. Use of the IMA in the Aorta-to-Coronary Artery Position. *Ann Thorac Surg.* 1973; 15:50–55.

Loop FD, Effler DB, Navia JA, Sheldon WC, Groves LK. Aneurysms of the Left Ventricle: Survival and Results of a Ten-Year Surgical Experience. *Ann Surg.* 1973; 178:399–405.

Loop FD, Cheanvechai C, Sheldon WC, Taylor PC, Effler DB. Early Myocardial Revascularization during Acute Myocardial Infarction. *Chest.* 1974; 66:478–482.

Loop FD, Christiansen EK, Lester JL, Cosgrove DM, Franco I, Golding LR. A Strategy for Cost Containment in Coronary Surgery. *JAMA.* 1983; 250:63–66.

Loop FD, Lytle BW, Cosgrove DM, Stewart RW, Goormastic M, Williams GW, Golding LA, Gill CC, Taylor PC, Sheldon WC, et al. Influence of the Internal-Mammary-Artery Graft on 10-Year Survival and Other Cardiac Events. *N Engl J Med.* 1986; 314:1–6.

Loop FD. Classics in Thoracic Surgery. F. Mason Sones, Jr., (1918–1985). *Ann Thorac Surg.* 1987; 43:237–38.

Loop FD, Lytle BW, Cosgrove DM, Mahfood S, McHenry MC, Goormastic M, Stewart RW, Golding LA, Taylor PC. J. Maxwell Chamberlain Memorial Paper. Sternal Wound Complications after Isolated Coronary Artery Bypass Grafting: Early and Late Mortality, Morbidity, and Cost of Care. *Ann Thorac Surg.* 1990; 49:179–186.

Loop FD, Lytle BW, Cosgrove DM, Woods EL, Stewart RW, Golding LA, Goormastic M, Taylor PC. Reoperation for Coronary Atherosclerosis. Changing Practice in 2509 Consecutive Patients. *Ann Surg.* 1990; 212:385–386.

Loop FD. Thoracic and Cardiovascular Surgery. Presidential Address. *J Thorac Cardiovasc Surg.* 1998; 116:683–688.

Loop FD. Coronary Artery Surgery. *Ann Thorac Surg.* 2005; 79:S2221–S2227.

Thomas J. Fogarty, MD

(b. 1934)

The thought of a balloon catheter occurred to me one day. I got some used ureteral catheters, took the baby finger of a rubber glove, tied it on with fly-tying techniques, put it in liquid disinfectant, and we used it. It was that simple.

— On the Fogarty catheter

Interviewed February 5, 2004

I grew up in Cincinnati, Ohio, a German town. I was an Irish kid in a neighborhood dominated by St. Boniface, a German saint, so I had a rather pugilistic upbringing, but it was a lot of fun. I went to a parochial school, Roger Bacon High School, in Xavier, Ohio. I got involved in medicine at an early age, in the eighth grade. There weren't many employment opportunities for people under the age of sixteen, but charitable and nonprofit institutions could hire underage people, and since many hospitals were nonprofits, young people could work in hospitals. I started working as the oxygen boy at Good Samaritan Hospital in Cincinnati when I was in the eighth grade. I rolled and cleaned oxygen tanks, and I also cleaned and repaired the Wangensteen stomach pumps, the old three-bottle machines. Through that process, I became exposed to medicine. I learned to run the sterilization machine, the big autoclave, initially in the central supply room, but because most of the instruments had to be cleaned and sterilized in the operating room, I started running the sterilizer there in the evenings. I got to know some of the nurses, and they felt that I could probably be a good scrub technician, so I became one in my sophomore year in high school, working part-time, mostly in the evenings. That was my introduction to medicine.

During the last part of my senior year in high school, I realized I had to be something other than a clown to get along in the world. I had not had a very distinguished academic career, and, in fact, I couldn't get a recommendation to go to college, because my grades were so bad. Finally, I got one of the priests to recommend that Xavier University take me on probation. Medicine had been of interest to me, so I applied for premed and majored in biology.

When I was working at the hospital as a scrub technician, I got to know Dr. Jack Cranley. He asked if I could scrub with him when I was available, and I worked with him a lot in the summers at the hospital. Also, if he had emergencies, he would call me to scrub with him in the evenings. He became my mentor and a significant source of income, and it worked out very well. I continued to work with him while I was in college, as a scrub technician and office assistant. I used to schedule the cases and line up anesthesia and even babysit with his children quite often. My father died when I was eight, and Dr. Cranley became a father figure to me. He always encouraged me and provided me with income by way of jobs, and I was able to get through college and much of medical school with his help. He was a great influence on my way of approaching problems, as he was always thinking outside of the box, about what works rather than what is tradition. I really owe a great deal to him.

Dr. Cranley was the first dedicated vascular surgeon in Cincinnati, and he started one of the first vascular labs. At first the procedures were rather crude. There was a lot of vein work, and that was pretty much the accepted way at the time, but arterial reconstruction was just coming into its own. We were beginning to do peripheral arterial reconstruction, simple procedures at the level of the inguinal ligament and aortoiliac bypass. Aneurysm surgery was still relatively new, and I remember the first aneurysm we ever did. It took twelve hours, and we scheduled it for a Saturday so that we could have the OR to ourselves. The grafts were lyophilized homografts, and one of my jobs was to go to the morgue, get the aortas, and lyophilize them. This involved exposing them to liquid nitrogen, freezing them, and putting them in a vacuum container. We had a whole bank of these lyophilized homografts, which were the first devices we used for bypass. We were also doing endarterectomies, but that did not serve all purposes, so we started banking the homografts. They weren't very durable and some became aneurysmal within a year. Later, they were replaced with Dacron grafts and various other things.

When I was a premed student, it occurred to me that a balloon catheter could be useful in embolectomies. The operation that you had to do for an embolus, particularly a saddle embolus, involved a major abdominal incision, plus two incisions in the groin and probably two in the popliteal region. It was a very prolonged, high-risk procedure under general anesthesia, and the patient usually had a significant risk of congestive heart failure because of mitral stenosis. I saw a lot of amputations and attempts at secondary operations, so the thought occurred to me that this was really a very cumbersome way to handle this problem. The thought of a balloon catheter occurred to me one day. I got some used ureteral catheters, took the baby finger of a glove, tied it on with fly-tying techniques, put it in some liquid disinfectant, and we used it.

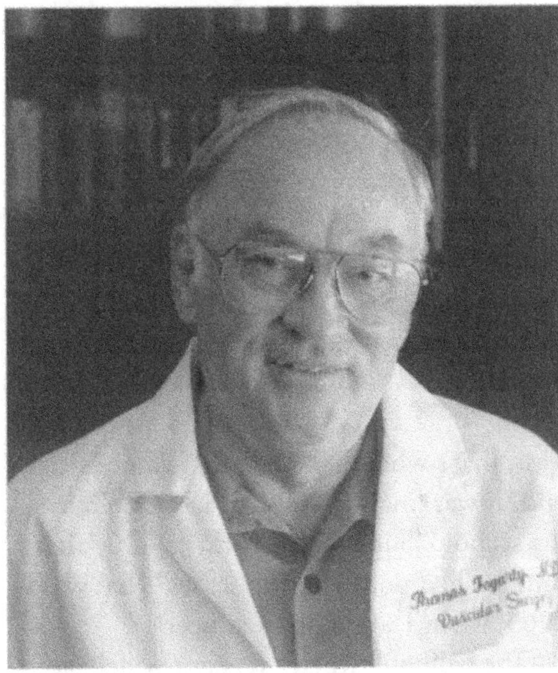

Thomas J. Fogarty

It was that simple, but it took a long time to be accepted. One of my criteria for a successful device is that it must be turned down by peer review journals, and the more peer review journals that turn it down, the better the idea probably is. The balloon catheter was turned down by three major peer review journals after we had done six successful clinical cases. As I recall, five of these were saddle emboli. To get through them successfully was an achievement, but *Archives of Surgery*, *Surgery*, and *Annals* all turned the paper down, simply because they felt it was dangerous and they didn't want people knowing about it; at

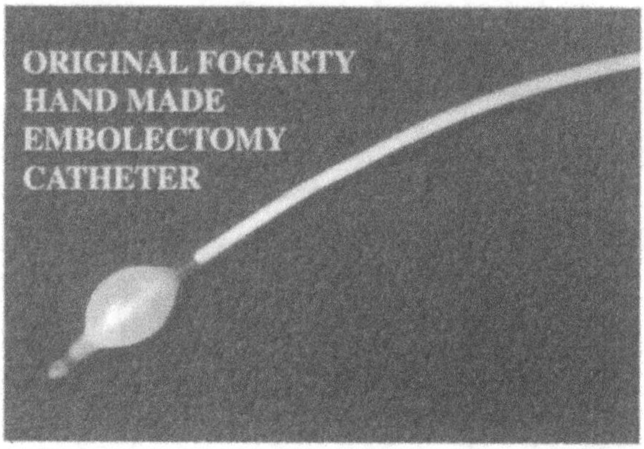

least, that's what the letters that came back said. It was finally published in *SG&O*, in the section "Surgeon at Work," and by that time we had done eighteen cases. That was in 1963, when I was a house officer.

The balloon catheter was not widely accepted. I will never forget Louis Hermann Sr., who was a senior vascular surgeon in Cincinnati. Dr. Cranley discussed the embolectomy at grand rounds at the Cincinnati General Hospital, and Dr. Hermann admonished me for indulging in such a dangerous procedure. Also, I went to England once, and I met Lord Brock, who invented the Brock commissurotomy device and who was an expert on emboli and rheumatic heart disease. He, too, had the impression that the balloon catheter was inappropriate and dangerous, and that only a very unknowing person would suggest it as a viable therapy.

In 1965 I went to the NIH and met Glenn Morrow. Glenn Morrow knew Lord Brock reasonably well, and he thought it was quite funny that Lord Brock had admonished me at the Royal College of Surgeons meeting. Glenn Morrow was a significant mentor in my life. He was painfully honest, to the point that sometimes his honesty bordered on cruelty, but he never really meant it that way. He always said that if you can't be honest, you will never really learn, because you will never admit to a mistake. He thought that you had to acknowledge that something had been done inappropriately in order to move forward. He was a strong advocate of self-assessment in a very honest way. He was based in physiology and taught clinical physiology. I think the teaching I received from him has served me very well over my career. As a technician, he wasn't flashy, but he always got the job done well and safely. He placed more of an emphasis on substance and on completion of the job than on appearance.

Before I was at the NIH with Glenn Morrow, I did my internship and residency at the University of Oregon, where I met Dr. Albert Starr. He was the person who made it possible for the embolectomy catheter to be commercially produced through his association with Lowell Edwards, an aeronautical engineer who knew a lot about valves. Dr. Starr and Lowell Edwards had collaborated on designing the ball valve. When I went to the University of Oregon from Cincinnati, the balloon catheter was just beginning to gain acceptance. Dr. Starr saw a lot of rheumatic heart disease, so he had a lot of patients with emboli. Whenever he had an embolectomy, he called me, so I got to do a lot of those very early in my career. Dr. Starr introduced me to the Edwards people, who agreed to take on the manufacturing of the balloon catheter. It was through Dr. Starr, then, that I expanded my interests from vascular surgery to cardiac surgery.

Once the development of the balloon catheter was mostly completed, I became interested in alternative valve designs, and I came up with the first tissue valve design. The Edwards Company helped me with the initial prototypes, but they decided not to pursue them. Dr. Starr, too, didn't think the biological valve was viable. That's why they agreed to let me develop it on my own with Warren Hancock, who was a marketing and sales director for both the valves and the embolectomy catheter. Warren and I pursued the development of the tissue valve with our own funds for about two years, while I was a first- and second-year resident at the University of Oregon.

Later, when I was at the NIH with Glenn Morrow, I did a lot of biological valve implants. We made the valves and treated them with different cross-linking compounds. At first we used formaldehyde and formalin, and then for various reasons we switched to glutaraldehyde. Warren went on to start Hancock Laboratories, and to produce the first commercial tissue valves, available in about 1966 or 1967. Johnson & Johnson eventually bought Hancock Laboratories, and they in turn sold it to Medtronic. The original valve is still around. Warren and I worked on a second generation of the valve, and that valve, which I call the blue valve, has just become commercially available in the United States. One of the problems with the original valve was that calcification could occur because of the glutaraldehyde. We came up with a process in the second generation that prevented calcification, and this valve also ended up in the hands of Medtronic.

We knew that device legislation was being considered in 1966, so we got the valve commercialized prior to the implementation of the legislation. At that time, we could test the valve and market it without too much difficulty. The public relied on the physician's integrity and the integrity of the company, and if you did something inappropriate, you were subject to malpractice. It was much simpler. There were no federal IRBs, and no FDA overlooking these things. It's not that there shouldn't be, but when you are considering putting a device on the market now, you have the IRB, the conflict of interest committees, the contracts committees, and then the FDA, so it is a much more burdensome path.

After my time at the NIH, I went to Stanford in 1968 to do my training in cardiac and thoracic surgery. I could have gone back to Oregon, but Dr. Starr thought it would be a good idea for me to learn something about transplantation, so I went down to Stanford and never went back to Oregon. I was at Stanford right after the very first heart transplants were done. I arrived probably a month after they did their first one, shortly after Dr. Christiaan Barnard did the first transplant in South Africa. I never heard Dr. Shumway say anything negative or critical about Dr. Barnard, but he was concerned about the spread of heart transplants all over the world to hospitals in different countries. He didn't think we knew enough about heart transplantation to be implementing these programs in many different sites. He thought that it should be focused in fewer sites, and he was critical of the rapid adoption of technology that still had a long way to go. I think he understood the seriousness of rejection issues more than others, who thought that there wasn't going to be much of a rejection problem. Obviously, Dr. Shumway knew better than that.

After I completed my cardiac and thoracic training with Dr. Shumway, I didn't pursue transplantation surgery as a career. For me, it wasn't a technical challenge any more, but rather a rejection challenge. Technically, a heart transplant is simple. If we were going to make any significant advances, it would be on the antirejection side, and I wasn't interested in that kind of research.

I was on the faculty at Stanford for three years with Dr. Shumway. We were part of the Department of General Surgery, but he wanted to create a separate, distinct Department of Cardiac Surgery. He thought that if he minimized the income of the division, other people in the department wouldn't care if he created it. He encouraged me and another faculty member, Pat Daily, to go into private practice. I had been offered a position at the NIH, and I was planning to go back there, but Pat Daily didn't want to be there alone in private practice, so he and Dr. Shumway convinced me to stay at Stanford.

Soon we became pretty busy, and Shumway stayed busy, so there wasn't enough room for all of the patients. There weren't enough ICU beds or standard beds. We were doing both cardiac and peripheral vascular surgery, so it was not unusual for us to have a census of sixty patients, and Shumway would have a high census also. There just wasn't enough room. It led to a conflict, and in the end I decided that he was there first. He strongly encouraged me to continue in my private practice, but somewhere else. At that time a certificate of need was still a significant hurdle in California, and he appeared before the governing body and said that we needed another open-heart center and that we were the best guys to do it. That started me at another institution, Sequoia Hospital, right outside of Palo Alto.

Venous thrombectomy has been a controversial procedure. If you look at its history, there have been many advocates of it, McHorner in Louisiana, Dr. Ochsner Sr., and my own mentor, Jack Cranley. If you can take an arterial thrombus or embolus out, you should be able to do a venous thrombectomy, and we developed a catheter system specifically for the venous system. The difference was that it had a tip that would bend back on itself so that you could get past the valves. It was similar to cannulation of the ventricle: If you had a catheter that bent back, you could flip the elbow through the valve. We designed that same system for the venous valves and did a large series of them with significant longitudinal follow-up, including venograms that demonstrated long-term patency.

As the procedure became more accepted, though, a problem arose. People failed to differentiate a chronic substrate from an acute extension of an established thrombus. The catheter was not designed to take out fibrotic areas in the venous system. People would do the thrombectomy, and then obviously they would have a recurrence. The procedure fell into disrepute, but if you differentiate the acute from the chronic and you use it for acute conditions only, it remains a good procedure.

It is interesting that now, with the percutaneous catheter approach, people are beginning to realize that the venous thrombectomy procedure has great utility over the thrombolytic agents. Thrombolytic therapy still has a significant number of complications, and the results are not that reliable. In the current environment, once again we are revisiting the concept of mechanical removal of the thrombus. The only difference is that we are figuring out ways to do it while minimizing blood loss and without an incision, thus avoiding the complications associated with thrombolytics. I think there is going to be a real resurgence in this area.

This is how it works. Imagine introducing something the size of a toothpick, then turning that toothpick into an eggbeater. The eggbeater would morsellate the thrombus, and then it could be withdrawn through a straw. You introduce something very low profile and deploy it into a thrombus so that you can morsellate it, and then aspirate it. You provide protection by means of a temporary filter. We are currently working on that technology.

Everybody thinks that I have planned my whole life, but I didn't plan anything other than being interested in innovation and making things work better. In the state of Ohio, when you graduate from medical school you are not required to take an internship before you get your license to practice. The Vietnam War was going on when I graduated, and I decided to go to Oregon to do my internship. I thought I wanted to be a cardiologist, but when I got there, I decided that was not what I wanted to do. I got interested in being a surgeon and was accepted for the surgical residency. About two weeks after I was accepted, I got a draft notice to report for duty right away. This was probably in March. I went to talk to Englebert Dunphy, who was the professor at the University of Oregon, and he said, "Well, I can probably intercede and fix it so that you can finish your internship, but beyond that, I probably can't help much." He asked them to let me finish my internship. They said, "Fine, but he's going to be drafted right after that," so I finished my internship and went back to Cincinnati, expecting to be drafted. I went to work for Dr. Cranley again as a surgical assistant, but I never heard from the army. They lost me. I called Dr. Dunphy and said, "You know, I haven't been drafted." He said that I should just keep my mouth shut, come back to Oregon, and finish my residency.

By the time I went back to Oregon, Dr. Cranley and I had already done clinical cases with embolectomy catheters. Dunphy knew about that because he and Jack Cranley were friends, and they kept in touch about my progress. In Oregon, Charles Dotter, who is an interventional radiologist, was developing the concept of coaxial dilatation of stenotic arteries. Essentially, he passed large-bore catheters down over one another in coaxial fashion to widen the arteries, but he had more problems than successes and would routinely call me to help him. He either had bleeding or thrombosis or both. He saw the balloon catheter being used, and he said, "Rather than using the coaxial thing, we have to use these balloon catheters." The balloon catheter was actually designed to deform in response to narrowings, so he said, "Tom, can you make one that won't deform, that will exert some lateral pressure?" I said I could, and I did.

About the same time, Dotter went to Dunphy and said, "I would like for this kid to take a year off and work with me." Dunphy called me into his office and said that if I wanted to finish my surgical residency, then I should quit messing around with that crazy Charlie Dotter. Obviously, I did want to finish my residency, but on the side I made catheters for Charlie. He would schedule a case at night, and I would go over and help him. The first iliac balloon catheter dilatation that Charlie did was with one of my handmade catheters. That was in 1963 or 1964, before I went to the NIH. Charlie studied that patient ten years later, and the artery was still patent. That was the first experience with angioplasty, and I continued to maintain an interest in it over the years. Charlie published it.

Andreas Gruentzig knew about the Fogarty catheter, and he asked me if I could work with Edwards Laboratory to make a catheter that had a noncompliant, fixed-volume balloon. Elastomer is compliant, and polyvinyl is noncompliant. One is like a balloon, which, when you blow it up, it only gets so big. That is an angioplasty balloon like the first one I made for Charlie. I went to Edwards and told him I thought this was a good idea. Once again, Albert Starr said it was a very bad idea. He had the surgeon mentality that if it wasn't a knife or a suture, he was not quite comfortable with it, but Gruentzig went ahead anyway and had it made by Bard, I think. Gruentzig was an angiologist, as they say in Europe. He was not a cardiologist and he was not a radiologist; he was somebody who studied angiology, which is the science of the vascular system. Most of those people were medically oriented, but he happened to be device oriented. It's important to understand that in addition to the medical literature about these devices, there is a whole commercial background to them, and these two backgrounds are truly not the same.

Atherectomy was a viable procedure that fell out of favor, but I think it will have resurgence. I worked on this device with the cardiologist John Simpson, who had the idea that rather than radially displacing the atheroma, as you do with dilatation, it would make more sense to remove it. This procedure was not an endarterectomy, because an endarterectomy would have a cleavage point. What Simpson wanted to do was debulk sufficiently so that you could return the artery to a normal lumen. We collaborated on the atherocatheter, as we called it. It had a somewhat short history because in the periphery there aren't many short segmental lesions, so you would have to do a long debulking. The catheter was not designed for that. In the coronary system, it actually performed reasonably well. When stents came along and it was possible to displace the atheroma and keep it displaced, atherectomy fell out of favor. What we're finding now is that recurrence can be reduced if you debulk, and then place a stent. That is the direction that we are going, at least in the coronary area. I think it's likely that you could go that way in the peripheral vessels as well, because we now have some pretty unique stents for the periphery that are really much more applicable than the first generation.

The radiologists, the cardiologists, or the surgeons could do this procedure, but I hope that soon we will have a hybrid physician who is trained to do mostly endovascular procedures such as this. From my perspective, that is what should happen, although I don't have a lot of confidence that it will happen, however, because of the way we train doctors. We are so oriented toward separate departments that we never get together and think about treating the pathology with the most appropriate technology and techniques that are available. We spend too much time promoting the traditions of each specialty, and this has to change, because the health care system won't be able to tolerate multiple specialties treating the same disease, which is a very expensive way to do things. You have a cardiologist who does six angioplasties on a patient, and then the cardiac surgeon finally says that it's time to operate. If doctors were working together more, there would be much less of that.

Charles Dotter, with whom I developed the balloon catheter, also suggested that endovascular grafts or stents were possible. He came up with the first Nitinol vascular stents in conjunction with a company called Raykin. Charlie and I maintained a friendship even after I left the University of Oregon, and since Raykin was located in Palo Alto, Charlie would stay with me when he came down from Oregon to visit them. He would always show me his latest Nitinol stent. Nitinol is a shape-memory metal. You can put it straight in a very low-profile place, and a temperature change will cause it to pull into a coil, turning it into a stent. He was working on that concept in the late 1960s and early 1970s, but the idea actually goes back to the early 1960s, when he began saying that we should be able to do an internal graft. He actually did it first in the portal vein system. Clinically, it was first used by a Russian surgeon named Votalos, and then later by Juan Parodi from Argentina. Parodi did some humans, with a stent graft that was straight, through the abdominal aorta, and then others began addressing the same issue, including me. We developed the bifurcated modular stent graft for the abdominal aorta. Still, credit for the original idea has to go to Charles Dotter. Volatos and Parodi and others did the first clinical implementations, but the first commercially available designs were different from Juan Parodi's. One is the Guidant graft, and the other one is the Medtronic graft, which I developed.

There is a graft for thoracic aneurysms also. It is a natural extension of the other grafts, but it is probably a more useful application because of the significant mortality and morbidity associated with surgical repair of thoracic aneurysms. The last thoracic endograft we did took thirty minutes, pretty good when you compare it with traditional surgery. For a thoracic aorta, the take-off of the descending aorta relative to the left subclavian becomes very important. You have to understand the anatomy, and usually it requires a 360-degree CT to figure that out. You need some purchase below the subclavian; but usually two centimeters are enough, and, of course, you have to end above the celiac. With the technology that is currently available, any thoracic aneurysm is a suitable candidate if it ends a couple of centimeters above the celiac and begins a couple of centimeters lower than the left subclavian. If they are markedly angulated, then you have to be careful about your stent graft selection.

We are starting to treat dissections now with endografts, and I think it's a very good application. I also believe that endografts for the ascending aorta will be developed; it would be relatively easy. The transverse aorta is going to be a challenge, but I believe you can do it. Maybe not everybody can do it, though. There are techniques and designs that could address those issues.

The abdominal aneurysm endograft is fairly complex. If you stick with simple anatomy it is OK, but as you begin to extend it to cases with a lot of tortuosity and with different areas of stenosis and occlusion, as in the hypogastric, then it gets more complex. If you take a straightforward aneurysm with a neck that is straight, three to four centimeters long, and the aneurysm ends a couple of centimeters above the bifurcation of the hypogastric, then technically it is fairly simple. It does take a fair amount of insight, knowledge, and planning on the surgeon's part. For the patient, the time savings are significant, but from the standpoint of the surgeon, you have to know a lot more than you do with a standard surgical repair. You have to know the images, the projections, when to get this, when to get that, when there's a problem, and when there's an issue. So in a way it's simple, but in another way, it's not so simple.

I think the Heartport system is not a good idea. The big advance was made when we went from peripheral cannulation to central aortic cannulation, avoiding the complications of peripheral cannulations, such as retrograde dissections and occasional embolization. I had previously tried to occlude the ascending aorta with balloons and figured out early on that it was not easy, and it was fraught with complications, so I was never enthusiastic about the Heartport system.

On the other hand, I was involved with off-pump coronary bypass procedures. I promoted that, by assigning technology and licenses that I had to one of the companies interested in beating-heart surgery, and I thought there was great value in it. Sometime in the mid-1980s, I visited Brazil and talked to surgeons there who had done a lot of beating-heart operations. I said, "Holy cow, this works!" I provided them with some shunts that they needed, and I became interested in it.

I do think that port surgery and robotics will happen, but I think it will evolve over a long time and is not going to happen soon. I have done enough of that kind of technology to know that it requires a major paradigm shift, which most surgeons will not accept quickly. They will accept components of it, but not in one big gulp. However, I think that in five to ten years there will be more robotic heart procedures.

In general, I believe that surgically oriented procedures will be eroded by catheter-mediated and less-invasive procedures. The erosion will continue, because the technology is available to do it. The concept of a coronary artery bypass graft via a catheter sounds ridiculous, but it's not. It's just a matter of time. In fact, for that procedure, the change needs to happen sooner rather than later. I think robotics is going to take longer to arrive.

I also believe we will see changes in managed care, but for that to happen, physicians as individuals will have to be more proactive. We cannot sit back and allow things to occur that are not in the best interest of the patient. We have to be vehement about this, and we have not been. You see a lot of guys who say, "I can't do anything about it, the insurance company won't let me do it, and the administration of the hospital won't let me do it." I think we have to be very vehement and vocal and raise hell on behalf of the patient, and we haven't done that. You *can* do something; you just have to do it. It is not pleasant to enter into battle or be confrontational, but if we are going to make any headway, it is absolutely critical that we do it, particularly when we are being compromised and our patients are being compromised.

I think the opportunities now for a young person going into medicine are even greater than they were when I started, but unfortunately, nonclinical, nonmedical people are in control of much of what goes on in medicine now. It is our obligation to change that. The therapeutic decision should lie in the hands of those with the greatest knowledge and integrity—the physicians taking care of the patients, not an administrator. It is the physician who cares for an individual patient. We can't tolerate the fact that people who aren't responsible for the patient are controlling decisions about the patient's care, but of course we can't be stupid about it. All of those administrators have something to offer, but when it comes to decisions about the treatment of the individual patient, the more that nonclinical people influence the clinical decisions, the worse off the patient is going to be, and the worse off we physicians are going to be. The person who talks to the individual patient is the individual physician, not somebody in the insurance company.

I have invented many devices in my career, the best known probably being the Fogarty catheter, but my first invention was not related to medicine, and that is the automatic clutch. I had a Cushman motor scooter, and it had two gears, a low gear and a high gear. If you were in high gear going up a steep hill, as you slowed down you switched to low gear, but what would happen was that your butt would be on the street and the scooter would be about twenty yards ahead of you. I thought about how this transition could become smoother, while working part-time in a motor scooter repair shop, and a friend and I came up with the concept of the centrifugal clutch with which the belt would automatically go down to a lower sprocket, and the driver would get more power without suddenly shifting. That was the concept of the centrifugal clutch, and it was soon incorporated in most small motors. I don't have a patent on that though—the company I worked for had what was called shop rights. Anything that was invented in that shop was owned by the shop, including the patent on inventions. That was my first lesson in patents.

The balloon catheter invention was something I take great pride in, because not only was it an endovascular procedure, but it was also the beginning of less-invasive surgery in general. It eliminated or minimized anesthesia, so that we could use local anesthesia. It also minimized the magnitude and number of incisions, and recovery time was shortened. Did I think that was what I was doing when I invented it? No. It just so happened that that was the beginning of minimally invasive approaches in surgery. It happened to be in the vascular system because that's what I was involved in. The use of balloon technology was extended to thrombectomy, biliary stones, and angioplasty, so I feel good about that.

The atraumatic clamps came about as a result of an observation that I made when I was a scrub technician, that the clamps were crushing tissue. The so-called atraumatic clamps were really metal, and I wanted to replicate pinching something between your thumb and finger, but in clamp form. I feel good about that invention also.

When I developed the tissue valve, I was thinking about whether we could find something less thrombogenic. I thought, "Well, our own valve doesn't clot, so why don't we just use something very much like it?" The tissues that we tried were pericardium, dura mater, fascia lata, and the valve from an animal, chosen simply from a sizing and manufacturing standpoint. We thought we had the angiogenicity problems fixed with glutaraldehyde, and we documented that, with the technology that was available at the time for measuring angiogenicity.

I was also involved with oxygenator technology, not so much by inventing anything but by identifying what didn't work. Lowell Edwards was very interested in a membrane oxygenator, and I used to work with him on that at a laboratory in Oregon where we would make silicone membranes, which actually worked extremely well, but we couldn't figure out a way to mass-produce them. Simultaneously, Dick DeWall was working on the bubble oxygenator, so he and Edwards were pursuing parallel courses. DeWall came to Edwards about the bubble oxygenator, but Edwards wanted to pursue the membrane oxygenator. Jim Bentley and I wanted to pursue the bubble oxygenator, so we actually bought that invention from Edwards, and Bentley and I started Bentley Laboratories in conjunction with DeWall. That was the origin of the Bentley oxygenator. I contributed by recognizing the clinical opportunity and recognizing that the bubbler would get better, although we didn't know how to improve it at that time. As we continued to develop and manufacture it, we made it long-lasting enough to get somebody through an operation as long as he was on the oxygenator less than five hours. Most of the pump times when we started out were pretty long, but they quickly got shorter, and, simultaneously, we identified the problem with the bubbler that caused it to lose its efficiency during the operation.

After that, I contributed to further variations of the clamp and the various devices that removed thrombus and clot beyond the first generation of Fogarty catheters. My involvement with beating-heart coronary revascularization was more from a commercial side, helping the developers identify the opportunity and the appropriate instruments. I also helped them to collaborate with physicians who could make a clinical judgment about its worth. When I look back on my involvement with technology, I can see that it is not the inventor who ultimately determines the value of an invention, but the people using it who determine its value. Over the years, one of the things I have learned is the importance of having your concepts, innovations, and technology validated by others. The endograft we developed, I think, is going to cause a major paradigm shift. Some of the design ideas that we put into it will persist.

I came up with another invention that is less well recognized, called the Mammotome, an instrument that takes core biopsies of breast lesions. That technology came out of our Fogarty group and is based on our experience with atherectomy. The original atherectomy device was essentially biopsying the arterial wall, so we redesigned it in such a fashion that you could not only biopsy the arterial wall, but also all of the tissue. You could get multiple biopsies through one stick and take the biopsies over 360 degrees instead of taking directional biopsies. If you put in a two-millimeter needle, you would end up with an eight-millimeter core by simply rotating it, and that did change the way we managed breast pathology. I am most proud of the inventions that people don't know I was involved with.

I owe a lot to the many great mentors I have had in my life. Medicine is kind of a science and kind of an art, and manners are critically important. Manners are something that you cannot teach to students in a classroom; they must be learned through one-on-one exposure, and in that regard, I will forever be indebted to Jack Cranley. Later, at the University of Oregon, Al Starr was certainly a mentor, encouraging me in my efforts in embolectomy and putting me in touch with a company that would finally make the product. On the general surgical side, J. Engelbert Dunphy, who was a very prominent surgeon at the time I knew him, encouraged me and was helpful to me in getting grants for laboratory and clinical research. After that, Charles Dotter was a mentor, and I learned a lot from him. He was an interesting guy, not technically talented, but he had great vision and concepts, and he was smart enough to know that he had to have others implement them. That's important. I had stumbled onto the broad therapeutic applicability of the catheter, but he contributed his own vision to it. At the NIH, I met Glenn Morrow, who had the greatest integrity of any person I've ever known. He was painfully honest not only with others, but with himself, and at the same time he had great empathy with the patients. He understood them and knew how to relate to them. He was a real human being. Norm Shumway, too, was a very substantive person. He was more interested in communicating his ideas than he was in his own stature. He often said, "If I surround myself with people who are smarter than I am, I will be that much better," and I think that is true. He strove to make people better and committed himself to helping people become well. Over the years I have been really fortunate to have been exposed to some of the giants of cardiovascular surgery.

Bibliography

Fogarty TJ, Cranley JJ, Krause RJ, Strasser ES, Hafner CD. A Method for Extraction of Arterial Emboli and Thrombi. *Surg Gynec Obstet.* 1963; 116:241–244.

Fogarty TJ, Krippaehne WW. Catheter Technique for Venous Thrombectomy. *Surg Gynec Obstet.* 1965; 121:362–364.

Fogarty TJ, Kinney TB, Finn JC, Hermann GD. A New Vascular Clamp. *Surg Gynec Obstet.* 1985; 160:264–265.

Burbank F, Parker SH, Fogarty TJ. Stereotactic Breast Biopsy: Improved Tissue Harvesting with the Mammotome. *Am Surg.* 1996; 62:738–744.

Fogarty TJ. Presidential Address: Who We Are, What We Do, and Where We Are Going. *J Vasc Surg.* 1996; 23:887–893.

St Goar FG, Fann JI, Komtebedde J, Foster E, Oz MC, Fogarty TJ, Feldman T, Block PC. Endovascular Edge-to-Edge Mitral Valve Repair: Short-term Results in a Porcine Model. *Circulation.* 2003; 108:1990–1993.

Mehran R, Leon MB, Feigal DA, Jefferys D, Simons M, Chronos N, Fogarty TJ, Kuntz RE, Baim DS, Kaplan AV. Post-market Approval Surveillance: A Call for a More Integrated and Comprehensive Approach. *Circulation.* 2004; 109:3073–3077.

Fogarty TJ, Arko FR, Zarins CK. Endograft Technology: Highlights of the Past 10 Years. *J Endovasc Ther.* 2004; 11(Suppl 2):II192–199.

Hill BB, Faruqi RM, Arko FR, Zarins CK, Fogarty TJ. "Over-the-Wire" Inversion Saphenectomy: A Simple, Minimally Invasive Vein Harvesting Technique for Arterial Bypass. *J Endovasc Ther.* 2005; 12:394–400.

Fogarty TJ. Is the Future Here and Now and Passed You By? *Am Heart Hosp J.* 2006; 4:172–173.

Transplant—Artificial Heart

Norman E. Shumway, MD, PhD

(b. 1923)

No one had any concept of the amount of media interest that heart transplantation would create. Soon transplants were being done in India and places where you would not want to have any kind of a heart operation. All those programs were discontinued because the results were so poor. We went from something like a 40 percent five-year survival before cyclosporine to 75 percent survival.

— On the effect of cyclosporine on rejection

Interview conducted on October 16, 1997

I was born in Kalamazoo, Michigan, in 1923 and was an only child. In those days the economy was so bad generally that most families had as few children as they could possibly manage. I had a lot of fun growing up in small towns in Michigan. After graduating from high school, I went to the University of Michigan and was a prelaw student for one year. World War II was starting, and I signed up for the enlisted reserves, but we were called up pretty quickly and sent for basic infantry training. Since we would be lawyers, of course, it was a good idea to get us into the infantry as soon as possible.

After we completed infantry training, they sent a certain number of us back to college. That was 1943 and nobody knew how long the war would last, so they anticipated needing more specialists in various areas, such as engineering. They sent me and many of my colleagues who had some education into engineering schools scattered around the country. I was sent to John Tarleton Agricultural Junior College in Stevenville, Texas, where I had two semesters of engineering. They then took another handful of us and said they were going to make doctors out of us, and that is how I got into medical school. I did not plan it at all, it happened by chance. There were five hundred of us in the engineering course at Tarleton College. One day they marched us into an auditorium and, as the army does, they said, "All of you will take a medical aptitude test." We all took the test and I will never forget the very last question. It said if you are chosen or pass this test, are you more interested in medicine or dentistry? Since it was wartime and I knew a little about the infantry, I was pretty sure they were going to need more doctors than dentists, so I marked medicine. Sure enough, a little later the dental part of the program was folded, and those poor guys who checked the wrong box were back in the infantry while the rest of us continued in premed. One of the failures of my education is that I still do not have a bachelor's degree because I was never in one school long enough to graduate.

Next we had three quarters of premed at Baylor University in Waco. There were thirty-five of us who finished, and this was from a group of five hundred. The thirty-five of us had admissions in six or seven different medical schools, none of which was Vanderbilt. They divided us up into groups of four and told us which schools would take us. Each four would have to decide which school among themselves. I flipped a coin with one of my colleagues and the winner would go to the University of Tennessee and the other would go to Arkansas, which, at that time, was a Class B medical school, and I do not think it was fully accredited. I won the coin toss and went to Tennessee. By the time I got to Memphis there were too many for the class that was about to start, and they took the last two of us to arrive, which was another chap and me, and they said they were going to send the two of us to Vanderbilt, which was not even on the original list. It was just by chance that I had the opportunity to come to Nashville. It is a murky story.

The chief of surgery at Vanderbilt was Dr. Barney Brooks, one of the great teachers of surgery, and a spectacular individual in his own right. If there ever was somebody who was a man for all seasons, it was Dr. Brooks. He was such a strong teacher that when he conducted grand rounds once a week, his great student and faculty member, Alfred Blalock, would be in the front row to listen to him. He was a fabulous individual, and in many ways a delightful man, and he had a tremendous influence on all of us. He would go into a patient's room, and if he did not like the dressing, he would turn to the nurse and the resident, "Go out there and get me an audience, and I will show them how to put the dressing on properly." They would go out and get the orderlies, secretaries, and students and fill the room with people, then he would proceed to revise the dressing. He was a remarkable person.

There were other great teachers in the Department of Surgery. Cobb Pilcher was just emerging as one of the most capable and best-known neurosurgeons in the United States. As a matter of fact, in my senior year we developed a Cobb Pilcher Lectureship because we thought so highly of his teaching ability. The first lecture was given by George W. Thorn, who had just been made the chief of medicine at the Peter Bent Brigham in Boston. Thorn was an endocrinologist and they were just beginning to talk about ACTH and cortisone and all of those interesting areas. The honorarium was $100, and we all chipped in to establish the Cobb Pilcher Lectureship; one of the best things we did while we were there.

When I finished at Vanderbilt I went to the University of Minnesota for my internship. I had spent a lot of time in the old medical library, run by Mrs. Cunningham, and I had discovered that a lot of the literature in surgery came from either the University of Minnesota or the Mayo Clinic. I always thought that a university would be a better place to train than one of the large clinics, since, at that time, Mayo did not have a medical school. When the time came for applications, I applied to several other places, Yale, New York Hospital, and Rochester, all of which had ties with Vanderbilt, but I decided to go to the University of Minnesota largely because of what I perceived at that time to be a large number of contributions to surgery.

Dr. Owen Wangensteen was the chairman of the Department of Surgery and was quite different from Dr. Brooks. One of Wangensteen's greatest attributes was that he had a total lack of envy. When I first arrived in Minneapolis as an intern, people were coming from all over the world to watch Dr. Wangensteen operate. When open-heart surgery got started there in 1952, they were not coming to see Wangensteen anymore. They were coming to watch Lillehei, Lewis, and Varco. Did this bother Wangensteen? Not a bit. He was so proud of what was going on with these young men that he just basked in the reflected glory of their contributions, and helped to advance and develop them. In no way did he say they were usurping his fame or position or whatever, and he was very supportive. He would try to get financing or whatever else it took to support a resident who might have a new idea. He was a marvelous individual. He always referred to himself as the regimental water carrier, and his job was to be sure that the troops had enough support. It was a remarkable attitude, particularly for those days.

When the Korean War started, I was called back into the service since I had had so much of my education at the expense of the government. I went into the air force and was stationed in Lake Charles, Louisiana, for two years. After that I returned to the residency program at Minnesota. Not all of the surgical residents were in the PhD program, but there was great emphasis on research. During my five years as a resident, I had one full year in the Department of Physiology and another year and a half working in the surgical laboratories. I had precious little training as a junior resident in clinical surgery. In fact, we pretty much went from the laboratory to chief resident status. The program was extremely liberal by the standards of today. Although many places had very rigid programs, it was freewheeling at Minnesota, and I think that was a good idea.

In medical training, we frequently selected a specialty or an area of research because of admiration for one of our mentors. One of the best surgeons at Minnesota was John Lewis, who did the first successful open-heart operation in 1952 using general hypothermia and inflow occlusion. Hypothermia was the principal theme of all of his research activities, and I started to work with him and help with that activity. The use of total body hypothermia was the subject of my PhD thesis.

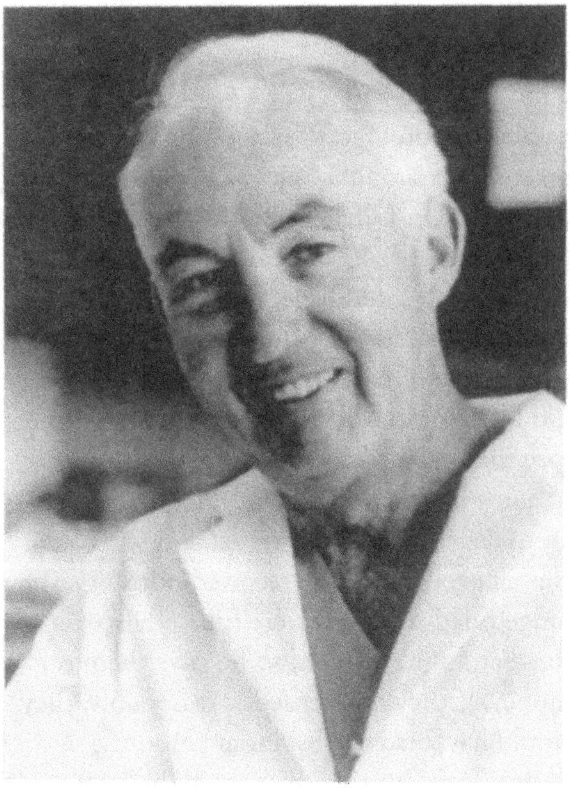

Norman E. Shumway

Dr. Lewis's first patient was a five-year-old child, with an atrial septal defect, who is alive today and a grandmother. From 1952 to 1954 all open-heart surgery was done with immersion hypothermia and brief inflow occlusion obtained by clamping the superior and inferior venae cavae. Lewis's colleague and best friend was Walt Lillehei, who developed the technique of cross-circulation with his two younger colleagues, Herb Warden and Morley Cohen. They used the mother or father as the oxygenator to support the circulation of the patient, which was usually an infant or small child. Lillehei did forty-five patients using this method. They liked to point out that it was the only operation that had the risk of 200 percent mortality.

In fact, there was only one accident involving the donor throughout the entire series, a mother who had an air embolus, which caused a neurological defect that was not too severe. This brought about an interesting set of events. Dr. Lillehei told the patient that he had malpractice insurance and advised them, "I think you should sue me and get some money for whatever future rehabilitation or anything you may need." They reluctantly did this, but once the lawyers developed the case they decided to sue for millions instead of a few hundred thousand. Lillehei had to go to court rather than settle, and when it was all over the family received nothing. The judge ruled that they were fully advised as to what might happen, so he gave them no money. If they had settled it reasonably, they would have had a substantial amount.

It was at this time that the bubble oxygenator was developed at Minnesota, the work of a young man named Richard DeWall. The pump-oxygenators had a lot of problems with blood clotting when exposed to glass surfaces, rubber tubing, and metal connectors. We would siliconize these materials, which made them friendlier toward blood. Dick DeWall developed a bubble oxygenator that consisted largely of plastic tubing, which got away from the problems of glass surfaces. It replaced the cross-circulation technique and was a much better arrangement, fairly simple and allowing longer periods of cardiopulmonary bypass. It worked very well, and DeWall went all over the world demonstrating it. He later had a very enviable career in heart surgery in Dayton, Ohio. I cannot remember exactly where he obtained the plastic tubing, but it was set up so that the blood was oxygenated by bubbling oxygen through the blood in a vertical cylinder. The blood then flowed down through tubing arranged in a helical fashion. This allowed the blood to debubble so that when it collected at the bottom it could be given back to the patient free of bubbles.

In May of 1953 John Gibbon used his screen oxygenator and pump to close an atrial septal defect of an eighteen-year-old at Jefferson Medical College in Philadelphia. His pump-oxygenator was developed with the assistance of several engineers from the IBM Company. He used the same pump on four or five other patients without success, so he became discouraged and did not do any more cases. He shared all of his information with John Kirklin, who built a similar device at the Mayo Clinic and began a successful program there in 1955. It is really interesting that the only two places in the world doing open-heart surgery were in Minnesota: Minneapolis and Rochester. It was a very exciting time, and surgeons from all over the world came to see what was going on.

In 1955, Walt Lillehei was mostly doing congenital heart defects. He would tackle some of the most difficult problems, such as atrioventricular canal, and he had some success but, of course, not always. He had very good results with patients with tetralogy of Fallot. It was not until 1956 or 1957 that he began to do valve patients. At the same time Lewis was still closing atrial septal defects with just hypothermia, no pump.

We, at the University of Minnesota, used to joke about the Mayo Clinic. We called it a charm school. There was such a contrast between the atmospheres at the University of Minnesota, which was truly laissez-faire, and at the Mayo Clinic, where everything was carefully regulated. There was little deviation, whether in the dress code of the residents or the methods of doing open-heart surgery. Everything was all carefully prescribed, and

I think this is true even today. They were not particularly innovative, but they could take somebody's innovation and perfect it to a degree that the originator probably never thought was possible. They were extremely good at polishing ideas and techniques. The Mayo-Gibbon pump-oxygenator is a perfect example.

When I finished my training at Minnesota in 1957, they were very busy, usually doing one or two open-heart cases a day, just beginning to do adults as well as children. They had moved into open repair for mitral valve disease and also some operations for aortic valve disease, and were just beginning to develop some of the valve replacement devices. When I left Minnesota, they had several men at my level who had worked with Lillehei and who were closer to having a faculty position than I could ever be. Wangensteen always wanted to keep everybody there and would go out to all of the neighboring hospitals and set up a Minnesota presence by making one of his trainees the chief of surgery there. He did this to nearly all of the smaller private hospitals scattered around Minneapolis. The place he wanted me to go was St. Joseph's Hospital in St. Paul. Well, I went over there to look at the situation. There was no possibility for laboratory research or anything, so it clearly was not a viable option.

Actually, I did not know quite what to do at that point. At one of the national meetings, I ran into a man who was trying to do thoracic and cardiac surgery in the little town of Santa Barbara, California; it is one of the most beautiful places you can imagine. I went out there and spent six weeks in private practice. I cannot remember if I quit or if he fired me, but it was one or the other or maybe both. Just by chance, one of my friends from Minnesota residency days was in San Francisco, so I went up to see him and he introduced me to Victor Richards, who was the chairman of surgery at Stanford. Dr. Richards hired me. It was very simple.

At that time Stanford was still in San Francisco. I started out as an instructor in surgery, and my principal job was to help run the artificial kidney. I worked on the artificial kidney with a man who was available only at night, because he was busy all day in his private practice in his office. In the middle of the night we would put these patients on the old Kolff drum artificial kidney and run it all night long. I would do that at night, and in the daytime I worked in the experimental surgery laboratory. It was our good fortune that the young resident assigned to the laboratory at that time was Richard Lower, so he and I began to work together, and that is really how heart transplantation started.

When we started we were not thinking about heart transplantation, but about a second open-heart surgery program. Frank Gerbode had the heart surgery situation very well in hand at the Stanford University Hospital, but there were other hospitals, like Children's Hospital in San Francisco, where I thought there was a chance to get another open-heart program started. We began to look at better methods of operating on the open heart instead of working on it while it was beating, trying to develop a technique in which the heart would be stationary and viable with a dry field. We began to do experiments using local cooling of the heart. We had an old Kay-Cross disc oxygenator. We would put dogs on bypass, clamp the aorta, and cool the heart suspended in the pericardium for an hour. This was topical cooling with no coronary perfusion. The usual technique used for valve operations involved coronary perfusion, which was very cumbersome because the coronary cannulas were always in the way.

Topical cooling seemed to work uniformly for periods of about an hour. The only trouble was that we were just standing there for that hour doing nothing. So I said, "Why don't we just take the heart out. We can cut it out at the atrial level and put it in some cold saline and then suture it back in place. We will get some experience in anastomotic surgery at the same time." We were just beginning to get some swaged-on suture material that we would steal from the operating room. So this is what happened, but we had very little success because in an autograft the suture lines were very tight because there was no excess tissue. Also, the atrial tissue of the dog is so fragile that it is like wet tissue paper, so Lower said, "Why don't we use the heart from a different dog? Then we will have more tissue that can be bolstered. We can bolster the suture lines and there won't be so much hemorrhage." I said, "Fine. We will just see if it works." We would take the heart from another dog and put it in with the same technique. With the extra atrial tissue that was available to bolster our suture lines, we were able to get some success. It started as sort of an accidental technique.

At first, we were not even sure that a denervated heart could perform satisfactorily. I think that of all the experiments that Lower and I did, the most important one showed that you do not need an innervated heart. It is true of course that livers and kidneys can be transplanted without any worry about innervation, even the bowel, but the heart is so importantly governed by physiology and its innervation that we were surprised, and of course very pleasantly so. A day or two afterward we found that the dogs had normal cardiac output and would be running around the laboratory beginning to look very normal indeed.

This was also just about the time that chemical immunosuppression was starting up. The earliest drug was 6-Mercaptopurine. I think it was Dameshek and Schwartz in 1962 who found the immunosuppressive properties of azathioprine. Steroids were also beginning to be used in renal transplantation. First of all, we did not know what the homograft rejection pattern would be for heart transplants, but that was readily established after a number of experiments. Some animals would live for two or three weeks, but others would die of rejection in just a few days. Rejection was inevitable, so we needed to blunt the immunologic reaction. We found we needed to use these chemicals in a different pattern from renal transplants. A heart transplant is a bigger procedure and the preparation is so fragile and delicate that when we used the same menu of immunosuppression that others were using for kidney transplants, our animals would all die of drug toxicity. There would be no rejection, for sure, but the animals were still dead.

Lower hit upon the idea of not giving immunosuppression until there was evidence of rejection of the heart. Well now, what would that evidence be? Then he had this great idea that diminution of the R wave of the EKG would indicate that there was the threat of rejection because of the edema and hemorrhage in the wall of the myocardium. These changes would cause the R wave to diminish. So what Lower would do would be to give no immunosuppression until he saw these changes in the EKG. This would roughly be around the fourth or fifth day, maybe sometimes later on the seventh or tenth day. He would then start the immunosuppression, and as soon as the R wave came back up toward the baseline, he would back off the drugs. With this we began to have animals living for protracted periods of time. It was then that we thought that maybe this did have some ultimate clinical applications. This was worked out in the middle 1960s.

By this time Stanford had moved to its new location in Palo Alto. We would be doing cardiac cases Monday, Wednesday, and Friday and then working in the laboratory on Tuesday and Thursday. Everything we were working on in the laboratory was also being used in the operating room, so they were complementary. We were cooling the heart with topical hypothermia, which made our surgery results very, very good. This was ideal protection for both congenital and valvular patients. It was a great time.

With the exception of Alexis Carrel, I think that Dick Lower was probably the greatest experimental surgeon that I have ever known about. I will tell you what else he did during that time. Using the same method of cooling the heart, he did the first of what is now called the Ross procedure, where he would transplant the pulmonary valve into the aortic position. He would take the pulmonary valve, along with some of the pulmonary artery and some right ventricular tissue, and would use that to replace the mitral valve or the aortic valve, either one. Then we would restore the right ventricular outflow tract with just a segment of homograft aorta, a conduit without a valve. The theory was that you did not really need a pulmonary valve. The replacement of the valve worked fine in the aortic or mitral position, but we found before long that you do need a pulmonary valve. It was not until homograft valves became available commercially that the Ross operation became a useful clinical procedure. Unless you have had some experience with cardiac operations on dogs you just cannot understand how difficult this operation can be. Lower could do this with 90 percent success. That is why David Hume recruited Lower, and he left in 1965 to become the chief of cardiac surgery at the Medical College of Virginia in Richmond. Of course, it was there that he encountered Christiaan Barnard, who was there looking into the techniques of kidney transplantation, of which David Hume was one of the leaders. During the summer of 1967 while he was there, Barnard would go down to the laboratory and see Lower doing these heart transplants with the same facility and success that he had had at Stanford. Barnard had one of his technicians with him on this trip, and the technician told Lower, "You know Barnard is going to go home and do that operation." Lower just shrugged it off as ridiculous, but of course, lo and behold, four months later in December of 1967, he did do the first human-to-human heart transplant, so it was pretty funny.

I knew Barnard slightly when he and I were residents in Minnesota. He worked mostly with Wangensteen on abdominal surgery, but later on, after I had finished, he saw that heart surgery was the wave of the future. He abandoned the general surgery research that he was doing, went over to work with Lillehei, and was Lillehei's chief resident for at least six months. When he went back to South Africa, Wangensteen gave Barnard $10,000 to buy a heart-lung machine so that they could start open-heart surgery at the Groote Schuur Hospital in Cape Town. He had substantial backing, and it worked out great. It is probable that Barnard never really got back into cardiac surgery on a full-time basis after those first few transplants, since, I think, he was consumed by the celebrity of the situation. In many ways it is too bad because he was a very capable and innovative cardiac surgeon. He had so many other interests by then that he did not particularly pursue it. I think his contribution was awakening the neurosurgical community to the concept of brain death, and, I think, if we want to give him some kind of credit, we can say in that sense he was a true pioneer.

In 1967 we were ready to begin a clinical trial. One of the main problems was the interpretation of brain death of the donor, and this was a difficult problem. As a matter of fact, when we did our first patient about a month later, our first donor came not from our academic neurosurgery department but from a private neurosurgeon in town, and it was through his auspices that we were able to get started. The donor was a relatively young woman with a ruptured cerebral aneurysm who had become brain-dead. Our own neurosurgeons were very slow to come to grips with the brain-death situation. For a long time, death was declared only when the heart stopped, which I used to call the Boy Scout definition of death. The neurosurgeons would come by in the morning, and if a patient was brain-dead they would remove the ventilator and then continue their rounds. They would come back a half-hour later when the heart had stopped, and they would then say that the patient was now dead. This tradition, or whatever you want to call it, was very slow to change. In fact, in the state of California it was not until 1973 that we had a state law that recognized brain death. For the first five years, we were technically in violation of state law as far as donor utilization was concerned.

A heart transplant is obviously a pretty simple surgical technique, so some surgeons were attracted to the publicity and personal aggrandizement. Soon transplants were being done in India and places where you would not want to have any kind of a heart operation. Houston, of course, jumped in with both feet as soon as possible. Then all those programs were discontinued because the results were so poor. During the 1970s, with the exception of Dick Lower's program, we were pretty much alone with a continuous program of clinical heart transplantation. In Europe, Terrance English began a program at Papworth Hospital near Cambridge in 1977, and Chris Cabrol started up in Paris. Both of them were very good friends of mine, we all worked together, and we helped them as much as we could; these programs continue today. The Houston programs both folded completely and did not begin again until we started using cyclosporine in 1980. The results were immediately so much better—we went from something like a 40 percent five-year survival before cyclosporine to 75 percent survival after cyclosporine.

No one had any concept of the amount of media interest that heart transplantation would create. It was, in many ways, a blessing that the focus was on Barnard, because it allowed us to continue our work without so much folderol. That was truly an important thing for us, because there were still many more things that had to be done, such as the percutaneous endomyocardial biopsy.

We used the EKG as our only method of interpreting rejection until 1971. We were pretty good at it, as we had had a lot of practice in the laboratory, but then we used endomyocardial biopsy. We had another wonderful visitor from the U.K., Philip Caves, a British-American Heart Association fellow who was working at the Brompton Hospital in London. Matt Paneth, who was a surgeon and an old friend of mine from Minnesota days, wrote that he had this very bright young man who wanted to come out and spend some time at Stanford. Caves came out and was absolutely brilliant: a hardworking, dedicated, highly motivated guy and just a wonderful doctor. For the first three or four weeks he was at Stanford, he stayed in a little cubicle in the library and we did not see him for a while; he was there all of the time. I kept thinking this guy is supposed to be so good, but I do not see anything along those lines. It then turned out that he had looked up this early work of Konno from Japan. They had a bioptome that could be introduced from the sapheno-femoral region into the right ventricle and could take a snippet of the heart. It was not developed to any extent but they did publish their method. Philip Caves and a little old German instrument maker crafted a bioptome with the handle of a forceps and some piano wire. This could be introduced into the external jugular of the dog and directed into the right ventricle. In patients, they used the internal jugular. He was able to take little pieces of the right ventricle that we could look at and determine the immunologic health of the transplant. This was a tremendous advance and was done entirely by Philip Caves and the pathologist Margaret Billingham, who is now world famous for her interpretation of cardiac biopsy material. They developed and perfected the technique, and it, of course, greatly helped survival. In 1971 we had a 20 percent five-year survival. By using the bioptome and myocardial biopsy, this moved up to around a 40 percent five-year survival.

Our principal drugs at that time were Imuran and steroids. We also did have rabbit antithymocyte globulin, made for us by Philip Oyer, who was, by that time, one of our staff members. He was an MD with a PhD in biochemistry, so he had the knowledge to make our own antithymocyte globulin, which was anything but standardized. We never thought splenectomy or thoracic duct drainage would be useful. We relied entirely on immunosuppression and it worked.

The donors at that time had to be in the hospital, so it was always difficult. We had a lot of problems also because the coroner for our county, Santa Clara County, did not subscribe to the concept of brain death. That was prior to 1978. The coroner and our hospital administrator had the agreement that, certainly, no murder cases would be used for donor purposes. One day I got a call from the district attorney in Oakland who had an individual with a gunshot wound of the head who was brain dead. His family wanted him utilized as a heart donor. It would have been impossible for us to do what we usually did, which was to bring the whole body over to our hospital, because of the local coroner's agreement with our administrator. So I said, "Well, I will tell you what we would like to do. We will remove the heart over in Oakland at the Highland Hospital and we will get a helicopter to fly us the fifty miles back to Palo Alto." We went over there that day and Buck Sampson, who was one of the leading older thoracic surgeons in California, was working in the operating room. I remember going into the surgeon's dressing room and he said, "Now what are you doing over here,

Shumway?" Well, I told him we were going to take the heart out of this donor and take it back to Palo Alto for a transplant operation. Of course, he thought the idea was quite mad. We flew it back and Randy Griepp, who was another one of our really excellent young men, implanted it. This was the first time that a heart had been removed from a remote location and used for a transplant. Although we had not planned to do this, I knew that there was experimental evidence that this should work. Lower had shown in dogs that he could remove the heart in the middle of the night from a donor and put it in cold solution in the refrigerator and then come in the next morning early and do the transplant. He found that if he did this within seven hours or less he would get uniform survival, but beyond seven hours the hearts were not really good enough to function immediately. So we felt that we could easily do this from Oakland. We gradually moved farther and farther away. The ischemic time was about two hours for that first remote retrieval.

Later we had a very long retrieval that involved a snowstorm in North Dakota. Vaughn Starnes was involved in that case; he was the chief resident at the time. We had chartered a Lear jet for the purpose of taking the retrieval team to Fargo, North Dakota. Ed Stinson went along because we thought we needed somebody who could evaluate the heart to be sure it was sufficiently strong, as we knew there would be a long period of anoxia. This was just before Christmas in 1986. I think there were four of them: Ed, the organ procurement nurse, the anesthesiologist, and the operating-room nurse. They left in their scrub suits and white coats, flew to Fargo where they removed a heart from a five-month-old donor and put it in the cold solution. They got ready to come back, but the engines of the Lear jet would not start; they tried everything. So somebody suggested that there was an Air National Guard in Fargo, so why not get a military jet to bring the heart back. Stinson talked to the colonel there who was in charge, and he said, "Well, we cannot do that. Our mission is to protect the United States against a sneak attack by the Russians over the pole, so we must keep all of our planes here." Well, that sounded a little far-fetched so Stinson called the governor of the state, a man by the name of George Sinner. He was up for reelection the next year and thought that this would be positive PR. So he instructed the colonel to let us have a F4 Phantom to bring the heart back to Palo Alto. The F4 Phantom is a two-seat plane, and only those two positions are climate- and pressure-controlled. The navigator was asked to hold the Igloo container with the heart in his lap in the seat behind the pilot. He said he did not want to do that because if they should have to eject, the Igloo container could create a serious injury for him. What they had to do was strap the container in the seat behind the pilot. The pilot then flew alone. The Phantom has a range of only one thousand miles, so he had to stop in Utah to refuel before continuing to Palo Alto. It finally got there and Vaughn Starnes put it in. The baby did amazingly well. He was six months old and, later on, had a lymphoproliferative disease which was not malignant but was very incapacitating. We had to gradually withdraw immunosuppression. He is now more than ten years old and is off all immunosuppression—the only patient in our whole series off immunosuppression. The total retrieval time was eight hours, which certainly validates the protective effect of local cooling of the heart.

Cyclosporine became available to us in December of 1980. This is an interesting story. The scientist working with Sandoz investigating cyclosporine was Jean Borel. He noted the immunosuppressive properties but found it was not useful for chemotherapy. Sandoz decided to abandon the drug, as they did not think it would have any commercial use, but a pathologist at Cambridge, David White, saw an article by Borel describing its immunosuppressive property. He was working at Cambridge with Roy Calne, who was their kidney and liver transplant man. White called Borel and told him he would like to try some of it in animal transplants. Borel said, "We are not making that drug anymore, but let me look around the lab and see if we have any left. If we do, I will send it over to you." Well, he did have a little bit, so he sent it to David White and Roy Calne, and, sure enough, they began to do renal transplants with success that they had never previously achieved, simply by using cyclosporine. When this news got back to Borel, Sandoz began to make cyclosporine again, and by the mid-1970s it had been introduced into clinical renal transplantation.

Borel was Swiss and, like most Swiss, he loved skiing. There was a meeting in Davos, Switzerland, on something to do with cardiac surgery. I was unable to go, but I told Phil Oyer if he would like to go skiing, we would send him to the meeting to see what it was all about, as there were some papers that he might find of interest. He met Borel on the ski slopes, they struck up a friendship, and largely on the basis of their interaction, we were given cylcosporine to use in our experiments. This began in the late 1970s. We started in the lab trying to find out what the dose would be for cardiac transplant. We knew it would be different from renal transplant because of our previous experience with Imuran. We finally got it worked out in December 1980, and the FDA permitted us to use it in clinical heart transplants. The positive results were immediate and we began to have 80 to 90 percent one-year survival. This, of course, led to all of the other heart transplant programs coming back to life. Prior to cylcosporine we had most of the donors and we were in great shape as far as donor material was concerned, but that very rapidly changed.

Prior to cyclosporine we were trying to do one transplant each month, because we wanted to get more and more experience from each case, rather than to do five or six in two or three days and then have them all die, which unfortunately had happened in other centers. We would try to gain experience from one case to the next. With cyclosporine we began to increase our activity, and the results were very remarkable. It was an improvement of such magnitude that I think we will never see again.

Cyclosporine comes from a fungus found in Norway in 1969, and FK506—with a similar type of immunosuppressive molecule—was found in the soil at the base of Mt. Fuji. Another drug, rapamycin, being introduced clinically by Sandoz, was found on the island of Rapa Nui, also known as Easter Island. All three of these very strong immunosuppressive molecules come from natural material. Cyclosporine made it possible for us to do heart-lung transplants. What had made these difficult was the postop breakdown of the tracheal or bronchial anastomosis because of the necessity of using high levels of steroids. Only three had been attempted, one by Barnard, one by Lillehei, and one by Cooley, and all had failed. We felt, now that we had cyclosporine, we could go ahead, and this work was started in the laboratory by Bruce Reitz in 1978. Lower and I had tried dogs in 1961, but dogs are very sensitive to pulmonary denervation. They develop a very slow Kussmaul-type of ventilation.

Aldo Casteneda and Watts Webb had found that you could denervate the lungs in monkeys and still have a normal respiratory pattern, so our dog lab became a monkey lab, and with the use of cyclosporine, Bruce Reitz was able to get long-term survival of monkeys after heart-lung transplantation. Bruce presented his animal results at a meeting of the AATS in San Francisco, and a woman journalist from Arizona, who had severe pulmonary hypertension, had read about this work in the newspapers. She was forty-five years old, on oxygen, in a wheelchair, and was terribly debilitated, but a very feisty individual. We told her we were very interested in her as a patient, but the FDA had not approved cyclosporine for use in heart-lung transplantation. She thought this was ridiculous and, of course, it was. Somehow she got hold of her senator, maybe it was Barry Goldwater, and within forty-eight hours cyclosporine was made available for her case. She had one episode of rejection, which was treated successfully, and she did quite well for five years. She fell at home and was hospitalized and died of an iatrogenic accident. During the insertion of a Swan-Ganz catheter, the superior vena cava was perforated, and she died as a result of this misadventure. Her heart and lungs were surprisingly normal.

Mechanical hearts are still a difficult problem. We have been working on them for over twenty-five years and have used the Novacor as a bridge to temporarily support patients until a donor became available. In a way, this intensifies the donor shortage, because these patients then go to the top of the list and are the highest risk. We hoped that the Novacor would become a permanent implant. It has been an electromechanical device right from the beginning, so it was never driven by pneumatic hoses and a refrigerator-sized console. We thought that it might have a future application as a stand-alone operation and that it would not necessarily be used only as a bridge to transplant. Baxter decided to buy it, and they have provided a lot of research money so we can continue. At present, a wire comes through the skin to a battery arrangement outside the body. Eventually there will be a subcutaneous coil, as it is possible to transmit enough energy through the intact skin to drive the device. These experiments are being done on sheep now, and so far they have been reasonably successful, although I think it will be some time before we reach clinical use. As you know, there are other problems too. We do not have a perfect heart valve, and clot formation is still a problem. I would hate to say that it will never happen, because I remember the early pacemakers. They were huge devices, and the first ones had wires coming through the chest wall. Maybe it will come about, probably not in the next decade, but as time goes by, it might.

The gene-altered xenograft is another interesting area. David White in Cambridge, to whom I referred earlier, is one of the leaders in genetically altered pigs. One of the young surgeons at Maryland, Robin Pierson, worked with us at Cambridge. At the time I saw him, he was simply perfusing these genetically altered pig hearts with human blood and getting a longer survival. Up to now, they have transplanted orthopically pig hearts into baboons or monkeys, and they have survived for a couple of weeks. They have been able to get away from hyperactive rejection, but the rejection that occurs thereafter is still of a severity that requires heavy immunosuppression. The toxic effects of that immunosuppression have prevented any real long-term survival. Whether this will eventually succeed, I do not know. It certainly is very difficult. I put the new genetic engineering programs and the artificial heart in a neck-to-neck race to see which will be useful in the future.

I have a slide that talks about the future, a quote of Linus Pauling. I attended some of his lectures, and, as you know, he was a two-time winner of the Nobel Prize. He should have had a third one for the double helix as well, because he had all of that laid out before Watson and Crick. He has this quote, which I think is wonderful, "I do not care to comment on the future of anything."

Bibliography

Lower RR, Stofer RC, Shumway NE. Homovital Transplantation of the Heart. *J Thorac Cardiovasc Surg.* 1961; 41:196–204.

Caves PK, Stinson EB, Billingham M, Shumway NE. Percutaneous Transvenous Endomyocardial Biopsy in Human Heart Recipients. Experience with a New Technique. *Ann Thorac Surg.* 1973; 16:325–336.

Griepp RB, Stinson EB, Shumway NE. Profound Local Hypothermia for Myocardial Protection during Open-Heart Surgery. *J Thorac Cardiovasc Surg.* 1973; 66:731–741.

Moreno-Cabral RJ, Shumway NE. Double-Patch Technique for Correction of Complete Atrioventricular Canal. *Ann Thorac Surg.* 1982; 33:88–91.

Reitz BA, Wallwork JL, Hunt SA, Pennock JL, Billingham ME, Oyer PE, Stinson EB, Shumway NE. Heart-Lung Transplantation: Successful Therapy for Patients with Pulmonary Vascular Disease. *N Engl J Med.* 1982; 306:557–564.

Haverich A, Miller DC, Scott WC, Mitchell RS, Oyer PE, Stinson EB, Shumway NE. Acute and Chronic Aortic Dissection—Determinants of Long-term Outcome for Operative Survivors. *Circulation.* 1985; 72:II22–34.

Grattan MT, Moreno-Cabral CE, Starnes VA, Oyer PE, Stinson EB, Shumway NE. Eight-Year Results of Cyclosporine-Treated Patients with Cardiac Transplants. *J Thorac Cardiovasc Surg.* 1990; 99:500–509.

Starnes VA, Griffin ML, Pitlick PT, Bernstein D, Baum D, Ivens K, Shumway NE. Current Approach to Hypoplastic Left Heart Syndrome. Palliation, Transplantation, or Both? *J Thorac Cardiovasc Surg.* 1992; 104:189–194.

Shunway SJ, Shumway NE (Editors). *Thoracic Transplantation.* Cambridge, MA: Blackwell Science; 1995.

Robbins RC, Barlow, CW, Oyer PE, Hunt SA, Miller JL, Reitz BA, Stinson EB, Shumway NE. Thirty Years of Cardiac Transplantation at Stanford University. *J Thorac Cardiovasc Surg.* 1999 May; 117:939–951.

Christiaan Barnard, MD, PhD

(b. 1922)

> *During my stay in Richmond, I heard that Dr. Richard Lower was doing heart transplants on dogs, and I went to the experimental lab to watch him do a cardiac transplant on a dog.*
>
> — On how he became interested in cardiac transplantation

Teleconference on September 15, 2000*

I am often asked, "What are the ingredients for success?" My reply is that I think there are four. They are opportunity, imagination, ability, and the last one is luck. I have been fortunate to have a little bit of each, but I have been especially lucky in that I have had many opportunities, and I have had a lot of luck. Let me explain to you what I mean by this. Let's take opportunity. Often when young surgeons from Europe or some other country are trained in the United States and they go back home, the head of the department finds it very difficult to give them opportunities to explore what they have learned and what they can do. Usually the head of the department wants to be the one to do the heart surgery. I have seen this happen in many parts of Europe and it has really retarded programs of heart surgery, this attitude of the head of the department. I was fortunate that my head was Professor Louw, and when I returned from Minneapolis in 1958 I said to him, "Professor Louw, we can do the heart surgery together," and he said, "No, no, I am not going to do it. You have been trained to do heart surgery; you go ahead." He gave me all the opportunities to explore certain aspects of heart surgery in the laboratory, and then when I thought I was ready, he approved our clinical program, so I have had ample opportunities to do what I had learned in Minneapolis in Dr. Wangensteen's department.

As far as luck is concerned, my whole career has been guided by unexplained and unexpected events. I will give you a few examples. I was studying general surgery at the University of Cape Town in 1957. I came back from lunch and I bumped into Professor John Brock in the parking lot. He said to me, "I have just come back from Minneapolis. I met Professor Wangensteen and he was very impressed by the training of South African doctors." He was referring to Alan Thal. He told me that Professor Wangensteen said that he would like to have another South African surgeon in his training program, and he asked me if I would like to go to Minneapolis and train there. I didn't even know where Minneapolis was, since I knew so very little about the United States, but I went home that night and talked with my wife, Louwtjie, and we decided we would go. It was so fortunate that I went there because, as you know, it was one of the first centers in the world where open-heart surgery was developed. At first, after I arrived in Minnesota, I was doing general surgery, working in the laboratory on intestinal atresia. One day I walked past an open door and saw some-

* Reprinted from a talk given by Dr. Barnard at Foxwood, Connecticut, on September 15, 2000. Used with the permission of John A. Elefteriades, MD, and the Yale University School of Medicine.

body working at the operating table. It was Vince Gott. He looked up and asked, "Have you something else to do right now?" I said, "No." He asked that I scrub and give him a hand. I scrubbed immediately and helped him as best I could. He was working with the heart-lung machine, using a bubble oxygenator, and for the first time I saw what extracorporeal circulation could do. One could exclude the heart and the lungs from the circulation and work inside the heart. I was immediately fascinated by this and decided that this was the direction that I would like to take. I went to see Professor Wangensteen and told him that I wanted to give up my work in general surgery and change over to cardiac surgery. He was not very happy with this but eventually allowed me to change. I was very fortunate to work with Dr. C. Walton Lillehei and his associates for the next few months, and also to learn how to run the heart-lung machine.

Eventually I was one of the senior residents, and I was able to participate in a number of heart operations. During that period, I completed my work on my PhD degree, with a thesis on intestinal atresia. At the same time, I worked on a master's degree in surgery, and the thesis was the aortic valve. I was fortunate to get an NIH grant to support my aortic valve work. When I decided to leave Minneapolis at the beginning of 1958, Dr. Wangensteen was so kind. He got enough money for me to buy a heart-lung machine to take home with me, so I was immediately ready to start a program of open-heart surgery in South Africa.

I think cardiac transplantation became a technical reality because of two discoveries, one at the beginning of the twentieth century, and the second in the middle of the twentieth century. The first was when Alexis Carrel showed that vascular tissues could be safely joined by just carefully suturing them end-to-end. The other was the development of the pump-oxygenator, which made it possible for the surgeon to exclude the heart and lungs from the circulation, and to remove the heart. The introduction of extracorporeal circulation brought about many advances in congenital and acquired heart disease. It also brought new surgical techniques and new complications. Cardiac transplantation was the same. It was the introduction of a new surgical technique and dealing with the problems inherent in that new technique. The first problem was the use of a human donor for the heart, and the second was the problem of rejection, especially the diagnosis

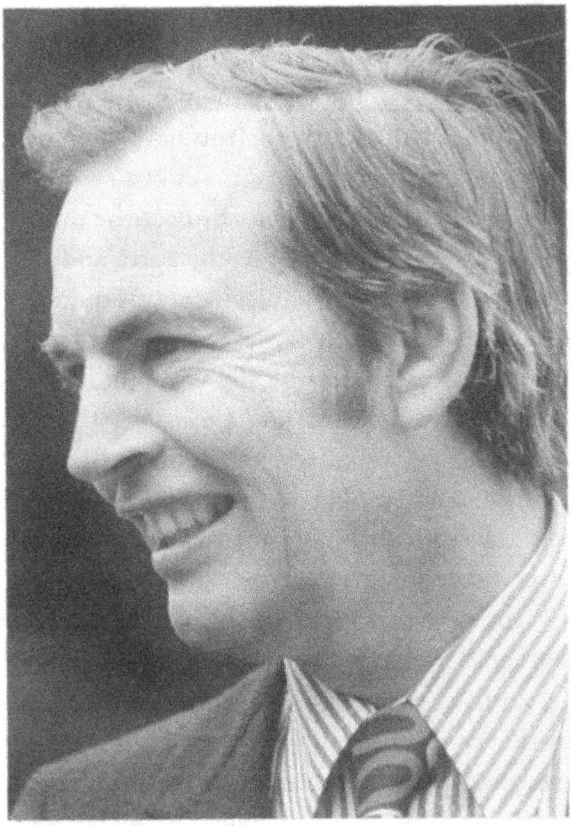

Christiaan Barnard

and treatment of it. As far as the operation was concerned, this was easy, because we could learn it in the experimental laboratory, and it is not that difficult. You have to join the pulmonary and systemic venous systems to the new heart and then connect the output of the two ventricles to the aorta and pulmonary artery. Technically, it was quite easy. We studied it in the laboratory until we were satisfied that technically we could do an orthotopic transplant, and I must say that in my career in cardiac transplantation, I have never had a complication with the technique itself, and we never lost a patient due to an error in technique.

The next thing was, of course, the use of a human donor and the problems of rejection. In cardiac transplantation, we were fortunate in that others were already doing kidney and liver transplants, and many of the problems are similar. In 1967 I managed to get a position in Richmond, Virginia, with the late Dr. David Hume. He was very kind to me, gave me a position to study kidney transplantation for a few months, and actually also gave me a very good salary. I learned about the use of human donors for the procurement of a vital organ, and also about the problems of rejection and its management. In our first cardiac transplant, we used the same immunosuppressive regimen that Dr. Hume used for kidneys. During my stay in Richmond, Dr. Richard Lower was doing heart transplants on dogs, and I went to the experimental lab to watch him. I spent about half an hour with him, and I had never seen any other cardiac transplant procedure done. I had never seen Dr. Shumway work, and I had never worked with him, not even as a fellow resident at Minnesota. The only experience in cardiac transplantation that I had outside of South Africa was the half hour that I spent with Richard Lower. During that same time, I visited Tom Starzl in Denver, who was also very kind. In those days, he was working with antilymphocyte serum, and I spent a few days with him observing its production, in case we wanted to use it in South Africa. I then returned to South Africa and prepared a transplant team. We did a kidney transplant, the first in South Africa, and it gave the team the opportunity to explore the moral and legal problems related to a human donor. We were very fortunate in South Africa in that the law was quite modern. A patient could be considered as a donor for a heart, kidney, or liver if two doctors pronounced that patient dead. One doctor had to be qualified for more than five years, and the two doctors were not to be part of the transplant team. We could use the diagnosis of brain death as the moment of death for a donor, and this was a necessary concept, brain death.

The first kidney transplant patient did very well, living twenty-three years with that kidney, so I have always said I had the best result with kidney transplantation of anyone in the world. I have a 100 percent twenty-three-year survival rate.

The next problem that confronted us was which patient we should select as the recipient for the first transplant. I spoke to other doctors in this field, and they said they thought they would only do a transplant on a patient who could not be weaned from the heart-lung machine after a heart operation. With an available donor, they would do a transplant, but we realized that this set of circumstances would be very unlikely. How often would you have a suitable donor at the same time that you could not wean a patient from the heart-lung machine? That situation is not planned ahead of time, and it rarely happens that the heart is damaged so much that you can't stop the pump support. I discussed this with our cardiologist, Professor Schrire. We reviewed the problems of selecting a recipient patient and decided to use the following criteria. First, the patient must have extensive irreversible destruction of the heart muscle. Second, he must be in total heart failure, no longer responding to medical treatment. Lastly, his situation must not be amenable to an already practiced surgical procedure. The first patient, as you know, was Mr. Washkansky, who was fifty-three years old and who had extensive heart damage from multiple attacks. He was diabetic and needed Southey's tubes to drain the edema from his legs. Now, I don't know how many people today know that Southey's tubes were sterile metal tubes introduced subcutaneously in the lower legs. The patient sat up with his feet in a bucket, and the edema fluid would drain out through the tubes into the bucket. He had been treated in that way, and unfortunately had had cellulitis of the wounds in his legs, from which we cultured both pseudomonas and klebsiella. I think we made a mistake in not treating him more vigorously with antibiotics before we did the transplant, as you will see later.

We all thought he would benefit from a heart transplant, so he was chosen as the first patient. We waited for a donor, and actually got one in November, three weeks before we did the transplant, but he was a black donor and both Professor Schrire and I decided that for the first transplant we would not use a black patient or a black donor. This was not because of the political climate in South Africa, but because of the fact that some might say we were experimenting on black people. We waited three weeks (December 3, 1967) for a white donor, a young girl knocked down by an automobile while she was crossing the street. Her mother was killed also. The girl sustained very severe brain damage and was eventually declared brain-dead by the neurosurgeons. We decided to put the donor on bypass with the heart-lung machine, and cool her heart down before removing it. We also decided not to begin the operation on the donor until the heart had stopped beating, because we were concerned about criticism if we took a beating heart. Once we had the recipient and donor in adjacent operating rooms, we opened the recipient's chest and prepared to start cardiopulmonary bypass. When all of this was ready, I then walked across to the donor's room, disconnected the respirator, and waited until the donor went into ventricular fibrillation. Only then did I ask my assistant surgeons to open the chest and remove the heart. In the meantime, we put Mr. Washkansky on cardiopulmonary bypass and at that time we nearly had a catastrophic event.

I had decided to cannulate the femoral artery, since we wanted the aorta clear for the anastomosis there. When we started on bypass, we always monitored the pressure in the arterial line, and the pump technician told me that the pressure was very high. I assumed there must be some obstruction in the pelvic vessels and that we would have to change the arterial site to the aorta. I clamped the arterial line before I told the heart-lung technician to switch off the pump. The arterial line pressure shot up and blew the arterial line off the connector, and now we had air in the arterial line. To correct the situation, I connected the arterial line to the venous line, and ran the arterial blood through the heart-lung machine, clearing it of air and bubbles. We cannulated the aorta and started bypass again, and the patient suffered no damage because his heart was still beating.

The operation went quite smoothly. The only part that I can remember is when I removed the patient's heart, and for the first time in my life I saw a living patient with a totally empty pericardium. There were only the back walls of the left and right atria, and the distal aorta and pulmonary artery. I realized that this was really the point of no return. They brought the heart across, cooled down by extracorporeal circulation, and we perfused the coronary circulation throughout the rest of the operation through the aortic stump left for the anastomosis. We only stopped the coronary perfusion long enough to do the aortic anastomosis. When the technical side of the operation was completed, we rewarmed the heart. It did not start in a sinus rhythm, but we defibrillated it, and it contracted very well. We rewarmed it further and then the time came to stop the support of the heart-lung machine. The first time we came off bypass, the heart failed; the blood pressure went down and the venous pressure went up. We went back on bypass, and again when we turned it off, the heart failed. I was in serious doubt as to whether this was going to be a successful operation, but, thank God, the third time we stopped the heart-lung machine, the heart took over. It was like music in my ears when the anesthesiologist called out the arterial pressure saying it was now fifty, then fifty-five, sixty, sixty-five, seventy, and eighty. We realized that technically this operation was successful, and the rest of it went quite smoothly.

I would like to point out that we did not take any pictures of the operation. We did not invite the press to the hospital. In fact, I didn't even tell the head of the hospital that I was going to do a transplant. When I called him after the operation and told him that I had done a heart transplant, he was quite annoyed that I woke him so early in the morning, because he thought I was referring to a dog. I said, "No, it was a human." I drove home and then, of course, it all started. The media heard about this operation, and we had reporters arriving from all over the world. As far as our patient was concerned, the one thing that we learned from this operation was how well a patient that is in total heart failure will do when you give him or her a new heart. The heart failure disappeared very rapidly over three days, and there was no evidence of pulmonary edema anymore. The severe swelling of the legs went down, and he passed lots and lots of urine. At first, he was doing extremely well, and we realized that heart transplantation, done successfully, would give the patient a very good quality of life. Subsequent experience with heart transplantation told us that assumption was correct.

Unfortunately, on the ninth day, Mr. Washkansky developed some chest pain. We took X-rays and there were shadows in the lung. I made a very bad mistake by saying that the shadows were evidence of rejection. Dr. Young believed that one could get "transplant lung" and the lung changes on X-ray could be evidence of rejection. I was wrong. It was an infection, and I made a mistake by increasing the immunosuppression drugs. I should have decreased immunosuppression drugs. Eighteen days after surgery, he died of a pseudomonas and klebsiella infection of the lung. The same organisms that we grew from the wounds in the legs eventually spread to his lungs and caused his death. At autopsy, we were very fortunate to see that the heart was in good condition, and there was very little evidence of rejection. Although the patient died, we were not totally disappointed by the operation. We realized that we could do it successfully, and, on the second of January 1968, I did a second transplant, on a dentist, Philip Blaiberg. He was the first patient to leave the hospital with a transplanted heart, and showed the world that such a patient could live a successful and good life afterwards. It was an extremely important operation, because if we had failed with Dr. Blaiberg, I think that transplantation would have ceased for a while, certainly in our hospital. Dr. Blaiberg lived eighteen months before dying of accelerated arteriosclerosis and severe chronic rejection. We continued our work on transplantation, and in the first group of patients that we did, we had a 50 percent one-year survival—the third one lived for twelve years and the seventh one lived for twenty-three years—so not only did this improve the quality of life, but it also prolonged life.

Because of the problem of acute rejection, I changed to a different technique, heterotopic cardiac transplantation. With this method, the recipient's heart is not removed and the donor heart is connected in a piggyback configuration. In theory, if the donor heart fails, the native heart would still be functional. However, immunosuppression improved, and the technique of heterotopic cardiac transplantation never became very useful or popular.

Bibliography

Barnard CN, Schrire V. The Surgical Treatment of the Tetralogy of Fallot. *Thorax.* 1961; 16:346–355.

Barnard CN, Schrire V, Goosen CC. Total Aortic Valve Replacement. *Lancet.* 1963; 2:856–859.

Bosman SC, Terblanche J, Saunders SJ, Harrison GG, Barnard CN. Cross-Circulation between Man and Baboon in Hepatic Coma. *Lancet.* 1968; 2:583–589.

Barnard CN. The Operation: A Human Heart Transplant: An Interim Report of a Successful Operation Performed at Groote Schuur Hospital Capetown, 1967. *So Afr Med J.* 1967; 41:1271–1274.

Barnard CN. What We Have Learned about Heart Transplants. *J Thorac Cardiovasc Surg.* 1968; 56:457–468.

Barnard CN. Human Heart Transplantation. The Diagnosis of Rejection. *Am J Cardiol.* 1968; 22:811–819.

Barnard CN. Medicine and the Mass Media. *Am J Cardiol.* 1972; 30:579–580.

Barnard CN. Advice on Heart Transplants. *Br Med J.* 1973; 2:363.

Barnard CN, Losman JG, Curcio CA, Sanchez HE, Wolpowitz A, Barnard MS. The Advantage of Heterotopic Cardiac Transplantation over Orthotopic Cardiac Transplantation in the Management of Severe Acute Rejection. *J Thorac Cardiovasc Surg.* 1977; 74:918–924.

Lanza RP, Cooper DK, Barnard CN. Effect of ABO Blood-Group Antigens on Long-term Survival after Cardiac Transplantation. *N Engl J Med.* 1982; 307:1275–1276.

Barnard CN, Cooper DK. Heterotopic versus Orthotopic Heart Transplantation. *Transplant Proc.* 1984; 16:886–892.

James D. Hardy, MD

(b. 1918)

We worried most about the ethical questions, of course, because obviously after all of those years, I didn't want to look like a screwball that was willing to do anything, although I'm sure that most people thought I was.

— On the heart transplant operation using a chimpanzee heart

Interviewed August 10, 1999

I was born in 1918 in Birmingham, Alabama, but I grew up in a little town called Newala, Alabama. My father actually named the town when he went there. He named it "New" for New York (his hometown) and "ala" for Alabama. So it was Newala. My father manufactured lime calcium oxide, using the very pure strain of limestone that ran through Shelby County. Newala was close to Montebello, about thirty miles south of Birmingham. My mother happened to deliver me in Birmingham because our family physician decided she was too large to have a normal delivery, and, to the surprise of all, she had twins; I was named James and my twin was Julian. Before she married, my mother's name was Julia Ann Pointer, and she taught Latin at a college in Montebello, where my father met her. There were five boys and two girls in my family, but, unfortunately, only two of us remain.

The lime powder was used in construction, farming, and water purification. Construction was the main use; the lime was used to make cement. During the Depression, my father's business had some hard times. At the lowest point, our enterprise was advertised in the county newspaper for nonpayment of taxes, but as children we didn't really know how bad things were. I have always admired my father enormously for the fact that he didn't believe in having his children worry. He didn't mention his financial problems and never complained, but spending money was extremely limited. That experience convinced all of us boys that we didn't want to be in the lime business when the Depression was over. I was considering farming.

I played tennis with some older friends (they beat me consistently, of course) who were premed students at the University of Alabama. They urged Julian and me to take premed, and, since we had nothing else in mind, we took their advice, but then they dropped out of premed. One of them became a physicist and the other was a full colonel in the army after World War II. Julian and I went on and finished in medicine. He practiced ob-gyn in Birmingham, and I went elsewhere.

I was interested in music and had a dance band. There had always been music in the family; my mother came from a family where the girls were all expected to learn to play the piano, to sew somewhat, and to cook somewhat. She played the piano most days and played at church if necessary. The one thing we did have at our high school was music. Ms. Selinsky came from Chicago; she was of Polish extraction, and she could play several of the instruments in the little band in our junior high school. I played the clarinet at first, but when a dance orchestra was organized, I changed instruments, because I saw a chance to make a little money. My younger brother Taylor played trumpet in the band, and my twin Julian played the saxophone. I went to Birmingham and bought a trombone for $20 in a pawnshop. I learned to play the trombone with Mother striking the notes on the piano.

The University of Alabama was a land-grant college, so every able-bodied male had to take military training or physical education. Of course, the ones who took physical education were sort of looked down on, so almost everybody, including myself, took the military. One day I was out there with a rifle, and the army captain who was drilling our company said he had an announcement to make. He asked if anybody wanted to swap his rifle for a musical instrument, because they needed instruments in the band. He said it very sarcastically, as if to say, "Who would stoop so low?" but I held up my hand. I was thoroughly familiar with weapons, as we grew up with them, and I didn't need any further instruction. I volunteered to play the trombone, and I played it right on through college. When I was in medical school, actually in my internship, I saw that a trombone was not a solo instrument for close quarters in the dormitory, so I took up the piano, and I play the piano now.

We had never had a soul of any medical persuasion in our family, so when I was in premed, I didn't know where to go to medical school. I knew I wanted to go to a four-year school though, and not the two-year program at Alabama. I ate with the football players, three meals a day and seven days a week. (It was $45 for three months.) One of the men at the table was a second-year medical student on campus, and I knew him well.

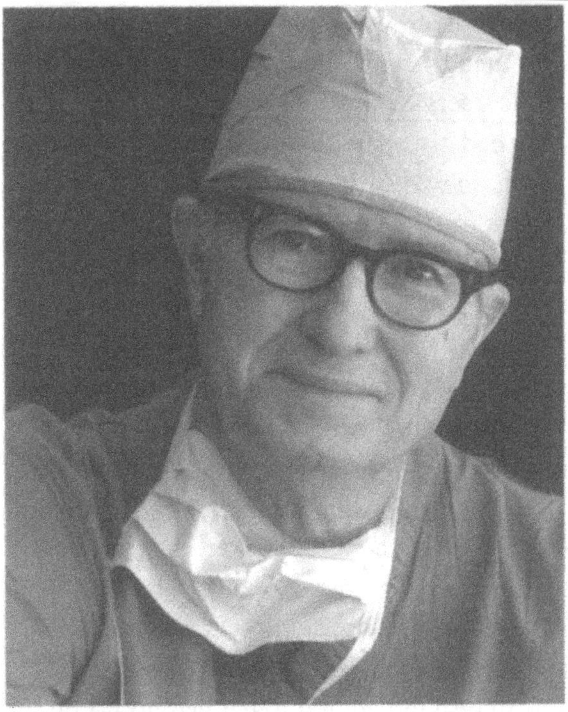

James D. Hardy

He said, "Why don't we go over and talk to James Donald? He could go anywhere. He's a superb student and he's going to the University of Pennsylvania." So I went over and talked to him. He was part of a whole clan of Donald doctors in Alabama, and he said they thought the University of Pennsylvania gave a practical blend of research and theory, along with how to treat a patient. That's why he was going there, so that's why I went there, the only place I applied. My brother Julian decided to go to the University of Alabama for two years because he was courting a young lady, but he did take the last two years at the University of Pennsylvania.

In my opinion, no physician ever forgets his year of internship, and that's the case for me. The University of Pennsylvania's Twentieth General Hospital had been sent to Siam in Northern India. All of a sudden, volunteers were needed to start their internships in April. I rotated first to the laboratory and then the emergency room, but my first clinical service was neurosurgery. In the past, they had always had at least two interns, one of whom was supposed to be a second-year intern, but I was the only one they had, and I was on my first clinical service. I tell you, it was a tough row to hoe, because the mortality was substantial in those days. They were trying to do larger and larger operations, but they were still doing it largely under local anesthesia. Endotracheal anesthesia was available, but it wasn't being used. I came very close to losing a child. I asked the pediatric intern what the dosage ought to be, and he gave me what he thought was a safe dosage. I am sure he thought it was safe, but the child was so heavily sedated that I was afraid he wouldn't come out of it. He did come out of it fine, but just the same, it was a real problem for me. I don't mean it did me in, but nonetheless it was a close shave. After that, I did fine.

I enjoyed the internship; a wonderful group of people were with me in it, fifteen from our school and five from other schools. It was a rotating internship, and mine was a full year. Some people's internships were a little less than a year; everything was accelerated because of the war.

The next year, I did internal medicine. I applied for a medical residency even though I already had a commission in the military by virtue of having gone to training camp in the summer. I thought I would surely have to go and was willing to go, but I wanted to have as much training under my belt as I could before I went. You never knew when, if ever, you were going to get back. I did get the residency in medicine, which was much sought after at the time. Of all the jobs I have ever had in my life, that medical residency job was the one that pleased me the most. I recently ran across a letter I wrote to my mother about it, and in the letter I was absolutely delighted.

The job didn't last quite a year. About March or April, a man named Robin Loeb (he wrote a textbook of medicine) was charged by the military to round up a group to go out to Chicago and do research on malaria, which was doing in more American soldiers than the Japanese were. The chairman of medicine called me up to his office and said, "Jim, you know, this is not the world's best plum, but it will keep you in touch with medicine and the laboratory while the war is on, so I advise you to take it. Loeb knows who you are." I had done some research already, so I said I would do it, but the army didn't agree. Loeb sent my name to Washington and the army said, "Look, he's been trained with the ground forces, he has a commission, and he's going with the ground forces." Three weeks later I was headed to the Carolina barracks. That's how it went. After the war, I came back and went into surgery.

By Christmas 1944 I was with the Eighty-first Field Hospital on a ship tied up in New York Harbor. We went to England, got the equipment set up, and went across the channel to Hamburg, Germany, at the end of the war. The field hospital had three units, and each one of them was equipped to take care of about a hundred patients, but if you kept the three units together, you could take at least four hundred. It was only a step below an Evac hospital. At one point, we moved Germans out of a hospital and moved our people in, but in general we were in tents, which were thirty or forty feet long, like the ones in the movie *Patton*. As for the patients, we always had some injured Americans, but we also had a lot of displaced persons who had been liberated from the work camps—Russians, Poles, even French and Italians that had been captured sometime back. About a third were injured Americans and the rest were DPs, as we called them. They had all sorts of diseases, particularly tuberculosis, with patients dying of it. They were malnourished to the extent that their immune systems were not working well, and some had typhus, typhoid, and so forth.

At the end of my military service, I went back to the University of Pennsylvania, but I asked to change to the Department of Surgery. During the war, I had decided I wanted to do surgery. I had had the feeling that if a person were really injured, I wasn't the one who could take care of him. I had done triage duty, where my job was to look over a group of patients and decide what could be done for each, send some to surgery and so forth. They had kept a job waiting for me at the University of Pennsylvania after the war, and I wrote them saying that I wanted a job in surgery, there or at some other place. I thanked them for keeping a place open for me, but I said I didn't need it unless it was in surgery. I didn't know it then, but those chiefs wrote Dr. Ravdin a very strong letter saying that he should take me, but he didn't take me for a long time. Finally, I decided to call his hand. I was at the Pentagon, only 140 miles from Philadelphia, and I told him I would be there on a certain day to get his final decision either way, because I had to know one way or another. When I went to his office, he looked across the street at the Wharton School of Finance and finally said, "When do you want to start work?" I said, "September first."

When I started the surgery residency, they gave me one year's credit for the medical residency I had done, as I had done a good bit of research and had published a number of papers, and they gave me a year for my almost three years in the army, so I had to have three more solid years of clinical surgery. After that I had two years of thoracic surgery with Julian Johnson, so I had five years of surgery training.

The residency in thoracic surgery was really more like an apprenticeship, because there wasn't enough thoracic surgery to have a formula for teaching it. I just asked the chief resident in general surgery if I could stay and get further experience in thoracic surgery. I was really the first thoracic surgical resident; although there was no formal residency, they agreed that I would work with Dr. Julian Johnson as his deputy.

You didn't leave the hospital in the daytime if you were a resident, but one day my wife wanted me to look at a piece of furniture downtown, so I went back out to our apartment. Julian Johnson (he could be a very sarcastic fellow) called me and said, "Jim, I wonder if you would favor us with your presence?" When I went back to his office, three or four blocks away, he threw a chest X-ray film on the viewbox and asked what I thought of it. I told him that somebody had a whopping big cavity. He said, "It's Charlie," meaning Charlie Curvey, who was sitting right there. I said, "You, Charlie?" He said, "Well, yes." It so happened that Dr. Johnson needed somebody to work with him because Charlie had to take PSA and streptomycin, and then have a lobectomy, but he died of tuberculosis later. I worked with Julian Johnson from 1949 to 1951 and got more exposure to thoracic surgery than I might have gotten otherwise; it worked out very well.

We treated patients with tuberculosis and carcinomas. Constrictive pericarditis and mitral valvulotomy had come in, and we also had coarctation and patent ductus, but that was about it. The tuberculosis operations were lobectomy or thoracoplasty or some combination of the two. We operated on people who had positive sputum in spite of prior treatment. We tried to sterilize them with drugs for say three months and hopefully to avoid spillover into an uncontaminated lung, and then we would do limited surgery, a small thoracoplasty. They brought the patients down from various sanitariums in the mountains of Pennsylvania. We only kept people in the hospital for a week or ten days of recovery after the procedure, because in those days people were scared of tuberculosis.

When I finished my thoracic training, I went on the staff at Penn, but I think I was number 11 on the door. If I managed to get a referral, I couldn't get my patient into the hospital because Dr. Ravdin had taken all the beds. Finally, I decided I needed to go to a place where I could operate more. I didn't have much of a practice, so I told Dr. Ravdin I wanted to move on. He didn't like that too much, but he did refer me to Mike DeBakey. Dr. DeBakey came by, lining up people for his effort in Houston. He was very honest and said he couldn't promise me a ward service. He thought he could eventually, but he didn't have it yet. I always appreciated his candor, but I didn't want to go down there and be no better off as far as doing surgery went. Then Carl Moyer said maybe I could work with him in Dallas, but I didn't think he would stay in Dallas, and he didn't—within six months he went to St. Louis. Harwell Wilson did need somebody in Memphis, and they had worlds of patients there. I told Jonathan Rhoads I was going to Memphis.

Dr. Ravdin had been a great boss, though. He would blow up sometimes, you know, but it was like a summer thunderstorm; thirty minutes later it was gone. It was fun really, working for him, one of the ablest fellows I ever worked for. He once operated on President Eisenhower. He went down to Washington very quietly, and they operated at night, and he never did say that he had operated on the president. Eisenhower had had a regional enteritis for some years, but nobody knew anything about it. He had eaten some celery and it had blocked off his intestine, so he had a small bowel obstruction. Dr. Ravdin and General Heaton, who was the surgeon general, I believe, were going to do the operation. Dr. Ravdin scrubbed with him, but he was very careful to give General Heaton the total credit and never mentioned that he was there. Others mentioned it, however, and Dr. Ravdin got a lot of criticism because he did a bypass instead of an end-to-end anastomosis, but Eisenhower did fine.

I went to work for Dr. Wilson at the University of Tennessee in Memphis. Actually, I barely saw him because he was in private practice, and he only came over to the university to dictate letters and make rounds once a day, at noon. I didn't have much contact with him, but I liked him. He was a fine fellow. The University of Tennessee never had a full-time surgeon until me, and there were only one or two in the Department of Medicine.

One of the first things I did at UT was

to ask Dr. Hyman, who was the vice chancellor, if he would put up some money for equipment and laboratory stuff. I had a bare laboratory, only a chair and a table in it. He said, "No, Hardy, we pay you to get the money." Well, I managed to get the money, a lot of money, in fact, more than I could use, so I proposed to send back some of the money. In any case, by the time I left, Dr. Hyman was strictly on my side. I think he had supported a lot of people that never produced anything, but we turned out stuff like a grist mill.

I was very busy during the three years I was at UT, publishing twenty-three papers, some of them with my friends from Pennsylvania though. I had been a Damon Runyon fellow when I was in Philadelphia; that was a research fellowship. I wrote them and asked if we could have some of their seed money, and they gave it to me. I promptly got the laboratory organized, and we moved right along.

We did research mainly on fluid balance and burns, basically to do with body composition. When I was in residency in Philadelphia, I worked very hard to set up the measurement of total body water with deuterium oxide—heavy water. That was the most exacting thing. You had to get the equipment fixed so that you could measure three parts per million. It took me a long time, but when I finally got it going, there was no place else that had it. Francis Moore had had it going, but he was using what was called a gradient two method, and it was too expensive because it used too much heavy water. We got a large contract from the army to research the cause of death in thermal burns, because at that time they were still talking about the toxemia of burns. We finally began doing frequent blood cultures on all burned patients, because it was obvious that most of them were due to infection.

We could also do cardiac outputs with the blue dye method, and the Balisto-cardiograph, on which I had worked while a resident in medicine, with Starr who invented it. As I tell the students, if you were ever lying in bed at night and had the sensation that the bed actually moved a little bit when you were worried about something, that's because it actually did. The principle of the thing is that you magnify that small movement of the bed, and you can calculate the cardiac output from it. We did a mouse study that was well received, wherein we compared the three methods of measuring cardiac output: the Fick method, the Balisto-cardiograph, and the blue dye method.

Of course, this was similar to the work that Dr. Blalock had done ten years previously with shock. We did the same thing with burns. As a matter of fact, I had him in mind all the time. He burned the dogs on one side and found that the burned side weighed a lot more than the other side. He basically solved the problem of fluid loss in burns. After he went to Hopkins, I was the president of the AOA at Penn, and had to get a speaker for our meeting. The head of medicine said, "Hardy, why don't you get Dr. Blalock to speak on his thymectomy for myasthenia gravis?" I was a student of course, but I wrote to Dr. Blalock and invited him to come speak. He wrote back that he would love to come, but he couldn't do it because he was going to Washington so much for the war effort and just couldn't take on anything else.

I stayed in Memphis for three years. Jonathan Rhoads, my colleague in Philadelphia, had been responsible for my going there, because his wife Terry and Harwell Wilson had been together at the University of Chicago, and he wrote to Harwell in Memphis, recommending me. When I was in Memphis, I related more to the physiologists and chemists there, because most of the practitioners were over in the old Baptist Hospital. I didn't want a private practice. I did have some patients, but I didn't want any more than the few I had. I went to the weekly meetings and seminars of the physiologists and chemists in Memphis, at one of which I gave a paper. People used to come up from Oxford, Mississippi, to attend the meetings in Memphis, and they got to know me, and I got to know them. When they were building their medical school, they invited me down to speak to the faculty at Oxford, which led to speaking in Jackson.

One day I was sitting in the lab at UT around graduation time. Tennessee used to graduate a class every three months, and people just dreaded having to go to commencement that often, so they sort of rotated it. I was there in the lab, and this fellow came in, introduced himself, sat down, and by Jove I do believe he put his feet up on my desk. I thought, "My heavens!" He talked all day. He said, "Well, Dr. Hardy, what do you plan to do with your life?" I said, "Well, sir, I'm going to work like the devil until I'm forty-five, and if I don't have a chair by then, I am going into practice." He said, "My, my, my. A lot of people are in your position, and I don't think you ought to set your sights so high." I said, "Well, that's my position." After he walked out, I realized he was from the University of Chicago and was down to give the commencement address that night, but no sooner had he gone out than the dean of the University of Mississippi came in and said, "Jim, the faculty voted to offer you the chair." Just like that, it couldn't have been more than thirty minutes.

In 1953 the medical school in Mississippi was not even built, but there was a huge hole in the ground of which I have a photograph. I was appointed in 1953 but declined to go down there until they had a place where I could operate. The people in Memphis were very generous in allowing me to go back and forth in the interim, and when they finally got the medical school built in 1955, I moved down with my family. The hospital opened on July 1, 1955. The nurses began to say, days ahead of time, that we just couldn't move in, it wasn't clean, and that it wouldn't be ready for another month or maybe six months. I said, "Look, we once admitted about three hundred patients to a field hospital in tents in one day. Don't tell me we can't open this place and take twenty patients from the old place downtown." So we got in. We had hardly been in there any time at all before they called and said they had a patient in the emergency room with an incarcerated hernia. It was a black man, and I think everybody on the staff put in one stitch, but we fixed his hernia. We were in business.

During the next few years I continued to publish lots of articles. I moved most of my research material to Mississippi from Memphis. Before I left, I asked Dr. Allen, the chancellor, and Dr. Wilson what they wanted me to leave in the lab. The man they were looking at to replace me was a dog-lab person, and he wasn't interested in the kind of work I had been doing, metabolic studies. Whatever they didn't want to keep, I got permission from the NIH to move down here. I also brought about six or seven people with me. Again, I told Dr. Allen and Dr. Wilson that these people wanted to come with me, but if they wanted to offer them more to stay, that was fine. They said, "Well, they really know what you do, so it suits us for you to take them." I brought four interns who were going to be residents, three technicians, a PhD, and a physiologist, and we moved right in. We applied for a heart grant to study various heart parameters and so forth, and Dr. Paul White came down with a group for a visit. They were surprised that we wanted to get started immediately, but all we had to do was set up and start. Anyway, the visiting group got down to the basement, and Dr. White indicated that he and I were going to the bathroom together, and the others were to stay outside. He looked around and said, "Dr. Hardy, how much money do you need?" I was afraid that if I asked for too much I would sound greedy, but if I asked for too little I would have to shoot myself. I told him an amount, and he said, "If that's what you need, that's what you'll get," and that is exactly what we got.

I was in the middle of writing a book called *Pathophysiology in Surgery*, and with everything else to do, there was just no way to write it but to get up and work on it early in the morning. I started going to bed about nine o'clock, right after the children, and getting up at three o'clock to dictate until I had to go down and operate. That's how I did it, and I carried on doing that almost all the time I was in the active chair. I did write some things out in longhand to get it as concise as I could. Even the part that I dictated, I sometimes rewrote later. Once you have a rough draft you can usually get on with it.

When I moved to the University of Mississippi in 1955, it was the time of the very, very beginning of open-heart surgery using the pump-oxygenator. Dr. Gibbon had done his first case in about 1953. I had been to Minnesota and seen them working on it when I was still a resident. Clarence Dennis was working with an oxygenator, so I got the Mississippi Heart Association to send a man who was going to be our first thoracic resident to Minnesota for a year. He was willing to go, to work in the dog lab, and then get all the parts for the bubble oxygenator. In July 1955, when the hospital opened, they brought all the parts for the oxygenator down here, and we got it set up in the dog lab, but it was really primitive. We didn't actually do a case on a patient until 1959.

The patients we started with were mostly people with congenital heart defects, and we did the first one on hypothermia. He was a little fellow, about two years old, named Sonny Crowe. With hypothermia, you don't run the risk of any of the pump complications. We just cooled him down to 94 degrees. He drifted on down, and we did the operation opening the pulmonary artery, putting the clamp on it, and rewarming him. About a week later, we used the pump and had one complication. We used the right leg for the arterial return and some hypothermia as well, and the patient developed frostbite of the heel. It all cleared up of course, but it gave us some concern there for a bit. I was talking to Rollo Hanlon about it a few weeks later and he said, "Join the club. If you haven't had that, you haven't operated." I said, "Well, I don't want to have it again, it scared the dickens out of me."

I decided before I came to Mississippi that transplantation was going to be important. We had done some skin grafting in Memphis because there was a lot of grafting to do with burns, and I planned that we were going to have an effort in the transplantation field. Not long after that, I began to work with Watts Webb, who was the prime mover with heart transplantation, whereas my group did the lung transplants. Watts started doing heart transplantation in 1956. He had come to see me while I was still in Memphis and said he would like to join the group. I had never heard of him, so I suggested that he stay at the sanitarium about thirty-five miles away. I said, "Why don't you just come up to the university an afternoon or two a week or something?" When I got to know him better, I said, "Why don't you go down to the sanitarium about one afternoon a week?" At the college forum the next year, we showed a movie of him leading a dog around the lab. Of course, we didn't have the pumps set up then, but he used hypothermia and rapid coupling devices. He put these coupling things in each tiedown and then sewed them at his leisure. He did a lot of work in the dog lab. We did the lung transplant first, and then we got permission to go ahead and look at the possibility of transplanting a heart in a human being.

We were also doing kidney transplants, but we never did really do liver transplants, although one was tried by the pediatric surgeon. There was a Turkish man named Alijohn who had worked with us for five years, and he got to the point that he could transplant livers and lungs every day in dogs with virtually no mortality. When he arrived, we had just had a patient, a young man, who had almost died of a gunshot wound to the left chest, pulverizing his left lung, which we had to remove. He had been drunk and aspirated probably, and his right lung was "whited out" as we say. I thought surely he was going to die, and I told the family so. As it turned out, he survived, but I thought to myself that if we could have transplanted a lung into the empty space, we would have been a lot safer, and he would have had ten days to clear up his remaining lung. We had begun to think about it and look at people who might need a lung transplant, and Alijohn and I worked on it together.

Our first patient for a lung transplant was a fellow who had a carcinoma of the left lung with a distal abscess, which had not cleared up with antibiotics. He was dyspneic, and we transplanted him. He did very well for three weeks and had almost no evidence of rejection. He had radiation to the mediastinum and Imuran and prednisone and so forth, but he was way down the hill from his cancer, and so he died with some renal failure too. He did very well, certainly, well enough to encourage the effort.

The news media were not nearly so interested in lung transplantation as they were in heart transplants. I remember I took the material and X-rays about lung transplantation to the American Medical Association meeting in New York. We had an exhibit, and I remember Mike DeBakey came over; he had an exhibit nearby. He said, "Now what's this about you transplanting a lung?" I remember him looking at the film and so forth. There wasn't much of a reaction as I recall.

In 1964 we began to get ready to do a heart transplant in a human. I told Watts, "Now you helped me to do the lung transplant, I'm going to help you do the heart transplant." I said, "Let's go talk to Dr. Marston and tell him what we've got and what we've done, and let's make sure that the university is with us." We went to see Dr. Marston and he agreed we could go ahead, but then all of a sudden Watts took the chair of cardiothoracic surgery at Southwestern in Dallas. We had a fellow who was a remarkably able technician who had worked with us a lot in the dog lab, and he just moved up into Watts's job. Ethical pressures weighed against heart transplantation. You had to have a patient who had been sick from irreversible heart disease for a long, long time, and who was really terminal, but we finally found one through one of our residents practicing in Laurel, Mississippi. He called and said he had a patient who needed a heart transplant and that it would certainly be ethical, but he was worried the patient was too far gone. That's how we found our first patient; it was in January, after Watts left the previous December.

The definition of death in 1964 was heart death rather than brain death, but that wasn't really a problem, because we couldn't count on getting a brain-dead heart. The problem was, if you put the heart in and it never beat a single beat, then that would be an awkward situation. Meanwhile, we were having as much trouble as anyone else getting donors for kidney transplantation. Keith Reemtsma and Oscar Creech had transplanted a number of chimpanzee kidneys at Tulane, so I went down there and looked over their situation, and I was very impressed. I saw two patients; one of them was a twenty-eight-year-old schoolteacher who had had a chimpanzee kidney for several months. She had a decent creatinine clearance. There was a man there also, about forty years old, and he was doing pretty well too, so I bought four chimpanzees to use here if we couldn't get a donor any other way. One of them eventually reached about 150 pounds, and I finally called down to the lab and had them put him to sleep, and we did a cardiac output. The heart wasn't huge, but it would have carried a relatively small person. We had one patient who was a potential recipient; we couldn't get a brain-dead heart because it wasn't allowed, so we used a chimpanzee heart.

Our plan had been, if we had had a donor patient, to wait until his heart actually stopped beating before we would remove it. With permission from the family, we planned to put the tubes in and heparinize the donor, and when the heart actually did stop, we would just start the pump, cool the patient, and then take the organ. That is what we were going to do, but it didn't work out that way.

The recipient patient had myocardial failure with numerous heart attacks over a period of years. He came to our place essentially comatose, but he got a little better. He had low cardiac output, so we transplanted the chimpanzee heart. It kicked off immediately and really had a very vigorous beat. It went for about an hour, and then gradually it began to slow, and then the blood pressure began to decline. I think the problem was that the patient had been in shock for about forty-eight hours. Anyway, it was obvious that he could be transplanted, and with a good organ and a better recipient, it ought to work, and of course it has worked.

One of the articles about our first heart transplant said that it raised ethical, moral, social, religious, financial, governmental, and legal questions. I think that is all correct. We worried most about the ethical questions, of course, because obviously after all of those years I didn't want to look like a screwball that was willing to do anything, although I'm sure that most people thought I was. One of my friends in Houston had called and said, "Jim, what's going on over there? Some newspaper man said that you had transplanted a human heart into a chimpanzee." I said, "Well, not exactly." In any case, I felt very comfortable with the one we did do, and I didn't worry too much about the criticism.

There was a tremendous amount of criticism, though. About three days later, the International Transplantation Society was meeting in New York City at the Waldorf-Astoria, and they called me and asked if I would join a panel for heart transplantation. I said, "Well, of course." We had something on the program anyway. The guy who was running the program said, "Now Dr. Hardy, before you start, I want to get one thing straight. As I understand it, they keep the black people in one cage and the chimpanzees in another, don't they?" Of course we were right in the middle of the civil rights movement at that time, and that set a poor tone for the meeting. Later that night he said, "Do you realize I was joking?" I said, "I'm not sure I do realize it, and I am not sure that the worldwide audience thought you were joking either," but, as a matter of fact, not one hand was raised to object. You would think that some fellow would have been crazy enough to, but not one. Norman Shumway said some positive things, and so did Bill Holden, but basically it was a grim day. That went on and on. Dr. Ravdin saw me and said that he had just come from a meeting upstairs, where he had heard that it was not merely immoral of me to transplant that heart, it was amoral. He said, "Now Jim, there's been enough of this stuff now; it's time to begin the counterattack." But where does one begin a counterattack? This went on for some years.

The government eventually had to get involved. What happened was that the NIH immediately began to pronounce all of these restrictions on clinical investigation. Now you have to have a committee for this and that. The heart transplant really started it. It became obvious that if we did another heart transplant before Shumway or somebody else did one to take the heat off of us, or at least share the heat, that they would take our grant money, so we just let it sit for a good long while. That was a difficult time.

In 1964 the main institutions doing serious work toward heart transplantation were our institution, Rollo Hanlon in St Louis, Shumway's group, and there was a fellow named David Blumenstock doing pretty well with the dog transplants. I don't think Blumenstock did any clinical work, but Hanlon's group could have done a transplant, and certainly Shumway's group could have done one. The first successful heart transplant was done in 1967. Dr. Barnard achieved a great deal of fame, but he was also criticized for not having done much basic research. I remember the exact time I heard that that heart had been transplanted. It was the night of the departmental Christmas party. I was coming in to the second floor of the country club, and there was a resident who met me at the head of the stairs and said, "Dr Hardy, I heard on the radio coming over here that somebody in South Africa transplanted a heart. We should have done that years ago!" I said, "Well, Jerry, it just wasn't the case that we could do it. Who was it?" He said that he had never heard of him, but it was Barnard. Chris Barnard had spent three

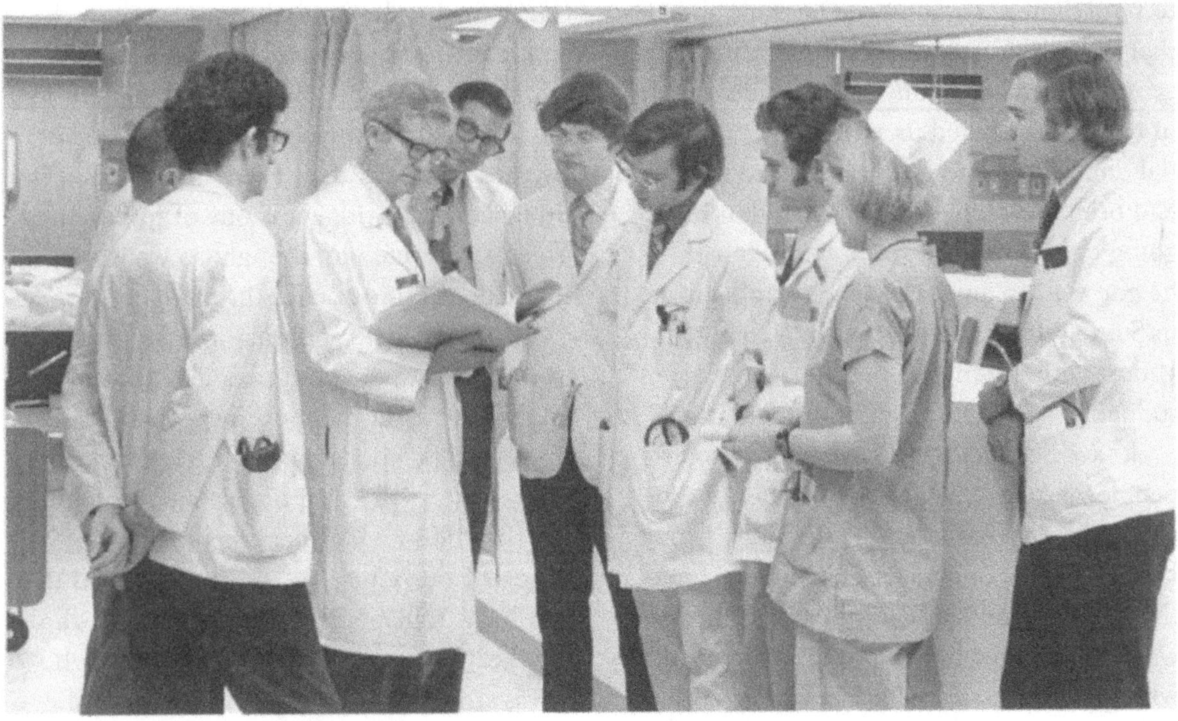

Dr. Hardy making rounds with his residents

months in Richmond, Virginia, with David Hume, learning the techniques of kidney transplantation. Dick Lower had gone from Stanford to Richmond by that time and was continuing to do heart transplant operations in the research laboratory. It was there that Barnard first saw a heart transplant operation on a dog. It turned out that Dick Lower had written me a letter about Barnard, but I hadn't gotten it yet because we had just sold our home, and the people who bought it would wait till they had a bundle of mail and then ship it to our place. Later I found the letter from Dick. He wrote that he knew Barnard and that Barnard had told one of his technicians, as he left to go home to South Africa, that he was going to go home and transplant a heart. Dick wrote, "We didn't really believe it, but he did do it, didn't he? We should have listened to him." Anyway, Barnard learned it from Shumway's and Lower's research.

After heart transplantation became accepted, we developed a cardiac transplant program here at Jackson. Within two weeks after the transplant in South Africa, the NIH called a meeting at O'Hare Airport in Chicago, for everybody who transplanted hearts. They had been threatening to take away grants before, but two weeks later they were urging everybody to get into it. They had Barnard there at the meeting, as a matter of fact. John Kirklin was there, and Lillehei. The people from Houston were there. Cardiac people from all over the country were there who had any interest in transplantation. Overnight the attitude of the NIH had changed: It was, "Get with it, buster, we're behind." The definition of death was changed very rapidly, and brain death began to be accepted. I was a little nervous about that though. Once we had some neurosurgeons in Canton, about twenty miles north of here, who offered us a patient as a potential donor who had a very bad head injury. It had been mentioned in his town that he was going to be a donor for the heart, but then he got well. In any case, after the operation in South Africa, the whole thing changed almost within a matter of days. The NIH suddenly was all for heart transplantation.

I have been lucky to have had so many people who have helped and influenced me in my career. That would include the people I trained with, of course: Dr. Ravdin, Jonathan Rhoads, and Julian Johnson. Then there was a biochemist by the name of Drabkin, who gave me space in his laboratory at the University of Pennsylvania. He was the head of chemistry in the graduate school of medicine there. Certainly my own father was a big influence on me, but that didn't have anything to do with medicine. I had great respect for the chairman of medicine at Penn; I hated to leave medicine because he had taken me under his wing. Also there was Dr. Miller, of the Miller-Abbott tube; he was a gastroenterologist. I think those are the main ones. After I was in Memphis, I was grown enough that I didn't really need mentors any more. If I think back to college, though, there was a man named Breckenridge who taught cat anatomy. He had a strong influence on me. I didn't do well in the first year of premed college because I was in four or five musical organizations and traveled with the football team every weekend. I wasn't sure I wanted to do premed anyway, but when I did decide, I wanted to dig in and show these people I could do it. By the time I did that, I was interested in it myself. Breckenridge was one of my teachers. The classes were big, though, so we weren't that close to our teachers in college.

Just a few days ago there was an article in the newspaper about people who were asked to vote on the most important scientific event in Mississippi in the last hundred years. One of the scientific events, which may not be so scientific, was the first bottling of Coca-Cola, but another one was the first heart transplant. Overwhelmingly, the first heart transplant won, so even though it was stressful and painful at the time, the world views it differently now. A man named Cooper is writing a book on early transplants, and I talked to him on the phone the other day for about an hour. He said, "Well, you know, Dr. Hardy, these things always come around," and it has come around. Actually, all we said was that we had shown that you could transplant a heart, and that it could support the blood pressure for a period of time. We thought that if you had a good heart and a good recipient, it would do well. That's all we ever said.

It is surprising to me that all that happened thirty-five years ago. I was visiting at the retirement home just yesterday, and the man across the hall said something about it. It surprised me that he remembered it. He was about my age.

Bibliography

Hardy JD, Godfrey L Jr. Effect of Intravenous Fluids on Dehydrated Patients and on Normal Subjects; Cardiac Output, Stroke Volume, Pulse Rate, and Blood Pressure. *JAMA*. 1944; 126:23–27.

Hardy JD, Eraslan S, Webb WR. Transplantation of the Lung. *Ann Surg*. 1964; 160:440–448.

Hardy JD, Chavez CM, Kurrus FD, Neely WA, Eraslan S, Turner MD, Fabian LW, Labecki TD. Heart Transplantation in Man; Developmental Studies and Report of a Case. *JAMA*. 1964; 188:1132–1140.

Hardy JD, Webb WR, Timmis HH, Watson DG, Blake TM. Patent Ductus Arteriosus; Operative Treatment of 100 Consecutive Patients with Isolated Lesions without Mortality. *Ann Surg*. 1966; 164:877–882.

Hardy JD, Timmis HH, Weems WL, Wesson RL, Moore JD, Langford HG. Kidney Transplantation in Man; Analysis of Eleven Cases. *Ann Surg*. 1967; 165:933–946.

Hardy JD, Chavez CM. The First Heart Transplant in Man: Developmental Animal Investigations with Analysis of the 1964 Case in the Light of Current Clinical Experience. *Am J Cardiol*. 1968; 22:772–781.

Hardy JD, Timmis HH. Repair of Intracardiac Gunshot Injuries: Report of Three Cases with Review of Literature. *Ann Surg*. 1969; 169:906–913.

Hardy JD, Beahrs OH, Anlyan WG, et al. Cost Containment: A Statement by the American Surgical Association. *N Engl J Med*. 1979; 301:283–284.

Hardy JD (Editor). *Complications in Surgery and Their Management* (4th Edition). Philadelphia: W. B. Saunders; 1981.

Hardy JD (Editor). *Hardy's Textbook of Surgery*. Philadelphia: J. B. Lippincott; 1983.

Sir Terence English, FRCS

(b. 1932)

To me, John Kirklin is the foremost cardiac surgeon of our generation. It was not only that he got involved in open-heart surgery so early, but it was his disciplined approach that has had a huge impact on everyone who has worked for him.

— On contributions to the evolution of cardiac surgery

Interviewed June 30, 2001

My background lies in South Africa, where I was born and brought up. My father was a mining engineer and died when I was only eighteen months old. When I was growing up, I decided that I wanted to follow in his footsteps, so I entered college planning to study mining engineering. Toward the end of my college years, I decided that I wanted to study medicine. I had an uncle that I greatly admired who was a surgeon and had done his training in Edinburgh. When I spoke to him about my decision to study medicine, he said he thought I ought to go to Guy's Hospital in London. I asked why and he said, "Well, it is a great London medical school, very strong on clinical training, and had a very strong South African tradition." So I applied to and was accepted by Guy's. I enjoyed my medical school years enormously. Initially I was attracted to cardiology. I think that may have had something to do with my engineering background, because I understood the concepts of flows, pressures, resistances, and so on. I was house physician to the cardiology unit at Guy's, and at the end of my time, Dr. Baker, who was the chief of cardiology, asked me what I wanted to do. I told him that I was interested in becoming a cardiologist. He said, "Well then, you need to spend a little bit of time with the surgeons, because you will be a better cardiologist if you have seen what they are up to." Well, that was a fine idea, but he had a lot of difficulty persuading Sir Russell Brock to accept me, a would-be cardiologist, on his surgical firm. Sir Russell did not think this was such a good idea, but Dr. Baker managed to prevail, and I joined the thoracic surgery unit in 1964 as a senior house officer. Within six weeks, it was quite clear in my own mind that I was never going to go back to cardiology, because there were so many fascinating things that were happening in the thoracic surgical unit at that time.

Sir Russell Brock became the president of the Royal College of Surgeons during the latter part of my residency. He was an amazing man. He was one of those driven souls who wanted to be completely perfect in his work, and he was not. He had a wonderful mind and was a superb clinician, but his technical skills were not of the highest order. He had grown up in an older school of surgery. He used to get very frustrated when he was operating, and those of us who worked for him suffered considerably as a result. At the same time, we all respected him enormously for his integrity, his great knowledge, and his vision. We especially admired his determination to persist with operating on patients with Fallot's tetralogy with very poor results initially but then gradually getting better. He made a huge impression on me. Donald Ross was also in the thoracic unit at that time. He had been Brock's senior registrar and was then a young consultant at Guy's. They were a wonderful, complementary couple because Donald was a much more lighthearted, less serious person. He was equally serious about his work and was a wonderful technical surgeon and a great innovator. It was a great joy working for those two, so I decided that I wanted to carry on in cardiothoracic surgery. I started in general surgery, and following that I did an extended locum at the Heart Hospital with Sir Thomas Holmes Sellors, who, like Brock, later became the president of the Royal College of Surgeons. He was known by everyone as "Uncle Tom" and was the archetypal English gentleman. He was terribly polite, he never got flustered, and was kind to all of his residents. He was a complete contrast to Brock, but both men made great contributions in their own way. "Uncle Tom" was the senior surgeon at the Heart Hospital when I worked there in the mid-sixties. There had been a controversy about precedence between him and Brock as to who had done the first closed pulmonary valvotomy. I think that the correct sequence of this was that Thomas Holmes Sellors did the operation first, and Brock followed within a week or ten days and was able to get it into the literature before Holmes Sellors. They were competing with each other at that time. During the early years of cardiac surgery, Holmes Sellors had a wonderful series of closures of atrial septal defects using hypothermia and inflow occlusion with superb results.

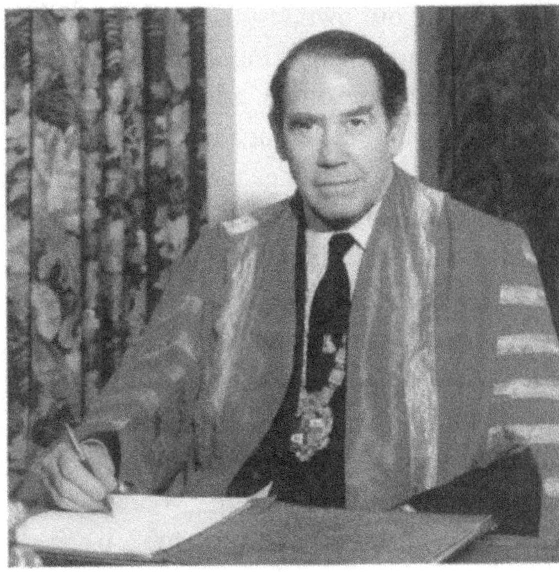

Sir Terence English as president of the Royal College of Surgeons

I then started on my senior registrar training in London. The great joy of the rotation between the Brompton, the National Heart Hospital, and the London Chest Hospital was that you worked for eight or nine London cardiothoracic surgeons and you could learn a lot from each of them. The most important year during my senior registrarship was spent in Birmingham, Alabama. I had heard John Kirklin give a lecture in London at the Hammersmith in 1967 or 1968, and I was enormously impressed by him. Subsequently I wrote to him and asked if I could do a year's research fellowship with him. He invited me to come, so I spent the year of 1969 there. To me, Kirklin is the foremost cardiac surgeon of our generation. It was not that he got involved in open-heart surgery so early, but it was his disciplined approach to the specialty that has had a huge impact on everyone who worked with him. His almost unreasonable desire to reduce operative mortality to zero, at a time when it was nowhere near zero, had a great impact on all of us. His insistence on analyzing our own results regularly and rigorously and then getting into the more sophisticated areas of risk-adjusted analysis of mortality has had a huge impact on most cardiac surgeons of my generation. Certainly I owe him a great deal.

After I left Birmingham, I completed my training on the London circuit. One day I was operating at the Brompton with my chief, Matt Paneth, and he said, "English, you ought to go to Papworth and work with Milstein." I said, "Who is Milstein and where is Papworth?" He said, "Well, there is a locum (temporary appointment) job for a consultant coming up. It is near Cambridge, Ben Milstein is a good man, and you should think about doing this job," so I did a three-month locum in the middle of winter at Papworth Hospital. Papworth had a long history as a tuberculosis sanatorium and then later as a hospital for diseases of the chest. Both Brock and Holmes Sellors had operated at Papworth on an interim basis before the war. The cardiac surgery service was added later and was a fairly small unit. There were only three surgeons—Ben Milstein, Chris Parrish, who was half time toward the end of his career, and I. I enjoyed both the hospital and working with Ben Milstein. He wanted to develop a completely integrated unit and that appealed to me. When the full-time job came up three months later, I applied for it and was appointed to the staff. I never went back to London.

About three months after I had started at Papworth, I went to Palo Alto, California, to visit my friend Philip Caves, who had been a registrar at the Brompton when I was a senior registrar. He was from Northern Ireland and was an incredibly able person. He had obtained a research fellowship with Norman Shumway, had worked in the lab there for a year, and had done some wonderful experiments which led to the introduction of percutaneous biopsy of the heart. This really allowed a sort of quantum development in the management of heart transplant patients, because for the first time you could detect early rejection by repeatedly taking small samples of heart muscle, looking at them under the microscope, and then treating the rejection. Having done that, he worked as Shumway's chief resident for the next year, which is when I went out to visit him. I was amazed when I was there to see relatively large numbers of heart transplant patients at Stanford coming back for checkups and looking very well. Philip, by this time, was incredibly enthusiastic about heart transplantation and wanted to start a program in Scotland, to which he was about to return. I got very interested because at the same time Roy Calne at Cambridge already had a large liver and renal transplant program, and it seemed that it might be possible to add a heart transplant program. I entered into discussions with him, soon after getting back, in 1973. Initially we had planned to do the work in the main teaching hospital at Addenbrooke's, which seemed logical because the immunology and the donors were there. As it turned out, it was not the logical place, because I realized after some time that this was very much a cardiac surgical operation and that you needed to have the patients at the same location as the anesthetists, the ICU nurses, and your whole team. Papworth and Addenbrooke's are twelve miles apart.

You will recall that Christiaan Barnard did his first heart transplant in December 1967, and then a lot of teams all over the world attempted to do them. Out of 160-odd patients that were transplanted between 1968 and 1970, only 11 percent were alive after two years, and indeed, only 50 patients were alive after one month. During this time, Donald Ross had done three heart transplants in London. His first patient died and his longest survivor in 1969 was 107 days. This experience, taken with the worldwide poor results, caused the Department of Health to impose a moratorium on further heart transplantation in the UK. We felt that if we could come close to approximating the outcome of transplantation at Stanford, we ought to be able to get that moratorium withdrawn. By 1978 Stanford was achieving these sorts of results. There were just better than 60 percent alive at a year and about 40 percent after five years, so this was a huge improvement from the initial experience. It was this sort of result that we were looking to achieve. The reasons for restarting the work in the UK were really threefold. One was the improved results from Stanford. The second, and very important, was that the diagnosis of brain death had been clarified in 1976 with a very authoritative report that had been accepted by the medical profession. It was now going to be possible to take donor hearts from patients in other parts of the country who were being maintained on a ventilator with their heart still working, but who were completely brain-dead. This was terribly important because until that time most kidney and liver transplants were cadaver organs from patients without any circulation, and clearly we could not use hearts from those kinds of donors. The third reason was that there was a lot of interest in heart preservation, and we were particularly interested in being able to have periods of up to four or possibly six hours to be able to take out a heart in the north country and bring it to Papworth for implantation. In our lab, we had been transplanting young pigs with donor hearts that had been stored in iced saline for sixteen hours without oxygen. The pigs were immunosuppressed and then three months later were sacrificed. They had grown at a normal rate from 25 kilograms to 50 kilograms, and the sizes and both the macroscopic and microscopic appearances of the heart were normal. That was the source of considerable support to us.

In January 1979 we did our first case. I have to say that we did it without the permission of the Department of Health because although I had submitted our protocols to them at the beginning of 1978, they had replied by saying that they would not be prepared to fund a heart transplant program in Britain, and they were not prepared to fund single cases that were done. Therefore, we organized it with our local health authority. I told the chairman what we were going to do and she said that we could use our facilities for two cases, and then we would have to find the funding for ourselves. The first case we did in January 1979 was a failure. The patient had been in the hospital for three months, had severe cardiomyopathy, and was extremely ill by the time the operation started. There was a period of cardiac arrest and resuscitation immediately before putting the patient on bypass. The anesthetist at Papworth felt that it was worth going ahead with the operation, because he could not be sure as to whether there had been any resulting brain damage. I was taking the donor heart out at Addenbrooke's. We did go ahead, the heart worked perfectly, and the patient woke up but never got off the ventilator and eventually died of infection seventeen days later. That was not a good start. We had been having a tremendous difficulty in getting donor organs, because by this time those involved in kidney transplantation were worried as to whether our entry into the field would make it more difficult for them to get donors, and we were not getting a lot of support from within Cambridge itself. We did get another heart in August, and this one went much better. Keith Castle was not an ideal patient for a transplantation because he was a heavy smoker and had quite serious peripheral vascular disease, but he was a wonderful man. He was a cockney, and his zest for life captured the imagination of the British public. He lived for five and a half years. I believe he did more to promote heart transplantation in Britain than any other factor.

We were relatively lucky with our early experience. There was the first failure, then Keith Castle lived for five years. Then we had another patient who lived for three years, one lived nine years, another failure, and then one who lived for eight years. This was important because there was a lot of criticism as to whether this was going to be cost effective, and whether the outcome was going to be worse than the disease. There was also a lot of antagonism within the profession itself. These survivors were very important to us.

In 1980 other cardiac surgery units around the world began to get interested. There was still controversy. The Massachusetts General Hospital decided not to embark on a heart transplant program, and the editor of the *New England Journal of Medicine* wrote a rather pompous editorial saying that the trustees' decision "demonstrates that physicians may not make independent decisions regarding what professional services they provide. If one considers that the medical profession has historically been fostered and supported to serve a societal need and not provide physicians with privileged status, one can find little argument with the course that MGH trustees thoughtfully and responsibly followed." Well, that brought a wonderful response from Norman Shumway, who wrote as follows: "Maybe it has to be considered (perish the thought) that the MGH is not the leading institution that it used to be. Apparently somebody feels they just do not have the horses." There was a lot of controversy within leading institutions as to whether this was worth doing or not.

The Department of Health watched all of this, but did not really want to get involved initially. About a year after I started, Magdi Yacoub started a program at Harefield Hospital, so the Department of Health decided that they would begin a research project to compare the programs at Papworth and Harefield and look at not only the cost, which was what they wanted to do initially, but also to look at the benefits as judged by extension of life and improvement in quality of life. This led to a publication in 1983, and it was this publication that led to the formal approval by the Department of Health for proper funding for both Papworth and Harefield and other units in Britain. This was the turning point as far as our hospital was concerned, because we then began to get quite generous funding from central moneys.

The first two and a half to three years, we used so-called conventional immunosuppression with azathioprine and steroids as was done at Stanford, but in the late 1970s, Sir Roy Calne introduced cyclosporine for kidney transplantation. Stan-

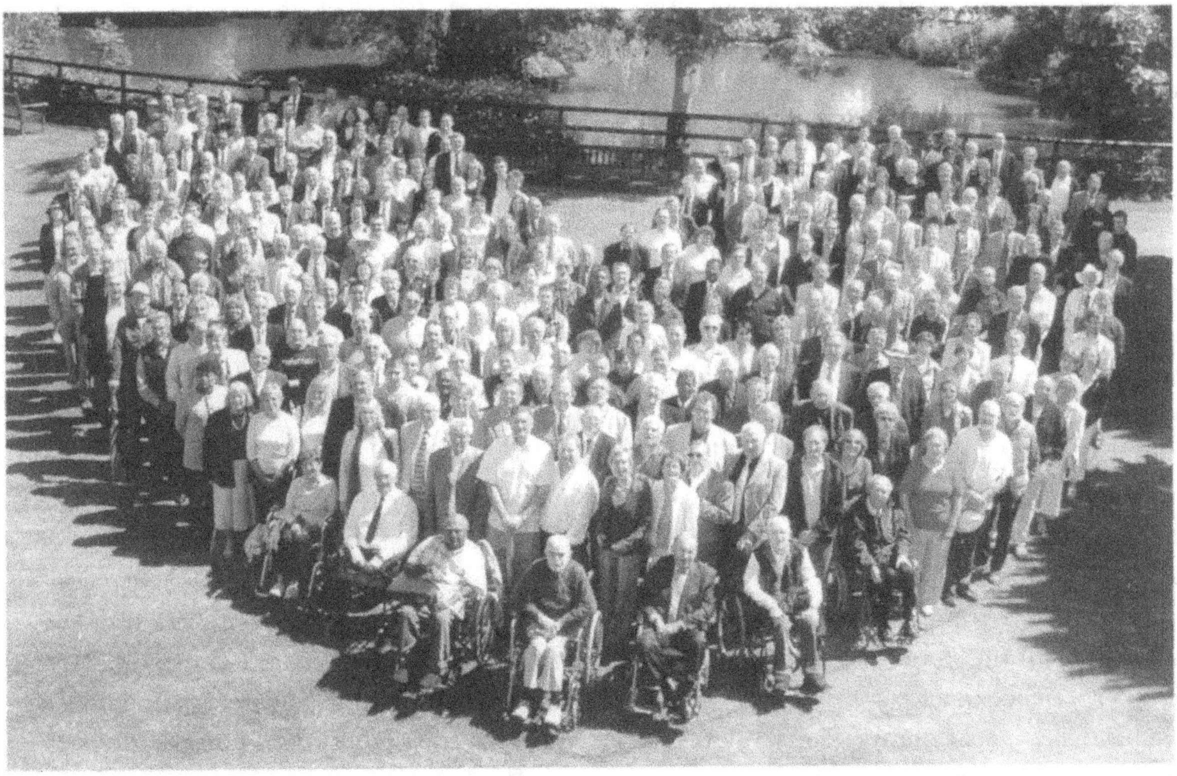

Heart transplant patients on the grounds of Papworth Hospital near Cambridge

ford used it for heart-lung transplants in 1981, and we introduced it to our program in 1982. This really changed the whole management of heart transplantation. Previously one could have a posttransplant patient who was well on day twenty-three and mortally ill on day twenty-five. What cyclosporine did was to really damp down the early rejection so that the patients could be managed much more effectively. A small number of heart transplants were done in the seventies and early eighties. There was a great increase in the mid-1980s, with up to nearly four thousand patients a year by the end of that decade. Then equally striking, there was a complete leveling off, and then the numbers even dropped a little. That meant that the number of available donor organs had been reached, and there could be no further expansion. This effect was mirrored at Papworth. Once we got the funding, the number of cases suddenly went up to doing about eighty heart transplants a year. We could have done more than that if we had had more donor hearts. That was, and is, the limiting factor.

From 1979 until 2003 we received twenty-five hundred referrals for possible heart transplants at Papworth Hospital. We could assess many of the early referrals either on paper or over the phone and determine that they were not suitable. About seventeen hundred patients were assessed, mostly at Papworth, and of those, a large proportion were accepted for transplantation. About one hundred patients were offered and underwent conventional cardiac surgery, coronary artery bypass grafting with or without aneurysmectomy. Eight hundred and forty-five patients were transplanted. The median waiting time was seventy-nine days. The group who died waiting had a median time, between acceptance and death, of only thirty-seven days, so they were a really sick group. The main causes of postoperative death in the first few months were rejection and infection. Like any transplant group, the patients are more susceptible to malignancy later on, particularly skin cancer and lymphoma, and most important of all, an accelerated coronary heart disease in the donor heart, which is immunologically mediated. The main causes of morbidity were kidney damage from cyclosporine and the side effects of the steroids. Looking at the total experience of all patients at Papworth, we have 80 percent one-year survival, 68 percent five-year survival, and 46 percent ten-year survival. The last seven hundred patients have had a much better long-term survival with 84 percent one-year survival and a ten-year survival of somewhere around 60 percent, but the main problem for all heart transplant groups at present is the limitation of the donor supply. Everything has been done to try to increase organ donation amongst the general population here; well, I say everything, but, in fact, everything has not been done. For example, Spain has a heart transplant rate of exactly twice that of the UK at present, and that is largely because they have a lot of transplant coordinators, one in each of their main hospitals, and they have lots of intensive care capacity. There will never be enough donor organs, and we have to think of other possibilities for improving the circulation.

Now I will just say a few words about the artificial hearts. Willem Kolff, who was responsible for developing the kidney dialysis machine in Holland during World War II, went to the Cleveland Clinic after the war and got involved in trying to develop artificial hearts. In a publication in 1963 he was very optimistic about the use of the artificial heart in calves. You could say, "today the calves, tomorrow man." It is now nearly forty years later, and we still do not have a successful artificial heart. The heart that Kolff worked on was subsequently taken up by Robert Jarvik in Utah. We became interested in the Jarvik heart in the early 1980s; it was an interesting device. The diaphragm inside the Jarvik heart moved by compressed air. A diagram of it makes it look very simple, but I assure you it was not. The drive lines came out through the patient's skin and activated the two ventricles by compressed air. There was a big console, which supplied the compressed air, next to the patient. Of course, it meant having to completely take out the patient's own heart and then sew the atrial cusps of the device onto the atrial cusps of the patient. For various reasons we got involved in this, and received some funding from the Humana Corporation to use the Jarvik heart as a bridge to transplant. My colleague, Frank Wells, and I used to fly to Utah to do these operations on calves and then go back three months later, take out the artificial heart and put in a new calf heart. All of this was a devilishly difficult procedure. It was an interesting time. Willem Kolff was still in Utah and was a fascinating man with whom to be associated. In November 1986 we eventually got a suitable patient in whom to use the Jarvik heart as a bridge-to-transplant. It was unfortunate that, within three days after we implanted the Jarvik heart, we were offered a great donor heart from Newcastle by a friend and colleague of mine, Chris McGregor, who thought he was doing me a great service. What we would have preferred was to have had the artificial heart in the patient for a much longer time so that we could have learned more from the procedure. Our patient was a big man. He had been a paratrooper, and he weighed about 250 pounds when we first met him. He was a little bit thinner by the time he left the hospital, but we needed a big heart and this was a big donor heart. We had to take the whole device out three days later and put in the donor heart. I never did another one of those operations, because it was clear that it just did not make sense to use a complete artificial heart as a bridge procedure. In fact, about three years later the Jarvik heart was withdrawn from use. Since that time, the whole field of left ventricular assist devices has been moving forward. Within the last three years at Papworth, we have inserted twenty left ventricular assist devices as bridges to transplant. It is a very difficult field in terms of how to select the patients. A few patients will recover while the left ventricular assist device is in place. In them, the assist device can be withdrawn, but overall it is very costly and is still very much at an experimental stage. At present there is no totally implantable artificial heart suitable for human use.

Xenografting has been a very interesting, but also a very frustrating story for the last five years. As early as 1995 a Cambridge-based company reported successful transplantation of genetically engineered pig hearts into monkeys. These were similar to the pigs that they had prepared to be future donors for humans. This caused a lot of controversy, so what the government did was to set up a regulatory authority called the Xenotransplantation Interim Regulator Authority. This meant that any unit that was going to embark on clinical xenotransplantation had to have their protocols approved by this organization before they could proceed. The two big problems at present are, first, the danger of new viral transmission from the pig organ into the human patient and then from the patient into the population at large. It is a slight risk, a very slight risk, but it is there, and that is causing anxiety. The other problem is the long-term immunosuppression of xenotransplants. Although the initial hyperacute rejection may be resolved by genetically engineering those pigs by putting bits of human protein into the endothelial cells of the donor pig, that is really just the first stage of the whole process. It will be interesting to see how things develop over the next five to ten years.

Bibliography

English TA, Cooper DKC, Cory-Pearce R. Recent Experience with Heart Transplantation. *Br Med J.* 1980; 281: 699–702.

English TA. What Price Excellence? *J Med Ethics.* 1982; 8:144–146.

Herrtage ME, Hall LW, English TA. Surgical Correction of Tetralogy of Fallot in a Dog. *J Small Animal Practice.* 1983; 24:51–62.

English TA, Spratt P, Wallwork J, Cory-Pearce R, Wheeldon D. Selection and Procurement of Hearts for Transplantation. *Br Med J.* 1984; 288:1889–1891.

English TA, Bailey AR, Dark JF, Williams WG. The UK Cardiac Surgical Register 1977–1982. *Br Med J.* 1984; 289:1205–1208.

Darracott-Cankovic S, Hutter J, Wallwork J, Wheeldon D, English TA. Biopsy Assessment of Myocardial Preservation in 160 Human Donor Hearts. *Transplant Proc.* 1988; 20(Suppl 7):44–48.

Hutter JA, Wallwork J, English TA. Management of Rejection in Heart Transplant Recipients: Does Moderate Rejection Always Require Treatment? *J Heart Transplant.* 1990; 9:87–91.

Stovin PG, Sharples L, Hutter JA, Wallwork J, English TA. Some Prognostic Factors for the Development of Transplanted-Related Coronary Artery Disease in Human Cardiac Allografts. *J Heart Lung Transplant.* 1991; 10:38–44.

English TA. Surgeons, Managers, and Politicians in the 1990s. *Royal Aust Coll Surg Bull.* July 1992: 12–17.

William C. DeVries, MD

(b. 1943)

I could be talking to a ladies' garden group or the American College of Cardiology, and they would ask the same questions. They always wanted to know what it felt like to have an artificial heart.

— On the first total artificial heart

Interviewed June 3, 1999

I was born in New York in 1943, but I lived most of my younger life in Utah. My mother was a nurse working in Salt Lake City, and my father was a rotating intern at the Latter Day Saints Hospital (LDS) when the war broke out. One night he received a telephone call from his father who said, "Henry, this is your dad and you are an embarrassment to me. The Germans have taken over our country (Holland). You are my oldest son, and you are the only son who hasn't joined the armed forces." My father explained to his father that he was trying to finish his internship, that he had just gotten married, and that he was waiting for a year or so to get on his feet, but his father said that he was to join the navy the very next day, and he did. He was a Dutch immigrant, and Dutch immigrants usually followed everything their father said. So I was born in the Brooklyn Naval Yards, and my father went away to war right after I was born. He never even saw me, for he was killed in action when I was about six months old. My mother gathered up all of our effects, and we went back across the country on a train. When she returned to southern California where her mother lived, she found out that her father had been killed in the war as well. Many times we do not understand what war is like. My mother and grandmother had a double funeral for my father and grandfather.

Later we moved back to Salt Lake City, and I was raised there. It was a safe haven for my mother, as most of her family came from that area. My mother remarried when I was about five years old, and I have nine wonderful brothers and sisters and a great stepfather. We had a great family. When time came for college there was not much money, as there were nine other children. I went to the University of Utah, basically because they offered me a basketball and track scholarship. I thought of college as a job, and so I ran and jumped my way through college. I went to medical school at the University of Utah as well. When I was in my first year, I walked into a lecture one day because I did not have anything to do at the time. The speaker was Dr. Willem Kolff from the Cleveland Clinic. Dr. Reemtsma was the chief of surgery at the University of Utah, and with his special interest in renal transplantation he was in the process of recruiting Dr. Kolff. In his lecture, Dr. Kolff talked about the artificial kidney and the artificial heart, and I was absolutely fascinated. The lecture lasted two hours, and I missed one of my gross anatomy classes because I lost track of the time. After the lecture, I went up to Dr. Kolff and said, "This is the most interesting thing I have ever heard in my life, and I would like to work with you if I could." He replied that there were some positions available for summer work at the Cleveland Clinic, and asked my name. (DeVries is probably the most common name in Holland.) He said, "You sound like

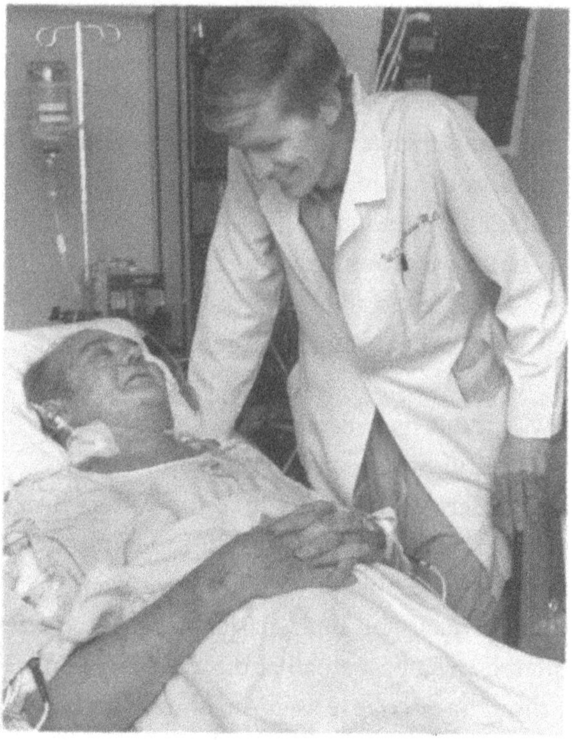

William C. DeVries with patient Barney Clark

a good Dutch boy. You're hired." That is how I got my start. I ran into Dr. Kolff during my freshman year, and he took me under his wing. I worked at the Cleveland Clinic that first summer, about the time Dr. Kolff was preparing to move his lab to the University of Utah. He had finished his work on dialysis and had started working on the artificial heart, and I continued to work under his supervision back in Utah.

I decided that I wanted to leave Salt Lake City after medical school. I was just an old western boy, and in the West you look to the East and the South as the centers of culture. I thought I would eventually come back to practice medicine in the West, and I wanted to get a new viewpoint on life.

I first interviewed in Boston and saw a stabbing five minutes before I arrived at the hospital. I also visited Johns Hopkins where they had armed guards to escort people in and out of the medical center. I did not want to subject my family to that type of environment. Stanford had a neat program where they were doing all heart surgery, but somehow that just did not seem right, because I wanted to do some general surgery too. I decided to go to Duke, because it was in a fairly safe, Southern town, and I thought it was a great institution.

I started my residency at Duke in 1970, and it was a wonderful nine years. I fell right into the system of rules and behavior, and it was captivating. It was a kind of macho thing. We were on call every other night, and we were expected to give undivided dedication and support to those above and below us. Everyone was fighting for the same cause, and you knew that you were getting the best education in the world. You knew what you had to do. It was all programmed, and you just did it, and you got there. One of the surgeons at Duke that influenced my training was Dr. Sealy. He was the most terrific guy, like a father to me. He was from the University of Michigan, and he was trained in many of the lost arts of thoracic surgery. He was one of the few remaining surgeons who really knew a lot about fungal diseases, tuberculosis, and other lung infections, and the other surgeons would come to him for advice. Every Wednesday when you were on his rotation, he would drive you down to Wilson, North Carolina, in his '56 Chevy, to a TB sanitarium. We would do eight rigid bronchoscopies under local anesthetic, and it was amazing to see how he worked. He knew the radiographic literature better than any of the radiologists.

When coronary bypass grafting came along, Dr. Sealy was near the end of his career, and he made an interesting decision. Coronary bypass surgery required a very fine, delicate technique using loupes and working on moving hearts, and Dr. Sealy decided, based on his own surgical abilities, that it was not for him. He said, "I don't want to get involved. I'm past that." Even though he had done a tremendous series of mitral commissurotomies, open and closed, he decided that he wanted to find something else he could do in heart surgery, and so he started surgery for the Wolff-Parkinson-White arrhythmia. He did that as a conscious effort, because he felt that coronary surgery was going to pass him by, and he was willing to let that happen. He knew his own talents, and he found something that he could do in the lab and put it right into clinical use. He was a visionary to do that, and had obviously been thinking about it for a long time.

Louis Pasteur said, "Discovery comes to a prepared mind," and Dr. Sealy was prepared at that time. He had a great dog lab where I worked for a while during my residency. He always enjoyed finding a surgical procedure to solve a medical problem, and he liked the idea that a precise surgical cut could end the need for the patient to take lots of pills. He was a wonderful gentleman to work with.

Dr. Sabiston was the chief of surgery at Duke when I was there. I had never met anybody like him. He was the absolute, ultimate professional, with great ideas about what it means to be a doctor. We worked in public hospital services where one patient might have many different doctors, and Dr. Sabiston always made sure the patient knew which doctor was taking care of him. When we would go on rounds he would say, "Now, Mr. Jennings here is a peanut farmer. Mr. Jennings, who is your doctor?" The patient would point out which intern was his doctor, and if he did not know who it was, there was hell to pay. Dr. Sabiston also pushed very hard on academics and appearances. Everything had to appear and go exactly right. He set up everything so you could succeed.

Things were always done on time and exactly the correct way. I could not have had a better residency or better teaching. Dr. Sabiston was just an ideal role model for me on how you should do things in those early days of my training.

During my last year of residency at Duke, I contacted Dr. Sabiston and explained that I needed a job. He said, "Well, you've got a job in Utah." Unbeknownst to me, when I finished medical school, Dr. Kolff had called Dr. Sabiston and said, "I have a medical student here who is promising, but I want him back. You take him for seven years and after that you send him back to me." I had no idea that this had occurred. I said to Dr. Sabiston, "They don't even do heart surgery there!" The medical center in Utah was doing one case per month. Dr. Sabiston replied, "You go there and help Dr. Kolff, and get the VA to help you get your program started up. If you don't like it in five years, I will get you another job." That is how I got back to Utah.

Dr. Kolff was a fascinating guy and a Dutch immigrant like my father. He was finishing his medical residency in Holland when the Germans took over. The hospitals had large numbers of patients with hepatitis and tuberculosis, for which they frequently blamed the Germans. There was also a lot of renal failure, and because Dr. Kolff had a lot of time and worked right next door to a sausage factory, he began to experiment with a way to treat those patients. He wound cellophane sausage skins around drums, put them in an old Maytag washing machine, and agitated the blood. He dialyzed seventeen patients this way, and they all died. Finally one patient lived, and that was the first successful artificial kidney. After the war, his method became well-known, but there was a lot of economic resistance to the artificial kidney in postwar Europe, so he came to Mt. Sinai Hospital in Brooklyn, and later to the Cleveland Clinic. At the Cleveland Clinic he also became interested in the artificial heart.

Kolff left the Cleveland Clinic toward the end of his career. He had taken up bird watching, and he wanted a slower life. He came to Utah with a promise from the chairman, Dr. Keith Reemtsma, that he would have some money and some laboratory space. Utah was the right place. It was quiet, and there were some military barracks that he took over as laboratory space. He wanted to establish a biomedical institute with electronic people, a polymer chemist, engineers, and doctors. I happened to be there right when all that started and crystallized under his power. He is still there now. He is eighty-six years old, a professor emeritus, and he is still just as active as can be. He is really the father of the artificial heart and the artificial kidney.

Dr. Kolff's first artificial heart operation was done at the Cleveland Clinic. With a Japanese fellow called Akutsu, he developed a heart that was air driven, made of polyurethane rubber with two chambers, and it supported a dog for ninety minutes before the dog died. In the beginning, their animal trials were dismal; all of the animals would die right away. He had not developed the whole concept of control of the heart.

By my senior year in medical school, we were putting artificial hearts in sheep and cows, mainly because there were a lot of them in Utah, and also because they have the same size heart as humans. I worked with him and actually implanted hearts with him, as he was unable to convince the older surgeons to help—they were not interested in this, and they thought it was crazy. He had a man named Jarvik, me, and a few other younger guys helping him. We were excited about the opportunity and excited that we were doing heart surgery.

Dr. Jarvik was an engineering student before he went to medical school, and Dr. Kolff brought him to Utah to help with the development of the artificial heart. Jarvik was also a fascinating guy. He first studied engineering at Syracuse, and then when his father, who was a general surgeon, died of a heart attack, he decided that medicine might be a good thing to do. He had terrible grades from engineering school and could not get into medical school in the states, so he applied to a medical school in Bologna, Italy, where all of the instruction was in Italian. At the end of the second year, he had to take competitive tests, but he could not pass. Dr. Jarvik met Dr. Kolff when he came to give a lecture at the school, and Dr. Kolff offered him a job at his biomedical lab in Utah because of his engineering background. Then one of the medical students at the University of Utah died of Hodgkin's disease, and Jarvik was able to take his place in the class.

He had a horrible time in medical school, because he was always thinking about other things. He had a totally untethered mind. The teacher would ask him to name the twelve layers of the retina and Jarvik would write down, "This is a useless question. I'm never going into ophthalmology. Why should I have to memorize this?" Of course,

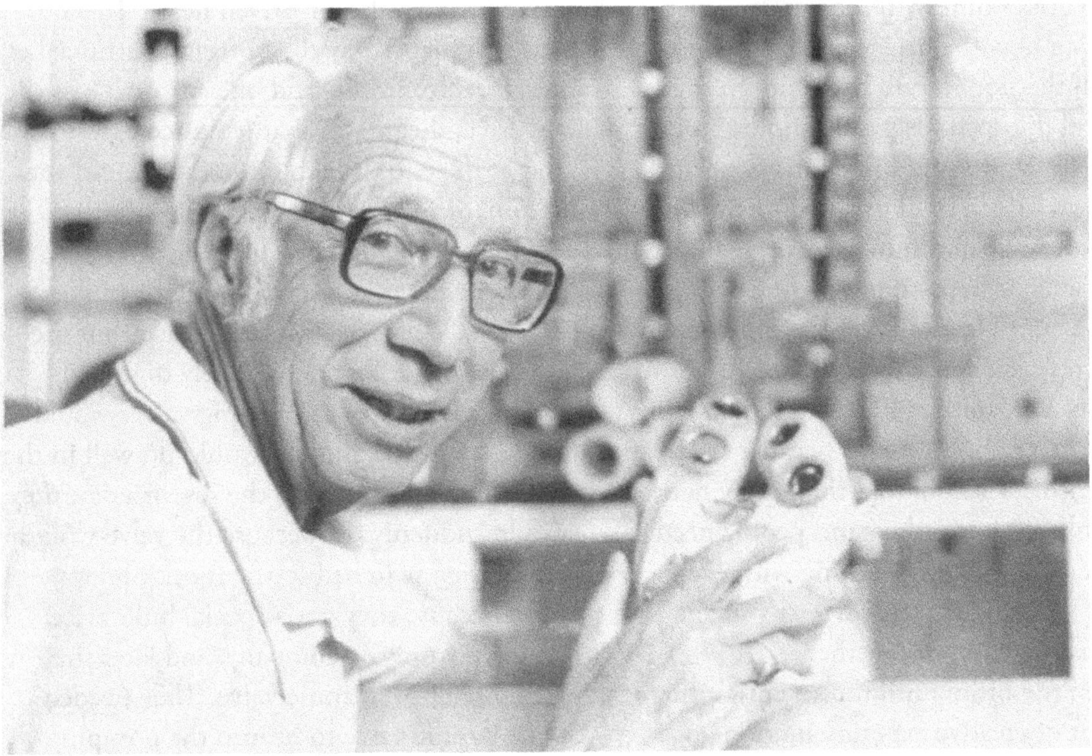

Dr. Kolff with artificial heart

the teachers would immediately give him an "F." I would say to myself, "There are only twelve things to remember; it's easy for me to do," so I always had very good grades. A question on a test would say, "Diagram the neurosensory pathways; a table might be appropriate." Jarvik would draw a picture of a table with forks and spoons on it. He nearly flunked out of medical school, and he decided not to do an internship. He wanted to do biomedical research, and he believed that he would get paid more and be taken more seriously if he had his medical degree.

Jarvik and I were exactly the opposite in just about every way, and it taught me an important lesson. He had all these great design ideas, but he did not know how to test them in animals. By the time we would develop a protocol and test it in a few animals, he would have changed the design four times. The work required a team effort with different people doing different parts, and then they all came together. The important lesson was that no man is an island, particularly in biomedical research. We all had to get along with each other, and we had to take each other's strengths and forget about their weaknesses. Dr. Kolff fostered this environment in which everyone's contribution was worthwhile. I was just a medical student working with these big-time hitters with big egos, but we were all part of the team. We had synergy. We never fought nor argued, and it was amazing.

It was also interesting because Dr. Kolff actually never got along with Jarvik; they were too much alike. They both did things their own way. I remember one time we were in a big classroom, with men and women, discussing how the drive system should come through the skin. Jarvik stood up on the table and dropped his pants, and he stood there is his shorts and pulled his pants up and down his leg to illustrate how the Silastic would move up and down the drive lines. All of the cameras were taking pictures of him up there, and Dr. Kolff was the only one in there who even appreciated that. We learned later that Dr. Kolff and Dr. Jarvik had gone to see a marriage counselor because the dean of the medical school told them they needed to be able work together, and people needed to perceive that they got along with each other. Dr. Kolff liked the diversity of the team that he had put together.

From the fifties until the seventies, there was a lot of creative experimentation going on in cardiac surgery. People may think that it was all systematically decided and that a careful scientific method was used, but it was really more like something out of *Popular Mechanics*. People would find what they could and make things in their garage to see if they worked. The artificial heart was air-driven, in part because NASA had a large aerodynamic center in Cleveland. Dr. Kolff was the type of visionary person who would, for example, stop and watch a road grader for an hour to study how it worked. When he was working at the Cleveland Clinic, he just walked into a NASA building to see what they were working on, and at that time it happened to be a system to pulse air. He took what he learned there about pulsatile air systems, and he and Adrian Kantrowitz, who worked with Dr. Kolff in Cleveland, developed the intra-aortic balloon pump. Later Dr. Kolff and Akutsu took the same concept he had used in the intra-aortic balloon and came up with the air-driven heart. There was no reliable way to control the artificial heart electronically, and one advantage of the air-driven heart was that it vented externally, and at the end of each diastole it would vent automatically and level itself.

They decided, based on their animal experiments, that they would use a biological valve. They tried pig valves first, but the artificial heart has an extremely high end diastolic pressure, and the pig valves would blow apart. The animals would do well in the beginning and then, on the seventh day, they would suddenly die because the valve would blow. They switched to the Björk-Shiley valve because they got a special bulk price on them from the company, and later they used a Hall-Medtronic valve. They needed a low-profile valve to fit into the pumping chamber.

They spent years determining the material to use for the heart, and thousands of animals died in the process. They started with Silastic, went to natural rubber, and finally ended up with polyurethane for the diaphragm, because it was the most inert with blood. The rubber would bend easily but would leach chemicals out into the blood, and the animals would hemolyze. The polyurethane was tough, durable, and easy to mold. They argued about whether the ventricle should have a smooth or rough surface. It was finally made up of seven layers with graphite between the layers of the pumping diaphragm, which helped it to move and flex without tears or stress lines occurring. It was an extremely crude yet ingenious device, its strength in its simplicity. They named it the Jarvik 7 because that was just the number Dr. Jarvik gave it. It wasn't the seventh one he designed, he just liked the name. Later he made a smaller one that he called the Jarvik 3. There were no other numbers in between. The name was a little joke for him; it was his own logic.

None of the animals were anticoagulated when we put the hearts in, and none of them ever had a stroke. I later learned that you can tie off the carotid arteries in most dogs and pigs, and it won't make a difference because of their circulation. We had a lot of bleeding with the animals, so we did not want to anticoagulate them, and we only anticoagulated them when on the pump. We were surprised when we had the first stroke in a patient. It does not make sense now that we could have been that stupid, but we really were a little stupid about it. Our first big problem with the artificial heart in patients was strokes versus bleeding, and it took ten years to work out the right combination of aspirin and coumadin, but the device itself remained the same for those first ten years. Now it is exciting because people are starting to use electric hearts and to develop the idea of transcutaneous transmission of power, but from 1979 to 1990, it was all air-driven hearts, which was the simplest way to do it.

When I first arrived back at the University of Utah after residency, I was on the faculty to do both thoracic and cardiac surgery. They only did one heart operation during the first two months I was there, and I became very involved in thoracic surgery, doing lots of lung nodules instead. I was becoming a noncardiac thoracic surgeon. I remember operating on ten solitary lung nodules, and they were all tuberculosis. Not many people smoked in Utah. There was a VA hospital across the street. I love VAs because they helped me a lot during my residency and kept me busy after residency as well. There was a patient at the VA that had cancer of the esophagus. I had seen a lot of that at Duke, so I became the local esophageal cancer expert.

My thoracic surgery kept me alive that first year in Utah. I had not yet passed my boards. At Duke you finished your residency in general and thoracic surgery at the same time, and then you applied for your general surgery boards, so I was taking them at that time. There was not a lot of cardiac surgery going on at the medical center at the university. LDS Hospital was across town, and the medical center was doing cardiac catheterizations and then sending their patients to the private hospital for their surgery. Dr. Russell Nelson had an excellent service at LDS, and Kent Jones, who was a year ahead of me at Duke, went to LDS as well, although Dr. Sabiston thought he was going to the University of Utah. You did not go into private practice from Duke. Kent Jones kept an office at the University of Utah, but he did all of his work across town. When I arrived in Utah, he more openly went to LDS, but I still had to keep his name on the letterhead so he could write to Dr. Sabiston.

I had a lot of time on my hands, because there was nothing to do. Dr. Kolff was the only contact I had with the cardiac surgery program, so I got involved with him and the artificial heart again. That was how I got into heart surgery. We did artificial heart implantations two and three times a week in animals that would live anywhere from six months to a year. When I took my boards for thoracic surgery, I think I had done eighty lung cases and about thirty esophagus cases that year in Utah, and I had done five hearts and one total artificial heart implantation.

We did the first human artificial heart

implantation in 1981. When I came back to Utah in 1979, I was amazed at the progress they had made during the nine years I had been at Duke. The animals only lived forty hours or so when I was in medical school, and when I came back they were living for almost a year. They had an excellent veterinarian who was able to help them keep the animals alive, but all they did was put the hearts in the animals and then watch to see how long they lived. It was kind of a "dead end." Nobody, amazingly, had thought about putting the artificial heart into a patient. When I suggested it, after being there about six months, I looked around the room and felt like I had a huge horn in the middle of my head. They could not understand why in the world anyone would want to do that. Nobody, including Dr. Kolff and Dr. Jarvik, was very interested in pursuing the next step.

Putting the heart into a patient was always the goal in the back of everyone's mind, but they still had not made any plans to do so when I returned to Utah. A man named Tom Kessler made the polyurethane hearts, taking him four days to make each one, and you could tell he loved doing it. One morning I told him, "Tom, I want you to make me a heart to put in a person." I can remember the look on his face, as if he was thinking, "What do you want me to do that for?" I said to him, "Well, we're going to put this one in a patient, and we need the lines to come off the artificial heart at a different angle." He told me he couldn't do that. I explained that it was the same way he made the hearts for the cows, and he said, "But if it breaks, it's not a cow that dies, it is a person that dies." I said, "Well, Tom, the person is going to die of heart disease if he doesn't have this," but he just couldn't understand.

Dr. Kolff was a little reluctant as well, because the NIH was supporting this project, and he was afraid of losing a large amount of his funding if it did not work. I think there was a tremendous lack of courage to risk failure. They had been working and working at it, and they just weren't willing to step out and put it to the final test. They were not ready to jump off the shore. Their work was obviously ready, and I eventually convinced them to move on to a patient. The situation was not unlike the circumstances of the first heart transplant. I once had a long talk with Christiaan Barnard, and he told me about his visit to Richmond, Virginia, in the summer of 1967 where he watched Dick Lower doing heart transplants in dogs with very good results. Norman Shumway and Lower had worked out all of the problems in the experimental lab, but they had not done a human transplant. Barnard said, "I saw all of this great technology. I am going to go back home and do a heart transplant." He thought Shumway was not ready to take that last step. "That was the contribution that I made: the final step."

Deciding what kind of patient we needed was an interesting problem. In 1979 there were three heart transplant centers in the United States, Shumway at Stanford, Dr. Copeland who had just moved to Arizona, and Lower at the Medical College of Virginia, and that was about all. We decided we needed a patient who had heart failure but who was not a candidate for a transplant, and we threw out all those at the hospital in Utah who met the criteria for a transplant, even though Utah did not have a transplant program. Although they did not have cyclosporine yet, the transplant patients could get Imuran. Another criterion for transplant was age. They would not transplant patients over the age of fifty, so we started looking for older patients, because we did not want to compete with the transplant programs. We also did not want to be accused of ending someone's life prematurely and of leading a patient away from some other more successful therapy, like a transplant or a drug.

When I first went to the institutional review board, I had three possible groups of patients. The first group was patients who could not come off bypass after other heart surgery; the review board said no to that group, although Dr. Cooley did his first two artificial heart operations on patients like that. The second group I suggested was the so-called bridge-to-transplant group, the patients who were going to die before they were able to get a transplant, and could possibly have the artificial device to keep them alive while they waited. The review board said no to that group also. That left me with one narrow group, people with end-stage cardiomyopathies who were not candidates for any other treatment.

The size of the patient was another problem. Dr. Kolff wanted to develop a life-size heart, and his initial cadaver studies were on a big man, but the Jarvik 3 and the Jarvik 7 had gotten increasingly bigger, and my cadaver trials showed that we needed a patient who weighed over 180 pounds, so we eliminated women as candidates.

When we got approval from the FDA to go ahead, it took almost a year to find what we needed, a big man with heart disease. Then Barney Clark's cardiologist sent him to us because he was dying of cardiomyopathy and they could not do anything for him. I took him in to see the animals, he watched us operate on them, and he decided at first that it was not for him. He said he was sicker than the animals, and he did not think he would survive. He went home, but he came back about a month later. At Thanksgiving dinner, his family had to carry him downstairs to the table. He could only eat a couple of bites of cranberry sauce, and then had to be carried back up. He said he told his wife that night that he realized he was not going to live much longer, and he had decided to have the surgery. We operated on him December 1, almost the same date in December as the first heart transplant. He lived 112 days with the artificial heart.

Barney Clark had an idiopathic cardiomyopathy; he did not have coronary disease, he just had a big dilated heart. He was sixty-one years old. He signed a thirteen-page consent form, and we had some people try to talk him out of the operation, and he had to wait a day after signing the consent. We even showed him some gory pictures of Dr. Cooley's failed artificial heart, and then we had him sign the consent again. Then we had to wait until he was so sick that he was about to die. When we wheeled him into the operating room, he was in ventricular tachycardia with almost no pressure. I thought he was dead, and that we would never get him on the heart-lung machine.

He had renal failure as well. I can remember sitting around watching the monitors before the operation. His wife would walk in and his pulse would go up and his pressure would go down, and he would go into supraventricular tachycardia and have premature ventricular contractions because his pressure was so low. We couldn't give him lidocaine because it dropped his pressure. Finally Barney just said, "Look, I've had enough of this. You either do it or you don't." So we took him right into surgery.

The technique of replacing the heart with an artificial heart is not too difficult. There are, of course, four connections: the left atrium, the right atrium, the pulmonary artery, and the aorta. The aorta and pulmonary artery of the Jarvik heart are standard woven Dacron grafts. The only problem here is that they come in only one diameter. You can't ask for a larger or smaller graft size, so the grafts sometimes have to be tailored if the aorta or pulmonary artery is unusually large or small, and the pulmonary artery is usually more fragile than the aorta so care has to be used to insure a suture line that does not leak. When the native heart is removed, the technique is similar to that used for heart transplants. The patient's atria are preserved and only the ventricles are removed. The coronary sinus is ligated, and the atrium trimmed right at the edge of the tricuspid and mitral valves. The aorta and pulmonary artery are divided just distal to their respective valves, preserving as much length as possible. The left atrial anastomosis is completed first. Each Jarvik ventricle has a large Dacron cuff attached to a polyethylene ring, which can be snapped off the ventricle. The cuffs are then anastomosed to the two atria with continuous sutures. Each ring then snaps back onto each ventricle. The two ventricles are separate, but after the aortic and pulmonary artery suture lines are completed, the two ventricles are joined with Velcro. The final step is to de-air each chamber through a nipple at each apex, where a needle can be introduced to vent the air. This is a little more difficult than with a normal heart, since once the Jarvik is sutured in place, it cannot be lifted or rotated very far.

I wanted to use Medtronic valves, because Björk-Shiley valves were occasionally coming apart in animals. I called the Shiley Company and asked them if they were having any of the problems in patients that we had seen in the animals, but they said they had never heard of anything like that happening, and so we ended up using the Björk-Shiley valve. Two weeks after the surgery, they called to say that Barney Clark suddenly had pulmonary edema. I went over to examine him, and he had lost sound of the artificial valve. The strut on his Björk-Shiley valve had ruptured and the disc had broken loose, so we took him right back to the operating room. We disconnected the left ventricle and popped a new valve. This time we used the Hall-Kaster valve and continued to use them in future cases.

The heart drive lines that had to cross the skin were similar to polyurethane vena cava catheters, and they were long. We needed a way for the tissue to grow into a button where the catheters crossed the skin. We tried putting a Dacron ring around the catheter and sewing it to the skin, but when the animal stood up after surgery, its lungs would drop down and everything would change position, causing the catheter and ring to move out of place. We solved that problem by making an accordion-type skin button, which was sewn under the skin, and then intussuscepted down to the attachment to the driveline, allowing for movement back and forth when the patient sat up or lay down. The growth of dense tissue into the Teflon button was critical in preventing bacteria from entering along the drivelines, and thereby avoiding infection. Most of the infections we had were probably blood-borne, and not from the skin buttons, as they were not skin bacteria.

We started Barney Clark's surgery around midnight and finished about seven o'clock in the morning, and it went pretty well. It had been snowing, and the University Medical Center was up on a hill. After Barney Clark signed his first signature, we waited twenty-four hours for his second consent, and during that time I kept the operating team at the hospital, concerned if they went home, they would be unable to return because of the snow.

About two o'clock in the morning, I came out of the operating room and asked the circulator how everything was going. She said, "You won't believe it, Dr. DeVries!" I thought she was going to tell me there was more snow, but she told me that she had gone downstairs to get a cup of coffee, and there were seven reporters there. Most of them ended up staying for the whole 112 days, which was great for the hospital cafeteria service, but for all the other hospital employees it was miserable. The news media never really remarked on the fact that we had done very little heart surgery at the University Hospital and that most of the heart surgery in Salt Lake City was done across town at the LDS Hospital. They were really interested in the artificial heart, and it was the first time I realized how much more there was to deal with, other than the technical aspects of the surgery. The medical decisions were easy, but this was a different world. The news media had a big impact on how we did things, things we would normally take for granted, the X-rays, for example. Did the patient own them? What if the family wanted to sell their story to a tabloid? How much information do you give the press, or do you just pull away from them? People were trying to sneak into intensive care to see him, so we had to ban everyone from going in. Some of the surgeons were very upset when they could not get into the intensive care unit to see their patients without an identity badge. They had never worn one in their lives, and they were not going to start then. There were a lot of complicating factors that we had not thought about ahead of time.

The news media attention was difficult for me. I was thirty-five and just then taking my boards, and suddenly I was dealing with a lot of new things. People had begun talking a lot about medical ethics, whereas before nobody had talked about them much. I would go to a meeting and someone would stand up and say, "Dr. DeVries, who has the right to turn the key off?" and I would say, "Well, I have a key, and I can turn it off, and so does the patient." Then they said, "Well, isn't that murder?" They asked me if the money spent on these operations wouldn't be better spent on antismoking campaigns, or "Dr. DeVries, aren't you playing God?" People would ask me these kinds of questions everywhere I went. I could be talking to a ladies' garden group or to the American College of Cardiologists, some of the most profound minds in the world, and they would ask the same questions. They always wanted to know what it felt like to have an artificial heart and if the patient can hear his heartbeat. Even Eugene Braunwald asked me these questions. I would come prepared to talk about cardiac physiology and hemolysis, but they wanted to talk about replacing the seat of the soul and the site of love with a piece of plastic. We would think to ourselves, "What is this all about? We are just trying to save a man's life."

I was on the cover of *Time* and *Life* magazines and several others. That made my mom real happy and it was an honor. I later went to a twenty-five-year commemoration ceremony for people who had been on the cover of *Time* magazine. It was fascinating, but you know, I did not get to see Mussolini, Hitler, or Milosevic. None of those people were there.

One of the best side effects of this fame was that I learned a lot more about my father. My mother did not want to talk much about him while my stepfather was alive. I knew he had been a navy doctor and had died six months after I was born, but when my mother remarried, she explained to me that life was much different now, with a large family and not much money, and she did not want to talk about my dad and what might have been. She wanted me to treat my stepfather like my dad, and I did. He was a great father and I feel good about that.

After Barney Clark's operation, he began receiving as many as five thousand letters a day. Lots of the letters were from schoolchildren from all over the world, so many that his family could not answer all of them. I started getting letters as well, and some would say, "Are you William DeVries, Hank DeVries's son?" People who remembered my father from when he was in the navy wrote. They would have these great stories about their captain and how he treated them. It was fascinating, and this was how I learned a lot more about my dad. For example, I learned how and when he died. A lot of different people corresponded with me: a bank president in Tampa, an internal medicine physician, and a policeman in Memphis. One time I was at a meeting at the Hyatt Regency in New York, and there was a man in the front row who was crying as I was speaking, and afterwards I went over to talk to him. His name was Bosman and had been on the destroyer with my dad, and he had come just to hear me talk. He said, "You have a voice exactly like your dad. I was shutting my eyes and hearing your dad talk." Later when I left the University of Utah to go to Louisville, my mother made an appointment in my office and came in and said, "Well now, your stepfather is dead, and I want to tell you about your father." It turned out that I knew more about him than she did because of all the people who had got in touch with me. That was the best part of the fame: getting to know about my father.

The FDA initially approved the use of the artificial heart, on a case-by-case basis, for six other patients besides Barney Clark, but after his surgery, when we were eager to do another case, the university began to have concerns about the cost. Barney Clark's hospital bill was around a quarter of a million dollars, which was a lot of money at that time. The heart itself cost about $20,000, and the drive system was another $20,000. One of the main costs of the heart was the valves. Each of the four was between $500 and $1,000. The FDA also required that you have a second drive system as a backup. I was asked to raise money and spent the next two years trying to do that. A few companies—HCA, Humana, and one other—had invested $5million early on toward the development of the artificial heart. We needed more money to do another case, and I was having trouble finding it, especially since there was a big fundraising campaign going on in Salt Lake City at the same time to build a new medical center. Humana finally approached me one year when I went to the Kentucky Derby and said they were interested in funding this research, but they wanted me to move to Louisville. Bill Frist had just come to Utah from HCA to train on the artificial heart. I moved to Louisville, and the first case I did there was Bill Schroeder, in 1984, and he lived about two years with the artificial heart. The next case was on a man named Murray Hayden, who lived about a year and a half, and then we did Tom Burcham from Illinois. When we put in the artificial heart, it was too large for us to close his chest. From all of our measurements it should have fit, but it just didn't. We eventually did get the chest closed and he lived about seven days, but we finally just turned it off. That experience created the impetus for the Jarvik 3, a smaller version, which had a one hundred cubic centimeter stroke volume. It opened the door for the development of the bridge-to-transplant device, which could be used in both women and smaller men.

The complications we had with these patients were mostly strokes and infections. We thought that the strokes were related to the anticoagulation and also to the subacute bacterial endocarditis (SBE), which had occurred in about 30 percent of our animals. Bill Schroeder, who lived for almost two years with the artificial heart, had SBE, and Murray Hayden also had it. They picked it up about forty to fifty days out from their operations, and it was related to their strokes. We treated them off and on with antibiotics. With Bill Schroeder, we could tell when he was going to have a stroke. He would develop an ileus and start to get nauseated, but his cultures would be negative. Then all of sudden his cultures would turn positive for staph, aureus, and then he would have a stroke. You could tell it was coming.

We began increasing his aspirin when he started to have these signs and prevented some of the problems. He had a number of bacterial vegetations on his heart valves. All of the patients were managed with coumadin, but when we thought they were having a stroke, heparin worked better. We did not want to leave them on heparin all the time, and it was very complicated deciding when to use it. They also had platelet disorders and gastrointestinal bleeding. Several of the patients had excessive bleeding right after surgery, and we would have to stop the anticoagulation for a day, but I only had one patient whom I had to take back to the operating room for postop bleeding. Managing all the variables was very complicated.

Altogether I did four permanent artificial heart patients and three temporary bridge-to-transplants, the first in Utah and the others in Louisville. I expected that other cardiac centers would want to jump on board as well, but it just did not happen. Dr. Shumway, for example, was very critical of the artificial heart. Once when I was sitting with Shumway, Cooley, DeBakey, and two or three other more senior surgeons on a panel of the American Thoracic, he just ripped me apart. He called the Jarvik heart a "clot machine" that was just going to cause strokes. I tried not to be hurt by it, but it really offended me. There was a good bit of criticism of the artificial heart after Barney Clark, who became a kind of medical curiosity. Most other surgeons sat back and watched and waited for the stamp of approval. We received the stamp of approval a couple of years later when Bill Schroeder did well, called the president of the United States on the phone, and asked for his Social Security benefits to be reinstated. At that time, we had three patients alive with artificial hearts, and they were doing things like going to ball games and participating in physical therapy.

Later the bridge-to-transplant device became available and other people starting using it, Dorman in Minneapolis and Copeland in Arizona, and it just took off. Left ventricular assist devices were being put in almost every month. The bridge-to-transplant device is four-chambered, like the artificial heart. The surgeon took the heart out right at the annulus, and sutured it in the same way as the Jarvik. The only difference was that it was replaced with a transplant as soon as a heart was found. There were a lot of patients on waiting lists who needed the device for only a month or two until they got a heart. If you left it in for a short time like that, it greatly reduced the long-term complications, so during the first year after Bill Schroeder's surgery there were about fourteen bridge-to-transplant devices put into patients in the U.S. Christian Cabrol in Paris had a series of over sixty of them at one time.

Another reason the bridge-to-transplant devices began to be used more widely was the failure of left ventricular assist devices (LVAD). When I was developing the criteria for patients who could receive an artificial heart, one of the things I had to prove was that an LVAD would not work. I reviewed the early data on LVAD, and they were not good. Many patients died. John Norman did a series of twenty-seven patients at the Texas Heart Institute, and all of them died, so I used his criteria and argued that these patients were already likely to die and therefore would be candidates for an artificial heart. Some of the excitement about the artificial heart stimulated the use of LVADs. The technology was similar, being essentially half of an artificial heart, and its use really helped set up the industry for the bridge-to-transplant artificial heart. Jarvik later made an LVAD called the Symbion, but by then there was a good bit of competition from other companies like Novacor and Thoratec, and they had better devices.

The artificial heart program continued until about 1986, when Symbion, the company that made it, got into trouble with the FDA. There were fourteen different principal investigators at that time, and we were all notified that we had to stop. I think Bill Frist had gotten a license to use it in Nashville, the Texas Heart Institute was using them, and so was the University of California Santa Barbara and San Diego, but we were suddenly told we could not do any more. Symbion had not been giving their data to the FDA and had not answered some of the FDA's concerns, so the FDA just smacked their wrist. I had to destroy all of my artificial hearts, and I had to document that I went through my inventory and punctured the diaphragm of each one. It was the saddest day of my life.

Senators Orrin Hatch of Utah and Teddy Kennedy of Massachusetts really fought the FDA to lift the ban (there was a company called Thermodynamics making artificial hearts in Massachusetts), but they were unsuccessful. Later Cardio West bought out Symbion, and Copeland started building artificial hearts with a new concept, which the FDA approved. The bridge-to-transplant device continued to be used successfully until cyclosporine came out. After that, transplant programs began to multiply until there were over 150 centers in the U.S. People over sixty years old began receiving heart transplants. Louisville had two transplant centers competing with one another for cases. The artificial heart as a permanent device just became unnecessary.

The artificial heart had a lot of potential for helping patients, and in the beginning I believed it would eventually replace transplants. There would be enough for everyone who needed them, and they could be sized to fit different people. However, it was very expensive as some of the biotechnology was not quite ready, and the complications—strokes and infections—were bad. Then cyclosporine came along and heart transplants became a much more user-friendly technology.

The one question people ask me at meetings is, "Why is the artificial heart program dead?" It is not dead. I was on an elevator in a big office building with about five other people, and a man got on the elevator holding a briefcase with wires coming out of it and going up under his sleeve. I could hear his artificial valves. He was an artificial heart patient waiting for a transplant. He got off a few floors later and no one else noticed. It wasn't news anymore. Nobody hears about it even though every major transplant center in the world has an artificial heart program and is implanting them, either left ventricular assist, right ventricular assist, or total heart devices. The Texas Heart Institute has done a lot of them, and Utah's program is still very strong. In Louisville today, there are six or seven patients walking around with artificial hearts. I think the one that ends up being the most successful will be the Novacor, an electric heart. Thermomedics is a nice program too. They are all very expensive, and different surgical centers are loyal to different devices. The hospitals are shopping around to find the least expensive and the best. It is almost like buying a car. I think a workable artificial heart is still possible, and it is just a matter of time until it happens. Other technologies started out the same and later became common. In the beginning, pacemakers were considered cost-prohibitive and cumbersome, but when they improved the technology and came up with better batteries, suddenly thousands of people had them. The total artificial heart is starting out the same way with its foot in the door with LVADs.

In the meantime, there are people who are investigating the use of animal organs, and that would really change things, but there is still a big demand for different therapies. Forty thousand Americans die each year of heart failure. We only transplant around two thousand people each year, and there are several geographic and economic issues with transplantation. It is a difficult problem.

Today I am in private practice, doing coronary bypass and valve surgery. I do miss the academic atmosphere and teaching the residents. I am fifty-five now, will probably practice for about five more years, and then get back into academic medicine. The artificial heart has had a tremendous ride. It was all very exciting stuff to be thirty-five years old and meeting the pope and the president, but really it also consumed me and changed everything about me. I was a candle burning at both ends. I really value being a doctor; I went into medicine to treat sick people, and I really enjoy doing that now. I was kind of evangelical about the artificial heart for a while, and when it didn't take off, I kept asking myself why it was not working better. I was very focused on it. When it did start taking off and developed a critical mass of data, then I could step back from it more easily and let someone else come in and take over. I was really pleased to put it down, because it ate me alive. It was not the only thing that I wanted to do, it was not what I was trained to do, and it was not what my mother wanted me to do, so it was time to move on.

Cardiac surgery is changing. Some cardiologists say that in ten years there won't be any more cardiac surgery. I remember in 1975 during my time at Duke, Dr. Clagett from the Mayo Clinic came to speak to us and said that soon there would be no need for coronary surgery, that all the patients with rheumatic heart disease would have had their valves fixed, and that all there would be left to do would be pediatric congenital defects. We all looked at each other and thought about how hard we were working, and how hard it was on our families, and we were thinking to ourselves that maybe it was all for nothing, and there would be no cardiac surgery for us when we were done with our training. Dr. Sabiston spent a lot of time doing damage control after Dr. Clagett went back to Minnesota. I think there will always be heart surgery. The cardiologists will start doing more invasive procedures and more multivessel angioplasties, and the coronary cases in the future will be riskier patients, older patients with diabetes for example. I think we also have an excess of surgeons fighting over fewer cases, but this will balance out in time. The artificial heart will still be there, young people interested in biometrics will be there, and there will be more transplants. There will always be work, but it will be less, not like when Dr. Cooley did twenty cases a day and filled up planes with patients from Holland. Those days are over, and I think the days of doctor adoration are over too. We have had to market ourselves more, and the public is a little less intrigued with us.

When my son graduated from medical school and chose not to go into cardiac surgery, I asked him why. His answer was, "Dad, get a life." I asked him what he meant, and he said he remembered when I was not at his Cub Scout meetings and his swim meets. He asked me, "Can you cure heart disease? Can you cure cancer?" When I answered no, he asked why then would I work so hard at such personal expense. I told him I'm a professional, and I enjoy it. I enjoy getting up in the middle of the night to treat sick people; it means a lot to me. He wants the easiest job with the most pay and the least hours. He wants to work for an HMO or the VA and have regular hours. That attitude discourages me, and I worry about the noble profession of medicine changing. I would probably be a surgeon even if I was not being paid. I love going to work, and sometimes I have trouble leaving work to go home.

Bibliography

DeVries, WC, Kwan-Gett CS, Kolff WJ. Consumptive Coagulopathy, Shock, and the Artificial Heart. *Trans-Am Soc Artif Inter Organs*. 1970; 16:29–36.

DeVries, WC, Seaber AV, Sealy WC. Unilateral Pulmonary Emphysema Created by Ligation of the Left Pulmonary Artery in Newborn Puppies. *Ann Thorac Surg*. 1979; 27:154–160.

DeVries, WC, Joyce LD. The Artificial Heart. *Clin Symp*. 1983; 35:1–32.

DeVries, WC. The Total Artificial Heart. In Sabiston DC, Spencer FC (Editors). *Surgery of the Chest* (4th Edition). Philadelphia: W. B. Saunders; 1983. 1629–1636.

DeVries, WC, Anderson JL, Joyce LD, Anderson FL, Hammond EH, Jarvik RK, Kolff WJ. Clinical Use of the Total Artificial Heart. *N Engl J Med*. 1984; 310:273–278.

Joyce LD, Johnson KE, Pierce WS, DeVries, WC, Semb BK, Copeland JG, Griffith BP, Cooley DA, Frazier OH, Cabrol C, et al. Summary of the World Experience with Clinical Use of Total Artificial Hearts as Heart Support Devices. *J Heart Transplant*. 1986; 5:229–235.

DeVries, WC. The Technological, Economic, Social, and Ethical Questions Raised by the Artificial Heart Program: Hearings before the Subcommittee on Investigations and Oversight of the Committee on Science and Technology. U.S. House of Representatives, 99th Congress 2nd Session; 1986. 218–255.

DeVries, WC. Surgical Technique for Implantation of the Jarvik-7 100 Total Artificial Heart. *JAMA*. 1988; 259:875–880.

DeVries, WC. The Permanent Artificial Heart. Four Case Reports. *JAMA*. 1988; 259:845–859.

DeVries, WC. The Physician, the Media, and the "Spectacular" Case. *JAMA*. 1988; 259:886–890.

Arrhythmia Surgery

William C. Sealy, MD

(b. 1912)

In my lifetime, the control of tuberculosis was the greatest benefit to humanity that has happened. You can't imagine what a terrible and devastating disease it was.
— On the early operations for tuberculosis

Interviewed April 18, 1998

I grew up in Reynolds, Georgia, which is in Taylor County about forty miles west of Macon. My father was a small-town country banker. My mother was from a large family in Coweta County, which is close to Newnan, Georgia, now on the outskirts of Atlanta. They both came up in the post–Civil War depression in the South, and only had the education that was given in their local communities. My father went off to Atlanta at some time or other and took a business course. From that he became a bank officer and he finally ran the bank in Reynolds, a town of about twelve hundred people. Its entire economy was tied up with agriculture. We were relatively prosperous for a small town in the South because it was a good agricultural area. We had good schools, and everyone who finished high school was expected to try to go to college. Most of us made it, and it was from this background that I went to Emory in 1929. Very shortly thereafter the Depression started. I actually entered medical school in 1933, which was pretty much the bottom of the Great Depression, and finally finished in 1936 about the time that recovery from the Depression was beginning. Since that time, Reynolds has changed from poverty-stricken Depression to a relatively prosperous area.

Our family doctor was well educated for a doctor of that period. He graduated from Vanderbilt Medical School and started family practice the same year. He was a very smart gentleman, and he kept up with changes in medicine. I admired him very much and used to stay around his office even before I went to medical school. I cannot say that he was the one that influenced me to go to medical school, but he was one of the people in my little community that I admired very much.

Medical school at that time was probably different from today's schools. In 1933, instead of students looking for medical schools, I think medical schools were looking for students, so they admitted a large number to the freshman class. We had eighty students, but by the time we were sophomores, there were only fifty left. Freshman medical students had almost a 40 percent mortality rate, so to speak, and gross anatomy was a big stumbling block. We had a very tough man that taught anatomy. We had one cadaver for every two students and we dissected all nine months of the school year, every afternoon. Biochemistry and histology were given in the mornings. Those that failed usually failed anatomy. The anatomy professor was very strenuous in weeding out the people that he did not think had the necessary equipment to become good doctors. We called him Blinco. It was quite tough, and we worked hard to show that we could finish. It seemed that the philosophy of the faculty was to

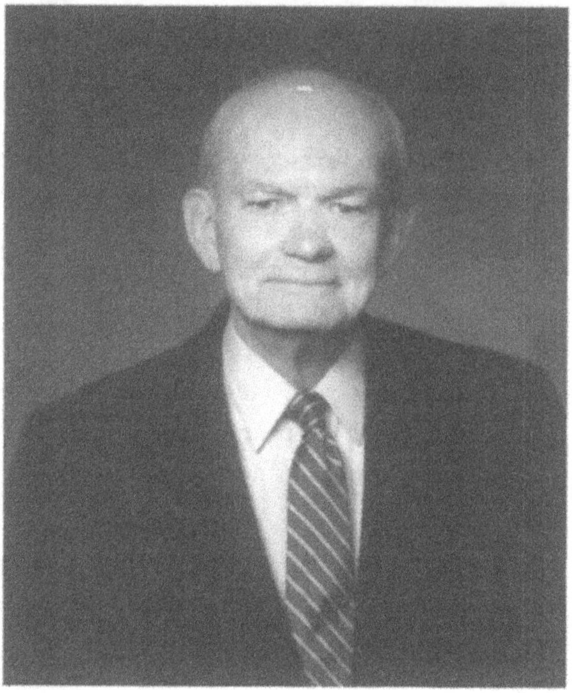

William C. Sealy

identify those, as early as possible, that were not going to finish , so they would not have to spend time and money on them. That was the way the unfit were eliminated. Of course, they were not all unfit, but Blinco thought so anyway.

Our clinical work was done at Grady Hospital, which was segregated. On one side of the street were black patients and on the other side of the street were white patients. The teaching service was almost entirely in the hospital for black patients. As it turned out, the faculty was made up of several very interesting people, and the medical care given on that side of the street was infinitely better than care given on the side for the white people.

The chief of surgery was Dr. Elkin, who had trained at the Brigham, and the chief of medicine was from Hopkins. They were very diligent and received practically no pay for running the service at Grady Hospital. They were all in private practice. We had one gentleman who ran the obstetrical service who got a public health salary. It was a very, very good hospital and we received a lot of good clinical training, but not as much academic training as students get now. It was a good practical medical school.

I had always liked internal medicine very much, and for a time I could not decide whether I wanted to be a surgeon or go into internal medicine. This is how I finally decided on surgery. Dr. Deryl Hart, the first chairman of the Department of Surgery at Duke, was a Georgia native born in University, Georgia. Many members of his family lived in a little crossroads not very far from where my family lived. Two of my uncles and an aunt were friends with Dr. Hart when he was a young boy, and it was through this connection that I became interested in surgery. When I was a junior medical student, I wrote to him asking about the chance to come to the new medical school at Duke as a surgical intern. He encouraged me to apply, which I did, and fortunately I was accepted.

It might be of interest to say a word about what it was like going to medical school during the Depression with no money. My first year, I obtained a room as a night watchman for a local high school. The room was in the boys' locker room, and I lived there one year. The next summer, I got a job working for H. M. Patterson and Son, which was the biggest undertaker in Atlanta. They had three medical students who lived at the funeral home. We would take calls two nights and be off one. We got our room rent and $7.50 a week, and that was my room and board for the next three years. In 1933, my father's bank went bankrupt, and I was pretty much on my own for finances from that time on, but I was able to borrow some money to pay my tuition from a church in Atlanta, which was very kind of them.

The only ambulance service in Atlanta was through the undertakers, so that was one of our duties. We also used to go pick up dead people and bring them back to the funeral home, and all sorts of other chores. We would sometimes have to help with funerals. I started at a different end of the profession, as an undertaker, and wound up as a doctor.

Dr. Hart came from the little town of Buena Vista, Georgia, which was very much like the place I came from. He went to Emory College, and after graduating stayed on another year and obtained a master's in mathematics. Johns Hopkins always made an effort to be a national school and they took students from all over the country, not just from Baltimore and Philadelphia. That was one of the things they stressed. Deryl Hart was accepted at Hopkins in 1915 or 1916. I know that he was not from a wealthy family, so he had a financial struggle to finish. He finished high in his class and was accepted as a surgical intern. They only took interns from the top 10 percent of the class. He stayed on as a surgical resident, and I believe it was eight years before he finished. During that time he became an accomplished neurosurgeon, plastic surgeon, and general surgeon. They were really well trained at that time, they could do almost everything in surgery. The last year that he was a resident, Duke Medical School was established and the dean was Dr. Wilbur Davidson, also a Hopkins person. He recruited Dr. Hart to be the first chairman of the Department of Surgery at Duke when it opened in 1931. I think it was 1928 when he received the appointment. He moved to Duke in 1929 before the hospital was finished so he could give advice about how he wanted the operating rooms arranged. He really went from chief resident at Hopkins to chairman of surgery at Duke.

During his last four years there he was the president of the university. They got into a big hassle about who would be the next president, and they asked him to be on a committee to resolve the various issues and look for a new president. The committee was so impressed with Dr. Hart that they said, "We have so many problems, why don't you just take it over?" So he was the president for four years and then finally retired, I believe in 1961 or 1962, so he was there for fifteen years after I returned from World War II.

When I went to Duke as an intern, I really had no money, and interns did not receive a salary. They provided room, board, and laundry, and it turned out to be a very pleasant experience. We had excellent food in a nice dining room, and for the first couple of years the food was served by waitresses. We had a menu and the dining room was run like a first-class restaurant. It was possible to have four meals a day if you wanted. We had the use of all of the university facilities because we were right on the quadrangle. We could use the swimming pool, gymnasium, tennis courts, or whatever. The problem was we had eight interns but only two were selected to stay on the second year. I was fortunate enough to be one of the two, and I spent the second year in the virology laboratory, which was one of the great periods of my life. I had a good time for the entire twelve months. I wrote a couple or three papers and I learned how to do research, although virology research was a long way from surgery.

I first worked on a papilloma virus and then equine encephalomyelitis. It is interesting how we got into this. The chief of the virology lab, Joe Beard, came to Duke from the Rockefeller Institute and was a most interesting fellow. He knew that equine encephalomyelitis was a widespread disease among horses, so if you could make a vaccine that would protect them, it would be a moneymaker. It turned out that the man who paid Joe's salary and supported his laboratory was a Mr. Bell, who was the president of American Cyanamid Corporation and was on the Board of Trustees of Duke Medical School. With this financial help, we decided to try to make a vaccine. We used the technique that came from Vanderbilt. Dr. Goodpasture of Vanderbilt was one of the great pathologists of the first half of this century, and he had devised a way to culture viruses on chicken embryos. You drilled a little hole in the top of the egg, dropped the virus in there, sealed it off with a cover slip and Vaseline, and the virus would grow in the chick embryo. Later we would take the embryo out, grind it up, and harvest the virus. I have forgotten how we killed the virus, but I think it was with formaldehyde. We then found that a vaccine made from the killed virus would, in fact, immunize guinea pigs against equine encephalomyelitis.

Lederle Laboratories, a subsidiary of American Cyanamid, was anxious to get this vaccine ready so it would be available to immunize horses before the next season, which would be spring and summer. In the middle of winter, we went up to Lederle Laboratories in New York and showed them how to grow and harvest the virus from chick embryos. We came back home, and four months later we learned that three or four people from Lederle Laboratories had died of encephalitis. During the previous six months I had been working with the virus every day. We then looked for antibodies in the people that had been working with the virus at Duke; of the four of us, I was the only one who did not have measurable antibodies. I guess I dodged the bullet. The vaccine patent was owned by Duke and a fair amount of money was accumulated, which endowed a surgical research laboratory. I saw that the Joe and Dorothy Beard Laboratory received over $6 million from NIH grants last year. It is still a great viral laboratory.

Joe Beard was a surgical resident at Vanderbilt under Alfred Blalock, and his name is on many of Dr. Blalock's papers on shock. After Joe finished the four-year surgical residency, through the advice of Dr. Blalock, he went to the Rockefeller Institute as a trainee, or fellow. He and Dr. Blalock had an agreement that whenever Dr. Blalock became chairman at some place, Dr. Beard would come and run his laboratories for him. When Dr. Blalock went to Hopkins, he offered Joe a position, which Joe declined. Joe Beard was one of the brightest people I have known in my life, and he did a lot of top-notch virology research, but he started out as a surgical resident. When he first went to the Rockefeller Institute, he went to work with Peyton Rous, the one that isolated the virus that could transmit chicken sarcoma. That was the first incidence of a viral relationship with cancer, and for this Rous received the Nobel Prize in 1966. However, Joe was a hot-tempered fellow, and after a year in New York, he left Rous and went down to another Rockefeller Institute lab for large animals in

Princeton, where he began doing really big-time viral studies.

The surgical residency at that time was six years. The chief resident had responsibilities involving teaching the junior residents and, of course, looking after the patients. We did a surprisingly large number of plastic surgery procedures, and I have done harelips and cleft palates. We also did a lot of radical neck dissections for lip and tongue cancer. We would do four or five thyroidectomies a week, maybe not quite that many, but it seemed like it. Two years before I became chief resident, the drug that suppressed hyperthyroidism, propylthiouracil, came into use. Before that, there was not much to do for patients with hyperthyroidism except surgery, and the patients were exceedingly difficult to handle. If the patient was a real "red hot" one, we would first remove one lobe and then bring the patient back to the OR in ten days and remove the other lobe. We would always give them iodine drops for ten days or so to cool them off, so they would not have a thyroid storm, which was a very dramatic and terrible event. The patient would simply burn up out of control with temperatures reading 105 or 106 and the heart rate racing. If they lived long enough they would develop hepatic failure and everything else that goes with a huge systemic insult. I did some studies in the laboratory on this and wrote a couple of papers. I would produce thyrotoxicosis in rabbits and then give them staphylococcus toxin, which would induce hepatic necrosis. It worked as a demonstration of what a serious problem this could be. Now, of course, we don't have it anymore. We also had a lot of patients with nontoxic nodular goiters, sometimes very large, extending down the neck beneath the sternum.

We began to do a lot of stomach resections for peptic ulcer disease, introduced in this country around 1936; before that time we only did gastroenterostomies. Cancer of the stomach then was almost as common as cancer of the lung is now. Most of the stomach cancers were far advanced, so in many patients it only involved confirming the diagnosis, and that was about all we could do, but on occasion we would find a resectable one. We would divide orthopedic patients between general surgery and orthopedics, but by the time I was chief resident, the two services were separated. The only thoracic surgery was thoracoplasty for cavitary tuberculosis, and lots of patients with lung abscesses. Believe it or not, many of them were post-anesthetic, and they could be difficult to handle. We also had a lot of post-pneumonic empyemas, which we would drain. That was a large part of the thoracic service, but we didn't do much in the way of definitive surgery. In 1937, when I was an intern, a patient came in with what was thought to be carcinoma of the lung, and Dr. Hart did a pneumonectomy. The patient survived, developed an empyema afterwards, but in the 1970s I saw her again. It turned out she had had a big bronchial adenoma obstructing the left main bronchus, so actually for that time it was a good operation. That was only three years after Evarts Graham did the first successful pneumonectomy for lung cancer. Dr. Churchill had come down to Duke in 1938 and gave a nice talk on bronchiectasis, and we did a few after that. Strangely enough, when I came back after the war, one of my first patients was the man that Dr. Churchill had operated on for bronchiectasis. It turned out that what he really had was a bronchial adenoma about as big as a lemon.

When I finished my residency training in July of 1942, I went into the service with a unit that was established by Duke faculty members and ex-residents, called the Sixty-fifth General Hospital. There were many similar units, and Vanderbilt, Emory, and Johns Hopkins had one. At one time we were in an area in England where there were six hospital units, each affiliated with a medical school.

During my time in the military there would be occasions when something good would happen. The first thing that was pleasant was that I was sent from Ft. Bragg to the University of Pennsylvania graduate school to take a six-week course in thoracic surgery. I had a great time in Philadelphia. We went to all of the hospitals in the city. About the only thoracic surgeons remaining were old Dr. Muller, who was well-known in the early part of the century, and Charles Bailey. Charlie Bailey became famous for his early heart surgery procedures after the war. We spent a lot of time with him during those six weeks.

We went to Ft. Bragg first, for organization and training to go to the Mediterranean in October of 1942. We got all ready to go—equipment, train reservations, who was to sleep in which bunk, in what car—and then they cancelled it all. We stayed at Ft. Bragg and worked at the station hospital until September of the next year. Again we got ready to go to the Mediterranean, but they changed our orders. We went to Massachusetts for two months, and then finally to England. At first we were in the Midlands, but we did not have very much to do because there were two hospitals close together, one from the University of Rochester and ours. The air force was not a separate arm of the service but was part of the army, and they complained that they were not getting proper medical care. Fortunately for us, the Sixty-fifth General Hospital was moved to the Wash around Norfolk and Suffolk to establish a hospital for the Eighth Air Force. They were doing those terrible daylight bombing raids over Germany, and we would get anywhere from ten to thirty casualties from each big bombing raid, poor guys shot up, and also with cold injuries and frostbite. The waist gunners on the B-17 fired their guns through an open window at twenty-five to thirty thousand feet, where it would be 25 to 30 degrees below zero, and the only protection against the cold was a heated flight suit. If the B-17 got shot up, they would sometime lose that source of heat and be exposed to the cold for several hours. Their face and hands would freeze, and they would come back in a terrible mess. We saw and treated a fair number of casualties in that regard, and it was a busy time. It was a really good hospital, and we had great people in every division.

I was then transferred out in August of 1944 to be the chief of surgery in a new hospital in southern England. Until the war in Europe ended the following April, I was really busy, as there wasn't anyone else there with any sort of surgical experience. I was the orthopedic surgeon and the general surgeon, but finally I got an orthopedic surgeon to help. I would have fifty to sixty compound fractures of the femur that were waiting to stabilize enough to be sent back to the States. The people we got had been wounded three or four days before, and we would get them in batches of 100 or 150. Usually, there would be ten or twelve who would be very sick that somehow or other got by the original surgery team. I had a rough time, but I did more good in those ten months than any time during the rest of my life, and I am still very attached to it. We had a lot of admissions for frozen feet, and there would always be this poor little eighteen-year-old that had come apart, so we had a bunch of psychiatric problems too. Interesting times.

When I was in England, I was fortunate enough to be sent down to the Brompton Hospital. Mr. Tudor Edwards was the thoracic surgeon there, and it was the leading thoracic institution in the British Isles. Mr. Edwards was one of the real pioneers in the development of thoracic surgery, and I spent six weeks there. I met Mr. Price Thomas, who later did a pneumonectomy on the king, and a half-dozen other people who were famous thoracic surgeons in the years after World War II. Mr. Brock, who later became Lord Brock, was on the staff, but was a junior surgeon and did a bronchoscopy every once in a while, but that was about all he got to do. I saw Mr. Edwards do a patent ductus operation and many operations for bronchiectasis. The most interesting man that we met was an anesthesiologist who was instrumental in the technique of using endotracheal tubes as a safe way to give anesthesia, and we spent a fair amount of time with him. Dwight Harken from the Brigham looked after us and arranged our schedule. He had spent a year or so at the Brompton as a resident before the war, so we got to know him very well.

Anesthesia was a more advanced specialty in England than it was in the U.S. At Duke, we did not have an MD anesthesiologist until right in the middle of World War II, and I believe this was true of all the major teaching hospitals. One exception was Hahnemann Medical School, where they had an MD anesthesiologist, and there must have been others during the 1930s, but mostly it was nurse-anesthetists. They worked for the surgeon, and he was responsible for what they did. It was a real experience to remove a substernal goiter with only mask anesthesia. World War II had a great deal to do with the development of anesthesia as a specialty.

The war ended in 1945, but I had to stay in the service for a year afterwards. I was married but had no children and had no combat stars, so I didn't get out until a year after the war was over. I spent a few months doing nothing, and then the last six months I spent first at Camp Butner General Hospital and finally at Lawson General Hospital, as chief of surgery in both places. I got back to Duke in 1946. Because I had done some research, and also because I had been promoted to lieutenant colonel for the last two years that I was in the army, Dr. Hart gave me a job as a very junior faculty member in the Department of General Surgery. I had by then made up my mind that I wanted to do thoracic surgery, and this is how that worked out.

When I was still a resident, I assisted Dr. Hart with an operation on one of our assistant residents, Dr. Joe Trent. Dr. Trent had married into the Duke family during his last year in medical school and, therefore, could not be on the Duke house staff, so he went to the Henry Ford Hospital, which had an excellent surgical program, and they took married residents. Not long after that, the marriage prohibition at Duke was dismissed, so he came back. He was then found to have a tumor and I helped operate on him. It was a lymphoma, and he responded reasonably well to treatment. Just before I got back, he had gone to Michigan as a thoracic surgery fellow under Dr. John Alexander, and about a year and half into his two-year fellowship, he developed a recurrence and came back to Duke. It was in his brain. Strangely enough, the chief of neurosurgery, Dr. Woodall, removed a significant part of his nondominant cortex, and he was able to return to work at Duke doing thoracic surgery. I asked Dr. Hart if I could work with him, and he agreed. For the next year, I learned a lot of thoracic surgery while Joe was still active. After he died, Dr. Hart told me I could have the job as chief of thoracic surgery, but I didn't really know a lot about tuberculosis. Dr. Hart made arrangements for me to go to Michigan for six months where I worked with Dr. Alexander and Dr. Haight. It turned out to be a great experience. I had no operative responsibility and no patient responsibility. I just went around with them, and I really did learn a lot about tuberculosis and chest disease. I was also able to read a lot, and, after that, I became chief of thoracic surgery at Duke.

Tuberculosis surgery was the main thing that thoracic surgeons did at that time. Many patients had stable cavitary tuberculosis with positive sputum, and if the cavity would not close, then we did a thoracoplasty to close it and get the sputum negative. Dr. Alexander thought that anyone who was admitted with fresh tuberculosis should have a phrenic nerve crush, so I did a lot of phrenic nerves. Dr. Alexander scrubbed on every bronchoscopy that was done, and I learned to do bronchoscopies with him.

When I returned to Duke, I made contact with the two or three county TB hospitals in the area as well as the state hospital in the eastern part of the state. I would go to these places once a month and see patients and talk to them about surgery. As the hospitals in the sanitarium system run by the state increased, we established a firm connection with the one in the eastern part of the state, and later on the one in the mid-state. At the time of the transition from thoracoplasty to pulmonary resection for tuberculosis, we began doing lung resections, and we had lots of patients. We did not have to do a large number of thoracoplasties, we did lobectomies and also decortications for patients that had been on long-term treatment with pneumothoraces. This was the basis for our resident training program in thoracic surgery, and actually each resident was able to do a relatively large number of operations.

In 1954 or 1955 three of us at Duke began to talk about doing open-heart surgery: Dr. Ivan Brown, Dr. Glen Young, and myself. I had a big laboratory with a lot of help and so did Ivan Brown. We began investigating various methods of cardiopulmonary bypass and tried to develop our own oxygenator, but that was not successful. We finally adopted the DeWall bubble oxygenator, tried it in the lab, and then took it to the operating room. It was not yet available commercially, and we made it from tubing that we ordered from Minnesota. Dr. DeWall and Lillehei had started using tubing that was from a dairy manufacturing company, I think.

There were still two ways to do open-heart surgery. One way was to immerse the anesthetized patient in a tub of ice water and lower the body temperature to 33 or 34 degrees Celsius. The patient was taken out of the tub, moved to the operating table, the chest was opened, and after occluding the superior and inferior vena cava (inflow occlusion), the atrial septal defect was closed or a pulmonary valvotomy was done. This technique allowed only six or seven minutes of open-heart operating time, and the patient was then rewarmed by being put in a tub of warm water. The second technique was to use the pump-oxygenator. The problem with the early bubble oxygenators was that they allowed only a relatively low flow, about twenty-five hundred cubic centimeters per minute maximum, and often as low as fifteen hundred or two thousand cubic centimeters a minute, about one-third of normal adult cardiac output. We thought that by combining hypothermia, which allowed six minutes of open-heart operating time, with a low-flow bubble oxygenator, which gave about twenty minutes of safety, we could put them together and have additional time needed to do a complex intracardiac operation. We immersed the patient in an ice-water tub, getting the temperature down to 34 degrees Celsius, used the pump-oxygenator to do the open-heart procedure, and then back into the tub to rewarm. We decided that it was quicker to rewarm just the blood. We made a wooden trough with stainless steel tubes in it, filled the trough with warm water, and circulated the pumped blood through the tubes and back to the patient. This would slowly rewarm the patient using the pump-oxygenator, and we didn't have to go through the long period of immersion, which could contaminate the wound. From this concept, Ivan Brown developed the first heat exchanger for use with the pump. He had lots of ideas and was a very, very bright man, and also had good luck. He went home on vacation to Lockport, New York, where his parents lived, and met a Mr. Emmons, the chief engineer for the Harrison Radiator Corporation. He told him about this problem and that we would like to be able to warm and cool the blood in the pump-oxygenator circuit with a relatively low flow of twenty-five hundred cubic centimeters per minute. In about six weeks, Mr. Emmons sent us a heat exchanger which was very efficient and would warm or cool the blood in a reasonable amount of time. It was a great advance.

At this same time, the late 1950s, there was a lot of interest in using potassium to arrest the heart. In the dog lab, we could stop the heartbeat by fibrillating it, using a 110-volt current. That did not seem to be a very nice thing to do to human hearts. We thought it would be helpful to stop the heart without contraction or fibrillation, and then we could do whatever was necessary with a good bit of comfort and ease. We read some of the old publications of Howell and his colleagues from many years ago on the effects of potassium on the heart and eventually developed a solution containing potassium, magnesium, and prostigmine, with the help of our good friend, Dr. Jerry Harris, who was professor of pediatrics. When this solution was perfused through the coronary arteries, it put the heart in cardiac arrest, and with the aorta cross-clamped, we could work inside the heart with a bloodless and quiet field. The problems with this technique were related to ischemia of the myocardium, not so much due to the concentration of the potassium as was originally thought. We did publish a paper about low flow, hypothermia, and cardioplegia, and I think we coined the term "cardioplegia." However, cardioplegia was soon discarded because it was thought that the potassium was harmful to the myocardium, and it was said that the concentration of potassium was too high. Sometime later, potassium cardioplegia was revived when coronary artery bypass procedures began to be done in large numbers, and Bill Gay and Paul Ebert were responsible for reviving it, at least in this country. By this time, much better methods of myocardial preservation were available during periods of aortic cross-clamp. A similar thing occurred with hypothermia. Viking Björk is a very capable cardiac surgeon, but he reported some microscopic changes and damage to the brain after profound hypothermia with circulatory arrest. This put deep hypothermia into the background for almost ten years before it was adopted again.

I became very interested in the surgical repair of coarctation of the aorta, one of the causes of hypertension. In the 1930s, there was as much money spent trying to find the cause of hypertension as we spend now trying to find the cause of breast cancer. It was a tremendous research challenge and work was being done all over the world. One very important experiment was done by Goldblatt around 1929 or 1930, showing that if you took out one kidney and then partially occluded the renal artery going to the remaining kidney, you could produce typical hypertension in the experimental animal. This just set the work of experimental hypertension on fire, and everybody was trying to do something in that regard. When Dr. Blalock was at Vanderbilt, he published a number of papers on that subject. When I came back after the war, I was reading and thinking about hypertension, and I became interested in coarctation. Actually, the first congenital heart operation, if you can call it a heart operation, was repair of a coarctation of the aorta. I made a plastic venturi-like tube that could be fixed in the descending aorta of dogs, duplicating the changes of coarctation: hypertension above the constriction and diminished pressure below. In the following few years, I spent a lot of time working with that preparation.

The most interesting thing that ever happened to me in my whole life occurred after coarctation resection and repair. It is a forgotten story now, as we never see it because it is now prevented. This is how it occurred. We had a big healthy patient who had a combination of coarctation and aortic insufficiency, before a suitable prosthetic valve was available. We had repaired a coarctation in other patients with some degree of aortic or mitral valve disease; fortunately all had survived. However, after the coarctation was repaired in this man, he began to complain of abdominal pain on the third postoperative day. At first it was not severe, but it became more intense and finally we were aware that something serious was going on. We explored his abdomen and found that his entire intestinal tract from the pylorus to midcolon was gangrenous, and there was nothing in the world that could be done. He died two or three days later. The interesting thing was that at autopsy it was found that he had a very severe arteritis that was confined to the arteries beyond the coarctation. This was an occlusive inflammatory change throughout the wall of the artery and some arteries were thrombosed, causing his intestinal gangrene. The pathologist removed some blood vessels from his neck and none of these vessels was involved. I think that this was the most unusual thing that I had ever seen. We then had another patient, a little boy about seven years old, that developed the same problem. We repaired his coarctation and about the third day he began to complain of abdominal pain. We got X-rays of his abdomen, and we could see gas in his small bowel, so we felt certain he had the same problem. Twenty-four hours later, we operated on him and removed two segments of gangrenous small bowel. The tissue had the same vascular changes that we had seen in the first patient. Fortunately he survived, but we were worried that he could have more problems. Dr. Harris, who was the chief of pediatrics, suggested that we give him a sympatholytic drug, resperine. We did, and he had no more problems. Over the next few months, we had several more patients with similar symptoms after coarctation repair. We went back and reviewed all of our coarctation patients and found that there were two types of response. One was immediate hypertension, which usually would resolve after twelve to eighteen hours. The second type of postop hypertension would start the second or third day, and at first the elevation would be more apparent in the diastolic pressure than in the systolic, but then they would get severe hypertension with diastolics in the 120 to 130 range and systolics over 200. It was in this group that abdominal symptoms and bowel ischemia could occur, although some patients with this pattern of hypertension had no abdominal symptoms at all.

We were then able to describe a syndrome which we called paradoxical hypertension. As time went on, we moved from resperine to shorter-acting drugs, which made it easier to control the blood pressure. No one ever sees this today because early treatment of hypertension is a routine part of postoperative care. We also measured twenty-four-hour urinary epinephrine and norepinephrine, and found a marked elevation of norepinephrine in some, but not all, patients. Without much success, I did a lot of work up until the seventies trying to prove what caused this response.

I became interested in arrhythmias when I started doing large numbers of atrial septal defects. Now and then a patient would develop an atrial arrhythmia that would be difficult to control, and it would make you wonder how this was related to the repair of the ASD. I tried to draw some conclusions by reviewing our ASD patients but was not able to find any answers. I began to study atrial conduction in the laboratory, and about the time we were getting started, a former Duke resident, Dr. Andrew Wallace, came back from two years at the NIH with Dr. Stanley Soronoff, a physiologist, where he had become very interested in electrophysiology. At that time, no one was doing clinical electrophysiology. I agreed to let him use my laboratory if he would help us with our atrial arrhythmia problem and at the same time train some of our fellows in pure science, to go along with my practical science. We began some experiments on atrial conduction by dividing the so-called preferential pathways from the SA node to the AV node. We were able to show that dividing these tracts produced a nodal rhythm, and that the pacemaker was somewhere other than the SA node after we divided these tracts. We were also able to show that these preferential pathways, which at that time were not thought to be specialized tissue, actually were specialized conduction tissue. These studies did not really help us to understand the atrial arrhythmias after ASD repair, but they did put me in contact with Dr. Wallace. It also brought me into contact with Dr. John Boneau, who was interested in right bundle branch block. He had been mapping the surface conduction on patients with right bundle branch block before heart surgery. The mapping equipment recorded the sequence of activation on the surface of the heart, and we had the mapping equipment available in the operating room.

A commercial fisherman from the outer banks of the North Carolina was admitted with congestive heart failure and an intractable supraventricular tachycardia of 150 to 160 beats per minute for weeks and weeks. They knew he had Wolff-Parkinson-White syndrome, and since they could not control it, they asked if we could divide what was then called the bundle of Kent. The only two reported experiences with a surgical approach to this problem had been at Salt Lake City and by Dwight McGoon at the Mayo Clinic. McGoon had been able to do mapping, and the epicardial mapping sequence showed that by injecting procaine in the region where they thought the pathway was, they could block the abnormal conduction. They made some incisions, but the operation was not successful.

A group in Philadelphia had described a similar patient, and showed a microscopic picture of the bundle of Kent. We had read Kent's original work, which described an abnormality around the AV ring that he thought was conduction tissue. We now know that it is not, but that is the source of the definition of the Kent bundle. Anyway, we went to the operating room and were able to map the area of earliest contraction of the ventricle. We found it in the right anterolateral area of the right AV junction, where Kent had noted abnormalities and where the Philadelphia people also had suspected. We had decided beforehand that we were going to divide the connection between the right ventricle and the tricuspid ring, and it was successful. The patient had normal conduction down through the AV node and no longer had tachycardia. We had divided a pathway that was in the anterolateral aspect of the atrioventricular junction, which we now call the right lateral pathway. That patient did very well and lived for another twenty years.

The probable reason people have died with this problem is that they go into atrial fibrillation and conduct rapidly from atrium to ventricle through the abnormal pathway. They then get ventricular tachycardia, which would degenerate into ventricular fibrillation, and this may be one of the causes of death in young athletes.

Electrophysiology has now become a practical specialty, and I think that one of our former residents, John Gallagher, did as much as anyone to develop it. Many of the people who have done a lot with arrhythmias were trained at Duke. Shineman, who first used a catheter electrode to disrupt AV node conduction, was a fellow at Duke, and many others, now all over the country, trained there in those early days. We had a great group of people working on arrhythmias, not only basic scientists, but also clinicians and surgeons. However, it is difficult to explain, but all of that disintegrated and disappeared.

Now almost all patients with WPW (Wolff-Parkinson-White) can be corrected with catheter ablation, so surgeons don't have much of a place in the treatment. I imagine that Jim Cox and Tom Ferguson's son, who is in New Orleans, have had experience enough to do the complicated patients that the cardiologists can't do.

We used to do a lot of AV node ablations. We would put the patient on cardiopulmonary bypass and then ablate the node with cryptherapy. One time Robert Anderson and I were doing a patient with persistent supraventricular tachycardia, but when we froze the AV node it did not ablate the tachycardia. I had been doing some work in the lab in which we had to practically separate the atrium from the ventricle to produce AV block, and there could still be conduction if we left any of the septum intact. I had done two patients where we divided the atrial system completely to produce AV block, and that is what this man needed. As I started dividing the atrial septum, his AV nodal reentry trachycardia stopped, and they could no longer produce it by stimulation. Because we had been on the pump for a long time and he was very much overweight, we decided to stop and not divide any more of the septum; he was cured. This patient, and a subsequent series of patients done in Australia, proved that AV nodal reentrant tachycardia was a process not in the compact node that you see so beautifully on microscopic sections, but in the area around the compact node. If you divide that, either posteriorly or anteriorly, you can interrupt the reentry tract. AV nodal reentry tachycardia is much more common than WPW, and this opened up another field of surgery. By now, this can also be done by catheter, by placing lesions close to the AV node.

The MAZE operation is a very complicated procedure and demonstrates that Jimmy Cox is a really fine electrophysiologist. He has had a lot of experience, beginning when he was a medical student. I don't know if anyone other than he and Guiraudon would have enough background to figure out how to do it. It is hard for me to see how it can be done by cardiologists with a catheter, but I never thought that they would be able to do all of the WPW patients, particularly posterior septals, because we sometimes missed those after cutting the atrium half in two. I am not sure if the MAZE is the best operation to do on a patient who has mitral valve disease and atrial fibrillation or flutter. I always thought that you should do an AV block and then control the rate with a pacemaker. Sometimes you can't control atrial contraction and rhythm, but you can control ventricular rate and therefore increase efficiency.

For the past few years I have lived in Macon, Georgia, and have been working at the Mercer University Medical School. After I retired at Duke in 1983, I piddled around working for an insurance company, a job that I didn't like. My younger brother is a cardiologist here in Macon, and I would come down here on my way to Florida or Sea Island and visit him. On one visit, I found out that they were having problems with the residency program at Mercer, so I asked him to see if he could get me appointed to the staff to help with the residency training. One thing led to another until finally I was offered the job as chief of surgery to run the educational part in the medical center. I agreed to come even though we had just moved into a brand-new home in Durham. My wife had always been on my side, so she agreed to move to Macon, thinking we would stay two or three years and then leave. It turned out that after I had been here a year, the doctor in charge of surgery, Dr. Hatcher, retired, we began looking for a successor, and I acted as temporary chairman. The first person we got was not satisfactory, and we had to let him go, and I was chairman for two and half years. By good luck, we found Rob Dalton at the University of Mississippi. After he was made chairman, I stayed on for another two years full-time, and then part-time for a year or so. Now I am really part-time, with no salary. They have been very kind to me, and it has been a great experience. I keep telling them I did not realize that general surgery could be so complicated. Since I was always a heart and lung surgeon, I thought that what the general surgeons were doing was pretty simple, but I have found out that sometimes it isn't simple. I did not do any general surgery, but I participated in the rounds and patient care, and I have really enjoyed it.

I think that I have been a promoter of lost surgical causes, since the three things that most interested me are no longer being done by surgeons. The three were tuberculosis, coarctation of the aorta, and the Wolff-Parkinson-White syndrome. When I was a junior faculty member, I was given a six-month leave of absence to go to the University of Michigan to work with a thoracic surgical group whose main function was treatment of pulmonary tuberculosis. I did a lot of reading and studying on tuberculosis, more than on any other subject I have ever done, and I thought that I was a real good tuberculosis doctor. The custom at Duke was that once you operated on a patient, he or she was yours from then on. It was a real challenge, and I got very good at it. From the mid-fifties to the mid-sixties, tuberculosis really disappeared, and in my lifetime the control of tuberculosis was the greatest benefit to humanity that has ever happened. You can't imagine what a terrible and devastating disease it was. Just as tuberculosis disappeared, heart surgery began; they almost overlapped. Some of us thoracic surgeons became interested in cardiac surgery, but many never did get interested, some that tried it didn't like it, and a few of those really did not have very much to do. I got into heart surgery and developed this tremendous experience with coarctation of the aorta. There was, of course, a backlog of patients, two or three generations, who had never been treated. After we caught up the backlog, it was not that common a problem. I did about 250 coarctation repairs, which I think was a lot, and I found this nice clinical aspect about it, paradoxical hypertension. Finally, I became interested in arrhythmias. What we did—the WPW operations, AV nodal reentry operations, and AV nodal ablation procedures—are now obsolete, no longer a sensible way to do it. We now have an easier and much more practical way, part of a revolution in surgical treatment that involves catheters, endovascular grafts, and laparoscopes. It is a tremendous revolution in surgery, and probably is not going to stop for a while yet. It may be that the surgeon using a knife may not have very much to do in the future.

There were several men who had a positive influence on my life. One of the most important was Dr. Deryl Hart. Without him, I would not have gone to Duke, and I don't know where my life would have gone. He was an unusual person and a great surgeon. He did everything. He had a very large neurosurgical practice, he did a lot of plastic surgery, and he did just everything and did it well. I have never seen anyone who was more efficient in the operating room. He was not a buddy-buddy person, but he was aware of everything that the residents did. He had some of the highly competitive spirit of

Hopkins when he first started at Duke. Hopkins people are the most competitive people in the world. After the war he changed a bit and became much more personable in that regard. He was always 100 percent honest, he never did anything underhanded, and never went behind one's back. He always told you where you stood. He was always the best person in the department to go to when you needed help. He made a statement once that if a junior resident didn't know enough to ask for help, then he would never become the chief resident. He had this great attribute, which is rare in surgical chairmen, that when he selected someone to do a job, then it was his without interference. He never questioned what we were doing and let us do what he had selected for us to do. This was the reason that we had great neurosurgical, orthopedic, and plastic surgery departments. When he brought Dr. Woodall in as chairman of neurosurgery, he stopped doing neurosurgical cases and turned them all over to Dr. Woodall. He did the same with plastic surgery and with thoracic surgery. As soon as I started doing thoracic surgery, he never did another chest case. He never interfered unless we asked him to. That was his great administrative policy, which was unique, and I think it takes a very strong person to do that. He helped me become what I am today.

Joe Beard was the other person who had a big influence on my career. He was head of experimental surgery at Duke and the brightest man I ever knew. He was a tremendous basic scientist, and he knew a lot of things other than biology. When he came to Duke, I was his first fellow, and I spent about half of my time knocking down walls, building mice cages, and doing all sorts of things. Somehow he couldn't make arrangements to get the dogs fed in the lab, so he bought a great big wash-pot kind of thing that he could heat up. We would then cut up horse meat, add black-eyed peas and brewer's yeast and cook dog food. He was just that kind of a fellow. Other than Dr. Hart, he was the one who influenced me the most during my years as a resident.

When I came back from the army, Keith Grimson was on the faculty. He had trained in Chicago and had spent two years in Belgium as a fellow with a surgeon interested in the sympathetic nervous system. He had a very active clinical laboratory and was interested in the surgical treatment of hypertension. He would remove all of the sympathetic ganglia from the stellate ganglion down to L2. He was probably the best clinical investigator that I have ever been associated with, and I learned a lot from him.

One influence was not positive. After Dr. Hart retired, the second Duke chairman was Dr. Clarence Gardner, who had moved to Duke from Hopkins with Dr. Hart. He was very bright and a very good surgeon, but never published very much. He was chairman for four or five years, and then David Sabiston came down from Hopkins as the third chairman. Right away he and I did not see things eye to eye. Most people that came from Hopkins felt that they had a great interest in congenital heart disease, and Dr. Sabiston considered himself to be a heart surgeon. Pretty soon I was sitting out there with a title but without much control or interaction with the house staff. Prior to that time, residents spent time on my service and I taught them a lot. I always had one or two working in my lab, so from that point of view, it was not very pleasant. At the same time, I had good laboratory projects, coarctation and various studies of arrhythmias. We did some work on atrial pacemakers, which I think is some of the best laboratory work that I have ever done. Actually, I received a lot of NIH support and then got into clinical arrhythmia surgery, so I never bothered him and he never bothered me, except he wasn't too pleased that it didn't come from his part of the department. Other than that, I had to take the good with the bad. At the time I thought it was pretty bad, but when I got away from it and looked back, it was just part of what you had to do. It became a highly competitive atmosphere. I think that is the Hopkins heritage to surgery: a highly competitive atmosphere. I don't see that among the trainees that I have now and the ones that I have been responsible for since I have been here at Mercer University Medical School.

Bibliography

Sealy WC, DeMaria W, Harris J. Studies of the Development and Nature of the Hypertension in Experimental Coarctation of the Aorta. *Surg Gynec Obstet.* 1950; 90:193–198.

Sealy WC, Harris JS, Young WG Jr, Callaway HA Jr. Paradoxical Hypertension following Resection of Coarctation of Aorta. *Surgery.* 1957; 42:135–147.

Sealy WC, Brown IW Jr, Young WG, Smith WW, Lesage AM. Hypothermia and Extracorporeal Circulation for Open Heart Surgery: Its Simplification with a Heat Exchanger for Rapid Cooling and Rewarming. *Ann Surg.* 1959; 150:627–639.

Sealy WC, Farmer JC, Young WG Jr, Brown IW Jr. Atrial Dysrhythmia and Atrial Secundum Defects. *J Thorac Cardiovasc Surg.* 1969; 57:245–250.

Sealy WC, Wallace AG. Surgical Treatment of Wolff-Parkinson-White Syndrome. *J Thorac Cardiovasc Surg.* 1974; 68:757–770.

Sealy WC, Seaber AV. Surgical Isolation of the Atrial Septum from the Atria. Identification of an Atrial Septal Pacemaker. *J Thorac Cardiovasc Surg.* 1980; 80:742–749.

Sealy WC. The Case of the Fisherman with the Fast Pulse and the Beginning of Arrhythmia Surgery. *NC Med J.* 1983; 44:489–490.

Sealy WC. The Wolff-Parkinson-White Syndrome and the Beginnings of Direct Arrhythmia Surgery. *Ann Thorac Surg.* 1984; 38:176–180.

Sealy WC. An Account of How Deep Hypothermia was First Used to Increase the Safety of Open Heart Surgery. *NC Med J.* 1984; 45:795–799.

Sealy WC. Paradoxical Hypertension after Repair of Coarctation of the Aorta: A Review of Its Causes. *Ann Thorac Surg.* 1990; 50:323–329.

Sealy WC. The Obsolescence of Surgical Operations: Causes and Effects. *Bull Am Coll Surg.* 1995; 80:25–29.

Sealy WC. Reminiscences of the Beginning of Clinical Electrophysiology at Duke. *Pacing Clin Electrophysiol.* 1997; 20:382–387.

James R. Jude, MD

(b. 1928)

Dr. Kouwenhoven was working there at Hopkins, with Guy Knickerbocker, and I got to know them. We started defibrillating my dogs with paddles. Then one time in 1957, I came to the lab, and Guy Knickerbocker said, "I found out that when we compress the chest, we can increase arterial pressure." It was Guy Knickerbocker, by serendipity, who came across this technique of external cardiac compression.

— On the development of closed chest resuscitation at Johns Hopkins

Interviewed May 5, 1998

I was born in 1928 in Maple Lake, Minnesota, the fifth of six children. I was a child during the Great Depression, of course, and by the mid-1930s I pretty well knew what was going on. My father was in the mercantile business, but he went into bankruptcy in 1935. Mercantile stores sold everything from food to clothing to all the farmers, but they had no money, and my father would give them credit, but his creditors were not as accommodating. He started jobbing candy and tobacco. Jobbing good tobacco in those days wasn't considered to be as bad as it is today. He built that up into a business that one of my brothers ultimately took over.

Maple Lake was a small town with only five hundred people. I went to a small school, with twenty-five students in my class. It was a great way to grow up at a time when the population of the United States was only around 124 million instead of our 265 million today. There was a lot of space and not a lot of inflation. People worked hard. There were people who came by our house because they didn't have any food. They would knock on the back door and my mother would give them something to eat, no money, but something to eat. These were real people, not the kind of homeless people of the type we have today. It was a different era.

This wasn't necessarily a bad time to grow up as we didn't really suffer any. I remember that there were Saturday afternoon movies you could go to, short features or cowboy movies, and they cost a dime. If your parents gave you a dime and you lost it, you didn't get a second dime, and you didn't get to go to the movie. Money was not easy to come by, and it meant something.

My father was of Irish descent. His ancestors came over during the potato famine, 150 years ago. They arrived in Maine first and gradually migrated to the Midwest. Of course, Minnesota is largely Scandinavian; people tend to migrate to an area similar to where they came from. The Scandinavians are all great people. Other groups also came to the Midwest, and there were a few Irish. My mother's family was from Luxembourg. Her father was born in the German section of Luxembourg, which is a very small country. He died before I was born, so I never knew him. My mother was really a first-generation immigrant, unlike my father. So I am kind of a mixture, of Luxembourg-Irish descent.

I went to a Catholic college called St. Thomas in St. Paul. Minnesota, like most of the Midwest, has a lot of liberal-arts colleges like St. Thomas. Most of the Catholic men's colleges had a women's college next door, and in the case of St. Thomas, the women's college was St. Catherine. There's St. John's in Saint Cloud, Minnesota, and there's a St. Benedict. Then there is Gustavus Adolphus, which is also a church school but not Catholic, and Hamline, and a whole group of them, all very good. St. Thomas is now the University of Saint Thomas, as it gives advanced degrees and is a sizable school.

I missed World War II because I was a little bit too young, although I was eager to enlist, and I joined the Naval Reserve. I used to go to a meeting once a week; you had to do something. When my older brothers came back from the war, one went to St. Thomas and one went to St. John's. I was eager to go to one or the other, and I picked St. Thomas.

I don't know why I went into medicine. There was no tradition of studying medicine in my family. I came from a small town, and most people didn't go to college; people had very little money even after the war. My parents gave each of us $500. Somehow they had scraped that together, and that was it. So we got scholarships and different things. I guess we thought of going to college as an escape, an escape from whatever class you were in to the next class up. You could do that with the help of your family. The opportunity was there if you wanted it.

When I got to college I just kind of picked premed, but I had a backup plan to be a farmer if I was not successful in premed. All of my uncles were farmers, and I used to milk cows and do things for my uncles. My father also had a farm and raised some cattle on it, but most of his business was mercantile, as I mentioned. Anyway, I thought if I failed at premed, I would go to the university and learn scientific farming, and I think I would have enjoyed that. As it turned out, I found medicine and science to be interesting, and I switched to medical school after three years at St. Thomas, as you could do in those days.

I applied to several Catholic medical schools, but the University of Minnesota was right there in St. Paul, and it was the most economical. It cost $300 per quarter, and you could get a scholarship. There were a lot of scholarships available then, just as today. Some of them are for the children of World War I or World War II veterans and the like, but a lot of them go unclaimed. The Minnesota Medical Foundation is part of the medical school, and you could apply for a grant of $500 there. You could also work. I had worked at St. Thomas on the switchboard, the old kind where you plugged the cords in and out, not like the modern electronic switchboards we have today. When I was in medical school, I worked at a fraternity washing dishes, and that's how I paid for my room and board. You could get by with no problem at all. I was even able to save up $150 and buy a 1931 Model-A Ford. I wish I had kept it; it was a great car. There was nothing under the hood but four cylinders, but it drove grand. Maple Lake, my hometown, was only fifty miles outside the Twin Cities, so I could drive back and forth on weekends. I sent my dirty laundry home to my mother, who washed it and faithfully mailed it back to me all pressed. You could survive very nicely.

I was a pretty good student. I had been valedictorian in high school, and I was AOA in medical school, so when it came time to look for an internship, I thought I could probably go to Johns Hopkins. I was aware of the beginnings of cardiac surgery at Minnesota at that time; Varco, Lillehei, F. John Lewis, and Dr. Wangensteen were all there. Dr. Wangensteen was a great professor, a great historian and teacher, and the kind of teacher who wasn't all just about pure science. There was always a story that went with the science. He could remember patients very well, and the weather on such and such a day, and he made a story out of everything. I decided to go away from Minnesota because most medical students don't like to stay home; they want to go somewhere else. During my senior year, we had gone down to the Mayo Clinic, which was not a medical school in those days. It was private, so there wasn't much encouragement to go there. In fact, the biggest factor in my decision to go to Hopkins may have been that I married a girl from Baltimore in my second or third year of medical school. She was doing postgraduate work in Minnesota. We had a St. Thomas Aquinas Club for Catholic medical students, and I met her there. (Aquinas was a great medieval theologian.) Meeting her kind of ruined my second year of medical school because I was seeing her so much, but after we got married, I got back on track. We lived in one of the Quonset houses from World War II, where students who were veterans could live.

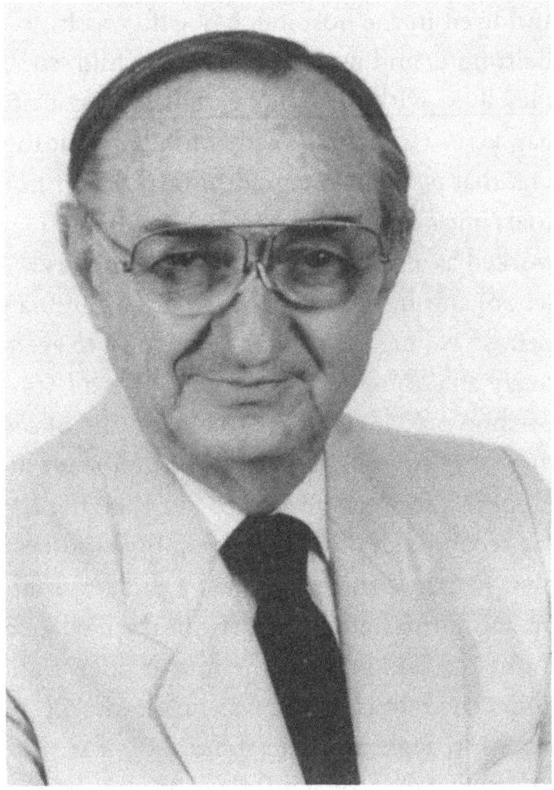

James R. Jude

In any case, I decided to apply to internships in the East. This was the second year of the intern-matching program. I talked to one of the advisors, and he warned me that the East was different. I thought, do they put their pants on in the morning one leg at a time, or do they jump into them? I didn't believe what he said, so I applied to Johns Hopkins, Massachusetts General, and Columbia Presbyterian. I went out to the East and had interviews at all of these hospitals, and also at the Brigham. I thought I could probably get into Hopkins, though. I had talked to Dr. Wangensteen, and he knew Dr. Blalock. Medicine was a smaller club in those days. Nowadays, it's enormous. In those days, it was a much smaller number, and transportation and meetings were totally different of course, in part because transportation wasn't as fast as it is now. I came out to the East by train, as there were no airplanes. I interviewed with Dr. Henry Bahnson, and also Francis Moore, and met Peter Vanbergen. I don't remember my interviews at the other two, but I went to them all. Anyway, I got matched with Johns Hopkins. I thought I would.

Hopkins took twelve interns, and you rotated every month, never got any time off, and lived in the hospital. My wife was from Baltimore, and we had a year-old child, so they lived with my wife's parents. We got no pay, zero. Hopkins provided food and clothing, that is, your outer clothing and a white coat, but not underclothing. My wife had worked as a teacher while I was in medical school and had saved her salary of $4,000 a year, so we had a little money. We were eventually able to rent an apartment over a barbershop on Monument Street, and the phone there was an extension of the switchboard at Hopkins, so we were able to live together for the second half of my first year, but not the first. For the first six months, I had a room up above the statue of Christ in the entrance to the old building, on the fourth floor, right under the rafters. There was no elevator. I would struggle up there about 2:00 A.M. and probably would be getting up in an hour or two, but it was all fine and worked out very well. We worked hard.

We were on call all the time, 365 days a year. If you wanted to go somewhere, like to a movie or something (we didn't have any money to go, but if we could scrape some up), you had to sign out to one of the other interns. Also, you got two weeks off, but only if you could get someone to take your place. There were a lot of senior medical students very interested in trying to earn a position as an intern, so as a consequence we did get a couple of weeks off, but I don't remember where we went. I think we went around looking at other possible jobs I might have after the internship. I remember going down to Charlottesville and a few other places to make sure I would have something to do the next year.

Hopkins had a fierce pyramid system, and only two interns were allowed to stay after the first year. I remember that Dr. Blalock called me in and asked me if I wanted to go to the laboratory, and I said I didn't know what to do in the laboratory. I thought, "Well, that settles that. I won't be sticking around," but I was asked to stay, luckily. In 1953 to 1954 I was an intern, in 1954 to 1955 an assistant resident, and then in 1955 to 1956 a Harvey Cushing fellow in the laboratory, where I met Dr. Kouwenhoven and a young fellow called Guy Knickerbocker, who was working on his PhD in biomedical engineering.

Before I went to NIH to do research, I did research in the laboratory at Hopkins, largely on hypothermia. Even earlier, at the University of Minnesota, I had done research for F. John Lewis on hypothermia, looking at how to preserve the body, work inside the heart, stop the heart, slow it down, or whatever. I was working with rats on whether you should warm them slowly or quickly after cooling, important because a lot of ASDs were operated on using hypothermia, and you had maybe six or seven minutes to do it. In 1952 I saw John Lewis and Mansur Taufic close the first ASD, in a twelve-year-old girl. John Lewis later went to Chicago, and I don't know what happened to Taufic; I guess he went back to Brazil or wherever he was from.

Anyway, when I got to Hopkins, I continued working on hypothermia in dogs, in the old Hunterian laboratory, where interns could do research. I rarely went during the day, but when I did go in the daytime, I remember that up on the next level was some old fellow who kind of waddled around and worked with electricity. You would hear big bangs like thunder, and lightning following it. I found out that it was Dr. Kouwenhoven, a professor and dean of the school of engineering at Johns Hopkins, who was very interested in the effects of electricity on the heart. I knew nothing about that. Usually I would go over to the laboratory in the evenings, all by myself. I would throw on the light switch and ten million cockroaches would disappear into the walls. I would get an animal and put on an ether cone and drop ether onto it. It depended on whether the dog or I went to sleep first, but if the dog did, then I would do some research on hypothermia and the use of some early heart-lung machines, specifically the bubble oxygenator. I had been doing this as an intern, and when I went into the lab as a fellow I continued it. The old surgical forum started by Wangensteen was a great thing, and I wrote a paper on how to prolong that period of hypothermia. It really wasn't the brain that was the problem, it was getting the heart to start again. It would slow down after six or seven minutes, and then what would you do? You could open the inflow, and that was fine, but the heart was very hypotensive and wouldn't start beating, so I was kind of hot-shotting the heart. I would take blood out, keep it warm, and then I would force it into the proximal end of the coronary arteries, and with this rapid rewarming, I was able to prolong the hypothermia time up to twelve or fourteen minutes.

I remember Hank Bahnson and Frank Spencer went to Australia, closing ASDs under hypothermia. They had a patient in Sidney, Australia, that fibrillated on the table while they were doing this. Dr. Kouwenhoven had been playing around with the defibrillator for years, as early as 1928, the year I was born. He wrote a paper with Booker and Langworthy on defibrillation. Defibrillation actually goes back to the turn of the century, but they were redoing it. He had a direct applicable alternating current, which he would put on the heart. We had used it experimentally in the dog lab, because in the hypothermia studies I was doing, the animals' hearts would be cooled down to 28 degrees Celsius. They would either go into ventricular fibrillation or a very slow rate with prolonged polarization; it was very dangerous to touch them during the T-wave because they would fibrillate. In any case, when Dr. Bahnson and Dr. Spencer were operating on the girl in Australia, that happened to them. They didn't have a defibrillator, so they created one with a couple of spoons, had somebody plug it into the wall, defibrillated the girl's heart, and saved her.

We used that kind of crude defibrillator too, experimentally. Claude Beck, at Western Reserve University Hospital in Cleveland, became interested in resuscitation in the 1930s and 1940s, and he was the first to successfully defibrillate a patient in the operating room.

Resuscitation actually goes back a long way, to the mid-nineteenth century and the introduction of anesthetics. Chloroform had a very close tolerance, and could cause ventricular fibrillation or asystole. There were actually some legal cases, including a famous one of a girl having her toenail removed under chloroform, who died, probably because she fibrillated. Even back then, they had lawyers in England, and the case ended up in court. Queen Victoria, I think, had some of her deliveries under chloroform, and had anything happened to her, it would have altered things a great deal. Anyway, these problems with chloroform stimulated research. A fellow named Schiff in Germany did some studies on cats, where he squeezed the heart directly, and also studied closed-chest resuscitation, but he did no human studies. As a result, nothing came of it, partly because we didn't have the communication that we do today.

Around the turn of the century, open-chest massage was occasionally being used, and used successfully, as in a case in Oslo, Norway, where a woman fibrillated during a hysterectomy. They were able to open the chest, massage the heart, and get her to recover. In the United States, George Crile Sr. was doing some work with pressure suits, like the suits that rescue people use today. They were antihypotensive suits, and the idea was to prevent cardiac arrest during surgery, which was not an unusual occurrence. Apparently Crile had a case in which he successfully used closed-chest compression, but it was not very well documented or disseminated. There was also some work being done on the effects of electricity on the heart, in ventricular defibrillation, but again, it seemed to get lost.

There was a big hiatus in the research until Dr. Kouwenhoven, an electrical engineer; Lanworthy, a psychiatrist; and Hooker, a physiologist, began to study defibrillation again. They wrote a paper at Hopkins on the effects of electricity on the heart, how it causes ventricular fibrillation, and how you could convert it. Out of that research evolved a very small alternating-current defibrillator, used only in the laboratory. A few people knew about it, though, including Claude Beck, who had one. Around 1942 during a colon resection a patient went into ventricular fibrillation, and Beck used an alternating-current defibrillator directly on the heart, saving his patient's life. That's how things stood until the post–World War II period.

Dr. Kouwenhoven received a small grant of $10,000 to $12,000 from the Edison Electric Institute, to study the effects of electricity on the heart, because of the problems of linemen being electrocuted. A couple of other things were evolving at around the same time, and one was artificial respiration. I had learned the prone pressure method in Boy Scouts, and the Sylvester arm lift chest-pressure method was another one. Neither method had any really good physiological basis, but they had some common-sense logic to them. In the mid-fifties, Peter Sapphire and Jim Elam, under a grant from the army, were studying mouth-to-mouth artificial respiration at Baltimore City Hospitals, now part of the Hopkins complex as the Bayview Medical Center. They were comparing resuscitation techniques with oximeters, crude oximeters, and they were doing these experiments on medical students, to whom they gave $100 to participate. They would anesthetize them and then paralyze them. With an oximeter on the student's finger to ensure that the oxygen level never got too low, they would do the Sylvester arm lift chest pressure or the prone pressure Shaeffer method. They tested mouth-to-mouth resuscitation too, and found that it worked very well. They published papers about it, and they made a movie about it.

As I said, Dr. Kouwenhoven was there in the Hunterian laboratory, where Dr. Blalock had given him space to study the effects of electricity on the heart under the Edison Electrical Institute grant. To avoid the problem of having to open the chest to defibrillate the heart, he was working on a capacitor defibrillator, one that could be off in the field and that could be charged up from automobile or truck batteries. He developed one that was mechanical; we didn't have the nice electronics that we have today. It was biphasic; you would pull a plunger out and push it back in, generating fifty watt-seconds or joules in each direction. It evolved from the alternating-current defibrillator, which of course was biphasic, sixty cycles, and it worked well on animals.

In any case, Dr. Kouwenhoven was working there at Hopkins, and Guy Knickerbocker worked with him, working on his PhD thesis in biomedical engineering. I went to that lab as a Cushing fellow, and I was doing research on hypothermia. I was having problems with the dogs fibrillating under hypothermia, so I went over and talked to them in the other part of the laboratory about my problems, and I got to know them. We started defibrillating my dogs with paddles.

In 1956 I went to NIH in Bethesda to work, but Baltimore wasn't far away, and I would come back to the Hopkins laboratory on the weekends to work with Guy Knickerbocker on the defibrillator. Dr. Kouwenhoven usually wasn't there. Then one time in 1957 I came to the lab, and Guy Knickerbocker said, "I found out that when we compress the chest, we can increase arterial pressure." The problem had been that we could only defibrillate a dog externally during the first minute and a half after onset. If you waited any longer than that, they wouldn't come back; they would have this idioventricular rhythm, but they wouldn't produce any pressure. But by compressing the chest, we found that we could extend that period of time. It was Guy Knickerbocker, by serendipity, who came across this technique of external cardiac compression.

You have to remember that this was a period when you could get drafted. The Korean War was winding down, but they were still drafting, and they were breathing down my neck, so I had to look for a position. After I left Hopkins, I went into the Public Health Service at the NIH where there were some Hopkins people. I didn't go to the Heart Institute, which was filled up already; I went into cancer research, but I still did a lot of research on the heart. I remember closing atrial septal defects. We put clamshell-like clamps in through the superior cava and just brought it together and closed it, experimentally. We never really did it on any patients. I also did a lot of research work on uropepsin production.

Dr. Glenn Morrow was there then; in fact, a steady stream of people from Johns Hopkins went to the NIH, where there was plenty of research money. The heart-lung machine was in its very early days. At the NIH, they had the old Kay-Cross type of rotating-disc machine, and it was one floor below the operating room. It all came up through the floor. Things were very complex. Later it was simplified; we took something very complex and made it very simple, but today we seem to be getting back to that complexity.

After I came back from NIH in July 1958, I started working with them again in the laboratory, and we began to further extend the cardiac arrest time. We got it up to ten and twenty minutes, practically as long as we had energy to do it, and we could still defibrillate them, using this capacitor external defibrillator. The dogs would be resuscitated, and they would be perfectly fine. There were no neurological changes, at least nothing you could detect in a dog, anyway, and we began hoping that maybe we would get an opportunity to use this on human beings. Paul Zoll was working on a defibrillator at the same time in Boston, and I think he was the first one to use it on a human being. The external one that Dr. Kouwenhoven had was on a big cart with a big transformer that you plugged in.

The first real case where we applied what we had learned about defibrillation didn't have anything to do with heart surgery; it had to do with cholecystectomy. Before laparoscopic surgery, an acute cholecystectomy would be done immediately, and we had a fairly obese woman having a cholecystectomy. There were some new anesthetics such as cyclopropane, which could cause explosions. I never saw an explosion at Hopkins, but I heard stories of them in other places. We had to wear special booties that conducted static electricity to a conductive floor. Cyclopropane was extremely expensive, so fluothane was also being used. Anesthesiologists were just learning about these new anesthetics, which have a very close tolerance. Anyway, this woman was having a general anaesthetic, fluothane, for a cholecystectomy, and suddenly there was no blood pressure. As usual we had no EKG hooked up, so what would you do? You would open the chest, but we didn't open the chest. We gave external cardiac compression immediately, plus pure oxygen, and after three to four minutes her blood pressure came back. We went ahead and did the gallbladder resection, and the patient was fine.

Later on, our case documentation was much better. The cardiac cath laboratory at Hopkins was called the Welcome Laboratory. That laboratory, which was given by Burroughs, Welcome, and Grant, was opened at Hopkins before I went there, and the thoracic surgeons, who were really general surgeons in those days, did all the cardiac cath procedures, but it was too much work and they gave it up, just as we gave up endoscopy because it was too much busy work. Surgeons like to cut. In the Welcome Laboratory, they used a little bit too much dye during a coronary arteriogram, and the patient had cardiac arrest. By using external cardiac compression, the doctors could see they were developing pressure because they had an arterial line in place, so they weren't taking any risks. Gradually the heart began to come back and the patient recovered. We had a lot of those kinds of experiences in late 1958 and 1959.

I remember another patient being dramatically resuscitated, and it was documented. We had surgical clinics, usually run by people in private practice, in return for the residents' looking after their private patients in the Marburg building. We had a lot of great men who were in private practice, good teachers and good clinicians, and one of them was Ben Baker. He had a patient come into the emergency room with chest pain, before the days of chest-pain clinics, and because the patient was not in any dire distress, he was sent home and told to come back to the cardiac clinic the next day. He did, but as he was being examined by Dr. Baker, he suddenly arrested. Dr. Baker called for an EKG, and he called me because he knew of my interest in cardiac resuscitation. I was senior assistant resident at the time, and I went over there and started giving cardiac compression externally. The EKG was the old type that had to be developed before you could look at the trace, but there was a little light that bounced up and down, and you could see that the patient was in ventricular fibrillation. Ultimately the EKG was developed, and we knew for sure. We got this alternating-current defibrillator, gave him a shock, he developed a pulse, and he came back. This was one of the first cases of resuscitation that was documented.

We also had a lot of documented cases

of children being resuscitated after cardiac surgery, and they were usually monitored at least with an EKG, and sometimes also with some kind of arterial line, so we knew what we were doing. We weren't taking any chances. In 1960 we went to Dr. Blalock and showed him all this, and he said, "Get more data." I think at that time we only had ten or twelve cases, but we went back and got more documentation, and when we went to see Dr. Blalock again, he said that he wanted us to submit an abstract. He refused to be a co-author, saying that he would support us but that we could only put something at the end of the article about his support, so Kouwenhoven was the lead author. It was presented at the American Surgical Association meeting in Boca Raton, Florida, in 1960. The next year, in 1961, we had an article in the *Journal of the American Medical Association* (*JAMA*), and that article documented a lot of patients. The first publication only had about twenty-eight patients, but the second one had a hundred.

That information disseminated pretty rapidly into medical centers. We had done this research under the Edison Electric grant, and we got a grant from the NIH for $20,000. In those days that was a lot of money, and it went a long way. After we presented the paper, the Maryland Heart Association got involved, gave us a grant, and started a resuscitation committee that included Leonard Shurless from the University of Maryland. Hopkins and Maryland were not competitive, so everybody worked together, and we produced slides and a teaching program. Marty McMahon and the fire department were involved, and they learned about mouth-to-mouth breathing. We had patients brought to the hospital in ventricular fibrillation, and some of those were defibrillated and resuscitated. I remember one patient by the name of Bertie Bush, who had had an MI, was resuscitated in that fashion, stayed in the hospital for three or four weeks, and then survived for several years thereafter.

All this happened while I was a resident. We started teaching CPR right there at Hopkins. We produced black-and-white films, and in fact there's one you can still get from Hopkins of Dr. Kouwenhoven, Guy Knickerbocker, and myself. Guy Knickerbocker is the patient, and we sketched a heart on him. After the *JAMA* article, the Heart Association meeting was in St. Louis, and Leonard Sherless thought we should have a session at the meeting. It was too late to get onto the regular program, so we had sessions in the hallway and taught a lot of people CPR in St. Louis at that time.

Dr. Kouwenhoven had actually retired in the mid-1950s, and then did full-time research. He must have been in his late sixties when I worked with him, late in his career, but he was very energetic and very good. He smoked a pipe. He did have hip problems, and would have done better with his hips replaced, but it was before hip replacement surgery. He was a great sailor with a sailboat at Gibson's Island, down on the Chesapeake, but gradually his hips got so bad that he had to sell his sailboat.

Vivien Thomas was at Hopkins then, a great fellow and a Nashvillian. Dr. Blalock had been at Vanderbilt in Nashville where he did a lot of research on trauma and how to prevent shock after trauma. He gained a lot of notoriety, was eventually invited to come to Hopkins as the professor, and brought Vivien with him. Vivien Thomas had extraordinary technical abilities, was a very nice guy, and ran the laboratory. We went to him as a mentor frequently, and he would help in any way that he could. There was also another fellow by the name of Claude Usta. Both he and Vivien Thomas were black, but that didn't mean anything to us, you know. When I was an intern at Hopkins, there were still signs on the doors that said "white" and "colored," and there had been separate wards for white and colored, but they weren't used any more. I came from the Midwest, and race didn't mean anything to me anyway. Claude and Vivien were great people, and Claude used to make great dandelion wine. Vivien was a great teacher, and he taught me a lot of techniques that were very important. He did a lot of work for Dr. Blalock and was part of the Blalock-Taussig Blue Baby operation.

Vivien Thomas and Dr. Kouwenhoven had something in common. Dr. Kouwenhoven was a doctor of electrical engineering, DEng. He had received that degree in Holland, as he was Dutch. Both he and Vivien received honorary degrees from Johns Hopkins and both deserved it. They couldn't go out and practice medicine, but they had made great contributions to the field.

Speaking of Dr. Blalock, he was a great teacher. He didn't want to take anything away from anybody. If you did the research, you were recognized for it. He knew that ultimately it would reflect well on him, and it did. He was open. If you had a good idea, he would support you. I remember one time I wanted to go to a meeting to present my research from my first year in the research laboratory. The research involved using a hot-shot type of prolonged hypothermia, and it didn't actually amount to much, but he gave me $500 to go to the meeting. I was actually at the NIH, and it was the only time I ever put on a uniform in the Public Health Service. I flew out to the meeting with the surgeon general in his airplane. It took three days to get there, but finally we did, and I stayed at the YMCA for $5 a night to save the $500. I needed the money.

Dr. Taussig was also a fabulous person, a pediatric cardiologist. She did not start out as that, but she became one. I remember as an intern rotating through cardiac surgery and going to her office to see the pediatric cardiac problems. Her examining room was surrounded by viewing boxes. We didn't have nice angiography in those days, but they had rapid film changers. They frequently jammed and were a pain, but they worked. They would inject these little children on the right side of the heart and follow the dye through. She would put all these films up, and it was like those flip books, you remember, where you would flip the corner and watch a moving picture. Here as you moved around quickly, you could watch the blood flowing through the heart, and that is where you learned congenital heart disease. That was a great learning period in our training.

Dr. Taussig had a hearing problem, so she had an amplifying stethoscope. Eventually Dr. Taussig had an operation on her ear, which improved her hearing. She continued to work even when she was supposedly in retirement until the day she died. She worked very well with Dr. Blalock.

Camaraderie was very strong at Hopkins, and it's one of the things Hopkins is known for. We were in competition, but with ourselves, not really with others. I remember when I went to see Dr. Blalock about what was going to happen to me after internship. He was very much a gentleman and helped in any way he could. I was lucky enough to stay, and he helped everyone else get placed. Nobody who was an intern from Hopkins had any problem getting placed.

It has been said that Dr. Blalock was

perhaps the most influential and powerful surgical chairman that ever was. There are many ways of gauging his influence. You could do it by looking at what he produced, and whom he produced, where they went, and whom they produced. He had people like Bill Longmire, Glenn Morrow, Frank Spencer, Henry Bahnson, and an enormous number of other people who went to excellent programs, and in turn produced more outstanding surgeons. Dr. Blalock stood out, but I think that was because of his humility and ability to get things done without taking credit for it. He provided the basis for good things happening, and then made sure there were good people there to make them happen.

Dr. Blalock was known for occasionally being a little whiny, though. On Friday afternoons, the medical men would be sending us all of their disasters, and he would say in an unhappy, whiny voice, "They don't all have to send them to us on Friday." We would have to take care of them over the weekend. If a patient was almost dead and was being sent to the operating room, he would whine, "They don't all have to die in the operating room." When we were doing the Blalock-Taussig operation, the nurse-anesthetist would anesthetize these kids with open-drop ether. It was very safe, and the stages are very definite. He would look in and say, "How is everything?" and the anesthetist would say, "Everything's fine," but Dr. Blalock would say in his whiny voice, "But the heart isn't beating." It was okay, though, because by then there were EKG machines hooked up, and you could see that there was electrical activity even though there was no mechanical activity. He took all this stuff in stride, though. He had a room where he would stay overnight when we were doing difficult cases. These patients would bleed, and we would tentatively knock on his door because we wanted to take the patient back and evacuate the clot. There would be a whiteout of the right lung from the blood that had accumulated, and we knew he didn't like this at all. He would say, "All right, take him back," so we would evacuate the hematoma, and the child would go home in a week or ten days, but if you didn't do that, they were sometimes in for four weeks—a long time.

To get back to the topic of resuscitation, though, in 1961 we published an article in *JAMA* about CPR and closed-chest resuscitation. We worked with a lot of others on that, to help people become aware of it. In those days, people worked to advance medicine, not just to advance their pocketbook, as so often happens today. It concerns me that nowadays so many people are more interested in making money than in advancing medicine; it seems like an ethical problem. Back in the early sixties, there was no money to be made in any of these things; our purpose was merely to advance health care in general. We worked with people like Chief Marty McMahon of the fire department. Peter Sapphire and Jim Elam were already teaching firemen mouth-to-mouth resuscitation, and they had one of the early rescue squads, with a few firemen who had been super-trained to do it. External cardiac massage combined with mouth-to-mouth ventilation became what we called CPR. We taught them, and then they applied it.

It was one thing to teach doctors CPR; it was another thing completely to teach it to people on the street, but we didn't jump to the street right away. First we went to other health care professionals, people on rescue squads, and the EMT technicians. We wanted to teach nurses too, but this wasn't very easy. The American Nursing Association thought that it wasn't within the scope of what an RN should do, but the RNs ignored their headquarters in New York, and they learned to do it pretty quickly. The internists and others who didn't wield a knife weren't about to do the open-chest compression, although Frank Spencer once said that everybody should carry a scalpel in their wallet so they could open a chest anywhere. I do remember one of the house officers at Hopkins opening a chest. He opened the chest, the lung, and the heart all at the same time, forgetting how sharp that knife was. Open-chest resuscitation wasn't a practical way to save a person.

Closed-chest compression was picked up quickly by health professionals, and also by the press. Testimonials about its effectiveness started to appear from nonmedical people, and so we saw that there was a need. We had taught people at the American Heart Association meeting in St. Louis, and then we got the Heart Association Resuscitation Committee in Maryland involved. Eventually the Red Cross got involved through the Heart Association, and we began to teach the public more about the procedure. This process was slow. We had a number of meetings in Washington, D.C., at the National Academy of Sciences, and it was gradually accepted that rescue squads should learn it. Seattle, Washington, was one of the first cities to teach the method to its rescue squads, followed by Jacksonville and Miami, Florida. In the early to mid-1960s, some cities in Scotland also began to use it. The procedure disseminated very rapidly because it was something anybody could do. As Dr. Kouwenhoven liked to say, "All you need are two hands and your lungs. You carry them with you at all times." The beauty of CPR is that you can keep the brain alive for a period of time without anything but yourself, until a defibrillator and the proper equipment and drugs can be used in the second phase of resuscitation. Anybody can do the first phase, and nowadays rescue squads and medical technicians are going ahead and defibrillating, usually with telecommunications.

The next generation of resuscitation came when people started asking the question, "What's really moving the blood?" We used to have meetings every three to four years, looking for new ways to improve CPR. There was some talk about abdominal compression and diaphragmatic elevation, but it requires a lot of extra equipment, and therefore it never became extremely popular. I think it could help, but it isn't the main ingredient, which is simplicity.

So we've pretty much swung back to phase one, the same CPR we've always had. Phase two, the second part of resuscitation with drugs and defibrillation, may vary a bit. Opening the chest still isn't a bad thing to do in certain circumstances if external compression doesn't work. If you don't have any blood and the heart is empty, external compression doesn't work. Internal won't work too well either, but it might work a little better. I think thoracic surgeons should still know how to do open-chest massage. I think that should be part of the training. These methods are rarely used now, but I do internal compression occasionally.

I stayed on as a faculty member at Hopkins through the mid-sixties doing all kinds of surgery. We were trained as general surgeons, but gradually we did more and more cardiac surgery. Those were the early days of valve replacement, although valve replacement had started in the late fifties. I advanced to assistant professor, and then Dr. Blalock retired. He was replaced by George Zuidema, who was very good, but he was a gastrointestinal surgeon and not cardiovascular, so I started looking for another job. I looked around and after three trips I decided to move to Florida, where I have been since, at first in an academic position, and then in private practice. In the three years I was a professor at Hopkins, I continued to do research in the laboratory. I worked on pacemakers and other things of that nature, but mostly I was involved with resuscitation. Some people now say we should have patented resuscitation, but it never crossed anybody's mind, and I don't think you could patent such a procedure.

There is a movement nowadays to patent operations such as the minimally invasive cardiac procedures. One of the ironies of this is that in the early days of coronary bypass surgery, we really did have minimally invasive surgery. We did operations without the heart-and-lung machine, but we didn't do a lot. We started very slowly in coronary surgery, bypassing first the right, later the LAD, and then finally the circumflex. We tried to simplify it. We knew you couldn't do a good job with the heart beating, and that's why we started using the heart-lung machine to have a quiet heart. Good anesthesia, cardioplegia, magnifying loupes, and good suture material made it all feasible. We really simplified it from a much too complicated operation. The reused pump tubing had pyrogens, which produced high fevers in patients. We got away from that with disposables, and now we dispose of everything except the nurses. We probably use too many disposables today. We have simplified the heart-lung machine, we have membrane oxygenators, and we don't mix the blood and oxygen. We have centrifugal pumps, so we don't compress the red cells and destroy them. Cardiopulmonary bypass isn't as complicated, we don't have as many neurological changes, and the patients always seem as alert as they were before the operation.

Now, it's true that there are some surgeons who have developed things for companies, and then the companies have made money, but the surgeons haven't. If that kind of research is done in a university, the university should benefit but not the individual researcher. You should not be doing this for the money, but for the benefit of mankind.

It's possible that some good will come out of the minimally invasive surgery idea, but the driving force behind it seems to be the ego of the surgeons, the marketing, and the competitiveness of the so-called health care industry. We used to call it the health care profession. It is more competitive because cardiac surgeons are getting less and less for what they do because of decisions made in Washington. They have to do more and more operations to make the same amount that they made before, which was probably too much anyway. When I finished my training in 1961, I stayed on at Hopkins for $12,000 a year. I had five or six children, so I got an NIH grant and got it up to $20,000. When I went to Miami University in 1964, I was paid $35,000 a year for an academic position. When I left there in 1971, I think it was up to $42,000. It hadn't really increased very much, and I was glad to be able to go into private practice.

Making half a million a year is totally absurd, and our expectations are too high. What we are doing has ethical implications.

We can look at it and ask the question, "Are you doing this just for the money?" You can read in the *Wall Street Journal* about these problems, which have come up repeatedly. People are looking after their own interests, and they are driven mostly by the bottom line, rather than by the real value of the procedure. In the case of minimally invasive surgery, keeping them on the heart-lung machine by some Mickey Mouse procedure is very complicated and takes away the real safety factors when you work through a keyhole incision to replace a valve. If anything goes wrong what would you do? Are you going to quickly slash them open? You risk making mistakes that way.

Now, if you can bypass the LAD with a left internal thoracic artery and if you can do a good job of that without using the heart-lung machine, then you don't have any physiological problems related to the pump. You have very good long-term results that have been proven, and the patient can get out of the hospital early. In fact, dividing the sternum isn't really a big thing, and you can see well enough to do a safe job. If you are going to work through a keyhole incision, you are going to have problems. Our patients now go home in four or five days after being on the heart-lung machine and after having five or six bypasses using both internal mammary arteries. Five days is the gold standard now, and four days is not unusual. If you send anybody home before four days, you're a sadist. You know it's just to boost your ego and to say that you've done it.

I do believe that there is a driving force in the public for smaller incisions, and that part of it is driven by publicity and advertising. Some patients are going to flock to New York or some other place where people really can do minimally invasive cardiac surgery, but the average surgeon is going to have trouble and is going to have a higher mortality rate, so we should rethink this and think about why we are doing it.

I did replace the aortic valve in a young female attorney recently, through a small seven- or eight-centimeter incision. You can undermine the skin and stretch it a little bit. The incision is all that the patient sees, and they have no idea what goes on underneath. I think some good will evolve, but we have to be very careful. Our national organizations should be speaking out about this, and there should be more debate about it at the meetings. People should get up and speak their minds. Some people say that the different opinions about minimally invasive surgery are just the result of the way different generations think, but I think it is more than that.

Bibliography

Kouwenhoven WB, Knickerbocker GG, Milnor WR, and Jude JR. Field Treatment in Electric Shock Cases-II. *Electric Engineering.* 1960; 79:500–503.

Kouwenhoven WB, Jude JR, Knickerbocker GG. Closed-Chest Cardiac Massage. *JAMA.* 1960; 173:1064–1067.

Jude JR, Kouwenhoven WB, Knickerbocker GG. Clinical and Experimental Application of a New Treatment of Cardiac Arrest. *Surg Forum.* 1960; 11:252–254.

Jude JR, Kouwenhoven WB, Knickerbocker GG. A New Approach to Cardiac Resuscitation. *Ann Surg.* 1961; 154:311–319.

Jude JR, Kouwenhoven WB, Knickerbocker GG. Cardiac Arrest. Report of Application of External Cardiac Massage on 118 Patients. *JAMA.* 1961; 178:1063–1070.

Jude JR, Kouwenhoven WB, Knickerbocker GG. An Experimental and Clinical Study of a Portable External Cardiac Defibrillator. *Surg Forum.* 1962; 13:185–187.

Spencer FC, Quattlebaum JK, Quattlebaum JK Jr, Sharp EH, Jude JR, Plication of the Inferior Vena Cava for Pulmonary Embolism: A Report of 20 Cases. *Ann Surg.* 1962; 155:827–837.

Wilder JR, Jude JR, Kouwenhoven WB, McMahon MC. Cardiopulmonary Resuscitations by Trained Ambulance Personnel. *JAMA.* 1964; 190:531–534.

Jensen JB, Humphries JO, Kouwenhoven WB, Jude JR. Electroshock for Atrial Flutter and Atrial Fibrillation. Follow-up Studies on 50 Patients. *JAMA.* 1965; 194:1181–1184.

Index

Page numbers in **bold** indicate pictures.

Illustration Credits

Many of the images in this book were supplied courtesy of the participants and their families. Grateful acknowledgment is made to them, as well as to the institutions that provided the images on the following pages: 3, 6, 7, 21, 24, 64, 126, 186, National Library of Medicine; 9, 10, 13, 17, Courtesy of the Alan Mason Chesney Medical Archives of the Johns Hopkins Medical Institutions; 15, Photograph © Yosuf Karsh, courtesy of the Alan Mason Chesney Medical Archives of the Johns Hopkins Medical Institutions; 25, Jefferson Medical College; 43, 51, 366, 406, Reprinted with the permission of The Cleveland Clinic Center for Medical Art and Photography © 2008, All Rights Reserved; 84, C. Walton and Katherine K. Lillehei Foundation; 149, Baylor College of Medicine; 198, Vanderbilt University School of Medicine, Medical Alumni Association; 245, Texas Heart Institute; 279, Edwards Lifesciences; 359, Photograph © Miguel Angel Generoso, courtesy of the Favaloro Foundation; 429, Stanford University Medical Center; 441, Retna and Camera Press / Maurice Henry; 447, 457, University of Mississippi Medical Center Department of Public Affairs; 465, Papworth Hospital; 470, 473, Special Collections Department, J. Willard Marriott Library, University of Utah; 490, Mercer University School of Medicine.

www.ingramcontent.com/pod-product-compliance
Lightning Source LLC
LaVergne TN
LVHW081942200926
848484LV00009B/2499
* 9 7 8 0 8 2 6 5 1 5 9 4 0 *